Nelson Yuan-sheng Kiang

Aphasia

Under the advisory editorship of
Hayes A. Newby

Aphasia

SELECTED READINGS

edited by

MARTHA TAYLOR SARNO
NEW YORK UNIVERSITY SCHOOL OF MEDICINE

ACC
New York

APPLETON-CENTURY-CROFTS
EDUCATIONAL DIVISION
MEREDITH CORPORATION

72 73 74 75 76 / 10 9 8 7 6 5 4 3 2

Library of Congress Card Number: 78-185650

PRINTED IN THE UNITED STATES OF AMERICA

C-390-77739-0

PREFACE

During the last twenty-five years, the study of aphasia has engaged the interest of workers in many disciplines. Once the exclusive province of the neurologist, to whom we owe a great debt for pioneering work, aphasia is now studied as well by the speech pathologist, linguist, phonetician, psycholinguist, and psychologist in a roster that is by no means exhaustive. The sizeable body of literature created by this upsurge of interest and endeavor is the prime stimulus for shaping a book of readings on the subject.

A second and more practical reason for this collection is a direct outgrowth of classroom needs in a graduate course in aphasia for speech pathologists. Since aphasiology has yet to arrive at the stage where a single author can be expert in all of its areas of study, journal reading comprises a significant part of any course. Both the student and teacher should find this volume convenient since all the publications from which these papers were drawn are rarely on hand and easily accessible in a single library.

These articles should provide the student with a broad, basic introduction to the ideas and approaches that characterize the last two and a half decades of study in aphasia. This accumulated wisdom, however important though it is for him to digest, is no substitute for the student's own clinical and research experience. The phenomenon we know as aphasia is best studied in the patient who demonstrates it.

Those who are familiar with the field will recognize the editor's desire to avoid presentation of a unified approach to aphasia. The emphasis is rather on recent advances that point up important problems or raise provocative questions.

Selections were not restricted, however, to studies presenting hard data. Only eleven of the forty-four papers included were published before 1960, and some very recent ones will be missed because they appeared after the publication of this volume. Some early and excellent contributions to the literature are not included since the ideas and concepts they set forth are amply reviewed and refined in subsequent papers. In some cases a publication was chosen even though its author does not elaborate his ideas fully or support them as persuasively as one might wish. In such instances the virtue of a fresh or ingenious approach was thought to outweigh deficiencies in argument or documentation.

Another burden on the conscience of an editor who prepares a volume such as this is the quantity of good material which must necessarily be excluded. In part, his background and experience dictate, consciously and unconsciously, the principles applied in making choices.

Because of limitations of space, articles on the history of the study of aphasia, though often of great practical value, are omitted. One is mindful all the same of the injunction of Arthur Benton, a leading historian of aphasia, who reminds us of the continual possibility that something described fifty years ago may be "discovered" anew. Aphasia, whose history dates back at least 2,500 years, has generated a substantial literature over the last 150 years. Great names like Broca, Wernicke, Dax, Hughlings-Jackson, Marie, Head, Freud, and Goldstein (*Language and Language Disturbances*, 2nd edition. New York, Grune and Stratton, 1965) signal the main courses of a diversity of thought on the nature of aphasia and the organization of language which is still relevant today. Unfortunately, no single volume traces in detail the history of the study of aphasia; chapters in Head (*Aphasia and Kindred Disorders of Speech*, New York, Hafner, 1963), in Schuell (*Aphasia in Adults*,

New York, Harper, 1964), and in Weisenburg and McBride (*Aphasia: A Clinical and Psychological Study*, New York, Hafner, 1964) do provide a good overall survey. Additional references on the history of aphasia are listed in the appendix.

Had space permitted, papers on the classification of aphasic disorders might also have been included. Even so, the reader will encounter many papers that presuppose or make use of classificatory distinctions and labels.

Problems in classification reflect the fact that the pathophysiology as well as pathological anatomy of aphasia are still poorly understood, whatever the abundance of theories. Depending upon the pathologist's background and experience, he may or may not postulate an anatomical classification. Schuell, Wepman, Weisenburg and McBride, and Bay devised systems based on the clinical observation of large numbers of patients. Luria (*Human Brain and Psychological Processes*, New York, Harper and Row, 1966), who expresses the multidimensionality of aphasic symptoms, arrives at a classification based on the correlation of symptom complexes with specific sites of brain damage. A discrete lesion, however, usually interrupts, as Luria emphasizes, only one link in a complicated function chain.

For a review of current thought on some psycholinguistic theories of aphasia, the reader should consult Chapter 5 of *Approaches to the Study of Aphasia*, edited by Osgood and Miron (Urbana, University of Illinois Press, 1963).

Finally, a large number of studies by neurologists and psychologists, which relate aspects of aphasia to a variety of brain functions—all in an attempt to elucidate further the nature of aphasia—are omitted. Many of these titles are listed separately in the appendix along with some suggested additional readings. A comprehensive review is the paper by Malcolm Piercy ("The Effects of Cerebral Lesions on Intellectual Function: A Review of Current Research Trends," *British Journal of Psychiatry*, **110**: 310–352, 1964). Chapters in Millikan and Darley (*Brain Mechanisms Underlying Speech and Language*, New York, Grune and Stratton, 1967), Head (*Aphasia and Kindred Disorders of Speech*, Volumes I and II, New York, Hafner, 1963), Penfield and Roberts (*Speech and Brain Mechanisms*, Princeton University Press, 1959), and in Russell and Espir (*Traumatic Aphasia*. London, Oxford University, 1961), contain excellent material on this subject. An outstanding collection of chapters written by distinguished authors is contained in the Ciba Foundation Symposium, *Disorders of Language*, edited by De Reuck and O'Connor (Boston, Little, Brown and Co., 1964).

An important work in press at the time of this writing which should be noted is *Assessment of Aphasia and Related Disorders* by Goodglass (Philadelphia, Lea and Febiger, 1972).

We have come a long way from the time when aphasia was viewed as a motor deficit of the tongue. We now recognize that the study of aphasia and the wider subject of normal brain function demands multi-disciplinary participation. This volume will, I hope, contribute to that ongoing process.

I am deeply grateful to the authors and publishers who consented to give permission to reprint their papers, to the many staff members of Speech Pathology Service, Institute of Rehabilitation Medicine, who assisted in the details of assembling this volume, and to Lita Elvers for the final preparation of the manuscript.

I am especially grateful to my husband, John, for his keen interest and incisive criticism.

M.T.S.

CONTENTS

LIST OF JOURNAL ABBREVIATIONS

Acta Neurol Psychiat Belg	Acta Neurologica et Psychiatrica Belgica (Brussels)
Acta Otorinolaring Iber Amer	Acta Oto-Rino-Laringologica Ibero-Americana (Barcelona)
Acta Psychiat Kbh Suppl	Acta Psychiatrica Scandinavica Supplement (Copenhagen)
Acta Psychiat Neurol Scand	Acta Psychiatrica et Neurologica Scandinavica (Copenhagen)
Ala J Med Sci	Alabama Journal of Medical Science (Birmingham)
AMA Arch Neurol Psychiat	American Medical Association Archives of Neurology and Psychiatry (Chicago) NOW CALLED Archives of Neurology and Psychiatry
Amer Arch Rehab Ther	American Archives of Rehabilitation Therapy (Montrose, N.Y.)
Amer J Ophthal	American Journal of Ophthalmology (Chicago)
Amer J Orthopsychiat	American Journal of Orthopsychiatry (N.Y.C.)
Amer J Phys Med	American Journal of Physical Medicine (Baltimore)
Amer J Psychiat	American Journal of Psychiatry (Hanover, N.H.)
Amer Sci	American Scientist (New Haven)
Ann Intern Med	Annals of Internal Medicine (Philadelphia)
Ann Otol	Annals of Otology, Rhinology and Laryngology (St. Louis)
Arch Gen Psychiat	Archives of General Psychiatry (Chicago)
Arch Intern Med	Archives of Internal Medicine (Chicago)
Arch Neurol	Archives of Neurology (Chicago)
Arch Phys Med	Archives of Physical Medicine and Rehabilitation (Chicago)
Arch Psychiat	Archives of Psychiatry (Chicago)
Arizona Med	Arizona Medicine (Scottsdale)
ASHA	Journal of the American Speech and Hearing Association (Washington)
Brain	Brain: Journal of Neurology (London)
Brit J Disord Commun	British Journal of Disorders of Communication (Edinburgh) INCORPORATES Speech Pathology and Therapy (London)
Brit J Psychiat	British Journal of Psychiatry (London)
Brit Med J	British Medical Journal (London)
Bull Hist Med	Bulletin of the History of Medicine (Baltimore)
Bull LA Neurol Soc	Bulletin of the Los Angeles Neurological Societies (Los Angeles)
Bull Menninger Clin	Bulletin of the Menninger Clinic (Topeka)
Bull Neurol Inst NY	Bulletin of the Neurological Institute of New York (N.Y.C.)
Bull US Army Med Dept	Bulletin of the U.S. Army Medical Department (Washington)
Canad J Psychol	Canadian Journal of Psychology (Toronto)
Canad Med Ass J	Canadian Medical Association Journal (Toronto)
Confin Neurol	Confinia Neurologica (Basel)
Cortex	Cortex: A Journal Devoted to the Study of the Nervous System and Behavior (Milan)
Dis Nerv Syst	Diseases of the Nervous System (Galveston)
Education	Education (Boston)

Encephale	Encephale (Paris)
Folia Phoniat	Folia Phoniatrica (Basel)
Hearing Speech News	Hearing and Speech News (Washington) FORMERLY Hearing News
Int J Clin Exper Hypn	International Journal of Clinical and Experimental Hypnosis (Baltimore) FORMERLY Journal of Clinical and Experimental Hypnosis
Int J Neurol	International Journal of Neurology (Montevideo)
J Abnorm Psychol	Journal of Abnormal Psychology (Washington) FORMERLY Journal of Abnormal and Social Psychology
J Abnorm Soc Psychol	Journal of Abnormal and Social Psychology (Washington) NOW CALLED Journal of Abnormal Psychology
JAMA	Journal of the American Medical Association (Chicago)
J Amer Geriat Soc	Journal of the American Geriatrics Society (Chicago)
J Aust Coll Speech Ther	Journal of the Australian College of Speech Therapists (New South Wales)
J Chronic Dis	Journal of Chronic Diseases (St. Louis)
J Clin Exper Hypn	Journal of Clinical and Experimental Hypnosis (New York) NOW CALLED International Journal of Clinical and Experimental Hypnosis
J Clin Psychol	Journal of Clinical Psychology (Brandon, Vt.)
J Commun Disord	Journal of Communication Disorders (Amsterdam)
J Consult Psychol	Journal of Consulting Psychology (Washington) NOW CALLED Journal of Consulting and Clinical Psychology
J Education	Journal of Education, Boston University School of Education (Boston)
J Gen Psychol	Journal of General Psychology (Provincetown)
J Hist Med	Journal of the History of Medicine and Allied Sciences (New Haven)
J Laryng	Journal of Laryngology and Otology (London)
J Learn Disabil	Journal of Learning Disabilities (Chicago)
J Ment Sci	Journal of Mental Science (London)
J Mount Sinai Hosp NY	Journal of the Mount Sinai Hospital, New York (N.Y.C.)
J Nerv Ment Dis	Journal of Nervous and Mental Disease (Baltimore)
J Neurol Neurosurg Psychiat	Journal of Neurology, Neurosurgery and Psychiatry (London)
J Neurol Psychiat	Journal of Neurology and Psychiatry (London)
J Neurol Sci	Journal of the Neurological Sciences (Amsterdam)
J Neuropsychiat	Journal of Neuropsychiatry (Chicago)
J Neurosurg	Journal of Neurosurgery (Chicago)
J Prog Inst	Journal of Programmed Instruction (West Nyack, N.Y.)
J Psychol	Journal of Psychology (Provincetown)
J S Afr Logoped Soc	Journal of the South African Logopedic Society (Johannesburg)
J Speech Dis	Journal of Speech Disorders (Danville) NOW CALLED Journal of Speech and Hearing Disorders
J Speech Hearing Dis	Journal of Speech and Hearing Disorders (Danville) FORMERLY Journal of Speech Disorders
J Speech Hearing Res	Journal of Speech and Hearing Research (Iowa City)
Lancet	Lancet (London)
Lang Learn	Language Learning (Ann Arbor)

Lang Speech	Language and Speech (Teddington)
Laryngoscope	Laryngoscope (St. Louis)
Ling Rep	The Linguistic Reporter (Washington)
Logos	Logos: Bulletin of the National Hospital for Speech Disorders (N.Y.C.)
Mayo Clin Proc	Mayo Clinic Proceedings (Rochester, Minn.)
Med Clin N Amer	Medical Clinics of North America (Philadelphia)
Med Hist	Medical History (London)
Med Rec	Medical Record (N.Y.C.)
Med Trial Techn Quart	Medical Trial Technique Quarterly (Mundelein)
Milit Surg	The Military Surgeon (Washington)
Nat Soc Prog Inst J	National Society for Programmed Instruction Journal (San Antonio)
Neurology	Neurology (Minneapolis)
Neuropsychol	Neuropsychologia (Oxford)
New York J Med	New York State Journal of Medicine (N.Y.C.)
NJ Speech Hearing Ass J	New Jersey Speech and Hearing Association Journal
NY Speech Hearing Ass Newsl	New York Speech and Hearing Association Newsletter (Great Neck)
Percept Motor Skills	Perceptual and Motor Skills (Missoula)
Postgrad Med	Postgraduate Medicine (Minneapolis)
Proc Roy Soc Med	Proceedings of the Royal Society of Medicine (London)
Psychiat Neurol	Psychiatria et Neurologia (Basel)
Psychol Rec	Psychological Record (Granville, Ohio)
Psychol Rev	Psychological Review (Washington)
Psychophysiol	Psychophysiology (Baltimore)
Public Health Rep	Public Health Reports (Washington)
Rehab Lit	Rehabilitation Literature (Chicago)
Science	Science (Washington)
Scot Med J	Scottish Medical Journal (Glasgow)
Slow Learn Child	The Slow Learning Child (St. Lucia, Brisbane)
Trans Amer Neurol Ass	Transactions of the American Neurological Association (N.Y.C.)
Word	Word (N.Y.C.)

part I

SYMPTOMATOLOGY AND PHENOMENOLOGY

Introduction

Since aphasia is, by definition, a group of symptoms, anything the student reads on the subject will contribute to his knowledge of symptomatology and phenomenology. Hence, the papers in this section are written by authors who represent many disciplines. The abundant literature which focuses on the symptoms of aphasia reflects in part the lack of an acceptable model of how language is organized in the brain and how it is lost by sickness or injury. Researchers can only describe as carefully as possible what they observe in the hope of providing some clue to the physiology and pathology of the underlying process.

While these papers will bring the student abreast of current concepts on the nature of aphasia symptomatology, his reading should also include some of the classical textbooks of aphasia. The works of Head (1), Schuell (6), Wepman (9), and Weisenburg and McBride (8) include a great deal of material relevant to symptomatology. Of particular value is the large number of case histories they contain. These texts are noted in the preface and listed in the bibliography at the end of this volume.

Most of the papers included in this section are of recent vintage, and many represent a trend toward describing the symptoms of aphasia from a psycholinguistic point of view. This perspective is particularly apparent in the work of Goodglass and his co-workers (Readings 3, 6, 8, and 14). Their studies provide a good sample of the kinds of research questions which can best be investigated by methods derived from psycholinguistic theory. Of particular interest is Reading 6, which presents objective data to support the diagnostic differences among Broca's, Wernicke's, and amnesic aphasics. The paper by Spreen (Reading 18) is an excellent review of the main course of thinking and research on the psycholinguistic aspects of aphasia and a strong argument for the value of studying aphasia from this vantage point.

The two papers by T. Alajouanine (Readings 2 and 22), the well-known French neurologist, were selected for their clinical as well as their theoretical interest. In each, the author concerns himself with special problems in aphasia: the loss or preservation of creativity in the professional artist and the interesting phenomenon known as verbal stereotypy. In addition to the excellent case descriptions to be found in these papers, the author presents stimulating and provocative material concerning the impact of aphasia on the creative process, the sparing of creativity in art forms not dependent on language (symbols) for expression, and the highly controversial subject of the relationship between language and thought.

Some of the classical symptoms of aphasia are studied in great detail in the representative papers selected; for example, the part includes Schuell on reduction of vocabulary (Reading 1), Geschwind on naming deficits (Reading 4), and Goodglass and Kaplan on disorders of gesture and pantomime (Reading 10).

Grewel's paper on acaculia (Reading 15) is to our knowledge the only one that focuses specifically on the clinical manifestations of calculation deficits, so commonly seen in aphasic patients.

The article by Benton on the Gerstmann Syndrome (Reading 16) is particularly valuable because it suggests a model on how to objectively approach the analysis of a behavioral entity, and especially in this case since a combination of symptoms were assumed for many years to belong together by virtue of anatomical propinquity.

Aphasia, which is generally held to be a disorder in the symbolic manipulation of language, seems also to implicate frequently phenomena in the motor expression of speech. The nature of these disorders and their relationship to symbolic functions is still unclear. Indeed, no dichotomy may exist. In order to expose the reader to this realm, the paper by Shankweiler and Harris on articulatory defects and phonetic disintegration (Reading 12) and the pioneer study of DeRenzi and others (Reading 13) are included. The latter explores the relationships between oral apraxia, articulation disorders, limb apraxia, and symbolic aphasia.

Some of the most interesting speculation on the nature of aphasia has centered on the perception or comprehension of language. Although one point of view holds that the totality of aphasia can be explained on the basis of disordered processing of language input, the mainstream of thought asserts either one of two perspectives: (a) that there are separate systems of comprehension and expression that are closely related but distinct entities; or (b) that there is a unitary system that binds together inextricably comprehension and expression. Two papers dealing with input or comprehension phenomena are included (Reading 11 by Spinler and Vignolo, and 19 by Efron). They are provocative, important papers advancing hypotheses based on sound experimental procedure.

The article "Language after Section of the Cerebral Commissures" by Gazzaniga and Sperry (Reading 17) is included because it seems to promise through the application of a new technique great importance for the study of language processes.

Although none of the renowned investigators represented in this volume can be singled out fairly as more preeminent than any other for his contributions to the field, certainly the collection would not be complete without a sample from the prolific work of Luria. His paper on brain disorders and language analysis, difficult as it is to categorize (Reading 23), provides an excellent example of his thinking on aphasia.

Because knowledge of the emotional impact of aphasia on the patient and his family is vital, we suggest some reading in this area. Ullman (7), a psychiatrist, has produced a volume of case histories which describe emotional sequellae in stroke patients, many of whom are aphasic. The personal account of Guy Wint (11) is most instructive, and the book *Stroke: The Condition and the Patient* (5) provides information that is often not included in papers and texts on aphasia.

We are still far from understanding the riddle of aphasia. And because our knowledge of the subject is largely descriptive, it is quite logical that the section devoted to this aspect should be the most extensive in the book.

REFERENCES

1. Head, H. *Aphasia and Kindred Disorders of Speech.* New York, Hafner, 1963.
2. Goodglass, H. Studies on the Grammar of Aphasics. In: Rosenberg, S., Koplin, J. E. (eds.): *Developments in Applied Psycholinguistics Research.* New York, Macmillan, 1968.
3. Jakobson, R. Towards a Linguistic Topology of Aphasic Impairments. In: de Reuck, A. V. S., O'Connor, M. (eds.), *Disorders of Language.* Boston, Little, Brown, 1964.
4. Luria, A. R. Factors and Forms of Aphasia. In: de Reuck, A. V. S., O'Connor, M. (eds.), *Disorders of Language.* Boston, Little, Brown, 1964.
5. Sarno, J. E., Sarno, M. T. *Stroke: The Condition and the Patient.* New York, McGraw-Hill, 1969.
6. Schuell, H. M., Jenkins, J. J. *Aphasia in Adults.* New York, Harper, 1964.
7. Ullman, M. *Behavioral Changes in Patients Following Strokes.* Springfield, Ill., Thomas, 1962.
8. Weisenburg, T. H., McBride, K. E. *Aphasia: A Clinical and Psychological Study.* New York, Hafner, 1964.
9. Wepman, J. M. *Recovery from Aphasia.* New York, Ronald, 1951.
10. Wepman, J. M., Jones, L. V.: Five Aphasias: A Commentary on Aphasia as a Regressive Linguistic Phenomenon. In: Rioch, D. M., Weinstein, E. A. (eds.), *Disorders of Communication.* Baltimore, Williams and Wilkins, 1964.
11. Wint, G. *The Third Killer.* New York, Abelard-Schuman, 1967.

1

Reduction of Vocabulary in Aphasia

HILDRED M. SCHUELL
JAMES J. JENKINS

HILDRED M. SCHUELL, Ph.D. (deceased), was director of the aphasia section of the neurology service of the Minneapolis Veterans Administration Hospital, and was with the department of neurology of the Graduate School of Medicine, University of Minnesota.

JAMES J. JENKINS, Ph.D., is with the department of psychology of the University of Minnesota.

This investigation was supported in part by Public Health Service Grant B 1948, from the National Institutes of Health, Public Health Service.

In the framework of present-day research it appears most meaningful to define aphasia as a reduction of language resulting from brain injury, which cuts across various language modalities, such as comprehension of spoken language, speech, reading and writing, and upon which specific perceptual, motor or sensorimotor deficits may or may not be superimposed.

Freud (1953) proposed regarding the speech area as a field, the peripheries of which were the primary motor and sensory areas. He suggested that if one imagined a movable lesion in this field, the closer the lesion approached one of the primary sensory or motor areas, the more observed symptoms could be expected to partake of the characteristics of the given area.

Penfield and Roberts (1959), from a ten-year study of language disturbances observed during seizures, sodium amytal injections, electrical stimulation of the cortex of conscious and co-operating patients, cortical excisions and other brain surgery, reached a similar conclusion. Roberts states that lesions in specific sites may result in specific clinical syndromes, although he points out that this does not mean that there is a center in Broca's area for the motor patterns of words, or one in the angular gyrus for recognition of letters, numbers or words. He adds that there is not a single case in the literature of "visual-verbal agnosia," for example, without other defects or without ability to recognize some word at some time, if the examination is detailed enough. This conclusion is compatible with findings reported by Head (1926), Weisenburg and McBride (1935), Wepman (1958), and Schuell and Jenkins (1959).

In a preliminary report of a study still in progress consisting of a factor analysis of test responses of 168 aphasic patients in 19 hospitals, Wepman and Jones (1958) have tentatively interpreted the major factor identified as "probably indicating a general ability of patients to manipulate verbal symbols." At the same time they found separate scores for visual and auditory stimuli, and oral and graphic responses extremely useful in characterizing individual patients. Both these findings are in essential agreement with the point of view expressed by Freud (1953), by Roberts (1959), and by Schuell and Jenkins (1959), that is, that there is a general language deficit in aphasia, but specific symptomatology differs from patient to patient. Both aspects of the clinical picture must be understood.

In a previous study by the present authors, responses of 123 aphasic patients to 18 lan-

From *Brain* 84:243-61, 1961. Reprinted by permission of the Editor of *Brain*.

guage tests which sampled various stimulus and response modes and covered a wide range of difficulty, were found to be scalable by the Guttman technique (1947). This means briefly that if tests were ranked in order of difficulty defined by the number of patients who failed each one, and if patients were ranked in order of severity of aphasic involvement defined by the number of tests failed by each patient, it was possible to predict from one scale to the other with about 90 percent accuracy. This is considered evidence of a single dimension of language deficit present in all these patients, at a statistically significant level, in spite of perceptual, motor and sensorimotor concomitants of brain damage present in some patients and not in others, and reflected in test responses. It means that nineteenth century theories of isolated disturbances of single language modalities resulting from circumscribed lesions of topographical cortical areas are no longer tenable, but neither are theories of cortical equipotentiality.

It is the purpose of this paper to explore one aspect of the general language reduction in aphasia, namely, reduction of vocabulary, and to present data showing some of the ways in which this reduction is manifested in various language modalities.

REDUCTION OF VOCABULARY IN COMPREHENSION OF SPOKEN LANGUAGE

It has been observed clinically that when aphasic patients were asked to point to objects or pictures named by the examiner, they tended to confuse (*a*) words which sound alike (goat, coat; lake, rake), an auditory perceptual confusion; (*b*) words associated in meaning or experience (sky, blue; chair, table), a semantic confusion; and that only a few patients, in general those most impaired, confused dissimilar unrelated words.

To explore these observations in a systematic manner, a test was constructed consisting of 15 picture cards. Each card contained four pictures: (*a*) the test object; (*b*) an object whose name rhymed with the test word; (*c*) an object closely associated with the test object, as evidenced by the fact that it was a popular response to the test word on the Kent-Rosanoff Word Association Test (Kent and Rosanoff, 1910; Russell and Jenkins, 1954); and (*d*) an unrelated object. The following are examples of the pictures contained on the first three cards, with the test word first:

(1) *Chair*, stair, table, apple.
(2) *Bread*, bed, butter, boy.
(3) *Man*, pan, woman, star.

A card was presented to the patient; the examiner spoke the test word only; the patient was required to point to the object named. Two presentations were made of the set of pictures. On the first presentation the stimulus was the word spoken by the examiner. This will be referred to as the auditory presentation. On the second presentation, a printed word on an individual card was presented at the same time the word was spoken by the examiner. This will be referred to as the combined auditory and visual presentation.

The test was administered to an unselected sample of 117 aphasic patients seen on the Neurology Service at the Minneapolis VA Hospital between March 1957 and November 1959. All patients had been previously examined by means of the Minnesota Test for Differential Diagnosis of Aphasia (Schuell, 1955*a*) developed at this center, and classified in clinical groups previously described by Schuell (1955*b*) on the basis of these findings. These classifications are briefly as follows:

Group 1.—Severe impairment, amounting to almost total loss of functional language skills in all modalities.

Group 2.—Reduction of vocabulary and retention span in all modalities.

Group 3.—Reduction of vocabulary and retention span in all modalities, with coexisting involvement of visual processes.

Group 4.—Reduction of vocabulary and retention span in all modalities with coexisting involvement of sensorimotor processes.

Group 5.—Simultaneous involvement of auditory, visual and motor processes with some functional language skills retained.

In addition 3 patients were classified as *Group* 6, a clinical syndrome characterized by auditory imperception with retention of some spontaneous speech. One of these patients was tested on two admissions, a year apart, making a total of four records for Group 6. This is the only such duplication in the series. 2 patients were unclassified because they were not considered physiologically stable when tested. These data are contaminated to some extent by inclusion of patients who had undergone intensive treatment for aphasia for varying periods of time, as well as patients who had received no treatment. 50 patients made no errors on either presentation, leaving data from 67 patients, of whom all made at least one error, to be analyzed.

Findings

Table 1-1 shows the number, the mean number and the percentage of each type of error, and the total errors made by patients in each clinical group, and for the whole sample, for both the auditory and the combined presentations.

Several findings are of interest here. The first is the relatively high frequency of association errors. When the auditory stimulus alone

TABLE 1-1. NUMBER, MEAN AND PERCENTAGE OF ERROR TYPES AND TOTAL AUDITORY RECOGNITION ERRORS FOR CLINICAL GROUPS

	Group	*N*	*Stim.*	*Aud. errors*	*Ass. errors*	*Ran. errors*	*D. K.*	*Total errors*
N	1	15	Aud.	27	44	19	2	92
M				1·81	2·95	1·27	·13	6·16
%				29%	48%	21%	2%	100%
N			Comb.	23	40	17	4	84
M				1·54	2·68	1·14	·27	5·63
%				27%	48%	20%	5%	100%
N	2	6	Aud.	2	9	0	1	12
M				·33	1·50		·17	2·00
%				17%	75%		8%	100%
N			Comb.	1	4	0	0	5
M				·17	·67			·84
%				20%	80%			100%
N	3	7	Aud.	3	10	1	0	14
M				·43	1·43	·14		2·00
%				22%	71%	7%		100%
N			Comb.	0	10	0	0	10
M					1·43			1·43
%					100%			100%
N	4	4	Aud.	3	11	0	0	14
M				·75	2·75			3·50
%				21%	79%			100%
N			Comb.	2	6	0	0	8
M				·50	1·50			2·00
%				25%	75%			100%
N	5	29	Aud.	12	46	2	18	78
M				·41	1·59	·07	·62	2·69
%				15%	59%	3%	23%	100%
N			Comb.	8	40	1	4	53
M				·28	1·38	·03	·13	1·83
%				15%	75%	2%	8%	100%

N	6	4	Aud.	1	9	0	1	11
M				·25	2·25		·25	2·75
%				9%	82%		9%	100%
N			Comb.	1	3	0	1	5
M				·25	·75		·25	1·25
%				20%	60%		20%	100%
N	Unclass.	2	Aud.	0	5	0	0	5
M								
%								
N			Comb.	0	2	0	0	2
M								
%								
N	Total	67	Aud.	48	134	22	22	226
M				·72	2·00	·33	·33	3·37
%				21%	59%	10%	10%	100%
N			Comb.	35	105	18	9	167
M				·52	1·57	·27	·13	2·49
%				21%	63%	11%	5%	100%

was presented, 59 percent of all errors were association errors, that is, confusion of words like chair and table, man and woman, house and car, nose and mouth and so on. 21 percent of the total errors were confusions of words which sound alike, such as chair and stair, bed and bread, house and mouse, and nose and rose. 10 percent were confusions of unrelated words such as chair and apple, bread and boy, man and star, and house and fish; 10 percent were "don't know" responses. There were about six times as many association errors as random errors. 86 percent of all the random errors were made by the 15 Group 1 patients, the most severe aphasics. Group 2 patients, who were in general the least impaired, made no random errors, and 75 percent of their total errors were association errors. One random error was made in Group 3 and two in Group 5. Since patients in both of these groups have involvement of visual processes, it is possible that these minimal errors could have been related to the pictures rather than the words. For example, it is possible that a patient might fail to see the correct picture and respond by guessing.

When combined visual and auditory stimuli were presented, the task became easier for most patients. The mean number of total errors decreased for all clinical groups, and the mean number of each type of error decreased for the total sample. The decrease in total errors was significant beyond the .001 level of confidence and the decrease in association errors beyond the .05 level. In other words, using combined visual and auditory stimuli helps most aphasic patients. The correlation between the scores of patients on the first and second presentations was + .84. This indicates that, in the main, the addition of the printed stimulus raised the frequency of correct identifications in a relatively uniform fashion. The subjects received about the same relative ranking on the two administrations. However, close examination of the data revealed that the combined stimuli were most helpful to patients in Groups 2, 4 and 6 who were presumably able to make the best use of added visual cues. Since the number of patients in some of the individual groups is too small for meaningful analysis, the percentage of error reduction with the combined stimuli is shown for patients in Groups 2, 4 and 6 combined, and compared with the reduction in Groups 1, 3 and 5. It is probable that in Group 1 the language reduction is so great that the printed word does not help much; in Groups 3 and 5 impairment of visual discrimination and recognition cuts down the effectiveness of the visual cue, although it still provides some help. The presence of the visual stimulus appears

TABLE 1–2. NUMBER, MEAN NUMBER AND PERCENTAGE OF ERROR REDUCTION ON AUDITORY RECOGNITION FOR GROUPS 1, 3 AND 5 COMBINED, GROUPS 2, 4 AND 6 COMBINED, AND FOR THE TOTAL SAMPLE

Stim.		*Aud. errors*	*Ass. errors*	*Rand. errors*	*D. K.*	*Total*
		Groups 1, 3 and 5 combined (N 51) (Patients with visual involvement)				
Aud.	N	42	100	22	20	184
	M	·82	1·96	·43	·39	3·61
Comb.	N	31	90	18	8	147
	M	·61	1·76	·35	·16	2·88
% reduction		26%	10%	18%	60%	20%
		Groups 2, 4 and 6 combined (N 14) (Patients without visual involvement)				
Aud.	N	6	29	0	2	37
	M	·43	2·07		·14	2·64
Comb.	N	4	13	0	1	18
	M	·14	1·14		·07	1·36
% reduction		33%	55%		50%	51%
		Total Sample (N 67)				
Aud.	N	48	134	22	22	226
	M	·72	2·00	·33	·33	3·37
Comb.	N	35	105	18	9	167
	M	·52	1·57	·27	·13	2·49
% reduction		27%	22%	18%	59%	26%

chiefly to reduce the number of "don't know" responses. These data are shown in Table 1-2, which simply indicates that all aphasic patients do not utilize visual cues equally, and that it is possible, on the basis of comprehensive clinical examinations to predict which patients will not be able to do so, since patients were not classified on the basis of the present test.

Table 1-3 shows the percentage of each kind of error made by patients grouped according to

TABLE 1–3. PERCENTAGE OF ERROR TYPES ON AUDITORY RECOGNITION FOR PATIENTS GROUPED ACCORDING TO TOTAL ERRORS

Stim.	*Errors*	*N. patients*	*Aud. errors*	*Ass. errors*	*Rand. and Total D. K.*	*Total errors*
Aud.	0	2				0
	1	19		100%		19
	2–3	24	21%	72%	7%	61
	4–6	13	15%	72%	13%	61
	7–9	5	22%	44%	34%	41
	10–12	4	39%	20%	41%	44
Total		67	21%	59%	20%	226
Comb.	0	15				
	1	24	8%	92%		24
	2–3	13	12%	85%	3%	33
	4–6	7	14%	67%	19%	36
	7–9	5	28%	45%	28%	40
	10–13	3	38%	38%	24%	34
Total		67	21%	63%	16%	167
Both presentations combined	1	14		100%		14
	2–3	17	7%	91%	2%	44
	4–6	19	19%	77%	4%	96
	7–14	8	15%	64%	21%	80
	15–25	9	31%	38%	19%	159
Total		67	21%	61%	18%	393

the total errors made on each presentation, and on the two presentations combined. Patients ranked as making zero errors made no errors on one presentation but did on the other. Here it can be seen again that association errors constitute the "best" errors; if a patient makes only one error it will almost certainly be an association-type error. In general the more errors a patient makes, the more random and "don't know" responses there will be. Auditory errors are less predictable on the basis of total score. The probability is that this kind of auditory confusion does not reflect a general language reduction in most cases, but rather a perceptual deficit, a partial auditory imperception found in some patients but not in others.

Findings reveal a reduction of vocabulary in auditory recognition. Errors are of three classes: (1) confusion of words closely associated in meaning; (2) confusion of words similar in sound; and (3) random and "don't know" responses.

When the stimulus is strengthened by the addition of a visual cue, errors decrease in general, but decrease most for those patients who are able to utilize the added visual cue to the best advantage.

Association errors are the most common, and constitute the greatest proportion of the errors of patients with mild impairment. Auditory confusions occur on all levels except perhaps the very mildest, and appear to represent a specific impairment of auditory perception. Random errors tend to occur only in the most severely impaired patients.

REDUCTION OF NAMING VOCABULARY

Previous studies have shown that naming, which involves recall, as well as a finely coordinated motor response, is a much harder task for aphasic patients than pointing to objects named by the examiner, which involves only recognition and pointing (Schuell and Jenkins, 1959).

A test was constructed consisting of 18 cards, each containing a picture of a common object, and the name of the object in print. Words were all taken from the first thousand most commonly used words in the English language (Thorndike and Lorge, 1944), and were all words used on the Kent-Rosanoff Word Association Test, for which the popular responses of normal populations are known (Russell and Jenkins, 1954). Words used were baby, bread, chair, yellow, hand, street, head, table, boy, green, house, sheep, window, girl, blue, bed, man and red. The patients were asked to look at the card and name the picture.

The test was administered to a non-selected series of 92 aphasic patients. 24 patients made no errors; 8 were judged untestable because no responses could be secured. Data consist of 487 errors, out of 1,080 responses made by the remaining 60 patients.

Errors were classified as association errors, approximations, and irrelevant and "don't know" responses.

Only errors clearly associated with the stimulus in meaning were classified as association errors. Most of these were popular responses, such as *boy* for *girl*, *green* for *red*, and *door* for *window*. A few were personal associations such as *Lisa* (the patient's daughter) for *girl*. Questionable associations such as *dig* for *girl* were classified as irrelevant.

Intelligible but defective responses (such as *dirl* for *girl*, or *boo* for *blue*) were classified as approximations. Mispronunciations which are recognizable attempts to pronounce the correct word are made by two groups of patients, those whose auditory feedback or auditory recall is imperfect, and those whose motor control is defective. Clinically these errors can be distinguished by the consistency of the motor errors (the same sounds tend to be consistently defective). For example, *wed* for *red* is an error which occurs frequently when patients have difficulty pronouncing initial "r." To take a different example from the present data, *timble* for *table* involves more complex coordinations than the correct word, and is probably an auditory inaccuracy. In addition to the inconsistency, auditory errors can usually be corrected readily by ear, while motor or sensorimotor errors tend to be more resistant. However, no attempt has been made to distinguish

TABLE 1-4. FREQUENCY OF ERROR TYPES IN NAMING FOR CLINICAL GROUPS AND TOTAL SAMPLE

Group	*N*		*Association errors*	*Approximation errors*	*D. K. and irrelevant*	*Total*
Group 1	5	N	5	20	52	77
		M	1·00	4·00	10·40	15·40
		%	6%	26%	68%	100%
Group 2	6	N	8	6	9	23
		M	1·33	1·00	1·50	3·83
		%	35%	26%	39%	100%
Group 3	6	N	18	3	3	24
		M	3·00	·50	·50	4·00
		%	75%	12·5%	12·5%	100%
Group 4	8	N	32	6	33	71
		M	4·00	·75	4·13	8·88
		%	45%	8%	47%	100%
Group 5	29	N	57	50	98	205
		M	1·97	1·72	3·38	7·07
		%	28%	24%	48%	100%
Group 6	4	N	16	5	43	64
		M	4·00	1·25	10·75	16·00
		%	25%	8%	67%	100%
Unclass.	2	N	7	2	14	23
Total	60	N	143	92	252	487
		M	2·38	1·53	4·20	8·12
		%	29%	19%	52%	100%

between the two types of mispronunciations here, since this involves detailed study of the overall speech pattern of each patient.

Irrelevant responses consisted of jargon, perseverative responses and occasional irrelevant words; these were combined with no response, for the purposes of this analysis.

Data here, like those for word recognition above, were contaminated by inclusion of patients who had received intensive treatment as well as patients who had received none.

Table 1-4 shows the number, mean number and percentage of each kind of error for the clinical groups previously described and for the entire sample. 29 percent of total errors were association errors, 19 percent were approximations, and 52 percent were irrelevant or "don't know" responses.

Comparisons between the clinical groups are not very meaningful because of the small number of patients in some groups. In general, Group 1 patients perform a little better than expectancy for this group, probably because patients who could not perform at all were excluded. Group 2, on the other hand, would be expected to perform more like Group 3 in this sample if this were a characteristic distribution of Group 2 patients. Here it included two patients who made eight errors each, one who made four, and three who made one error apiece. In Group 4 more approximation errors would be expected; these are probably obscured first by the fact that patients who had received treatment had mastered most common monosyllabic words, and secondly by the large proportion of unintelligible or "don't know" responses made by the more severe patients in the group.

Table 1-5 shows that if Group 6 is excluded, the order of severity for the clinical groups is about the same for naming as for auditory recognition.

Group 6 patients ranked third in order of severity (M = 2·75) on word recognition, and most severe on naming (M = 16). These are patients who have partial auditory imperception, with retention of some appropriate spontaneous speech. The extreme difficulty such patients have naming and giving specific information, even when they understand what is desired, is in marked contrast to their conversational speech, which must arise from complex patterns of environmental and internal stimuli. This discrepancy is found in no other clinical group. Theoretically, if Penfield and Roberts (1959) are correct in postulating a language

TABLE 1-5. MEAN NUMBER OF ERRORS FOR CLINICAL GROUPS AND TOTAL SAMPLE ON WORD RECOGNITION (AUDITORY STIMULUS) AND NAMING TESTS

	Word recognition mean	*Naming mean*
Group 1	6·16	15·40
Group 4	3·50	8·88
Group 5	2·69	7·07
Group 2	2·00	3·83
Group 3	2·00	4·00
Total sample	3·48	8·12

integrating mechanism in the thalamus which receives impulses from auditory and visual cortical areas, such a clinical picture could result from partial interruption of these pathways, while the thalamic nuclei could still be stimulated from other sources, producing some language. The spontaneous speech of these patients while frequently fluent, well-formulated and appropriate is by no means intact. One Group 6 patient receiving treatment at present frequently tells his clinician, "You tell me it's right, but I don't know what I said." At the same time he frequently knows when his response is wrong.

In Table 1-6, patients in Groups 1, 4 and 5, all of whom have a motor or sensorimotor defect are combined, and compared with patients in Groups 2, 3 and 6 who have no specific motor problems, although they mispronounce words because of defective auditory feedback and recall. In spite of this, patients in the first three groups make more approximation errors, as would be predicted, both when means and percentages of approximation errors are compared.

In Table 1-7 types of naming errors are compared with total errors ranked in order of magnitude. Here it can be seen again that in general there is an inverse relationship between association errors and total errors, and a positive one between total errors and irrelevant or "don't know" responses. Approximation errors, on the other hand, are less predictable on the basis of total score, since they reflect specific kinds of impairment which are present in some patients and not in others, and which may be of any degree of severity, from mild to extremely severe.

REDUCTION OF READING VOCABULARY

A test was constructed consisting of 30 sets of paired words. Ten pairs were popular associa-

TABLE 1-6. FREQUENCY OF ERROR TYPES IN NAMING FOR CLINICAL GROUPS 1, 4 AND 5 AND GROUPS 2, 3 AND 6 COMBINED

N		*Association errors*	*Approximation errors*	*Irrelevant and "don't know"*	*Total*
		Groups 1, 4 and 5 combined (Patients with motor involvement)			
42		94	76	183	353
	M	2·24	1·81	4·36	8·40
	%	27%	21%	52%	100%
		Groups 2, 3 and 6 combined (Patients without motor involvement)			
16		42	14	55	111
	M	2·63	·88	3·44	6·94
	%	38%	13%	49%	100%
		Total sample (58*)			
58		136	90	238	464
	M	2·34	1·55	4·10	8·00
	%	29%	20%	51%	100%

*Two unclassified patients omitted.

TABLE 1–7. FREQUENCY OF TYPES OF NAMING ERRORS COMPARED WITH TOTAL ERRORS

Total errors	*N*	*Association errors*	*Approximation errors*	*D. K. and irrelevant*	*Total*
1	12	9	1	2	12
		75%	8%	17%	M 1·0
2–4	9	12	10	1	23
		52%	44%	4%	M 2·25
5–7	7	19	5	15	39
		49%	13%	38%	M 5·57
8–10	11	44	15	37	96
		46%	16%	38%	M 8·73
11–15	11	37	35	76	148
		25%	24%	51%	M 13·45
16–18	10	22	26	121	169
		13%	15%	72%	M 16·90
Total	60	143	92	252	487
		29%	19%	52%	M 8·12

tions, such as desk-chair, window-door and stand-sit. Ten pairs were words which sound alike but do not look alike, such as pies-buys, bed-said and blow-sew. The last ten pairs were words which look alike but do not sound alike, such as horse-house, bear-hear and bank-bark.

Two presentations of the test were made to each subject. For the visual presentation each card contained a picture of the test object, with the two printed words below, and the subject was required to point to the word which matched the picture. For the auditory presentation each card contained the two words of the pair, and the subject was asked to point to the word spoken by the examiner. Association, visual and auditory pairs were randomized for presentation, and the two forms of the test were administered on different days.

The test was administered to 21 aphasic patients. This cannot be considered a representative sample. It consisted of 13 Group 5 patients, 4 Group 3 patients, 2 Group 6 patients, and 2 patients who were not classified because they were not considered neurologically stable.

Findings

Table 1-8 shows the number, mean number and percentage of each type of error made by 21 patients on each type of presentation, with combined errors for both presentations.

The fact that more errors were made matching words to pictures than matching printed to spoken words is considered an artifact of this sample. There is a similar test on the Minnesota Test for Differential Diagnosis of Aphasia, except that error types are not differentiated and precise discriminations are not required. Unpublished data from an exploratory study which tabulated results for 131 aphasic patients shows a reversal of this finding. 41 percent of this sample made errors matching printed to spoken words, with a mean error of 5.13, while 31 percent of these patients made errors matching words to pictures, with a mean error of only 1.65.

However the present data are sufficient to show a reduction of reading vocabulary, even on very common words, and the presence of both association errors and perceptual confusions.

TABLE 1–8. NUMBER, MEAN AND PERCENTAGE OF TYPES OF READING ERRORS

N		*Visual errors*	*Auditory errors*	*Association errors*	*Total errors*
		Matching Word to Picture			
21	N	17	12	31	60
	M	·81	·57	1·48	2·86
	%	28%	20%	52%	100%
		Printed to Spoken Word			
21	N	24	9	19	52
	M	1·14	·43	·90	2·48
	%	46%	17%	37%	100%
		Combined errors: both presentations			
21	N	41	21	50	112
	M	1·95	1·00	2·38	5·33
	%	36%	19%	45%	100%

TABLE 1–9. PERCENTAGE OF REDUCTION OR INCREASE OF READING ERRORS ON MATCHING PRINTED TO SPOKEN WORDS

	Word to picture				*Printed to spoken word*				*Combined errors*			
Type of error	*Visual*	*Auditory*	*Association*	*Total*	*Visual*	*Auditory*	*Association*	*Total*	*Visual*	*Auditory*	*Association*	*Total*
1. *Patients Who Made More Errors Matching Word to Picture* (*N* 8)												
No. errors	10	8	14	32	7	2	6	15	17	10	20	47
M	1·25	1·00	1·75	4·00	·88	·25	·75	1·88	2·13	1·25	2·50	5·88
%	31%	25%	44%	100%	47%	13%	40%	100%	36%	21%	43%	100%
% reduction or increase					−30%	−75%	−57%	−53%				
2. *Patients Who Made More Errors Matching Printed to Spoken Word* (*N* 6)												
No. errors	2	2	6	10	12	3	4	19	14	5	10	29
M	·33	·33	1·00	1·67	2·00	·50	·67	3·17	2·33	·83	1·67	4·83
%	20%	20%	60%	100%	63%	16%	21%	100%	48%	17%	35%	100%
% reduction or increase					+500%	+50%	−33%	+90%				
3. *Patients Who Made Equal Total Errors* (*N* 7)												
No. errors	5	2	11	18	5	4	9	18	10	6	20	36
M	·71	·29	1·57	2·57	·71	·57	1·29	2·57	1·43	·86	2·86	5·14
%	28%	11%	61%	100%	28%	22%	50%	100%	28%	17%	55%	100%
% reduction or increase					0	+100%	−18%	0				
4. *Total* (*N* 21)												
No. errors	17	12	31	60	24	9	19	52	41	21	50	112
M	·81	·57	1·48	2·86	1·14	·43	·90	2·48	1·95	1·00	2·38	5·33
%	28%	20%	52%	100%	46%	17%	37%	100%	36%	19%	45%	100%
% reduction or increase					+41%	−25%	−39%	−13%				

Table 1-9 shows that even in this small sample all patients do not perform alike. Eight patients made more errors matching words to pictures than matching printed to spoken words, which is a reversal of the usual finding. It can be seen that the spoken word helped the patients considerably to identify the correct word, reducing auditory errors by 75 percent, association errors 57 percent, visual errors 30 percent, and total errors 53 percent. This would seem to indicate that for these patients visual processes were too impaired to permit the necessary discriminations and recognitions to function adequately without assistance from another sensory modality.

Six patients made more errors matching printed to spoken words than matching words to pictures. Depriving these patients of the information presented by pictures and forcing them to depend on the spoken word *increased* visual confusions 500 percent, auditory errors 50 percent and total errors 90 percent, while association errors decreased 33 percent. The 50 percent increase and the 33 percent decrease are probably not significant, since they represent differences of only one and two errors respectively, spread over 6 patients. What is significant is that these patients made six times as many errors identifying words spoken by the examiner as matching the same words to pictures, pointing to more severe auditory than visual involvement.

Seven patients made an equal number of errors on both presentations. The number of visual errors remained exactly the same; auditory errors decreased by two, and visual errors increased by two when the spoken word was presented. The latter differences are probably not significant.

The sample was considered too small for further analysis.

REDUCTION OF WRITING VOCABULARY

The following 20 spelling words are a part of the Minnesota Test for Differential Diagnosis of Aphasia, administered to all patients on admission to the Aphasia Clinic: bed, car, chair, clock, house, table, boy, dog, bread, apple, paper, grass, man, has, rain, watch, yellow, country, business and necessary. For the first six words the patient is asked to write the name of a picture; the rest are written to dictation. Words were selected from grades 2 to 6 on graded spelling lists. From a test series of 157 patients tested on the Research Edition of the Minnesota Test (1955), all the original spelling papers contained in the files were extracted for patients in Groups 2, 3 and 4. To these were added the records of the first 10 patients in Group 1 and the first 15 patients in Group 5 whose original papers were on file, making a series of 79 papers for analysis.

All errors were tabulated and classified as follows:

(1) No response, or no appropriate response. Responses judged not appropriate were illegible responses, perseverative responses and meaningless combinations of letters such as NEL for clock.

(2) Association errors, such as *green* for *grass* and *home* for *house*. Recognizable approximations of associated words were also included in this category, such as *tabe* for *bed* and *flr* for *bread.*

(3) Visual confusions. These consisted of distortions and reversals of letter forms, confusions of letters with similar visual configurations, such as *bog* for *boy*, *match* for *watch*, and *howse* for *house.* Phonetic spellings were also included in this category, since these are characteristic of patients with visual impairment on a cerebral level (Schuell, 1954); examples from the data are *bisness* for *business*, *boe* for *boy*, and *bred* for *bread.*

(4) Auditory confusions, consisting of substitution of words which sounded like the given word, such as *red* for *bread* and *hair* for *chair.*

(5) Proprioceptive confusions. A tendency had been observed for patients with sensorimotor impairment to confuse sounds with similar articulatory positions and movement patterns, such as *pbm* made on the lips, *tdnl* with the tongue tip touching the teeth ridge, *fv*, *kg*, *rl*, and so on; therefore this category was included. Examples found were *apper* for *apple*, *bet* for *bed*, *taben* for *table*, *chail* for *chair*, et cetera.

(6) Approximations. These were misspellings in which at least a part of the given word was correct. Errors were omissions of letters, reversals of letter sequences, letter substitutions and so on. Examples of words classified as approximations were *buisness*, *grss*, *chur*, *yellew*.

Since it is impossible to know what was going on in the patient's mind when he wrote a word, it is of course probable that there are misclassifications. However, it was possible to consider errors in the context of the overall performance of each patient, which made judgments more reliable, since patients tend to show consistency in the kinds of errors they make.

Findings

The number, mean number and percentage of each error type for each clinical group and for the total sample are found in Table 1–10.

The high percentage of no response or no appropriate response is characteristic of severely impaired patients, as is indicated by the fact that 95 percent of the errors of Group 1 were of this class. It is also characteristic of some patients in other groups who have received no treatment for aphasia. Many aphasic patients can write so little at the time of initial testing that error patterns cannot be studied until more performance can be obtained. However, several findings are of interest in Table 1–10. Group 1 patients are chiefly notable for lack of performance on writing tasks. Patients in Group 2 perform a good deal better than patients in any other clinical group, as can be seen from a comparison of the mean number of total errors for all the clinical groups. They made three visual-type errors; one was a reversal, one a confusion of two similar letters, and one a phonetic spelling. Actually, any patient beginning to write with the nonpreferred hand may produce an occasional reversal. A diagnosis of visual impairment was not made unless such types of errors occurred frequently, were persistent and characterized all samples of the patient's writing.

Whereas on word comprehension and naming, Group 3 patients performed much like Group 2 patients, showing a comparable amount of language reduction, on writing comparatively easy words they averaged three and a half times as many total errors and more than 19 times as many visual errors. Group 5

TABLE 1–10. NUMBER, MEAN AND PERCENTAGE OF ERROR TYPES ON SPELLING FOR CLINICAL GROUPS AND TOTAL SAMPLE

		No response	*Association errors*	*Visual errors*	*Audio errors*	*Proprio. errors*	*Approx. errors*	*Total*
Group 1	N	190	0	2	0	2	4	198
(N 10)	M	19·00		·20		·20	·40	19·80
	%	96%		1%		1%	2%	
Group 2	N	23	6	3	1	1	17	51
(N 18)	M	1·27	·33	·17	·06	·06	·94	2·83
	%	45%	12%	6%	2%	2%	33%	
Group 3	N	92	15	75	3	3	41	229
(N 23)	M	4·00	·65	3·26	·13	·13	1·78	9·96
	%	40%	7%	33%	1%	1%	18%	
Group 4	N	56	10	8	0	5	27	106
(N 13)	M	4·31	·77	·62		·38	2·08	8·15
	%	53%	9%	8%		5%	25%	
Group 5	N	64	3	41	1	2	38	149
(N 15)	M	4·27	·20	2·73	·07	·13	2·53	9·93
	%	43%	2%	27%	1%	1%	26%	
Total	N	425	34	129	5	13	127	733
Sample	M	5·38	·43	1·63	·06	·16	1·61	9·27
(N 79)	%	58%	5%	17%	1%	2%	17%	

patients who also show some visual involvement, had the second highest mean number and percentage of visual confusions.

Group 4 patients who have sensorimotor involvement showed the highest percentage of proprioceptive confusions, but the number cannot be considered significant. This was predictable, for such errors do not usually appear until patients have acquired functional vocabulary, and been taught phonetic techniques as an approach to reading and writing. They tend to be striking through the learning period, then gradually decrease in all modalities.

DISCUSSION

Data have been presented which show reduction of vocabulary in aphasia appearing in all language modalities. The same kinds of errors tend to appear, whether patients are asked to point to objects named by the examiner, to name objects, match words to pictures, match spoken to printed words or write words to dictation.

Confusions of words which are associated in meaning or experience are common to all modalities. Aphasic patients who misname objects frequently use the same words that normals use when asked to respond to a word with the first word they think of (Schuell, 1950). These are, of course, learned associations. It would appear that as we learn language, verbal symbols become linked not only to specific objects of certain sizes, shapes, colors and other attributes, but generalized to some extent to total situations and to concepts of many degrees of complexity, to which many other verbal symbols also become linked. Hebb has tried to provide a neurological basis for this kind of learning with his theories of reverberating circuits and cell assemblages (Hebb, 1949). In children learning to talk, in states of fatigue and inattention, and much more severely in aphasia, it is as though given stimuli activate only parts of these clusters. Clinically this seems to be true. When patients are being trained to recognize individual sounds and hear them in words, they are usually able to give only one word which begins with a given sound at first; later the same stimulus may produce two or three, or four or five different words. The same kind of performance results when patients are asked to respond to a stimulus word with whatever they think of. One patient who had travelled in many parts of the world, was asked to respond thus to *India.* He said only *women.* Later, to the same word he said, "Ganges, river, stones, women washing clothes." Similar processes sometimes occur when patients are searching for particular words to convey their thoughts. One patient, trying to tell what kind of a car he had, went on something like this, "Ford, no, Dodge, no, Chevy, no, Plymouth, that's it, that's right. I got a new Plymouth."

While present knowledge does not permit description of the neurological mechanisms involved in such complex cerebral processes as language, it is becoming increasingly clear that simple associative processes such as those described here play an important part in many aspects of normal language behavior. Experimental studies performed in the last ten years have shown that a variety of functions such as recall (Jenkins, Mink and Russell, 1958), learning (Russell and Storms, 1955), transfer (Ryan, 1957) and generalization (Mink, 1957) may be mediated by such linkages. The importance of these processes in normal language is in close accord with the findings presented here regarding associative errors in aphasia. As vocabulary breaks down in aphasia, those association processes still intact serve to mediate the errors which appear. At more severe levels of vocabulary deficit, association processes themselves begin to break down, and errors of more remote origin manifest themselves. At the most severe levels of deficit, errors become even more irrelevant, finally becoming random or "no response" errors.

The effects of auditory, visual, sensorimotor and motor impairment on language can also be observed in aphasia. Some of these defects produce a much greater deficit in one modality than another; writing is more dependent on visual processes, for example, than is comprehension or speech; speech is more dependent upon complex motor coordinations than is comprehension or silent reading. In some aphasic patients visual processes are intact, but reading and writing suffer varying degrees of impairment from the effects of the general language deficit which is present, of which reduction of vocabulary is one aspect.

SUMMARY

Data have been presented which show that reduction of vocabulary in all modalities is characteristic of language impairment in aphasia. Further, the similarities between errors observed in recognizing spoken words, naming, matching printed words to pictures, matching printed to spoken words and writing words to dictation are considered evidence of a language deficit independent of modality and of the recurring patterns of clinical symptoms found in aphasic patients. At the same time, other kinds of errors reflecting specific perceptual, motor and sensorimotor involvement present in some patients and not in others, were found to impair performances differentially in various modalities and in the diagnostic groups described.

This research was done during the tenure of an NIH research grant by the senior author. Some of the computational work was done by Joanne D'Andrea, as a research assistant employed by funds from this grant. The reading tests were constructed by Lydia Landis, member of the staff of the Aphasia Clinic, Minneapolis VA Hospital. Tests were administered by the senior author, Amy Bricker, Virginia Carroll, Lydia Landis, Jayne Nelson, Ruby Simmons and Barbara Street, members of the staff of the Aphasia Clinic at various periods since 1955.

REFERENCES

Freud, S. (1953) "On Aphasia." New York.

Guttman, L. (1947) *Educ. Psychol. Measmt.*, **7**, 247.

Head, H. (1926) "Aphasia and Kindred Disorders of Speech." New York.

Hebb, D. O. (1949) "The Organization of Behaviour." New York.

Jenkins, J. J., Mink, W. D., and Russell, W. A. (1958) *Psychol. Rept.*, **4**, 127.

Kent, G. H., and Rosanoff, A. J. (1910) *Amer. J. Insanity*, **67**, 37 and 317.

Mink, W. D. (1957) "Semantic Generalization as Related to Word Association." Minneapolis.

Penfield, W., and Roberts, L. (1959) "Speech and Brain-Mechanisms." Princeton.

Russell, W. A., and Jenkins, J. J. (1954) "The Complete Minnesota Norms for Responses to 100 Words from the Kent-Rosanoff Word Association Test." Minneapolis.

——, and Storms, L. H. (1955) *J. Exper. Psychol.*, **49**, 287.

Ryan, J. J. (1957) "An Experimental Comparison of Response Transfer Facilitated by Meaningfully Similar and Associated Verbal Stimuli." Minneapolis.

Schuell, H. (1950) *J. Sp. and Hear. Dis.*, **15**, 291.

—— (1954) *Neurology*, **4**, 179.

—— (1955*a*) "The Minnesota Test for Differential Diagnosis of Aphasia." Research Edition, Minneapolis.

—— (1955*b*) *A.M.A. Arch. Neurol. Psychiat.*, **74**, 308.

——, and Jenkins, J. J. (1959) *Psychol. Rev.*, **66**, 45.

Thorndike, E. L., and Lorge, I. (1944) "The Teachers Word Book of 30,000 Words." New York.

Weisenburg, T. H., and McBride, K. E. (1935) "Aphasia, a Clinical and Psychological Study." New York.

Wepman, J. M., and Jones, L. K. (1958) "The Production and Demonstration of a Primary Language Abilities Test for Aphasia." Chicago.

2

Verbal Realization in Aphasia

THEOPHILE ALAJOUANINE

THEOPHILE ALAJOUANINE, M.D., is with the department of neurology and neuropsychology of the Hospital de la Salpêtrière, Paris.

The subject which I am going to discuss concerns verbal expression in aphasia and, more especially, oral expression. In other words, I am going to limit myself to that phase of language which concerns the transmutation of intellectual, or psycho-emotional processes into those sounds which constitute speech, that is to say, to what would have been called formerly the motor side of language. Of course, we know that the emission of sounds that constitute speech is always completely dependent on the mental conditions which initiated them: when we use the term verbal expression, it includes verbal stimulation.

The disorders of verbal expression in aphasia appear in many different aspects, the analytical study of which, alone, would require long explanation. How wide is the difference between patients who can use only a few elementary sounds which they repeat again and again at each attempt at speech, and those, in contrast, who have a rich oral expression, a volubility, the content of which is so foreign to us that we call their language a jargon. Between this extreme poverty of expression and this rich fluidity of speech without practical meaning, how many variations manifesting themselves in a wide diversity of verbal expression there are in aphasia! And yet by attentive study of these patients, one can see that each of these individual cases is closely related to the other. One discerns in them two principal poles of aphasic disorder: one, the disturbance of the power to produce words; the other, the disturbance of syntactic structure, and of the semantic value of words.

From *Brain* 79:1–28, 1956. Reprinted by permission of the Editor of *Brain*.

The clinical material of the present study consists in 317 consecutive cases observed from 1950 to 1954. These cases have been followed at least for several months, and many for years, with periodical examination conducted along the same standardized methods: neuro-

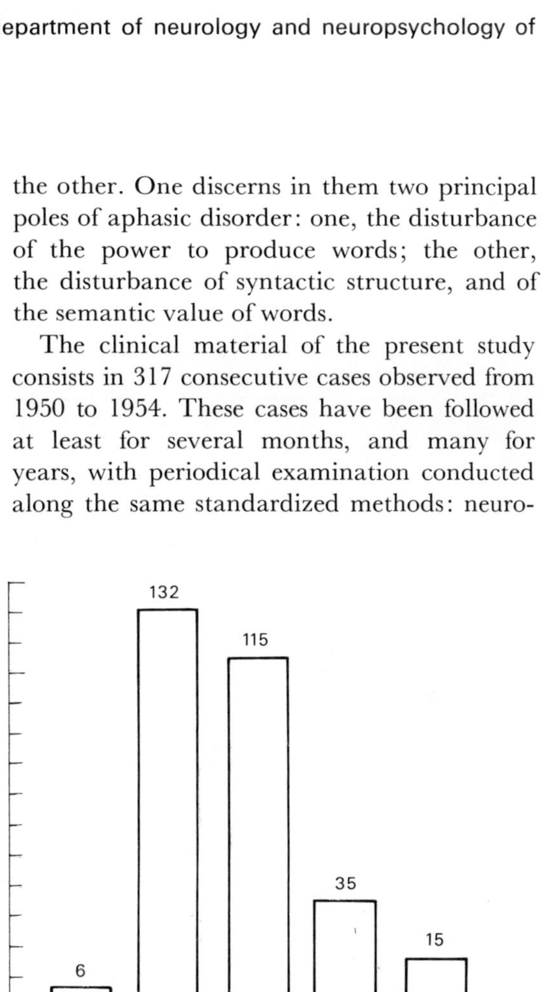

Fig. 2–1. Distribution of 303 patients with:
—disorders of speech
—disorders of visual or auditive perceptions
—purely articulatory defects
Beside aphasic disorders this figure includes alterations of both receptive and expressive poles of speech

logical examination; condition of speech; psychological examination with verbal tests and general intelligence tests (Figs. 2-1, 2-2, 2-3).

I must also make clear that my terminology is the one used by Pierre Marie and his pupils, which does not reflect any pathogenic considerations:

Wernicke's aphasia—formerly sensory aphasia;
Broca's aphasia—formerly motor aphasia;
Anarthria;
Agnosia (auditory or visual).

I must add that in the linguistic approach of verbal expression, I use the words: "phonemes" —sounds, and "morphemes" and "semantemes" as described by the great linguist, F. de Saussure, to differentiate the morphological structure (phonetic) and the meaning of vocables. This study being primarily a functional one, I have purposely neglected the location and the ætiology of the causative lesions, which are chiefly vascular.

Among the multiple aspects of the disorders of verbal expression, I shall limit myself to considering:

(1) Stereotyped verbal expression, especially the permanent one which I shall call *verbal stereotypy*.

(2) *Agrammatism*, which I consider, as I shall define it later, closely allied to the former.

(3) *Phonetic disorders* (pure anarthria or associated with aphasic disorders).

(4) *Jargon aphasia*.

The fixity, the lasting quality, and the homogeneous symptomatology of these four important varieties of disturbance of verbal expression, make it possible to form a definite idea of their character and to follow their evolution; I shall try also to identify the elements of the neurological disturbance which causes them.

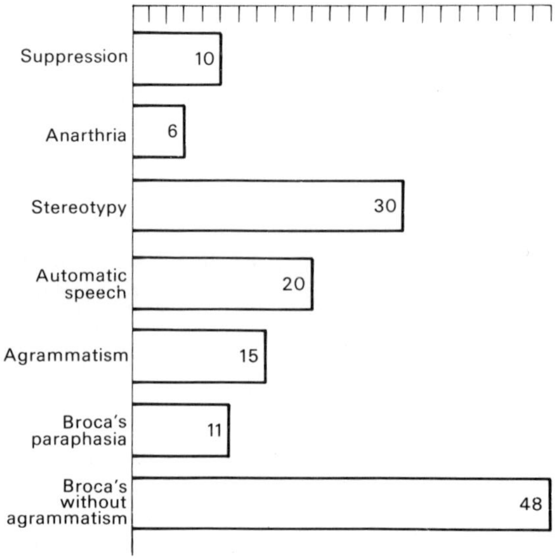

Fig. 2-2. Broca's Aphasia and Anarthria (138 cases). Patients are classified according to the principal disorder. When they successively showed several of these symptoms, we retained the most characteristic and durable.

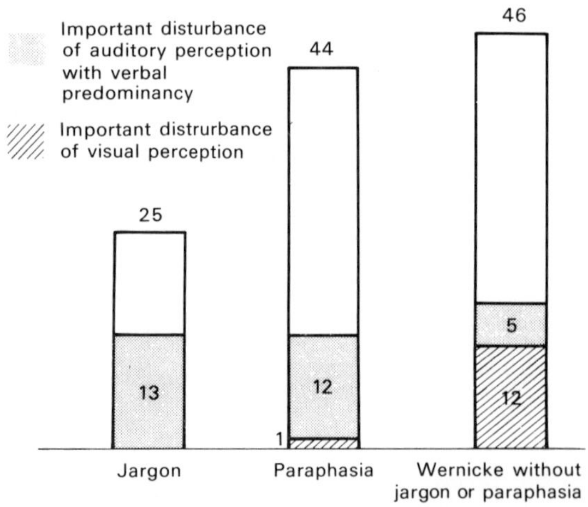

Fig. 2-3. Wernicke's Aphasia. Jargon and Paraphasia frequency (115 cases).

PERMANENT VERBAL STEREOTYPIES

Aside from a total suspension of speech, which is ordinarily only a transitory phenomenon, the verbal stereotypy is the most restricted aspect of verbal expression. Broca has given the first observation with his patient retaining only the stereotyped expression "Tan-Tan." But Jackson was the first who described its chief aspects; he called them first "stock utterances" and later preferred the term "recurring utterances": he gave four types of them: a fragment of meaningless jargon; a single word; a phrase; "yes" or "no" or both these words.

It is not necessary to recall the admirable analysis he has given of the way "yes" or "no" can be used on a propositional sense, or simply as a type of emotional interjection; for this is the key to his famous conception of the two uses of speech, and their dissociation in aphasia.

I propose without neglecting the important contribution of Jackson, to consider the verbal stereotypies according to: (1) their linguistic constitution; (2) their characteristics as utterances; (3) their association with other disorders of aphasia; and especially (4) their evolution. This study will also attempt to demonstrate their physiopathological and prognostic values.

I shall consider first the *permanent verbal stereotypies*, that is to say, those established from the beginning of the aphasia, and persisting for several months without apparent modification of their structure.

In the *first type* of permanent verbal stereotypy the utterance expresses no meaning; it consists either of one syllable, always the same, but repeated several times (iterative stereotypy) or of several syllables always connected in the same way and producing a vocable or a word unknown in any language (jargonized stereotypy). The "Tan-Tan" of the first Broca's patient, or the "Titi-Titi" of one of our cases are examples of iterative stereotypy; the words "Monomentif" or "Cousisi-Cousisi" of the classical cases of Trousseau, end the sequence "Me me commiti my, pittimy, lor, veah" of the well-known case of Jackson, are examples of jargonized stereotypy.

The essential fact in the above is the absence of linguistic meaning. The sounds to which the speech is reduced are phonemes or better only morphemes entirely devoid of sense: or else the sense can only be guessed at, as in the case of the expression "pittimy" cited by Jackson.

All this represents a very severe disintegration of speech, which destroys any language (French or English, for instance), and falls into a fixed and unvarying pattern, strangely restricted to one or a few utterances, the almost constant iterative character of which must be emphasized. This phenomenon is very far from being understood.

In the *second type* of permanent verbal stereotypy, the utterance has linguistic meaning, sometimes expressed in an isolated word; for example, one of my patients continually repeated only the word "volontiers = willingly," another "dire, dire = tell, tell" in which one finds again the iterative character emphasized before. This isolated word may be a curse or a coarse interjection. The great French poet, Baudelaire, the first translator of Edgar Allan Poe into French, retained only the word "cré nom," probably part of "sacré nom de Dieu."

Or, sometimes, the word "yes" or "no," the use of which Jackson has so well described, said in a purely automatic way and with no propositional value, is a stereotypy. However, such an expression loses its character as soon as the patient is able to use it in a correct manner adapted to the circumstance. This is the simplest and most definite example of the evolution of a stereotypy, as indicated first by Jackson.

Sometimes, again, it may take the form of a single sentence, generally a short one, presenting some grammatical construction, but not a perfect one, thus giving a first indication of agrammatism. For example, one of our patients said constantly: "Ai bien dit = have well told" which she always repeated; another always said: "faut écrire = must write," another in a curious way associated an affirmation and a negative expression: "je suis belle, je ne suis pas belle = I am pretty, I am not pretty." A man of letters whose case I described in my Harveian lecture on "Artistic realization in aphasia," published in BRAIN some years ago, could say only in a pathetic way: "Bonsoir, les choses d'ici-bas = Farewell, things of this world."

In the analysis of the other characteristics of permanent verbal stereotypy beside their structure and their linguistic aspect, upon which our classification is based (stereotypy with or without linguistic meaning), one notices first the *completely involuntary utterance:* verbal stereotypy shows up at every attempt at speech; this forced repetition is observed more frequently when the utterance is short. This utterance is rapid, almost explosive, in the manner of an interjection, and without any phonetic disorder. This mode of expression, as its name indicates, is always identical. The patient cannot free himself from this set form, within which he is forced to remain in any attempt at expression. At other times it is impossible to make him repeat the single or the few stereotyped vocables, or to make him write them.

Another aspect, not less important, is the patient's *unconsciousness* of the disorder constituted by his stereotyped verbal expression, in complete contrast to his full awareness of his defect of language; here is an extraordinary association of what one might call according to the Jacksonian terminology a positive disturbance, that is to say, an unconscious stereotyped utterance, and a negative one, the unawareness of his deficiency in speech. Hence the patients who go through varied gesticulations and suggestive mimic, and try to express themselves by gesture in order to show their lack of ability to express themselves in language, utter, without knowing it; at the same time they utilize a set form of expression devoid of sense, which they can neither interpret voluntarily, nor write, and which they do not recognize when they hear it, or when one has read it to them. They are no more conscious of their pattern of speech than are normal subjects who repeatedly interject some ready-made expressions annoying to their audience, but without noticing it themselves.

These intrinsic qualities of stereotypies suffice to define them in an exact way, and one can thus summarize them as a *permanent stereotyped verbal expression with or without linguistic meaning, unconsciously and involuntarily uttered* (a fact which will later require a comparison with the liberation of certain psychomotor activities).

THE EVOLUTION AND REGRESSION OF VERBAL STEREOTYPIES

It will be sufficient now to mention rapidly the phenomena associated with this special disturbance of speech. Fig. 2-4 is a résumé of 22 cases observed over a long period of time. In one-half (11 cases) the language disorder remained unchanged, and, having been so for several years, seems to be fixed. In the other half (11 cases) there was some degree of regression, the stages of which we shall discuss later on.

It will be noted that the naming of things and repetition of spoken words on request are impossible in such a condition; furthermore, the patient's writing is always poor; and his

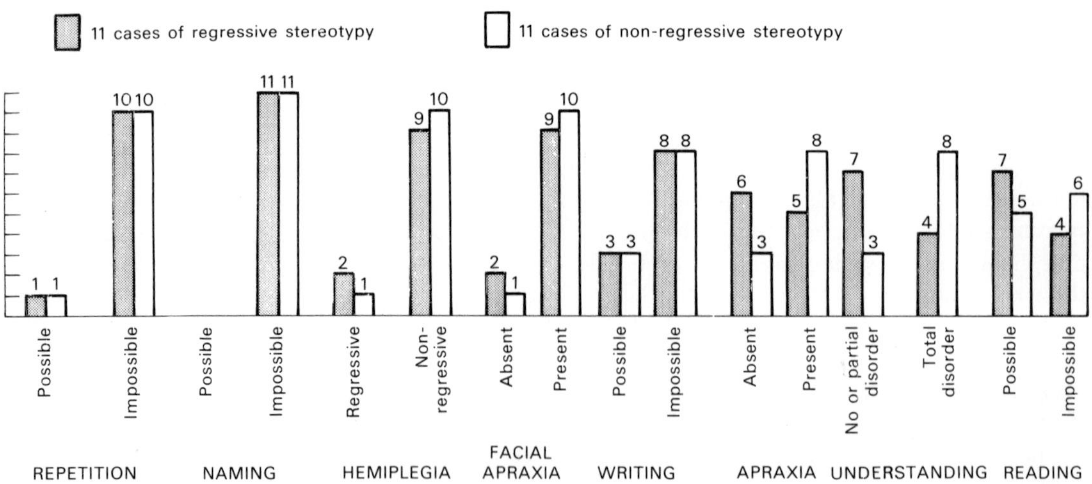

Fig. 2-4. Comparison between associated symptoms in regressive and non-regressive stereotypy.

understanding is always disturbed, for verbal as well as for written orders (the only way of appreciating reading ability). In our material, a severe hemiplegia was invariably present in this condition as well as bucco-linguo-facial motor disorders of apraxic type: indeed, a general apraxia is frequently found. In brief, here we are concerned with the very seriously affected patients of the Broca's aphasia type. In them, however, there are to be observed certain peculiarities which are interesting in relation to the study of the evolution of stereotypes which remains to be considered.

This study of the speech behavior of the aphasic patient over a period of time seems very important, yet it has not been given very much attention till now, as if it were thought of only as an insignificant spar remaining from the shipwreck of speech. Jackson, however, was the first to emphasize the importance of the transformation of the words "yes" or "no," uttered at first as interjections, into words used in a propositional manner. This point is of the greatest interest, for this transformation is, to my mind, one of the keys to their interpretation (Tables 2-1 and 2-2).

The *evolution* of the permanent verbal stereotypies which, as we have explained by our statistics, shows regression in half the cases, must be closely studied. Even when the condition remains permanent, it is far from remaining unchanged. Whereas, in the beginning there is the usual stereotypy, in these cases, an interjection may be uttered; generally an oath or a coarse word and usually in an outburst of anger. This was the case with Broca's patient, who sometimes replaced his perpetual "Tan-Tan" with a curse, always the same one. Another modification of the permanent stereotypy consists in a change in the manner of utterance, and of the intonation according to circumstances, the intonation varying according to what the subject tries to express, thus giving the stereotypy a variable emotional complement, which is of great importance.

But, what is more important is that after months of such relative fixity of verbal expression (and as a matter of fact in one of our patients after two years) one may see the disappearance of the stereotypy. How does it happen? In what way is the "mechanical barrel organ" (to employ the suggestive term given by Gairdner and adopted by Jackson) replaced by a more complex instrument? This change is usually not without transition, and these evolutionary processes reveal facts of the greatest interest. It is possible, according to our observations made with Pedro de Castro, of

TABLE 2-1. FOLLOW-UP OF VERBAL STEREOTYPY

(1) *General Follow-up*

Total number	*Definitive stereotypy*	*Regressive stereotypy*
30	11	19

(2) *Duration of the Stereotypy Before Improvement*

Total number	*Transient stereotypy (less than one month)*	*Long-standing stereotypy (from one month to two years)*
19	6	13

TABLE 2-2. RELATIONS BETWEEN TYPE OF STEREOTYPY AND MODE OF EVOLUTION

	No.	Wernicke's	Broca's	Agrammatism	Anarthria
Long-standing stereotypy without linguistic value	5	—	1	4	—
Transient stereotypy without linguistic value	0	—	—	—	—
Long-standing stereotypy with linguistic value	8	—	4	4	—
Transient stereotypy with linguistic value	6	5	—	—	1

Madrid, to distinguish, in this progressive liberation of verbal expression from the rigid and obligatory cast, several stages, which we shall study in a systematic way, but which do not always follow such a schematic order in each subject.

The change takes place in an orderly succession of four stages:

(*a*) A stage of differentiated organization of the stereotyped verbal emissions where the manner of utterance and the intonation are first modified.

(*b*) A stage of checking the involuntary utterance, which is at first partial and imperfect.

(*c*) A stage of fluctuating utterance in which there appears beside or in place of the residual stereotyped expression, either another stereotyped utterance, generally less fixed and less lasting, or some other expression, either in the form of a ready-made phrase, or even a highly volitional utterance.

(*d*) Finally, a stage in which the stereotypy is definitely checked and no longer occurs even occasionally. Then there is a volitional speech, which presents characteristics the opposite in every respect to the stereotypy, and of which one of the special aspects is agrammatism, which we shall study later on.

Of the different stages of regression of the verbal stereotypy we have observed definite examples, the analysis and the comparison of which furnishes an important physio-pathological explanation for the understanding of this type of speech of the dissolution of the activity of speech.

(1) The stage which I call the differentiated organization of the permanent verbal stereotypy may announce itself rather early, and remain for a fairly long time, the process of differentiation becoming richer little by little. The identical nature of the content continues as before, and it is only in the manner of utterance and intonation that the differentiation takes place. This change permits the patient to express with his vocable, uniform and unchanged, a whole scale of meanings colored by variations of emotion. What the subject, reduced to such poverty of expression, tried before to express by his gestures, or gesticulation, he now tries to render by the modification of his utterance and by the intonation of his stereotyped word or phrase. One of the best examples I have observed of this differentiated organization of a verbal stereotypy is that of a patient who did not say and could not say anything but: "Ai bien dit = have well told" which was uttered in iterative fashion. We saw this patient, while retaining her eternal stereotyped words, modify the utterance of the expression both as to speed and intonation. At one moment it was monotonous, although rapid, and then became faster or slower according to the circumstances and changed in intonation, which became sometimes sad, sometimes even tearful, sometimes on the contrary, satisfied or approving. This was true to such a point that each expression, though still identical in phonetic content, was enlivened by the addition of emotional expression —a fact which has much significance. It was astonishing to see this patient with such meager verbal means succeed in furnishing a quantity of information which, though certainly not explicit, was nevertheless sufficiently suggestive so that one should not misunderstand the general meaning it implied. "The melody of speech" to use Brissaud's expression, had come to superimpose itself upon the stereotyped utterance.

(2) The second stage of the evolution towards improvement of the stereotypy is characterized by the fact that the patient tries to check, then succeeds in checking, his involuntary utterance, announcing thus the first signs of the breaking-down of the stereotyped condition. It is very curious to see the patient set in motion as usual his pattern of verbal behavior, and, then, sometimes, suddenly try to slow his utterance (ordinarily rapid and even explosive, as we have marked) to the point of lowering a part of it and even of rendering the end of the utterance inaudible; or again, on the contrary, to see him hasten the utterance of it in an apparently volitional way, as if he wished to get rid of it, finally succeeding in stopping it, when it is no longer more than a suggestion of itself, in the way a person may cut short at the beginning a statement which suddenly seems

incongruous to him. There is undoubtedly at this point in the evolution of the stereotypy the reassertion of the consciousness of an abnormality by the patient and a somewhat successful attempt on his part to block or check it by the will. This is the first evidence of the appearance of a volitional phenomenon in the oral expression of such patients. It is difficult to say whether it is the reappearance of the patient's consciousness of the disorder which permits the action of the will, or whether inversely, the volitional activity causes the consciousness of the disorder, as we believe.

(3) Then there comes a stage which we describe as fluctuating because there occur in it verbal expressions very different in nature, and which, varying from one situation to another, come to accompany the original or initial stereotyped expression, the persistence of which is only occasional, and less and less frequent. There may then occur a transfer: a new stereotypy replaces the former one; this new stereotypy contains the same characteristics and is different, therefore, only as to its content and its shorter duration. It marks nevertheless a new step in the evolutionary regression of the stereotypy; the case of one of our patients may be cited as an example of this stage: one day on hearing the telephone ring at home, he exclaimed: "Telephone, telephone," and from that day he substituted this word, telephone, for this former stereotyped word. It was as if a new pattern had been established that day, inhibiting the use of the former one. Another whose stereotypy was a curse word, and who was often asked by his wife to say "pardon" did not succeed in so apologizing, but changed one day a part of his stereotyped rude word and mixed it with the word "pardon," so as to say only "mardon," at every attempt at speech. A certain number of our patients have thus changed their stereotyped expression once or even several times. This type of change usually indicated a more favorable outcome.

With others, after a more or less continual blocking, there appeared intercalated stock phrases, particularly formal expressions of politeness, their appearance testifying to the fragility of stereotyped organization, which because of the fact is less permanent. One of our patients stopped his leitmotiv to say: "After you, sir," or "Oh, pardon me," according to the circumstances. There is here, then, the appearance of the language Jackson described as "ready-made speech" which testifies to the fact of substitution for the stereotypy of another speech, still inferior, of an automatic sort, but which is no longer uniform, stereotyped like the first and indicates an adaptation to the circumstances.

Finally, there appear in an episodic fashion, volitional expressions, propositions, in the sense Jackson has given to this word. Although occasionally they have considerable interest; they announce at this stage of the evolution the break up, the failure of the involuntary stereotyped organization, of the automatic expression, and are the signs of the reappearance of a real language of volitional character.

(4) The last stage: the verbal stereotypy has definitely disappeared. The compulsory verbal expression, let loose or ejaculated suddenly and even recently, has given place to a willed expression which, however, is slow, and difficult of accomplishment, imperfect, in which there appear suddenly a ready-made sentence uttered with ease—a new aspect of automatic expression different from the first. That is, the characteristics of the verbal utterance now contrast with the initial stereotypy: the compulsory, involuntary character has given place to a willed expression, but accomplished slowly and with difficulty. The unconscious character of the disorder has disappeared also in great part. It is no longer only of his general deficiency of speech of which the patient is aware, but also now of the difficulty and the imperfection of his verbal accomplishment. The speech still lacks that spontaneity, that facility of utterance and that rapid rhythm which characterized the strictly stereotyped condition: it is slow, is produced with effort, as if the patients were groping for words. One sees appear, likewise, some phonetic disturbances which were totally absent in the stereotypy and which so often characterize the utterance of those suffering from aphasia of Broca's type.

At this stage, there are two principal types of aphasia considered according to the verbal expression of the patient:

(1) Those who, as we have just said, have this slow, difficult speech with imperfect phonetic accomplishment, mixed with ready-made language uttered with ease, the whole expression respecting grammatical organization.

(2) Those whose grammatical organization is faulty, whose language is infantile of the type "parler petit nègre." This is agrammatism, something which merits being set apart as an evolutionary mode of the stereotypy.

This evolutionary mode of the recovery from the permanent verbal stereotypy is not always identical with the picture we have traced. We have given, rather, four aspects of the dissociation of stereotyped organization, than of a fixed, obligatory succession of four stages; and besides, some patients remain at one of these stages. The evolution of this poor debris of speech—the stereotypy—too much neglected till now, affords us suggestive data on the importance of the dissociation of automatic and volitional uses of language to which we shall return. This evolutionary view has moreover a practical interest of a prognostic kind; it certainly is of great value to know whether a patient afflicted by aphasia will remain walled in this rudimentary parrot-like kind of expression, or whether he has a chance of freeing himself from it, and of regaining a true language, even if more or less imperfect.

From our study it appears that there are at least two elements of particularly bad prognostic value (Table 2-3).

(*a*) The non-linguistic character of the iterative stereotypy (54 percent of these cases of definite stereotypies).

(*b*) The importance of associated apraxia (nearly all our cases in which the stereotypy did not regress had an important apraxia).

One understands easily that the stereotypy devoid of linguistic meaning which represents the most profound disintegration of speech, is an especially severe disorder. But, I have no idea concerning the significance of apraxia in such cases, except for the part it plays in phonetic disintegration, as we shall see later.

THE CONTENT OF VERBAL STEREOTYPIES

There is finally a special aspect of verbal stereotypy which deserves our attention a moment more; it is its content. Is there a hidden significance behind this involuntary and unconscious utterance?

Jackson was the first to put this question to himself. He noted that, in a certain number of

TABLE 2-3. FUTURE OF STEREOTYPY

	Wernicke's	Broca's without agrammatism	Agrammatism	Anarthria
Transient stereotypy	5	0	0	1
Long-standing stereotypy	0	5	8	0

PROGNOSTIC VALUE OF THE TYPE OF STEREOTYPY

		Definitive No.	Stereotypy %	Regressive No.	Stereotypy %
Stereotypy without linguistic value	11	6	55	5	45
Stereotypy with linguistic value	19	5	26	14	74

cases, the words of the stereotypy (those, of course, having a linguistic meaning) seemed to be the expression of the patient's thought at the moment of his stroke; he supposed that they may have represented a fragment of the sentence which the subject wished to pronounce at the moment of losing consciousness and therefore described them as a stillborn proposition. He wisely emphasized besides, that, though it is not always possible to know what the patient's state of mind was at the beginning of his illness, one could even in these circumstances, from the content of the recurring utterance, infer something of the thought or feeling which had given rise to this form of expression.

Of such utterances some examples have become classical. I shall recall only the man whose recurring utterance was "Come on to me," and sometimes only, "Come on"; he was a railway signalman and was taken ill on the rails in front of his box. A woman could only utter "Gee Gee"; she was taken ill while riding a donkey. Jackson refers, too, to a case of Dr. Russell, a clerk who became paralyzed after hard work making a catalogue, and could only say, "List complete"; and to one of Sir James Paget's patients who was injured in a brawl and whose recurring utterance was, "I want protection."

Gowers believed that the terms used in the stereotypy were exactly the last the patient had said before losing consciousness. One of his well-known examples was that of a woman who was taken ill in a cab; on entering the vehicle she had asked to be driven to Mrs. Waters; her stereotyped word was "Missus, Missus," a part of the last words she spoke.

Critchley believes that Jackson's interpretation is not as close to reality as that of Gowers. He gives two examples: a patient with the recurring utterance, "on the booze," who had been overtaken by apoplexy in a tap-room brawl; and the case of "an attractive young lady of dubious morals," who, after a cerebral hemorrhage, could say nothing but the "revealing words": "Not tonight, I am too tired."

I am not convinced that the precise interpretation of Gowers is truer than that of Jackson, which is broader and with more nuances. Here are some of my own observations. It is unlikely that the writer, of whom I have already spoken, who kept repeating spontaneously as well as in reply to questions, "Farewell, the things of this world," had been pronouncing this sentence at the time of his stroke, which occurred in bed in the morning; but it corresponds doubtless to his impression of the imminence of disaster which he expressed in such a poetical way. The patient whose stereotypy consisted in the words, "Ai bien dit," was paralyzed as the result of an accident in an automobile driven by her husband whom she had told repeatedly that he was driving too fast, and doubtless wished thus to renew her warning which had not been followed: "Indeed, I told you so." One of my patients, a butcher-boy paralyzed when he was serving a customer, constantly repeated, "The customer, the boss, the customer, this evening." Another said only, "Must write, must write"; he had had his attack after having written reluctantly numerous letters at the New Year. Finally there was the case of a tiler who was on the roof of a school when he was taken ill and who constantly used the word, "School, school," in the way of occasional utterance.

In reality, the interpretations one may propose, to explain the exact way in which the stereotypy is installed admit of an important element of uncertainty. These interpretations are nevertheless close to one another in the sense that they refer to the expressions uttered just before the stroke, or at least, in conformity with the Jacksonian view, refer to the situation in which the patient was at the moment. They consequently point towards the end to which the verbal expression was directed; a pattern, one might say, which was ready for use and on the way to being organized, and because of the illness became a single pattern used in barrel organ fashion.

It would be interesting, too, to try to furnish an interpretation for the iterative speech of verbal stereotypy. I do not know any that is entirely satisfactory: I propose, however, the following explanation. As there is only a single kind of phoneme the patient is able to utter, perhaps this obligatory mould in which the verbal stimulus results, provides the necessity to say the word or words over and over. The verbal stimulus continues to take again and again the only free path, the only route, one might say; and the more obligatory, the more simple is the stereotyped expression. This is somewhat like what takes place in normal speech when a call is repeated several times, "Come, come," or a recommendation or an urgent warning. "Attention, attention" = "Be careful, be careful"; or even when a speaker repeats what he has just said, before he has found the form in which to cast what is to follow in his discourse. There is also an analogy which comes to mind: the similarity between iteration in aphasic stereotypy and in the condition called palilalia by Brissaud and Souques in Parkinson's disease and pseudo-bulbar palsy. In these cases the iterations affect an entire sentence which is repeated rather often with rapid utterance in a monotonous way and with a timbre which becomes gradually weaker until it becomes a mere whisper. But this unexplained phenomenon has, in common with iterative stereotyped speech of the aphasia, only its involuntary character, but not its fixity and especially the unawareness on the part of the patient. The muscular rigidity of these patients strongly suggests the idea of a motor disorder, partly of hypertonic nature.

AGRAMMATISM

We have seen that a certain number of patients go from the permanent verbal stereotypy to agrammatism. This word was coined by Kussmaul and has acquired its greatest importance with Pick who has devoted a monograph, unfortunately not finished, on agrammatical disturbances in speech.

Agrammatism constitutes a very special disturbance of verbal expression, of which the grammatical disorder is the chief phenomenon, but this deterioration of grammatical organization is not sufficient to define it in its most general aspect. This rather frequent disturbance belongs to very diverse categories of aphasia and therefore has no significant symptomatic value. Head wished to establish a special type of aphasia based solely on disturbance of syntax, but in our opinion he included under this heading many other disorders.

Entirely different from the variable and incidental impairment of the grammatical organization found in a number of aphasic cases, which are, may one say, "occasional dyssyntaxias," there is an agrammatism characterized by regularity, fixity, and permanence in the grammatical arrangement, which characteristics testify to its being a very special disturbance. As we shall see, its aspect and its evolution are always the same and it is always to be met in the same group of a particular variety of expressive aphasias. This fact causes one to infer in it a certain symptomatic value and gives it a particular prognostic value.

This type of agrammatism, which for me is true agrammatism, is rather difficult to define other than by the essential fact, which the talk of the patient immediately reveals, that there is reduction of the sentence to a skeleton of its construction; only nouns and verbs in the infinitive form are retained, and all of the little words, "the little tools of language," are suppressed. All grammatical differentiation, gender, number, and tense in particular, and also all subordination of clauses are lost. The more rich language is in such differentiation, the more pronounced appears to be the agrammatism. It may be compared to the elementary use of a little-known foreign language or to the systematic abbreviations used for telegraphic messages, or better to the stage of infantile speech which follows the phase of the "word-phrase." This style of speech is called either "telegraphic style," or "parler petit nègre" (piccaninny speech). These comparisons are of some value in the interpretation of agrammatism.

My study is based on 19 cases of agrammatism of this type observed in 145 cases of Broca'a aphasia; but it concerned only permanent cases, and not other patients who may have had a transitory agrammatism.

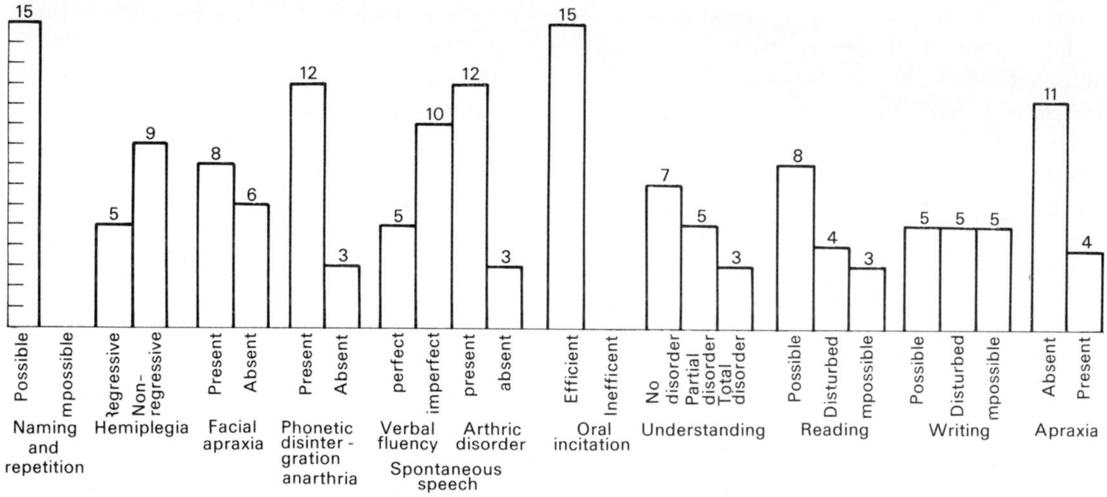

Fig. 2–5. Associated symptoms in agrammatism.

Fig. 2–5 shows the most important of the associated symptoms in the clinical picture of these aphasic patients. Among the symptoms which must be emphasized are, first, that all these patients have a subnormal ability to name objects; and they are likely to repeat all that one asks of them, something unusual and unexpected when one considers their mode of speech.

However, one is struck immediately by their articulatory defect which in the greater number of cases, is of a dysphonetic sort (of this we shall speak later). Their spontaneous language is emitted usually with a slow rhythm, hesitantly, and with pauses which occasionally suggest a certain scansion or element of stuttering. This amounts essentially to a difficulty in accomplishing sounds. Besides this difficulty of spontaneous speech, which exists as well in speech initiated by a question, one notices, especially in attempting to name objects or in pronouncing certain words, the extraordinary efficiency of oral incitation on the part of the observer. It is enough that the observer suggests the beginning of a word or sometimes that he simply makes the slight mimic gesticulation suggesting the word, whispering rather than speaking, for the patient to pronounce and repeat without any trouble. However, this is no longer the case with a sentence, especially a rather long one.

The understanding of many of these agrammatic patients is little disturbed, but it is so for reading and writing, as we shall see later on. There was in nearly all of our cases a hemiplegia which was always severe and only partially regressive. The greater number have also an apraxia which is not always predominantly in the brachio-facial region.

The essential feature of agrammatism is, above all, the special grammatical disposition of what the subject wishes to, or can, express. The laws of this are much more difficult to establish. The first fact is the predominant and capital place that nouns have in their language; then, the use of the infinitive of the verbs, without agreement or without tense; and, finally the disappearance of articles, pronouns, conjunctions, and often adverbs. As we said before, the grammatical organization is skeleton-like and because of this, language structure is rigid and impoverished and without any of the shades which make the richness of discourse. An example may be given. The writer whose pathetic stereotypy we referred to before, having become agrammatic, he whose language had been so rich and so delicate, received me with "To-day, Doctor. Good evening. Talk literature." There are, of course, many degrees in this grammatical alteration; certain subjects little by little enrich their speech at long intervals, here with an adverb, there with a conjunction in incidental and variable manner. Their written language has these same characteristics, quite the opposite from the fluctuating mobility of oral and written syntactical disorders of other aphasic patients. Many patients who are agrammatic, can read and write rather well, but in doing so omit articles, conjunctions, etc., thus rendering their text agrammatic.

A very remarkable fact, observed in many of these patients, is the normal grammatical arrangement in that part of speech which is no longer under volitional control, in other words is spontaneous: ready-made formulæ of salutation, exclamations, etc. The formulation of such phrases is correct and rapid. Thus the agrammatism does not extend to automatic language, which is in these subjects much reduced.

There is a last characteristic of this clinical picture which is not less curious, that is, the relatively slight awareness the patient has of his own disorder. He seems to believe that he has used language almost normally, and he is astonished, for example, to find himself incapable of conjugating the verb he has just used in the infinitive, when asked to do so. Already completely unaware of his trouble when he was at the stage of verbal stereotypy where he began, he is not aware, either of his difficulty in speaking or of the insufficiency of his grammatical accomplishment.

The evolution of agrammatism presents two important peculiarities: first, as we have already noticed, agrammatism is one of the essential modes of evolution of long-standing stereotypy. Of the 15 cases of our table, we see (Table 2-4) that 8 whom we were able to observe a long time, were first reduced to verbal stereotypy (almost always of the type with linguistic signification): 4 of our patients were not seen before the beginning of the agrammatic stage and 2 of them had had at first a complete suspension of ability to speak and had passed directly to the utterance of ready-made expressions. These 15 cases show the importance of the stage of verbal stereotypy as a pre-grammatical phase, a stage which has lasted from a minimum of several weeks to two or three months, and often for many months or even years.

The other evolutionary characteristic of agrammatism is its persistence: it seldom shows any very pronounced tendency to improvement, especially in cases in which it developed slowly, having become established little by little after a long phase of verbal stereotypy. Our 15 patients remained enclosed in an obligatory agrammatical framework, and, as shown in the table, 11 of these were unable to escape the mould of verbal stereotypy. Thus from our material it would appear that agrammatism has a poor prognosis, which accounts for the frequent failure of rehabilitation. I do not wish to say, however, that transitory agrammatisms may not exist, for such patients may not have come under our observation.

We shall not consider psychological or linguistic explanations of agrammatism in any detail because of their hypothetical nature. Perhaps this mode of speech represents a reduction in grammatical construction or a return to an initial infantile stage of grammatical organization, a dissolution according to the Jacksonian meaning of the word. We wish to emphasize the clinical point, which is that a pure agrammatism is a quite definite clinical state, always the same, permanent or long-

TABLE 2-4. PRELUDE TO AGRAMMATISM

	Symptoms various to agrammatism	Duration of aphasia before agrammatism
1	Stereotypy	1 month
2	Stereotypy	2 months
3	Stereotypy	9 months
4	Stereotypy	20 months
5	Stereotypy	15 years
6	Stereotypy	7 months
7	Stereotypy	2 months
8	Stereotypy	2 months
9	Automatic speech	11 days
10	Suppression of automatic sentences	Unknown
11	Unknown	—
12	—	—
13	—	—
14	—	—
15	Suppression	1 year

standing, often in association with a severe motor disorder, and, accordingly, has a precise prognostic signification.

THE SYNDROME OF PHONETIC DISINTEGRATION

There is a level of disintegration of speech, more especially that of elocution, which concerns the articulation of words rather than the formulation of language. Here, besides the alteration of the linguistic system, the main impairment involves the phonologic system which will now be considered in further detail.

We have noted that patients whose permanent verbal stereotypy disappears may have a speech which is slow, hesitating and deformed; we have described certain of these deformations as dysphonetic. The problem which is posed by this condition is whether there is a defective verbal accomplishment, due to perturbed verbal stimulation in the really aphasic manner, or whether there exists, on the contrary, a disturbance having to do only with the articulatory phase of the speech, i.e. an anarthria in the terminology of Pierre Marie? This conception of anarthria has been discussed, and the position of Pierre Marie has been attacked by Dejerine as well as by Head, who reserved for such facts the name of verbal aphasia.

It is certain that anarthria in a pure state is rare, especially in its very first phase. Nevertheless, the fact that articulatory disorders of this type may exist in isolated form is enough to indicate that they may occur in association with indisputably aphasic disorders. In the latter event, their interpretation must be different from that of the paraphasias. To be convinced of the reality of this type of disturbance of the elocution of spoken language there must be a complete integrity of written language. In such rare instances as we have observed, the patient is unsuccessful in pronouncing words he wishes to utter and capable of producing only incomprehensible sounds and such patients, always armed with a pencil are able to express their thoughts in writing without any difficulty. Does not Head himself point out that certain of his patients had such difficult oral expression that they constantly used paper and pencil. To a lesser degree, a discrepancy between the rareness of deprivation of words in written language, and such severe disturbances in spoken language, is not infrequent. Head notes it also. This type of disorder, in which articulatory disturbances are predominant, forms an important category within the group of Broca's aphasia. It was observed by Pierre Marie, who was led to the conclusion, which he later presented as an axiom, that Broca's aphasia is aphasia plus anarthria.

Having become convinced by such cases that elocution could be disturbed in selective fashion, we undertook with Ombredane and Melle Durand, some years ago, an experimental phonetic study of the modes and mechanisms of elocution, by recording the verbal emissions of the patient on Rousselot's cylinders. We were able to confirm by this means that there is a syndrome in which the primary disorder is in the process of elocution. The deterioration of the phonetic system was found to consist of a disturbance of both the possibility of uttering specific phonemes, and the power to link together the phonemes into elocutory series, the times of which are solidary or interdependent. There is, moreover, a difficulty in passing from one phoneme to another under specific conditions for the grouping of such phonemes, in the speed and tempo of this transition and in vocal modulation and accentuation (records).

Contrary to what one might have expected, these phonetic alterations present a remarkable homogeneity and consistency which permits one to reduce them to a certain number of characteristics described in our monograph. From this analysis, which cannot here be explained in detail it is possible to distinguish:

(*a*) *a paretic aspect* with insufficiency of breath as shown by spirometry and weakness of articulation; (*b*) *a dystonic aspect* with excessive movements of articulation, inordinate in their strength and length, the speech being dominated by hypertonia, postural rigidity and synkinesia; (*c*) *an apraxic aspect* with important simultaneous bucco-facial apraxia. There are, then, several degrees and several levels of the alteration of the motor speech mechanisms, from the disturbances of the elementary movements to the highest disorders of the psychomotor level.

It is our impression that there are strong analogies between the pathological phonetic alterations and the first manifestations of infantile language. The former, indeed, is distinguished by tonic characteristics of the primitive oral reactions and the existence of synkinetic associated movements is very clear in them. Numerous changes which can be observed during different stages of recovery in our patients are also found in the normal phonetic progress of a child, i.e. dissimilation, assimilation, metathesis, elision, etc., to use the terminology of phonetics.

Thus, in conformity with the Jacksonian principle of dissolution of function, the patient's speech is reduced to primitive levels, found in the first stages of the development of language. We have named the disorders due to alteration of the process of elocution, the "syndrome of phonetic disintegration."

Critchley, in his Semon lecture of 1953 on "articulatory defects in aphasia," while considering kindly our work as the most important of those having entered upon the problem of dysphonetic alterations, does not declare himself, however, entirely convinced by our demonstration, which to him seems to rest upon too restricted a number of cases, and which, on the other hand neglects fluctuation according to circumstances of the speech of the aphasic patients and according to the uses of language. These criticisms do not seem fully justified. First, as to the number of patients submitted to phonetic exploration, as noted in our monograph, we chose only certain cases in which there had been a complete and detailed study, about 50 records in all, from a much larger series that had been submitted to such exploration and which yielded identical results. Secondly, as for there being wide phonetic variations according to the diverse aspects or uses of language, our material does not substantiate this statement. Our objects showed a severe difficulty of utterance and a remarkable fixity of phonetic deprivation in all the experimental conditions of verbal evocation to which we submitted them. We are continuing this study, having at the present time an even more simple and easy method of oscillographic recording of both voice and lip muscles.

Admittedly, the interpretation of the disorder is difficult. We agree with Critchley, if we had not been already convinced of it before, that we must guard against a too mechanical conception of phonetic disturbances. We know by experience that it is not always easy to distinguish them from certain paraphasic deformations, which are usually less fixed and more fluctuating according to circumstances, and also of different utterance and rhythm.

JARGON APHASIA

The aphasic language, which we have been discussing, though reduced to one or several words without meaning, restricted to elementary forms of grammatical syntax, and altered by phonetic or paraphasic disturbances, usually retained some significance. One may discern at least some elements of appropriateness in emotional expression or some meaning which could be grasped, at least as a whole. But there is still another type of disturbance of verbal expression: the jargon aphasia in which the major element is the disappearance of that very quality which gives signification to speech. In other words there appears to be a suppression of the semantic values of language. Here we are concerned with a profound loss of the meaning of words which we had already found to be disturbed in stereotypy without linguistic meaning.

Although not easily defined, jargon aphasia is not difficult to recognize clinically, since it is an incomprehensible language, not because of abnormal utterance or defect of articulation, but simply because it is completely lacking in meaning. Indeed, the verbal utterance is often so facile and quick that to analyze this strange speech, one has to use a wire recorder: only in this manner is it possible to detect in this speech disorder several types of abnormality.

(*a*) First, there is what can be named an *undifferentiated jargon*, very close to verbal stereotypy without linguistic meaning. However, the latter was easy to distinguish because it was composed of only one or two phonemes, always the same, in contrast to jargon aphasia, where there is an almost incessant flow of sounds more or less varied and fluctuating from one moment to the next.

(*b*) Second, the jargon is composed of neologisms, i.e. new terms devoid of any linguistic meaning, which make it like some queer foreign language, since there remains in it some semblance of syntactic organization; we have called this *asemantic jargon*.

(*c*) Third, a jargon made of constantly misused words. This phenomenon of substituting one word for another is frequently observed in Wernicke's aphasia, particularly when the patient attempts to name objects. However, jargon aphasia is constant and results in series of non-understandable sentences. This state we have named *paraphasic jargon*.

These different types of disorganization of speech in jargon aphasia vary greatly. For instance the last one may eventually be translated, which is quite impossible for the others.

Here is an example of undifferentiated jargon in one of my patients: sanénéqueduacquitescapi. Asemantic jargon (used by one patient who had been asked to describe a picture) is illustrated by the following phrase: "les costelles qui se friment, ici un racrème, deux enfourches a janpié, deux zènes sobe, un chaudier qui met le clistone," etc. Paraphasic jargon is exemplified by the speech of another of our patients "Le bon est vieux du bon Dieu en servant à ces dames," which may be translated: "The good is old from Good God using to these ladies."

These different forms of jargon aphasia may be distinguished by analysis, but experience has taught us that they may appear together in the same patient, at different moments of evolution on recovery from aphasia.

If one studies the chief characteristics of jargon without lingering on the mode of disintegration of the speech (the syntax being not infrequently preserved, as could be seen in the last two examples), one may notice: First, ease and fluency of verbal expression; the quick utterance, the spontaneity, and the absence of delay of incited speech; all of which stands in perfect contrast to the difficulty, effort and slowness of the patients suffering from the preceding categories of Broca's aphasia.

Second, an unawareness on the part of the patient of his language disorder. The patient never doubts for an instant his speech is normal. It is amazing to see such a patient uttering in a confident and natural way utterly meaningless words or extraordinary sentences. For instance, one of our patients called on by a neighbour who wore splendid new shoes, told her admiringly: "Oh, what beautiful chemists you have." This interchange of words which, of course, surprised the neighbour, was the beginning of a paraphasic jargon and the first symptom of a left temporal tumor. The importance of such anosognosia among the symptoms of jargon must be emphasized, because it is one of the major phenomena.

Another curious aspect of this same phenomenon is that such patients criticize the physician when he uses the words taken from their own jargon, an observation which we have made several times. This fact emphasizes the contrast between their own anosognosia and their ability to criticize others, which is possible only because they retain, at least in part, some understanding of spoken language.

Of course, jargon exists not only in spontaneous speech or attempt at conversation, but also in the naming of objects, in the describing of pictures or simple narration. It is observed in written as well as in oral expression, even in reading. It is especially remarkable to see a written order be correctly executed while the patient describes at the same time his action in an extraordinary jargon.

The understanding of spoken language is, indeed, very often much less disturbed than one would expect from the patient's unawareness of his own jargon. There is, nevertheless, as our tests have shown, very often an auditory agnosia, a perceptive defect which must not be neglected. Then, too, many of our patients were found to have severe disturbances of hearing by audiometric study.

Tables (figs. 2-6, 2-7 and 2-8) show the symptoms associated with jargon aphasia in 25 cases. These we cannot consider in detail.

The outcome and eventual prognosis of jargon aphasia is of the greatest interest. In contradiction to the opinion of many authors who regard jargon aphasia as the most severe form of speech disturbance, there are, in our experience, jargons which undergo a regression often to the point of great improvement. Of course, in considering prognosis, one must take into account the ætiology of the aphasia, the extent of the causative lesion and the character of associated neurological abnormalities (auditory agnosia, hemianopia, motor or sensory defect). A permanent hemiplegia appears to be an ominous sign and the same is true of auditory agnosia. Even undifferentiated jargon is not necessarily permanent. It may be nothing but the beginning phase of aphasia and rapidly give way to one of the other forms. But if it continues for an extended period of time, the prognosis appears very poor.

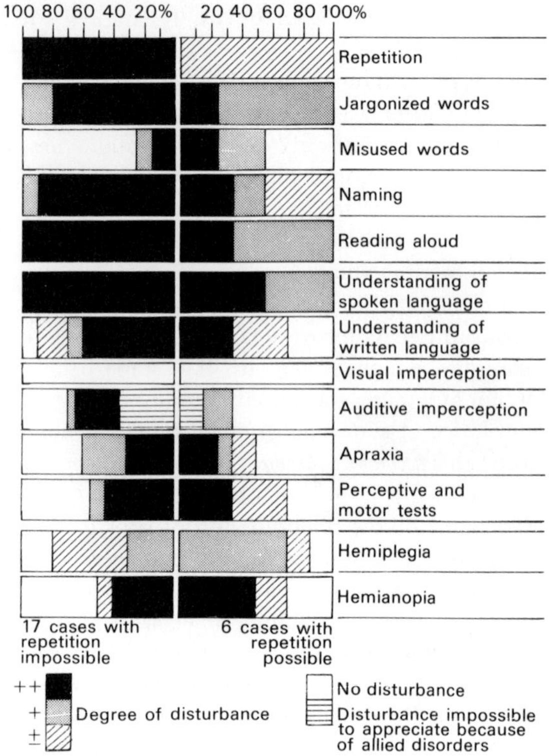

*Results are expressed in percentage but have no statistical value.

Fig. 2–7. Comparison of associated symptoms in 2 groups of jargon aphasia selected in respect of their ability to repeat.

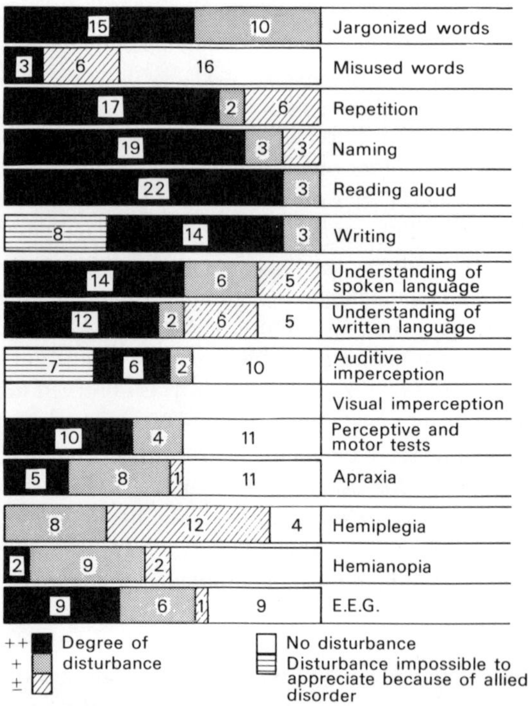

Fig. 2–6. Associated symptoms in 25 cases of jargon aphasia.

The evolution of jargon aphasia tends to be from an undifferentiated jargon to asemantic jargon and thence to paraphasic jargon of "one word for another" type. Moreover, one may observe various degrees of paraphasic jargon varying according to the lack of correspondence between the speech and the idea to be expressed, or, as Lotmar has expressed it, to the degree in which the verbal utterances belong to the same conceptual family. With improvement the severity of the paraphasia lessens.

Another proof of the potentially transitory character of some jargon aphasias may be obtained in some cases of aphasic seizure. Here the patient speaks for a shorter or longer period of time in jargon, and after the termination of his seizure his speech becomes normal.

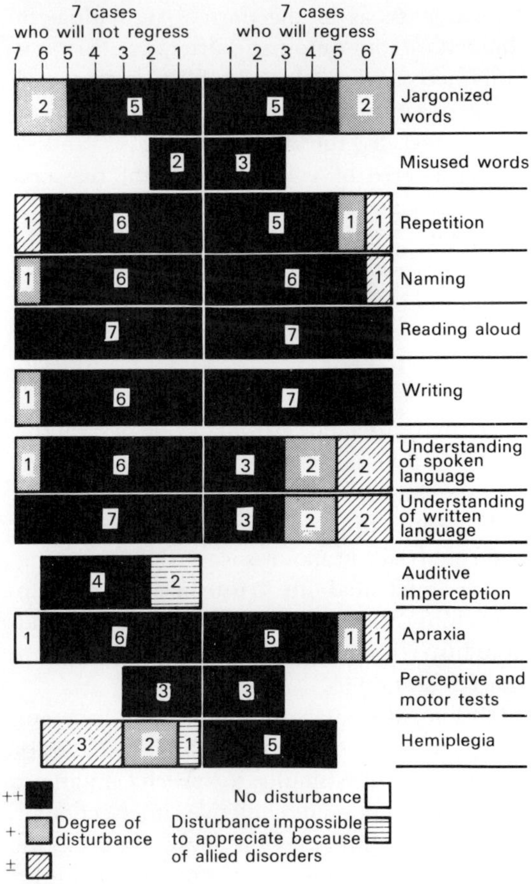

Fig. 2-8. Comparison of associated symptoms in 2 groups of jargon aphasia at the initial phase.

CONCLUSIONS

The facts we have just reviewed possess not only a clinical interest and a prognostic value, but also elucidate to some extent the two great problems of verbal expression in aphasia. The first is the interpretation of the disorders which involves the manner according to which verbal stimulation passes into its expression. This disorder causes a dissociation between the uses of speech. The key to its interpretation lies in what we have called, with Ombredane, Baillarger-Jackson's principle. The other, still more difficult to interpret, is the significance of the relative or complete anosognosia of this defect of realization.

(a) What we call Baillarger-Jackson's principle was named by Jackson himself, Baillarger's principle; but he has developed and described it in such a masterly way that it is necessary to associate their two names. Baillarger, who was a physcian at La Salpêtrière, while discussing in 1869, at the French Medical Academy, the paper of Dax dealings with localization of speech in left brain hemisphere, expressed the remarkable idea that the main disorder of aphasia was the suppression of voluntary verbal stimulation while spontaneous verbal stimulation remained.

Here is the text selected and quoted in French by Jackson himself. "Quand on lit des observations d'aphasie, on constate chez un certain nombre de malades ce phénomène singulier qu'il leur est impossible de prononcer certains mots quand ils essayent de le faire et qu'ils y appliquent toute leur énergie de volonté; au contraire, quelques instants après, ils prononcent ces mêmes mots sans le vouloir. Ainsi il y a chez eux perte de l'incitation motrice volontaire, conservation de l'incitation motrice spontanée."

In several of his papers, Jackson came back to this remark of Baillarger, which he considered, as we have seen, as a principle, and emphasized its value. He gave numerous instances in which he expressed also his views on the different uses of language, which he named propositional and emotional. I have myself, in various studies, found it necessary to revert to this valuable interpretation of the physiopathology of aphasia. In my opinion it provides the best explanation for the data which have been presented.

In *permanent verbal stereotypy* we have been struck by the character of involuntary speech, and, during its regression we have noted the increasing influence of will. During the first stage of verbal stereotypy all voluntary speech is abolished; it remains only a fixed and automatic verbal expression. Later, as speech comes more differentiated, the automatic utterance is checked by voluntary speech as the latter reappears. The more propositional and volitional forms of speech remain imperfect and difficult, while ready-made or emotional language becomes facile.

In agrammatism, which is only the end of such an evolution, the same dissociation is found: voluntary speech shows agrammatism; automatic speech escapes such a disorder.

In *pure anarthria*, which is an isolated disturbance of the material means of elocution, stable and regular in its character, no dissociation is left. The studies of "visible speech" also reveal that these articulatory troubles are to some extent related to the situation in which speech occurs. They seem to be less obvious in emotional speech, especially when they are associated with other disorders more clearly of an aphasic nature.

And lastly, in *jargon aphasia*, logorrhœa, quick utterance, uncontrolled expression show indisputably the lack of voluntary influence; the latter reappears clearly when jargon regresses. Furthermore, in the automatic language which is the jargon, there is something else, anosognosia and disintegration of the semantic value of the speech.

(b) As far as anosognosia is concerned, we must confess that the interpretation of that important element in the disturbances of verbal expression seems extremely difficult. Strictly speaking, it is not a true anosognosia, as is for instance the unawareness of a diseased state of the body i.e. Anton-Babinski syndrome. It is not of his disease that the aphasic patient is unaware, but only of a particular disturbance of verbal expression caused by the disease. It is a selective agnosia of a function, or better, the agnosia of the way in which the speech activity takes place. It is similar to what is observed in some patients with hemianopia or cortical blindness, who are unaware of their visual disturbance. Regardless of whether or not auditory imperception plays a part in the aphasic anosognosia, the essential point remains that the patient does not consider his speech as abnormal. Perhaps the relatively automatic character of his speech is the reason for this lack of awareness, as in the normal individual in whom the more automatic utterances are but dimly perceived. Such a possibility is suggested by the diminution or disappearance of aphasic anosognosia as the speech improves and a greater degree of voluntary control reasserts itself. Anosognosia may, then, be only the mark of distorted motor verbal activity and not a primary event in itself.

SUMMARY

In summary I would say that our analysis of the strictly oral verbal aspects of aphasia have led us to the following conclusions.

(1) Lesions of parts of brain concerned with language result in motor speech defect varying from complete inability to utter a single word to an inability to adequately express feelings and thoughts, despite volubility in the most complex situations.

(2) The adequacy of verbal accomplishment in any one patient, if properly tested, varies according to his stimulus to speech: situations leading to emotional, expletive, interjectional, automatic, habitual language are always more effective than those requiring volitional or propositional speech.

(3) The verbal residues, which often appear in a compulsive, almost involuntary manner, without the patient seeming to be fully aware of them, take several relatively uniform and easily recognizable forms. These which we have called verbal stereotypy, agrammatism, phonetic disintegration, jargon aphasia have been described in detail.

(4) Prolonged observation of these disorders of verbal expression reveals certain predictable evolutionary sequences, which are of value in prognostication of the outcome of the speech disorders, and which possess a certain pathophysiological significance.

3

Specific Semantic Word Categories in Aphasia

HAROLD GOODGLASS
BARBARA KLEIN
PETER W. CAREY
KENNETH J. JONES

HAROLD GOODGLASS, Ph.D., is director of psychology research at the Boston Veterans Administration Hospital.
BARBARA KLEIN (EFRON), M.A., was formerly with the Neurophysiology-Biophysics Research Unit at the Boston Veterans Adminstration Hospital.
PETER W. CAREY, Ph.D., is with the City University of New York.
KENNETH J. JONES, Ed.D., is with the department of psychology of Brandeis University, Waltham.
This work was supported in part by Grant MH 4187 from the National Institute of Mental Health.

Categories of aphasic symptoms based upon the status of visual, of auditory, or of articulatory processes are most acceptable to our habits of thought because they correspond to psychologically discrete modalities of sensation and motor expression, and to neurophysiologically understandable subdivisions. However, aphasia in its multiple forms, may present us with symptoms which do not follow the lines of preconceived categories. In this paper, we discuss those symptoms in which variations in performance must be defined along lines of semantic word category. There are a number of such symptoms, or combinations of symptoms, which are encountered clinically, among which are the following:

Loss of object naming, without impairment of letter naming or of number naming.

Impairment of auditory comprehension for body part names, but not for object names.

Impairment of color naming, without other anomic difficulties.

Impairment of repetition of all word categories except numbers.

Of the foregoing, only *color name aphasia* has been found to occur as the unique expressive disturbance in otherwise normal speech. It has been observed repeatedly as an accompaniment to pure alexia, and is also reported by Nielsen (1946) in association with visual agnosia for objects. Sparing of repetition of letters or of numbers is described by Goldstein (1948) in several cases of conduction aphasia (Goldstein's term is "central aphasia"), a syndrome marked by disproportionately severe disturbance of repetition, in a setting of good comprehension and fair articulation. In our clinic, dramatic sparing of number repetition has been repeatedly observed in patients who showed severe disturbances in repetition of other word categories.

Up to the present time there has been no systematic collection of data on the problem of differential capacity for word-finding and understanding of various semantic categories. This paper reports findings which indicate that systematic differences among these categories are a regular feature of aphasia and that the pattern of differences varies predictably with the major clinical types of aphasia.

PROCEDURE

Subjects. The total aphasic sample consisted of 135 consecutively examined patients who were

From *Cortex* 2:74–89, 1966.

seen between 1960 and 1964, chiefly in the aphasia program of the Boston VA Hospital. Of the total sample, 72 had their tape recorded conversations classified by judges as to the type of aphasia represented by their speech patterns. Of these, 37 were considered to be Broca's aphasics, 18 Wernicke's aphasics, and 17 amnesic aphasics. The speech characteristics on which this classification is based include articulation, fluency, retention of speech melody, variety of grammatical constructions, presence of paraphasia in running speech, prominence of word-finding difficulty, and level of auditory comprehension. Because Wernicke and amnesic aphasics have in common frequent production of long runs of fluently articulated words, they are also treated under the single heading of "fluent aphasics" in contrast to Broca's aphasics. Details of the method of classification are described by Goodglass, Quadfasel and Timberlake (1964).

Tests used. The Boston VA Hospital Diagnostic Aphasia Test was originally designed to include the possibility of making comparisons among several semantic categories in the comprehension and naming spheres. Auditory comprehension is assessed by the "Word Discrimination" subtest which is subdivided into separately scorable category sets each having 6 items: "Objects" (chair, comb, key, glove, hammock, cactus), "Geometric forms" (circle, square, triangle, spiral, cone, star), "Letters" (L, H, R, T, S, G), "Actions" (smoking, drinking, sleeping, running, falling, dripping), "Numbers" (7, 42, 15, 700, 1963, 7000), and "Colors" (blue, red, gray, brown, pink, purple). These are multiple choice tests in which the examiner names and subject points. An auditory comprehension inventory of 20 names of body parts is also part of the test. The naming subtest contains the same subdivisions as the comprehension subtest except for "Geometric forms" and "Body parts."

Scoring of comprehension and naming items includes credit for speed and accuracy. On comprehension items a subject can earn from 0 to 2 points per item, and a maximum of 12 points for any given category set. The Body part comprehension score range is from 0 to 20. On naming, a subject can obtain up to 3 points per item and a maximum of 18 points for each category set.

Treatment of test scores. Two statistical procedures were used in the analysis of the data. The first employed as basic data the determination, for each subject, whether any semantic categories were deviantly high or deviantly low in score, as compared to the other categories. In the word-comprehension subtest, where a subject could earn up to 12 points per category set, a category was considered deviantly high if its score was at least three points more than the score of four of the five remaining categories. (Body part comprehension is not included in this analysis.) The inverse operation determined a deviantly low score. In the naming subtest, a deviantly high category was defined as at least four points above three or all four of the remaining categories. All scores not meeting these criteria of "deviance" were considered to be "intermediate" and, of course, many subjects had only intermediate scores.

The first analysis described in this report is based upon nonparametric tests of the incidence of deviantly high, deviantly low, and intermediate scores in the several semantic categories, for both expression and for comprehension. The second analysis, described later in this report, is a *discriminant analysis*, utilizing the full range of scores in all of the tests.

RESULTS

Deviant scores analysis

Incidence of high, intermediate, and low scores on each semantic category. This set of results is essentially a reflection of the relative difficulty of the several semantic categories. This order of difficulty can be a function of the distinctiveness or of the number of class members per category, which affects their discriminability and their availability as responses. Those differences in difficulty which are uniform in both the receptive and expressive modalities may possibly be artifacts of the difficulty of the vocabulary chosen. Such differences are relatively trivial from the theoretical viewpoint.

Of greater interest, however, would be differences between expressive and receptive modes of performance, since these may reflect contrasts in the psychological processing of various categories of words.

Figure 3-1 summarizes the occurrence of deviantly high and low scores in each semantic category. Overall Chi Square tests, applied to the "Naming" and "Word Discrimination" distributions indicate that the disparities between semantic groups are well beyond the realm of statistical accident. Examination of Figure 3-1 shows that "Object Naming" was, by a considerable margin, the most difficult expressive category but, along with "Actions," the easiest of the receptive categories. This relationship is paralleled by "Numbers," but drastically reversed in the case of "Letters," which are by far the most difficult to decode and the easiest to encode vocally. For many subjects, color comprehension ranks as the lowest comprehension subtest but colors are relatively less difficult to name.

Comparing "Numbers" and "Letters" directly, it is seen that "Numbers" are more often a high-score category than "Letters" in auditory discrimination and less often a low-score category. In the expressive modality, however, this relationship is reversed. A Chi Square test applied specifically to the distribution of the extreme scores in these two semantic categories is significant beyond p = .05, for both naming and auditory discrimination.

Analysis by diagnostic groups. Up to this point, we have considered differences which apply to all aphasics, and which may be rationalized on a psychological basis. It remains to be seen whether any particular subgroup of the aphasic population is principally responsible for the observed differences. As we indicated above, the aphasic group was divided into the opposing diagnostic sub-groups "Broca's aphasics" and "fluent aphasics." Table 3-1 gives the distribution of high and low word-discrimination scores and high and low naming scores in each semantic category, for the two diagnostic groups.

Inspection of the auditory comprehension of the two groups shows essentially parallel performances. "Objects" tend to be the easiest category for 12 to 15 percent of subjects in both diagnostic groups. Both groups had more frequent difficulty with color names, but it was the comprehension of letter-names which was the most remarkably difficult for both categories of patients—deviantly low in about 25 percent of each group.

Inspecting the naming tasks, a number of

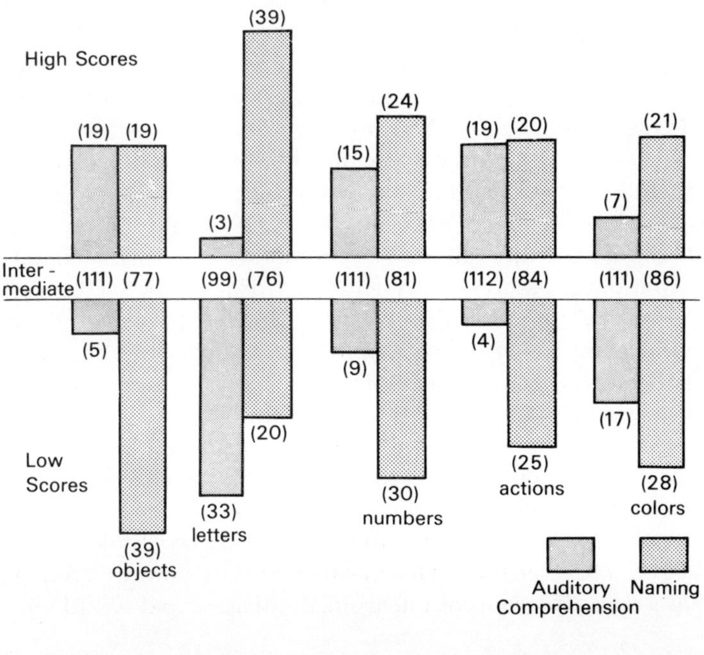

Fig. 3–1. Incidence of deviantly high, deviantly low, and intermediate scores in naming and understanding words of five semantic categories.

TABLE 3-1. INCIDENCE OF DEVIANTLY HIGH AND LOW SCORES IN EACH PERFORMANCE MODALITY FOR BROCA'S APHASICS AND FLUENT APHASICS

	Word Discrimination				Naming			
	Broca's		Fluent		Broca's		Fluent	
	High	Low	High	Low	High	Low	High	Low
Objects	5	2	5	1	6	7	3	18
Letters	2	8	1	10	5	6	15	4
Action Words	3	1	7	1	5	6	6	7
Numbers	6	2	2	2	4	10	9	8
Colors	2	8	2	5	4	6	5	7

interesting differences appear. We see that in no case does the concentration of high or low scores in expression parallel that for comprehension. The positions of "Objects" and "Letters" are completely reversed; "Colors" and "Actions" are now equally often high or low. When we examine the naming scores of Broca's aphasics, it does not appear that any semantic word-group is significantly more often deviantly high than deviantly low or vice versa. A tendency for "Numbers" to be on the difficult side is well short of statistical significance. The fluent aphasic group, however, is markedly deficient in Object Naming, relative to their other categories, and markedly superior in Letter Naming. When the combination high "Letter-Naming" and low "Object-Naming" is taken, we find that this identifies 13 fluent aphasics and only 4 Broca's aphasics. Interestingly, the absolute level of "Object Naming" is virtually identical for Broca's and fluent aphasics.

Discriminant analysis

In contrast to the above-described analysis, which is based only on the incidence of deviantly high or low scores, the method of *discriminant analysis* exploits the information contained in the full range of subscores. The essentials of this procedure are that the data are first grouped on the basis of an external criterion and then examined statistically to see if they are related to the external criterion. If there is a relationship, it becomes possible to predict from which group any subject's set of scores was drawn. As mentioned earlier, our data were 72 sets of scores from patients classified as Broca's aphasics (37), Wernicke's aphasics (18) and amnesic aphasics (17). The scores were submitted for discriminant analysis on an IBM 7094 computer, using a program developed by Dr. Kenneth Jones. The output of this program yields two "discriminant functions," which define the mathematical dimensions along which there is maximum separation of the groups' test scores.

Corresponding to each discriminant function is a set of "scaled vectors," which represent the weight—positive or negative—by which each standard score of any subject's set is to be multiplied. The sum of these terms then gives the subject's score on the discriminant function. Thus the magnitude of the scaled vector is a measure of the importance of a particular test, in context with the others, in determining the discriminant score. Since, in the present data, there are two discriminant functions, the position on each function can be computed for each subject's set of scores. Knowing these two positions, it is possible to determine the probability that the set belongs to each of the diagnostic categories. It is then possible to compare the total array of classifications calculated from the experimental variables with the a priori diagnostic classifications.

Table 3-2 shows how many cases of each diagnostic type earned the highest probability of membership in each diagnostic group, through the computation of discriminant scores. Fifty-four or 75% of the cases are "correctly" classified by the profile of their scores in naming and understanding the several semantic categories. This number is arrived at by adding the "correct" classifications (the diagonal elements of Table 3-2, 30 + 11 + 13 = 54). Significance test done on the discriminant functions indicated that this was considerably better than one could do by chance. This means that if we now are given a group of unclassified aphasics, and we admin-

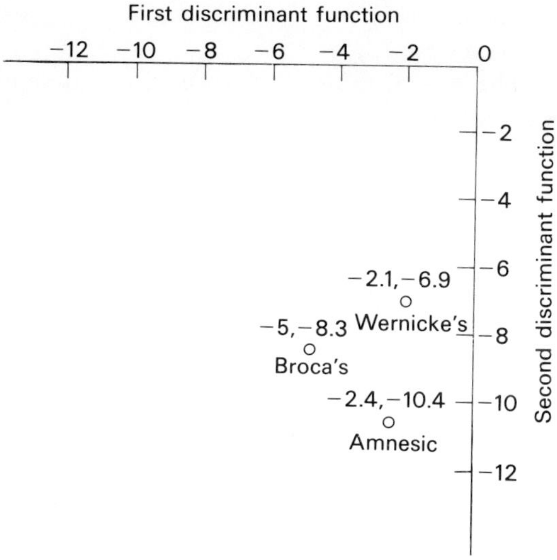

Fig. 3-2. Center of distribution of scores of each diagnostic class, plotted against two discriminant functions.

ister the 12 tests to each, we may expect to correctly assign them to their respective diagnostic groups 75% of the time.

When the two discriminant functions are treated as the axes of a pair of coordinates, it is possible to plot the center of distribution of each diagnostic type in terms of this pair of coordinates. This plot, reproduced as Figure 3-2, shows that the first discriminant function separates the Broca's from the fluent aphasics, while the two sub-categories of fluents are barely distinguished in terms of this function. The second function, however, distinguishes the amnesics from the Wernicke's aphasics, while the Broca's group are centered around the middle of the range of this function.

The interpretation of the discriminant function begins with the inspection of the vector scores (Table 3-3). These vectors represent the relative value of the scores as predictors, and do not necessarily reflect absolute differences between scores. Thus a high vector score for a test variable on the first discriminant function could be produced by deviantly high scores on the part of fluent aphasics or deviantly low scores on the part of Broca's aphasics, or by a combination of both. Figure 3-3 was designed to make the interpretation of the vectors easier, as follows. Taking the means of the five expressive subscores of Broca's aphasics (Table 3-4), we obtained the deviation of each from the grand mean of the five. This operation was repeated for the first six receptive tests (excluding Body Part Comprehension—a 20 point test). The deviations from the grand means were similarly computed for the combined Wernicke and amnesic groups. When

TABLE 3-2. MOST PROBABLY STATISTICAL CLASSIFICATION ON BASIS OF TWO DISCRIMINANT FUNCTIONS

A Priori Classification	Broca's	Wernicke's	Amnesic
Broca's	30	3	4
Wernicke's	6	11	1
Amnesic	2	2	13

TABLE 3-3. SCALED VECTORS FOR THE TWO DISCRIMINANT FUNCTIONS

Test Variable	Scaled Vectors 1st Discr. Funct.	2nd Discr. Funct.
1. Object comprehension	—.07	—.21
2. Form "	+.34	—.18
3. Letter "	+.33	+.16
4. Action "	—.19	—.08
5. Number "	—.12	+.01
6. Color "	—.05	+.17
7. Body part "	—.44	—.22
8. Object Naming	—.37	+.38
9. Color "	—.25	—.39
10. Action "	+.38	—.09
11. Number "	+.17	—.48
12. Letter "	+.44	—.22

it appeared, from inspection of these mean deviations, that a positive vector was determined entirely by a relatively high score in the given variable on the part of the fluent aphasics, the vector was represented in Figure 3-3 by a stippled bar, entirely above the line. When a positive scaled vector corresponds to a deviantly low mean score by Broca's aphasics, it is represented entirely below the line, with cross hatching. The converse applied to negative vectors. When opposite tendencies are found in the two means, the vector bar is divided in proportion to the contribution of each mean deviation to their absolute total.

Our results now are susceptible to comparison with those from the earlier reported incidence of deviantly high and low scores. As reported in the earlier results, we see that most of the variation in capacity to handle different semantic categories is found in the "fluent" and not in the Broca's aphasics. Moreover, the most outstanding specific finding is that the fluent aphasics are characterized by the combination high Letter-Naming with low Object-Naming. The discriminant analysis shows that to some degree, the Broca's aphasics actually reverse this finding, making the contrast between them and the fluent group more dramatic. This latter result was not apparent from the analysis of the deviant extremes.

The second discriminant function separates the amnesic aphasics from the Wernicke aphasics on the following characteristics: a) more consistently depressed Object Naming scores for the amnesic group; b) more frequent failures in Action and Number Naming by the Wernicke aphasics; c) more difficulty with Body Part Comprehension on the part of Wernicke aphasics.

DISCUSSION

Much of the literature on the psychology of language makes the tacit assumption that the "knowledge" of a word as a symbol is a unitary phenomenon; that in a sense there is a memory trace for any word which is activated when we say the word and which is isomorphic with a memory trace through which we understand the word on hearing it. This idealization of the concept of "knowing a word" is widespread in spite of contradictory evidence from child development and from aphasia. Young children, while understanding and beginning to use adult words in their speech, may hold on to a few idiosyncratic words of their own

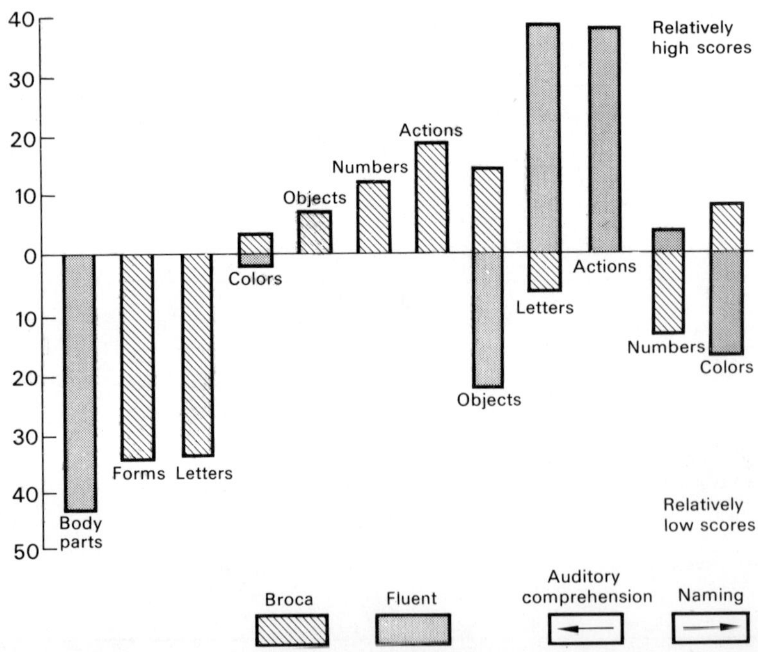

Fig. 3–3. Relative magnitude of scaled vectors for first discriminant function, showing contribution of high or low scores by either diagnostic class to the determination of the vector.

TABLE 3–4. MEAN SCORES IN EACH SEMANTIC CATEGORY FOR EACH DIAGNOSTIC GROUP, WITH SIGNIFICANCE LEVEL OF DIFFERENCES

	Broca's	Wernicke's	Amnesic	F	p
1. Object comprehension	11.35	10.06	11.76	4.09	.02
2. Form "	9.32	9.00	11.06	3.29	.04
3. Letter "	9.65	9.72	11.24	2.17	.12
4. Action "	11.22	10.39	11.76	3.72	.03
5. Number "	10.76	10.06	11.71	2.77	.07
6. Color "	10.70	9.72	11.35	2.20	.12
7. Body Part "	16.76	14.72	18.71	3.40	.04
8. Object Naming	11.76	11.11	11.94	.11	.89
9. Color "	11.22	10.50	14.35	2.56	.08
10. Action "	11.43	11.94	14.94	3.02	.05
11. Number "	9.15	11.78	15.35	6.74	.002
12. Letter "	10.43	14.22	16.29	3.40	.04

invention for certain concepts, and use them exclusively in expression. The senior author's daughter, for example, used the monosyllable "lah" for the concept "milk" exclusively, even after she had a considerable vocabulary of conventional English words. When the word "milk" was included in a short series of words for repetition she still used "lah" as the expressive equivalent of the perceived word "milk." Other examples are cited by Seth and Guthrie (1935).

In aphasia, a familiar, if not common phenomenon is for a patient to use a word appropriately in running speech, yet fail to demonstrate understanding of it when he hears it spoken out of context. The findings of this study reinforce the position that the operation of producing language is in surprising measure independent of understanding it—even where the *same* lexical content is involved. In addition, we found that there is a differential effect for different forms of aphasia on words from different semantic categories. From this we can infer that individually spoken words which are normally considered equivalent from an expressive viewpoint, may in fact be experienced differently psychologically and produced through different processes.

To summarize our findings, the relative difficulty for word evocation of five semantic categories was different from their order of difficulty in auditory comprehension. There are several striking reversals in these data: namely, that object names are the easiest category for comprehension and the most difficult for naming. Precisely the reverse was true for Letter-Naming. The relation of Letter-Naming to Number-Naming was the reverse of the relation of Letter Comprehension to Number Comprehension. It is apparent that these results cannot be explained by differences in difficulty of vocabulary, from one category to another. If vocabulary difficulty were a major factor, we would find the same order of difficulty for the semantic categories in both the expressive and receptive performance modalities, because the same words are used in both.

"Numbers" and "Letters" deserve close comparison because they share certain psychological characteristics. The word for a number, like the word for a letter, is simply a name assigned to one of a small set of arbitrary written symbols. A written letter or number (unlike an object), is experienced only as a visual configuration. It has no tactile or kinesthetic associations and few, if any, affective experiential connotations. Any response to an isolated number or letter is mediated by its name—either spoken aloud or experienced silently. One might object that since there are only 10 digits, but 26 letters, there are differences in difficulty introduced by the number of class members from which any item must be discriminated. However, in order to name all the possible numbers up to the thousands, one needs an additional vocabulary of at least 13 number-words (eleven, twelve, hundred, etc.) plus six combinational rules, making a total number vocabulary which is very close to the letter-vocabulary.

From the point of view of speech, however, the important difference between Numbers and Letters lies in the amount of phonological information given by the naming of each. Thus, in the English alphabet, nine letters have in common the vowel /i/ (B, C, D, E, G, P, T, V, Z), six the vowel /ɛ/ (F, L, M, N, S, X), and four, the diphthong /ei/ (A, H, J, K). Only a single consonant, inserted before or after the vowel serves to specify the identity of the letter. Thus, the listener (or decoder) must base his letter comprehension on a minuscule bit of phonological data. In the case of the numbers up to 10, however, only "five" and "nine" share a vowel, and all of the numbers except "two" and "eight" have more than one consonant. Multi-digit numbers, of course, are still richer phonologically. While the demands on the listener for decoding a number which he has heard are smaller than in the case of letter-names, this relationship is reversed in the naming of the visually presented stimulus. It is now the encoder who must concentrate a great amount of phonological information in each number name than he does for each letter-name. Thus, results predictable from an information theory point of view have been obtained.

If we attempt to apply the same line of reasoning to explain the subjects' superiority in comprehension of "Objects," in comparison to their low scores in "Object Naming," the result is less satisfactory. Considering phonological information alone, there is no obvious basis for regarding "Objects" as either more or less difficult than "Colors," "Actions," or "Numbers."

However, leaving aside phonological considerations, there is the relative cohesiveness within such categories as colors, letters, geometric forms, and numbers to consider. These are each well-demarcated semantic groups, whose members are not very distinct from each other with respect to experiential connotations. In contrast, Object Names and Actions each represent a potentially limitless variety of connotations. Object Names are treated as a single semantic group chiefly on the basis of their having a grammatical function in common. The same is true of Action Names. Hearing the name of an object or of an action, then, provides a cue which carries connotations very distinctive from the other object or action words. It is not surprising therefore, that "Objects" and "Actions" are the two highest scoring comprehension categories for each of the three diagnostic groups (see Table 3-4).

We have just seen that consideration of the informational qualities of object and action words appears to have explanatory value with respect to auditory comprehension. However, on examining the second group of findings, we find that a more complex explanation may be necessary in dealing with the *naming* of words by aphasics. Here, we find that the loss of object names, in combination with the preservation of letter names, is characteristic of only one segment of aphasics: the "fluent" aphasics, who comprise those with posterior temporal and temporo-parietal lesions. In contrast, Broca's aphasics showed a tendency to the reverse finding—i.e., inferiority in Letter Naming, in conjunction with superiority in Object Naming. The categories "Colors," "Actions," "Geometric forms," and "Numbers" contribute in a less dramatic way to the differences between the major diagnostic groups. We do not know the reliability of these lesser findings, which emerged only in the discriminant analysis and not in the inspection of deviantly high and low scores.

With respect to object naming, we have recently collected some evidence which indicates that the very quality which facilitates the appearance of nouns in the free conversation of Broca's aphasics inhibits them in the conversation of fluent aphasics. Specifically: the names of picturable objects constitute a larger than normal proportion of the nouns for the "fluent" aphasics. Exactly the reverse, however, is true for indefinites—i.e., the words "thing," "person," "time," "place," "one" and their compounds with "some-," "no-" and "any-." In this respect, the Broca's aphasics resemble young children. Brown (1957) has reported that both the nouns and verbs of young children are more concretely picturable than those of adults.

We can certainly not, however, explain away the speech pattern of the fluent aphasics as a "mature" one, because of the predominance of vague superordinate words in their speech. It seems compelling to recognize the anomic component of fluent aphasia as a specific deficit which is qualitatively different from the retardation and failures in word-finding which are found in nearly all aphasics. This qualitative difference is further highlighted by the present demonstration that letter naming and object naming are relatively dissociated skills, with a reversal in their order of difficulty between fluent and Broca's aphasics.

In view of the predominantly anterior location of lesions for Broca's aphasia and posterior site of the lesions in fluent aphasia, it seems natural to consider an anatomical basis for our findings. It is possible to postulate that the word-finding system is subdivided anatomically according to the psychological character of different word categories. Thus, we might assign letter naming to anatomic structures which are more likely to be injured or isolated in Broca's than in fluent aphasia. Another possible basis for anatomic subdivision of the word-finding system might be the principle sensory modality through which a nameable object is experienced. It is true that routine clinical testing of naming by touch vs. sight, or by sound vs. sight, only occasionally turn up a case with marked discrepancies between modalities. However, a carefully controlled study which includes reaction times, has not been reported. Research in this direction is currently being undertaken.

SUMMARY

This study was prompted by clinical observations that aphasic defects in naming or in auditory comprehension of words are sometimes disproportionately severe for certain semantic categories or are even confined to one category. The question was posed as to whether any regularities existed between such circumscribed deficits and other factors in aphasia. One hundred and thirty-five aphasics were tested for their proficiency in naming objects, colors, numbers, letters, and actions, and for their auditory comprehension of words in these categories, plus the additional categories of "geometric forms" and "body parts."

It was found that "Objects" were the most difficult category to name, but one of the two easiest to comprehend auditorily. In contrast, "Letters" were the easiest category for naming, but the most difficult for auditory comprehension. A further analysis by diagnostic class of aphasia was based on data from 72 patients, who had been classified as either Broca's, Wernicke's, or amnesic aphasics. It was found that for all classes of aphasics, comprehension of object names was most frequently the easiest receptive category and comprehension of letter names most frequently the hardest. Body part comprehension was most frequently depressed among Wernicke aphasics, relative to the other categories. The most striking distinction between diagnostic classes emerged in relation to the naming of objects and letters. It was the Wernicke's aphasics and amnesic aphasics whose scores accounted for the previously observed superiority of letter-naming and the inferiority of object-naming. The Broca's aphasics, in contrast, showed no significant differences between the various semantic classes in their naming proficiency.

It is concluded that the pattern of differences in naming and auditory discrimination among words of various semantic categories varies predictably with the major clinical types of aphasia.

REFERENCES

Brown, R. (1957) *Linguistic determinism and the part of speech*, "J. Abn. Soc. Psychol.," **55,** 1-5.

Goldstein, K. (1948) *Language and Language Disturbances*, Grune and Stratton, New York.

Goodglass, H., Quadfasel, F. A., and Timberlake, W. H. (1964), *Phrase length and the type and severity of aphasia*, "Cortex," **1,** 133-153.

Nielsen, J. M. (1946) *Agnosia, Apraxia, Aphasia*, Hoeber, New York.

Seth, G., and Guthrie, D. (1935) *Speech in Childhood*, Oxford Univ. Press, London.

4

The Varieties of Naming Errors

NORMAN GESCHWIND

NORMAN GESCHWIND, M.D., is chairman of the department of neurology of Harvard University, Cambridge.

Supported in part by Grants NB06209 and MH08472 from the National Institutes of Health to the Boston University Aphasia Research Center.

In this paper I shall be discussing anomia in the sense of the inability of the patient to name things shown to him, what can be called failure of naming on confrontation. This task makes up so large a part of the testing of aphasia that it deserves attention. It is sometimes even asserted that failure in this task occurs in all aphasics. While as a rough statement this may be true, it deserves modification before it can be accepted without reservation. Thus there are certainly aphasics in whom naming on confrontation is very good relative to the patient's abnormal spontaneous speech production, even if rarely fully normal. This is particularly true in some cases of Broca's aphasia, and Jakobson (1964) has made much of this in his description of polar types of linguistic disturbance in aphasia.

I would stress also that we are speaking of naming in the narrower sense and not of word-finding in the flow of speech. The reasons for the failure to find words in one situation while they can be found in another have not yet been adequately studied and will not be discussed here. Instead I shall simply confine myself to discussing four distinguishable varieties of failure of confrontation naming which may have some theoretical importance in considerations of aphasia, and are of significance in clinical diagnosis.

From *Cortex* 3:97–112, 1967.

The localization of anomia has often been a disputed point. In classical writings there were two opposing views, one which asserted that anomia resulted from a lesion of the left parietotemporal region while the other claimed that it was the result of diffuse disorder of the brain. The proponents of each localization had supporting data for their point of view. Gloning, Gloning and Hoff (1963) dealt with this question simply by accepting both types of localization. As I will try to show, this problem can be at least partially resolved by the demonstration that local and diffuse localization respectively correspond to different types of anomia.

One must of course be sure that the failure to name an object is not the result of failure of perception. This if a patient calls a "pencil" a "fork" it is conceivable that this could be the result of perceptual distortion. A test which is often used to rule out perceptual error is to offer the patient names and to see if he chooses the correct one. This test can, however, serve to exclude perceptual disturbance but cannot be used to prove that it is present. Thus, if the patient always selects the correct name from those offered to him he must in each instance have recognized the object. Failure to accept the name might, however, be due not to incorrect perception of the object but to incomprehension of the name. Other tasks must be used to insure the correctness of perception.

Correct pantomine of the use of the object proves correct perception. Similarly, matching tasks may be used. If a patient calls a "pencil" a "fork" but invariably matches a pencil to another pencil or a picture of a pencil, one must rule out perceptual difficulty. Similarly, if the patient is shown an object and misnames it but then draws it correctly, we must again exclude perceptual disturbance.

The classic form of anomia is characterized by difficulty in naming on confrontation, while the patient usually but not always accepts the correct name. The patient may also show by many of the other maneuvers listed above that he recognizes the object. He may simply fail to produce the name, or he may produce an incorrect name or a circumlocutory description. Almost invariably, when confrontation naming is impaired the patient's spontaneous language production is disturbed so that while speech is fluent, it may contain many paraphasias, circumlocutions or "empty" words (such as "thing," "place," "these"). The word-finding difficulty in spontaneous speech is not confined to the names of physical stimuli but also involves abstract nouns and adjectives and other parts of speech (Wepman et al., 1956; Howes, 1964). When in addition to these features the patient's comprehension and repetition of speech are normal we have the classical syndrome of anomic aphasia, the lesion of which usually lies in the left temporo-parietal region (the angular gyrus). If disturbances of either comprehension or repetition, or of both are present in association with the above picture of fluent, paraphasic speech, the localizations are somewhat different although in all instances the lesions lie behind the Rolandic fissure.

In this first group the anomic difficulty tends to be a rather general one. It involves all modalities and all types of stimuli. The intensity of the disturbance is not, however, necessarily equal for all stimuli, as has recently been shown in careful studies by Goodglass et al. (1966).

In contrast to the above type of anomia we have another more restricted form, of which I will cite two examples, both of which I have presented elsewhere (Geschwind, 1965) although I did not in my earlier discussion bring out some of the differences between this type and the classical form of anomia discussed in the preceding paragraphs.

An example of this variety of anomia was seen in the patient of Geschwind and Kaplan (1962) who had a proven infarction of the corpus callosum sparing only the splenium. He had no difficulty in naming objects visually and speech was normal. When blindfolded he misnamed objects held in the left hand. The misnamings were bizarre, e.g., "eraser" for a ring, "balloon" for a watch, "book of matches" for a padlock, "an elastic" for a nail, "piece of paper" for a screwdriver. Furthermore, he did not accept the correct name when it was offered to him. That there was no perceptual failure could, however, be proven by the fact that after feeling an object with the left hand while blindfolded he could, using the same hand, pick the object by touch alone out of a bag or select it with eyes open from a group. When blindfolded he would use the object correctly with the left hand simultaneously misnaming it. In addition he could afterwards draw the object correctly with the left hand. It is clear that perception was intact and that this must be a naming defect.

It might be objected that one could explain this disturbance as the result of a combination of a minimal sensory defect in the left hand with minimal general naming disturbance. This is similar to the explanation advanced by Critchley (1966) to account for cases of color-naming difficulty. This type of explanation can be shown, however, to be inadequate to account for the naming difficulty of our patient for objects held in the left hand. The patient had definite sensory loss in the *right* hand as manifested by position, vibration, and two-point testing. In the *left* hand he could be shown by non-verbal testing to have normal sensation. Yet he correctly named objects felt with the right hand but not those held in the left. This fact clearly rules out the explanation of sensory loss plus minimal naming difficulty since naming of objects held in the right hand should then have been more seriously involved than that of objects held in the left hand. I suspect that this type of explanation will rarely if ever be justified in any case. It is difficult to believe that a combination of two borderline disturbances could produce so dramatic and delimited a syndrome as this patient demonstrated. This case similarly cannot be accounted for by dementia or uncooperativeness since these would fail to explain the unilaterality of the disturbance.

A second example of this variety of anomia illustrates an even more delimited syndrome. This is the color-naming defect which accompanies some cases of pure alexia without agraphia. Geschwind and Fusillo (1966) have recently described such a case in detail. Consistent results were found on repeated careful testing over a nine-month period. This patient had a right hemianopia. He could not read, but he named objects normally (only one error in object-naming was made in all the testing sessions). He misnamed colors, but his misnaming always consisted of other color-words. The responses were not consistent in that the same red might on one occasion be called "gray," on another "green." The answer "gray" was, however, more common than any of the other color-words. The patient failed to select the correct answer from a group. Furthermore, he failed in the task of selecting a named color from a group presented to him. On the other hand, perceptual deficit was ruled out by the fact that the patient matched hues correctly despite wide differences in brightness or saturation, that he could sort colored chips correctly, even sorting into separate piles chips of slightly different shades of the same hue. He correctly matched colored pieces of paper to uncolored pictures of objects. Finally he performed normally on two pseudo-isochromatic tests of color vision, the Ishihara and the American Optical Company tests. Loss of memory for color-names was ruled out by the fact that he correctly answered questions such as, "What is the color of a banana?" Kinsbourne and Warrington (1964) in an earlier publication described a similar, although not identical, case.

It is obvious that this too is a naming disturbance. Critchley (1966) has suggested, as was noted above, the possibility that this disorder is not a specific entity "but rather a very mild disorder of visual perception coupled with a minimal dysphasia." This explanation is difficult to accept in the face of the powerful evidences of normal color perception I have cited above, and does not account readily for the highly delimited character of the syndrome. Furthermore, many patients with the combination of an obvious mild anomia and a hemianopia do not show dramatic difficulty in color naming, although one would expect this to be a common effect of this combination if Critchley were correct. Furthermore, since some degree of color-blindness is presented in about 7 percent of males, one would expect this percentage of mildly aphasic patients to show dramatic color-naming difficulties. Yet color-naming disturbances are rare and are most likely to occur in association with another rare syndrome, that of pure alexia without agraphia which has a characteristic pathological picture (Geschwind, 1962).

Both of the cases described above have come to anatomical examination, the brains having been cut in whole-brain sections, with alternate sections stained for myelin and cells. In the case of Geschwind and Kaplan the corpus callosum was infarcted and the splenium was spared. In the case of Geschwind and Fusillo the left visual cortex and the splenium were destroyed. The tactile naming difficulty in the left hand in the first case was interpreted as the result of disconnection of the right somesthetic cortex from the speech area, and the second case was interpreted as the result of disconnection of the right visual cortex from the speech area. Since I have discussed these explanations in detail elsewhere (Geschwind, 1965) I will return to our central interest at this moment, the character of the anomia in these cases.

Difficulties in naming, predominantly in a single modality, have been mentioned by many authors although these have frequently been treated as agnosias. Arguments against this interpretation have been summarized in Geschwind (1965) and will not be repeated here. Two excellent recent examples of dissociation between modalities are seen in the case of Ettlinger and Wyke (1961), who named better visually than by touch, and in the cases of Spreen, Benton, and Van Allen, who cited two patients with predominantly visual and three with predominantly tactile anomia. Kaplan and Geschwind (unpublished) observed one patient with a predominantly tactile naming disturbance.

Let us look at the features of this second form of anomia which distinguish it from the classical form. In the first place the second type of anomia is remarkably delimited, being confined to the tactile modality in the left half of the body in the first case and to color-naming in the second. The classical type of anomia is more global in its effect. In the second place spontaneous speech was normal in both of these cases and neither patient showed word-finding difficulty except on confrontation. Thus the second patient showed no difficulty in finding color words except when confronted with a color. This contrasts with the classical form of anomia in which even mild confrontation naming difficulty is almost always accompanied by word-finding difficulty in spontaneous speech as manifested by hesitation, particularly in finding substantive words (as against "grammatical" words), by an increased tendency to use "empty" words, by circumlocution, or by production of paraphasias.

A third difference is in the nature of the errors. The classic anomic may fail to name or may produce verbal paraphasias, combinatory paraphasias (e.g. "ring-key" for "key-ring"), phonemic paraphasias, or even grossly neologistic errors. Patients with the second variety of anomia usually produce no combinatory or phonemic paraphasias or neologisms. This is not the result of differential severity of naming disturbance since classic anomics even when mildly impaired may produce phonemic paraphasias while the cases of the second type of anomia discussed above produced no phonemic paraphasias despite gross naming failure in the affected spheres.

The errors of our patient with the tactile naming disturbance in the left hand were in general "wildly" incorrect and not errors in sphere (i.e., related by sound or meaning) such as are often produced by the classic anomic. It may be argued that in the case of color-naming deficit the patient did produce errors in kind since he always produced the name of some color. This, however, overlooks the fact that it was the method of testing which led to this result. We would ask the patient, "What color is this?" and he would therefore confine his reply to color-names. It is obvious that our first patient also used the information from the question "What do you feel in your left hand?" to give names of small palpable objects. This is a much larger class than that of colors and permitted therefore of apparently more random answers.

A fourth difference, one of major importance, is the fact that the patients with the second type of anomia showed not only disturbance in naming but also what might at first be thought of as comprehension disturbance. Thus, these patients failed to choose the correct name from a group. The second patient could not select a named color from a group. This special type of comprehension disturbance was not recognized classically since it was taken as evidence of "agnosic" difficulty. We have, however, already shown that these failures were not due to perceptual disturbance, but we can also see that they are not failures of comprehension in the usual sense. Thus these patients both perfectly understood the names of objects and colors in such sentences as "Tell me the name of something red" or "Are roses green?" A more accurate description would be to say that the patients could not match the sensory stimulus to the spoken name. The classic anomic is like the second variety of anomic in failing to produce the name when presented with the stimulus, but differs from the second variety in usually being able to choose the correct stimulus from a group when presented with the spoken name.

Another difference lies in the patient's response to his deficit. The classic anomic may admit to not knowing the name. On the other hand he may show various forms of denial. He may insist that he never knew the name, or that he has always called it by the term which he has just used, even when this is clearly incorrect. He may assert that he really knows the word, but I suspect that this "tip-of-the tongue" phenomenon is at least as often mistaken in the patient as it is in normals.

The second group of patients almost never admit to not knowing the correct name but will almost always produce a response. When pressed as to the reasons for the discrepancy between his response and the one designated by the examiner as the correct one, the patient may assert that he hasn't done this kind of thing in the past, or that things "look different" to him from the way they look to the examiner. In short the classic anomic acts as if his vocabulary and that of the examiner differ; the patient with the second type of anomia may act as if his perception and that of the examiner differ although perception can be shown to be intact by non-verbal methods.

We can summarize the two groups as follows. The classic anomic has difficulty in naming on confrontation which more or less involves all types of material and is more or less equal for all sensory modalities. The inadequacies of naming may consist of failure to produce a response, verbal paraphasias which are generally related by sound or meaning, phonemic paraphasias, or circumlocutory descriptions. There is usually difficulty in spontaneous speech, manifested by word-finding pauses or any of the other difficulties listed above. The patient can usually choose the correct name if offered to him by the examiner and can select a named object from a group. The patient ascribes his errors to differences in knowledge or usage of words. The lesions in these cases are in the dominant angular gyrus region.

Contrasted with this is the second type of anomia, best characterized as an *inability to match a stimulus to its spoken name*, i.e., the patient can neither produce the name when presented with the stimulus nor choose the correct stimulus when given a name. The difficulty is confined to a single modality, and even to a single class within that modality, and may be confined to one-half of visual space or one side of the body. Circumlocutory errors or phonemic paraphasias occur uncommonly if at all. The errors consist primarily of verbal paraphasias which are not related to the correct word by sound and are related only in the most general way by meaning. Spontaneous speech is normal even for the categories which are specially impaired in confrontation naming. The patient cannot usually choose the correct name of the item when it is offered to him; nor can he select a named item correctly from a group. Comprehension deficit in the usual sense, however, is ruled out because the patient shows normal understanding of the same words when he is obliged to give purely verbal responses. Perceptual deficit is ruled out by the patient's ability to carry out the various tests listed earlier in the paper. The patient may ascribe his errors to differences in perception between himself and the examiner. The lesions are those which produce disconnections from the speech area.

It is of some importance to consider the differences between these groups of anomic disturbances. To call one disturbance aphasic and the other perceptual or agnosic runs counter to the demonstrated fact that perception can be shown to be intact even in those patients suffering from the second group of disturbances who assert that their difficulty is perceptual. A point of great theoretical importance which arises out of a careful consideration of the differences between the two groups is that one can safely reject the thesis that classical anomic aphasia is the result of the accumulation of large numbers of separate naming disturbances. Since the isolated naming disturbances are likely to be of the second variety a large number of these appearing together in the same patient would produce a picture quite different from classical anomia as any consideration of the discussion above will clearly show. Thus phonemic paraphasic errors may be seen in classical anomia which is also associated with difficulties in spontaneous speech but without comprehension deficit; in all of these ways it differs from the isolated naming disturbances. Classical anomia appears therefore to differ not only in degree but also in kind from the isolated naming disturbances.

It seems clear, however, that occasionally one must encounter patients with classical anomia who also have the admixture of one or more isolated naming disturbances thus leading to an apparent selective impairment of certain types of naming. Unfortunately there is little documentation as to whether such patients show the specialized type of comprehension disturbances specified above for the second group. Thus in the studies of Goodglass et al. (1966) cited above it may be that the increased difficulty in certain naming tasks in classical anomics may reflect admixtures of "disconnection" anomias. If this is the case then one should find difficulties in comprehension of the specialized type I have described in these categories above. It will be important to investigate this further in the future.

How can one account theoretically for these two varieties of anomia? The second type, i.e., the "disconnection" anomia, appears to be more readily accounted for than does classical anomia. Thus if a lesion cuts off most of the connections between the cortical representation of a given sensory modality and the speech area, it is easy to see that the patient will name incorrectly since the sensory information will fail to reach the speech area. It is also easy to see that the patient will have difficulty matching a name spoken by the examiner to the stimulus since there is no path from the speech area to the association cortex of the modality in question. The patient will make no errors in matching *within* the affected modality, nor will he have any troubles in purely verbal tasks. Spontaneous speech would be normal. The patient will often refer to his errors *as if* they were due to perceptual difficulty since the speech area which is giving the account is indeed not receiving the perceptual information. As stated above, the lesion by disconnecting the speech area from some given sensory region prevents the matching of a sensory stimulus to a speech stimulus, regardless of the order of presentation.

Classic anomia implies, however, a lesion in a more complicated system. This system can be conceived of as one which receives the sensory information and finds the spoken word appropriate to it. It is a system which may be thought of as containing the rules for finding a word given some of its attributes. Obviously it uses information from all modalities since it can "find" a word when presented with the actual object in one or more modalities or on the other hand it can find the word when given its attributes in verbal form. As may have been noticed, this system is referred to as finding the *spoken* word corresponding to a set of attributes. It is my guess that it would act primarily to find the auditory form of words since it is this form which is first learned. Finding the written word would therefore be secondary to finding the auditory form.

It is reasonable that the region involved in the activity of finding a word given some of its attributes in one or more modalities is the angular gyrus since, as I have suggested elsewhere (Geschwind, 1964, 1965), this region is probably involved in the formation of associations between the various non-limbic sensory modalities (vision, somesthesis, audition). It is also easy to understand why damage to such a region should leave the grammatical structure of spoken language so well preserved. The "small" grammatical words depend little if at all for their evocation on attributes in different sensory modalities. More generally grammatical structure, e.g., rules of word order and their transformations are almost certainly not dependent on such intermodal interactions but probably develop, like the small grammatical words, almost entirely within the auditory system.

It is reasonable that such a set of rules would be formulated in the large region of gray matter which is probably more or less equipotential. It also must be so designed that it is easier to find the attributes given the word than to find the word given the attributes since patients with lesions in this system comprehend the word more readily than they can find it. The system is therefore in some ways like a punch-card system. It also seems reasonable, however, to assume that in the most extensive cases of destruction of the area involved in this activity significant comprehension deficit would occur although it is not seen in partial destruction. I have made the speculation elsewhere (Geschwind, 1965) that perhaps these more extensive cases correspond to the "syndrome of the isolated speech area" but I will not go further into this problem at this point. In any case, it seems clear that we need further study of the anatomical connections of the angular gyrus region and further investigation of the classical anomias in order to learn the rules by which words are encoded in this region. It would also seem reasonable that the delimited anomias ultimately depend on disconnections of a particular sensory modality from the left angular gyrus.

Having discussed these two types of anomia, each with localizable lesions (in the left angular gyrus or in connections to the left angular gyrus respectively), let us consider now a third variety. As was pointed out earlier, classically there was a disagreement as to the localization of anomic aphasia. One group attributed it to focal disease in the angular gyrus region while others claimed that diffuse lesions of the brain were necessary. As I have already noted, both groups were in fact partially correct. It is clear, however, that what was not realized classically was the fact that the anomias in the two types of syndromes were different. Edwin Weinstein and his co-workers (e.g., Weinstein and Keller, 1964) have made the most significant contribution in presenting the characteristics of anomia which may occur in acute diffuse disease of the brain. It is quite clear that many neurologists have overlooked this syndrome. On the other hand, it is necessary to avoid the reverse error, i.e., that of mistaking focal aphasic disturbance for this condition of "non-aphasic misnaming."

Non-aphasic misnaming typically occurs in disorders which diffusely involve the nervous system, especially when the disturbance comes on fairly rapidly. It is thus very common in head injuries, subarachnoid hemorrhages, rapidly increasing intracranial pressure, and in toxic or metabolic disorders such as intoxications, withdrawal syndromes, uremia or congestive heart failure. Thus in my experience the syndrome of non-aphasic misnaming has only rarely been seen on the Aphasia Unit in the Boston Veterans Administration Hospital, is occasionally seen elsewhere on the Neurology Service, but is more often seen in the medical or neurosurgical wards. By contrast, misnaming in the aphasic whether in classic anomic aphasia or as part of one of the other syndromes resulting from post-rolandic lesions can occur in chronic, stable form over months or years in patients having focal unilateral lesions without evidence of widespread diffuse involvement.

Non-aphasic misnaming is perhaps a poor term for the syndrome as a whole since it highlights only one feature of the disorder. Depending on the particular variation seen in any one case, the examiner may be deceived into thinking that the patient is aphasic, or that he is suffering from a disturbance of memory or of perception, or indeed that the patient is deliberately being facetious (Weinstein terms this "ludic" behavior, and it clearly corresponds in good part to the classical moria or Witzelsucht). This is illustrated in the sort of reply that one often gets from such patients when the question, "What do I do?" is made by the examiner. A typical response is "You're someone who asks a lot of questions" or "You're an investigator of some kind." Characteristically the errors tend to "propagate." Thus the patient being asked where he is may say "In a bus," and may then say that the examining physician is the driver, that those around him are passengers and that the bed he is in is used by the driver for resting. It is usually obvious once a sequence of questions is asked that ordinary aphasic misnaming is readily ruled out. Thus in aphasic misnaming there is no tendency to "propagation" although perseveration, i.e., repetition of the same incorrect word, occurs frequently. On the other hand perseveration can also occur in non-aphasic misnaming and may thus present a difficulty of interpretation. In aphasic misnaming the problem rarely arises that one has to consider the possibilities of memory loss, perceptual difficulty, or jocularity since these are easily ruled out. It is much more difficult to exclude these in non-aphasic misnaming since it often appears impossible to obtain the patient's cooperation. The aphasic with misnaming who has no comprehension deficit usually accepts correction by the examiner but in non-aphasic misnaming this is often difficult or impossible to achieve.

The "connected" or "propagated" character of the errors may show up particularly in relation to the hospital and the patient's illness. He may call the hospital a "hotel," the doctors "bell boys," the nurses "chambermaids," and will not accept correction. One man dying with terminal cancer said that the building in which he was located was a "slaughter house" where "they hang up bodies" and that the examiner was a "grinder." He denied specifically that it was a hospital. This example of what Weinstein calls "tragic ludic behavior" (equivalent to "gallows humor") illustrates another characteristic of the syndrome, i.e., that it is often possible to demonstrate that the patient in fact knows the correct answers since his errors are so clearly motivated. This is well illustrated by Weinstein's patient who asserted that she was in the "Mount Cyanide Rest Home." She could have produced this pun only with the knowledge that she was in fact in the Mount Sinai Hospital. This motivated misnaming is not a feature of aphasic anomia in which the patient will usually show no increased difficulty in talking about his illness or the hospital and may even perform at his best when the examiner turns to these topics.

One feature which often characterizes non-aphasic misnaming is that spontaneous speech is usually (but not invariably) normal despite gross errors in naming. In aphasic anomia errors in confrontation naming are almost always accompanied by a disturbance in spontaneous speech in which word-finding pauses, empty phrases, paraphasias and circumlocutions appear.

Some of the errors in non-aphasic misnaming may appear to be more "aphasic" than the "motivated" or "propagated" misnamings. In some instances rather bizarre errors occur, misnamings apparently totally unrelated by sound or meaning, but also not occurring in an obvious connected context. The differential diagnosis of these may be quite difficult. Thus while it is true that classic aphasic anomia usually leads to errors which are related in sound or meaning to the correct word it is clearly the case that such bizarre errors do occasionally occur, particularly in that group of patients with the syndrome of the "isolated speech area" which Goldstein (1917) discussed and which I have commented on elsewhere (Geschwind, 1965). In these cases, however, the patient suffers from a gross comprehension disturbance, often with echolalic repetition, and can thus be easily distinguished from cases of non-aphasic misnaming.[1]

It is not possible at this time to give a more detailed account of the pathogenesis of non-aphasic misnaming. While it typically occurs in situations in which there is diffuse involvement of the nervous system this does not neceserily rule out that it is some focal aspect of the diffuse involvement which is really important. It is true that a single stable unilateral lesion has not been shown to produce this syndrome. It is possible, however, that stable bilaterally symmetrical lesions in some particular area are necessary. Certainly many aspects of this syndrome are reminiscent of some of the features of chronic bilateral frontal disease, but it would not be possible with assurance to equate non-aphasic misnaming with frontal disease. Furthermore, it is possible that this syndrome may occur transiently with acute unilateral disease in some specific focus and disappears in time, but this would be difficult to disentangle from the more widespread effects of acute lesions. In addition the place of involvement may not be cortical but may be subcortical as Weinstein himself has suggested. Unfortunately our knowledge of well-defined chronic behavioral syndromes from non-cortical lesions is confined to a small number of disturbances such as Korsakow's syndrome or akinetic mutism. A further possibility is that the name-finding system of which we spoke earlier in this paper and which is located in the angular gyrus region may be very readily disturbed by diffuse disease because it depends so heavily on multiple connections from many regions.

[1] Dr. Ennio De Renzi has pointed out to me that the syndrome of non-aphasic misnaming is similar in many ways to that described by continental psychiatrists as disordered language in mental confusion. He points out that a further useful criterion is that aphasics will generally have more difficulty in naming uncommon as against common objects while the patient with non-aphasic misnaming may paradoxically do better in the naming of uncommon objects. This same association could of course be seen in patients with hysterical or malingered naming disturbances.

The diagnosis of non-aphasic misnaming presents many difficulties. While one may see a relatively "pure" example, e.g., the patient who is intoxicated, the differential is much more difficult when there is concomitant focal damage. The problem is compounded by the fact that the syndrome of non-aphasic misnaming may be superimposed on a mild focal anomic disturbance or on a Korsakow's syndrome. Examination is particularly difficult in such cases because the cooperation of the patient is often extremely difficult to obtain. Thus, we have seen cases in which once the non-aphasic misnaming had cleared, it became obvious that the patient was suffering from a classical Korsakow's syndrome. In other cases with clearing of the picture of non-aphasic misnaming we have observed a mild but definite aphasic anomia with an appropriate left posterior Rolandic lesion. This syndrome remains a major problem for students of the neurology of behavior and has been generally neglected except in the pioneering work of Weinstein.

We have now presented three situations in which misnaming may occur—classical anomic aphasia, those disconnection syndromes in which matching of a stimulus with its spoken name is impaired, and the syndrome of non-aphasic misnaming. We now turn to a fourth group of disturbances which includes hysterical and malingered anomias. In these cases the patient often fails to find the names of very simple objects presented to him. He usually shows great apparent concern over the failure. If the examiner insists that he is sure the patient can find the word, he often receives a response of annoyance or a protest that it is impossible to go on. These responses can also occur but are much less likely in aphasic anomia. The clue to the diagnosis in these cases is that despite a gross global defect of confrontation naming in all modalities, the patient's spontaneous speech is normal. Thus, one patient whom I examined would fail to name as common an object as a pencil presented either visually or tactually and yet could tell us with perfect fluency in her spontaneous speech that her husband was an electronics engineer who was working on the design of digital computers. The anomia may be the only obvious abnormality or may occur against the background of a more outspoken hysterical pseudo-dementia, e.g., an outspoken Ganser syndrome. This "functional" misnaming syndrome is rare but failure to recognize it may have serious consequences.

SUMMARY

Four syndromes are discussed in which there occurs failure of naming on confrontation. The first is the anomia of posterior aphasia-producing lesions. The second is a much more delimited disturbance produced by lesions which isolate certain sensory regions from the speech area (probably from the left angular gyrus in particular) and which may be best characterized as failure to match certain sensory stimuli to their spoken names. The third syndrome is that of non-aphasic misnaming which occurs in disorders which diffusely involve the brain. The fourth is anomia occurring as a manifestation of hysteria or malingering. The clinical syndromes are outlined as well as the distinguishing features of the anomia in each type. Some of the theoretical problems raised by each form of anomia are also discussed.

REFERENCES

Critchley, M. (1966) *Acquired anomalies of colour perception of central origin*, "Brain," **88,** 711–724.

Ettlinger, G., and Wyke, M. (1961) *Defects in identifying objects visually in a patient with cerebrovascular disease*, "J. Neurol. Neurosurg. Psychiat.," **24,** 254.

Geschwind, N. (1962) *The anatomy of acquired disorders of reading*, in Reading Disability, ed. by J. Money. Johns Hopkins University Press, Baltimore, pp. 115–130.

—— (1964) *The development of the brain and the evolution*

of language, in Monograph Series on Language and Linguistics, ed. by C.I.J.M. Stuart. Georgetown University Press, No. 17, pp. 155–169.

—— (1965) *Disconnexion syndromes in animals and man*, "Brain," **88,** 237–294 and 585–644.

——, and Fusillo, M. (1966) *Color-naming defects in association with alexia*, "A.M.A. Arch. Neurol.," **15,** 137–146.

——, and Kaplan, E. (1962) *A human cerebral deconnection syndrome*, "Neurology," **12,** 675–685.

Gloning, I., Gloning, K., and Hoff, H. (1963) *Aphasia—a clinical syndrome*, in Problems of Dynamic Neurology, ed. by L. Halpern. Grune and Stratton, New York, pp. 63–70.

Goldstein, K. (1917) *Die transkortikalen Aphasien.* Gustav Fischer, Jena.

Goodglass, H., Klein, B., Carey, P., and Jones, K. (1966) *Specific semantic word categories in aphasia*, "Cortex," **2,** 74–89.

Howes, D. H. (1964) *Application of the word-frequency concept to aphasia*, in Disorders of Language, ed. by A.V.S. De Reuck and M. O'Connor. Little, Brown, Boston, pp. 47–48.

Jakobson, R. (1964) *Towards a linguistic typology of aphasic impairments,* in Disorders of Language, ed. by A.V.S. De Reuck and M. O'Connor. Little, Brown, Boston, pp. 21–46.

Spreen, O., Benton, A. L., and Van Allen, M. W. (1966) *Dissociation of visual and tactile naming in amnesic aphasia*, "Neurol.," **16,** 807–814.

Weinstein, E. A., and Keller, N. J. S. (1964) *Linguistic patterns of misnaming in brain injury*, "Neuropsychologia," **1,** 79–90.

Wepman, J. M., Bock, R. D., Jones, L. V., and Van Pelt, D. (1956) *Psycholinguistic study of aphasia: a revision of the concept of anomia,* "J. Speech and Hearing Disorders," **21,** 468–477.

5

Effect of Word Frequency and Word Length on Aphasic Spelling Errors

AMY L. BRICKER
HILDRED M. SCHUELL
JAMES J. JENKINS

AMY L. BRICKER (HARRIS), M.A., is with the department of speech pathology and audiology of Emerson College, Boston.

HILDRED M. SCHUELL, Ph.D., (deceased) was director of the aphasia section of the neurology service of the Minneapolis Veterans Administration Hospital, and was with the department of neurology of the Graduate School of Medicine, University of Minnesota.

JAMES J. JENKINS, Ph.D., is with the department of psychology of the University of Minnesota.

This study was supported in part by Public Health Service Grant # NB-03364 from the National Institute of Neurological Diseases and Blindness.

We have defined aphasia as a reduction of language that cuts across various language modalities, such as comprehension of spoken language, speaking, reading, and writing, and upon which specific perceptual, sensorimotor, or dysarthric deficits may or may not be superimposed (Schuell and Jenkins, 1959). This definition suggests two broad areas into which research in aphasia may be directed. The first deals with the interrelations of various aspects of aphasic behavior. It is concerned with covariance of deficits, with specification of central and peripheral factors, and with identification of patterns of impairment that have diagnostic and prognostic significance. This body of research is in the tradition of differential psychology, and is represented in the literature by scaling studies (Schuell and Jenkins, 1959), factor analysis studies (Jones and Wepman, 1961; Schuell, Jenkins, and Carroll, 1962), and, of course, by the classical clinical studies of aphasia (Head, 1926; Weisenburg and McBride, 1935).

A second area of research deals with the study of variables associated with given dimensions of impairment. This research is in the experimental tradition, and deals with "process laws," or the relation of selected stimulus variables to resultant behavior, Schuell and Jenkins (1961) have reported reduction of vocabulary in all language modalities in aphasia. Other recent work has related reading difficulty (Siegel, 1959), reduction of vocabulary in free speech (Wepman, Bock, Jones, and Van Pelt, 1956; Howes and Geschwind, 1962), and errors in auditory comprehension of words (Schuell, Jenkins, and Landis, 1961) to the general frequency of usage of words in the language.

The present study is in the domain of the second research area, and deals with stimulus variables that determine written spelling errors of aphasic subjects. Two variables seemed to be major determinants. The first was frequency of word usage. Previous studies have shown word frequency is important in both visual and auditory recognition of words. This has been documented by Howes and Solomon (1951), King-Ellison and Jenkins (1954), Howes (1957),

From *Journal of Speech and Hearing Research* 7:183–92, 1964.

Postman and Rosenzweig (1956, 1957), Rosenzweig and Postman (1957, 1958), and by Solomon and Postman (1952). Howes (1952) found word frequency related to sentence intelligibility, while previously cited studies found a relationship between word frequency and auditory comprehension, visual comprehension, and free speech in aphasic subjects. One study (Filby, Edwards, and Seacat, 1963) found no relationship between errors and word frequency in either aphasic or normals, but the task was simply to determine which of two printed words matched the test word, with simultaneous exposure of all three words. The item-error ratio was extremely low for all subjects. When there are no statistically significant differences between the performance of aphasics and the performance of normals the task is obviously not a language task.

The second variable that seemed of interest was word length defined by number of letters. Several investigators have demonstrated the importance of word length in visual recognition (McGinnies, Comer, and Lacy, 1952; Postman and Adis-Castro, 1956; Rosenzweig and Postman, 1958). The longer the word the harder it is to recognize in a brief visual exposure. Bloomer (1958) found word length the single most important variable in the spelling errors of school children. On a purely statistical basis, the more letters there are in a word, the more opportunities there are for error. Retention span is commonly restricted in aphasia (Schuell and Jenkins, 1959), which adds to spelling difficulty for an aphasic population. Longer words present more opportunity to forget the exact form of the word, to confuse letters with similar visual patterns, and to make sequencing errors.

Zipf showed in 1935 that frequency of usage and word length are negatively related in English. It is clear, however, that length and frequency must be regarded as separate variables, because word length is negatively related to visual perception, and positively related to auditory perception. Longer words that are familiar to the subject tend to be easier to recognize by ear than short ones. This is understandable, since the auditory stimulus is transitory, and long words exceed short words both in duration and in the number of distinctive cues they present to the ear. Since in this study words were presented aurally for graphic response it was not necessarily obvious that length of word would have a simple relation to spelling errors in either direction.

The specific purpose of this study was to explore the relationship between (a) spelling errors of aphasic subjects, and (b) frequency of word usage in the language, and (c) word length.

METHOD

Subjects

Subjects were 64 aphasic patients admitted to the Aphasia Section of the Neurology Service of the Minneapolis Veterans Administration Hospital between April 1955 and February 1962, to whom the Wide Range Achievement Spelling Test (Jastak, 1946) was administered. This was a selective factor, since the Wide Range was a supplementary test used to determine spelling level in patients with some residual writing ability. All patients passed the first seven items of the test, which required printing or writing seven letters, indicating that subsequent errors did not result from motor impairment. In addition, subjects were eliminated from the research series who were not diagnosed as aphasic, or who showed psychotic or regressive behavior.

Sixty-three patients were male, and one was female. The age range was 18–70, with a mean age of 44.78 years. Education ranged from fourth grade through professional degrees, with a mean of 11.3 years of schooling. Testing occurred from 1 to 160 months after onset of aphasia, with a mean period of 13.8 months.

Forty-seven subjects incurred aphasia as the result of a cerebrovascular accident, 5 from trauma, 4 following an infectious process, 2 from tumor, 2 from carbon monoxide poisoning. Etiology was undetermined for 4 patients.

Procedures

The Wide Range Achievement Spelling Test was administered in standard manner. Each word was spoken by the examiner, used in a short sample phrase, then pronounced again. The subject then wrote the word. Stimulus words were dictated in standard test order until 10 consecutive failures were recorded. The number of errors was tabulated first for each word, and second, for each subject.

Frequency

The 100 test words were arranged in order of frequency according to the Lorge Magazine Count (Thorndike and Lorge, 1944). For further study, the words were divided into 5 lists of decreasing frequency, as follows:

List I: 22 words that occurred from 140,000 to 1,000 times per 4.5 million words, with a mean frequency of 13,404.91.

List II: 26 words that occurred from 999 to 300 times per 4.5 million words, with a mean frequency of 554.19.

List III: 21 words that occurred from 297 to 100 times per 4.5 million words, with a mean frequency of 203.52.

List IV: 22 words that occurred from 99 times to 1 per 4.5 million words, with a mean frequency of 36.77.

List V: 9 words that occurred from 3 times to 1 per 4.5 million words, with a mean frequency of 2.11. These words did not occur in the list of occurrences in 4.5 million words but were calculated on the basis of 4.5 million from reported occurrences per 18 million words. This count included the (T), (L), (J), and (S) counts for computations.

In addition, two words were classified arbitrarily *Proboscis* was included in List IV, since it occurred one time per million in the General Count. *Pulchritude* did not occur in the frequency count, and an assumed count of 3 times per 18 million words was used.

The mean frequency for the 100 words was 3,144.19 occurrences per 4.5 million words.

Length

Words were ordered by length determined by the number of letters per word. The 100 words were then divided into 6 lists of words of increasing length as follows:

List A: 11 words of 2 or 3 letters, with a mean letter length of 2.82.

List B: 17 words of 4 or 5 letters, with a mean letter length of 4.59.

List C: 17 words of 6 or 7 letters, with a mean letter length of 6.59.

List D: 13 words or 8 letters.

List E: 19 words of 9 letters.

List F: 23 words of 10 to 13 letters with a mean letter length of 10.78.

The mean letter length for the 100 test words was 7.44.

Subjects

Finally, to facilitate comparison of relationships at various levels of spelling ability, subjects were ranked in order of total test errors, and divided into quartiles of 16 subjects each, as follows: Q_1, 87 to 100 errors; Q_2, 71 to 86 errors, Q_3, 51 to 70 errors; Q_4, 3 to 50 errors. In addition, errors were analyzed for 15 subjects classified as having simple aphasia with no perceptual impairment, and 21 subjects classified as having aphasia complicated by involvement of visual processes. Classification was determined by the overall pattern of errors obtained on the *Minnesota Test for Differential Diagnosis of Aphasia*.

RESULTS

The mean number of errors per word was 42.90, and the mean number of errors per subject was 67.03 for the list of 100 spelling words. This means that the average spelling grade level for the 64 aphasic subjects was 3.8 on initial testing, although the range was from first grade to college level.

Table 5-1 shows the mean number of errors with the standard deviation for each of the five frequency word lists. It is readily apparent that spelling errors increase as frequency of usage decreases. To compute the correlation between these variables the frequency of usage of each word was converted to a common logarithm. The logarithm of the frequency is ordinarily found to be the best transformation of raw frequency in psychological studies (Howes and

TABLE 5-1. MEAN ERRORS PER WORD AND STANDARD DEVIATIONS OF 64 APHASIC SUBJECTS FOR FIVE WORD LISTS OF DECREASING FREQUENCY

List	Mean	S.D.
I	17.86	8.21
II	37.27	11.22
III	50.86	7.38
IV	59.00	4.11
V	62.44	1.83

Geschwind, 1962, McNemar, 1955). The correlation between logarithm of frequency and number of errors was −0.830. It is illustrated graphically in Figure 5-1.

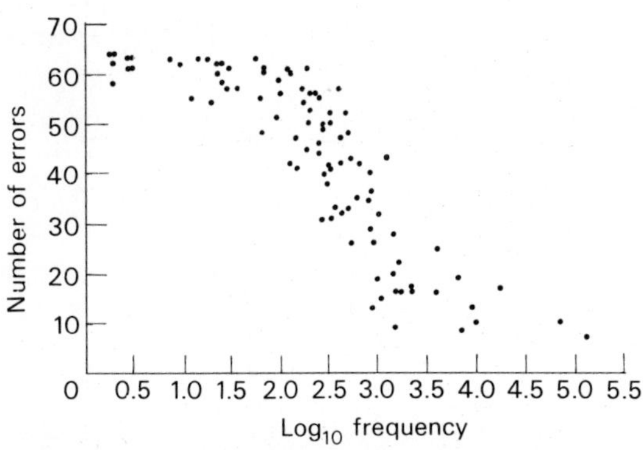

Fig. 5-1. The cumulative number of errors in relation to the logarithm of frequency of usage for each word per 4.5 million. The abscissa represents the logarithm of word-frequency, the ordinate the total number of errors.

TABLE 5-2. MEAN ERRORS PER WORD AND STANDARD DEVIATIONS OF 64 APHASIC SUBJECTS FOR SIX WORD LISTS OF INCREASING LETTER LENGTH

List	Mean	S.D.
A.	11.82	3.88
B.	24.06	8.53
C.	39.59	8.16
D.	50.54	7.32
E.	56.47	5.16
F.	58.61	6.13

Table 5-2 presents the mean number of errors and the standard deviations for each of the six lists of words ordered by length. The correlation between length and number of errors, as shown in Figure 5-2 was +0.899.

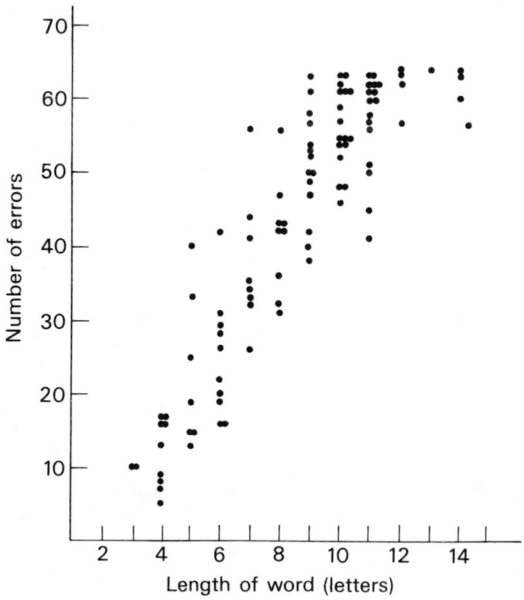

Fig. 5-2. The total number of errors in relation to word letter length for each word. The abscissa represents the number of letters in a word, the ordinate the range of errors.

The correlation between the logarithm of frequency and word length was −0.801. This relationship is shown graphically in Figure 5-3.

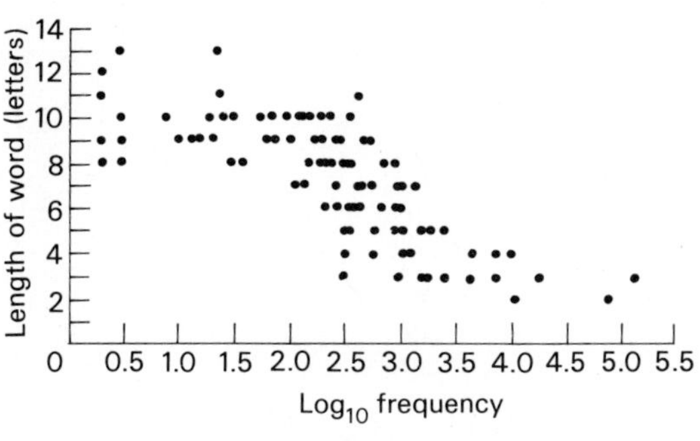

Fig. 5-3. Word letter length in relation to the logarithm of frequency of usage for each word per 4.5 million. The abscissa represents the logarithm of word frequency, the ordinate the word letter length.

The number of errors on a particular word may be accurately predicted from the logarithm of its frequency and its length, as is shown by the multiple correlation of 0.919.

The scatter plots in Figures 5-1 and 5-2 suggest that the relation between each of the predictors and the number of errors is curvilinear. To determine the extent of the relationship and to test the departure from linearity of regression, correlation ratios (McNemar, 1955, pp. 207, 262) were computed for each of these relationships. The correlation ratio between the logarithm of word frequency and number of errors was 0.894, while that between word length and number of errors was 0.924. Both of these correlation ratios are significantly greater than their product-moment coefficients ($p < 0.001$), indicating that the regression is indeed curvilinear. This means that even the remarkably strong relation indicated by the multiple correlation coefficient of 0.919, given above, is an understatement of the interrelation between these stimulus variables and obtained errors. We must conclude that word frequency and word length together account almost completely for spelling errors on any given word in this population.

Figure 5-4 shows the percentage of error by frequency for subjects in each quartile of the test distribution. The curves demonstrate that spelling becomes increasingly difficult for all subjects as word frequency decreases, regardless of level of spelling performance. Figure 5-5 shows a similar systematic relation between word difficulty and word length on all spelling levels.

Subjects classified as having simple aphasia without specific impairment of visual preception averaged 50.17 errors, while those with

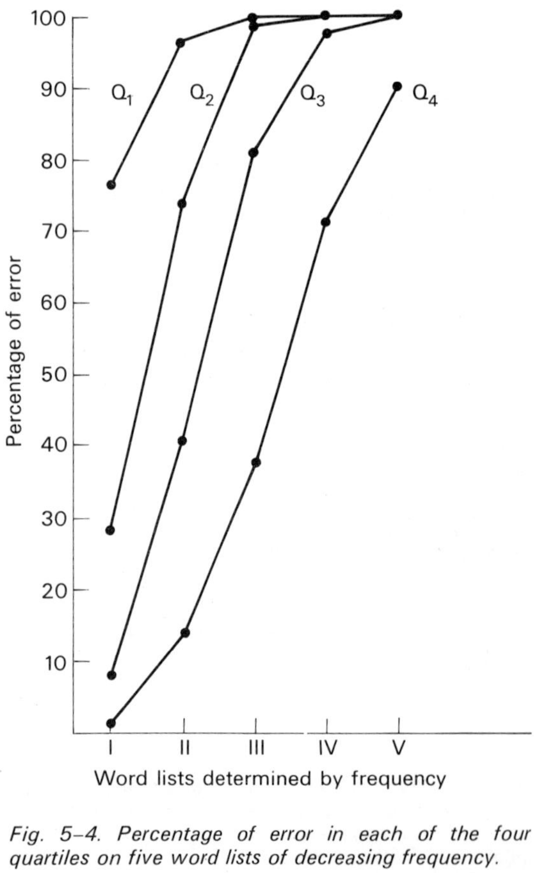

Fig. 5–4. Percentage of error in each of the four quartiles on five word lists of decreasing frequency.

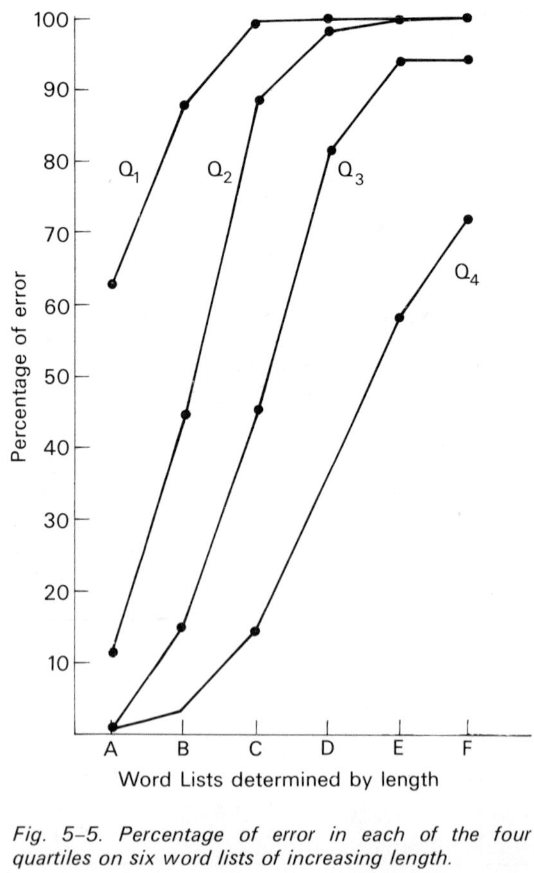

Fig. 5–5. Percentage of error in each of the four quartiles on six word lists of increasing length.

visual involvement averaged 73.92. This difference is significant beyond the 0.01 level. Within each of these groups of subjects essentially the same relationships between the predicted variables were found. For subjects with simple aphasia (N = 15) the logarithm of the frequency of usage of words correlated −0.851 with errors. For subjects with additional visual difficulties (N = 21) this correlation was −0.784. The obtained difference was not statistically significant.

Word length correlated +0.833 with errors in the first group, and +0.821 with errors in the second group. The multiple correlation was +0.888 in the first group, and +0.848 in the second. The correlation between errors made on each word by patients in the two groups was +0.883. Thus in spite of large differences in mean errors, the two groups showed essentially the same relationships between error rate, word length, and word frequency.

DISCUSSION

These data support Zipf's (1935) finding that frequency of usage is inversely related to length. The most meaningful question to ask is what happens when frequency and length are not so correlated, and we cannot answer this question conclusively. The significance of the present study lies in confirmation of the lawful relationship between the spelling performance of aphasic subjects and general language phenomena found in aphasic performances in other language modalities. Aphasic patients have more difficulty perceiving language and generating language responses in all modalities than nonaphasic adults, but their language behavior is not bizarre or idiosyncratic.

The curvilinearity of the regression of the logarithm of word frequency and number of errors occurred at both ends of the curves. The words of low frequency were too difficult, and all subjects missed *pyorrhea, daguerreotype, eleemosynary,* and *iridescence*. Conversely, the high frequency words were correctly spelled by almost all subjects, although a small percentage did not show success on even the most commonly-used words. The curvilinearity observed here, then, appears to be in large part, a function of the range of difficulty of the test words.

Since an unselected aphasic population is never homogeneous in pattern of deficit, the clear-cut effect of the dimensions explored is remarkable. Subjects included aphasic patients with specific impairment of discrimination, recognition, and recall of learned visual configurations (Schuell, Jenkins, and Carroll, 1962). These patients repeatedly spell a word aloud correctly and write it incorrectly, since they tend to confuse letters that look alike. The patient may print MATCH for WATCH, TRFF for TREE, or CO for GO, and at the same time spell longer and less frequently used words correctly aloud. Using lower case or script merely changes the probability of which letters the patient will confuse. This did not counteract the effects of length and frequency, even for this segment of the sample.

Spelling errors were markedly inconsistent with Lorge frequencies for seven words. Obtained errors on *cut, cat, correct, institute,* and *lucidity* were less than would be predicated from the frequency count. Length undoubtedly operated with *cut* and *cat*, which were the only three-letter words on the frequency list on which they appeared. *Correct* and *institute* may have been more familiar to subjects than the magazine count predicts. The comparatively good performance on *lucidity* may be partly a function of length, since the only other eight-letter word on the same frequency list was *pyorrhea*, which all subjects missed. Other words on the same list ranged from 9 to 13 letters, with an average length of 10.56.

On the other hand subjects made more errors on *believe* and *explain* than frequency can account for. Here length may also have been a factor, since these were the only two seven-letter words on the frequency list on which they appeared. The range of letters on this list was 2–7, with a mean length of 4.05 letters. We assume, however, that errors resulted in part from the low frequency symbol-phoneme equivalence of *ie* and *ai* in English.

There were also seven words for which spelling difficulty did not correlate with length. More subjects missed *ruin, brief, museum,* and *anxiety* than length would lead one to predict. Errors on these words were usually characterized by reversals of vowel order. In *anxiety* the low frequency *x* appeared to be a further source of error.

Subjects made fewer errors on *person, equipment,* and *reasonable* than length would predict. This is probably a result of the comparatively high frequency of these words compared to the words grouped with them for length, as well as the relatively straightforward phonetic spelling of these words.

Thus it appears that length affects spelling errors when frequency is controlled, and frequency affects errors when length is controlled. In addition there are words in which other factors, such as the probability of symbol-phoneme equivalence seem to enter.

SUMMARY

The Wide Range Achievement Spelling Test was administered to 64 aphasic patients on the Aphasia Section of the Neurology Service of the Minneapolis Veterans Administration Hospital. Total errors on each of 100 test words and errors made by subjects in each quartile, were analyzed in relation to word frequency reported in the Lorge Magazine Count and word length determined by number of letters. In addition, errors were analyzed for 15 subjects who showed simple aphasia with no complicating conditions, and for 21 patients with involvement of visual processes. Findings were as follows:

1. There is a predictable and orderly breakdown in the spelling performance of aphasic subjects.
2. Frequency of word usage is a significant variable in determining the spelling performance of aphasic subjects.
3. Word letter length is a significant variable in determining the spelling performance of aphasic subjects.
4. Regardless of level of spelling ability, spelling is increasingly difficult for aphasics as frequency of word usage decreases, and as word letter length increases. Other factors occasionally affect word difficulty, but appear to play a minor role. This was true for subjects who showed involvement of visual processes, as well as for those with simple aphasia uncomplicated by specific perceptual impairment, and for the total population.

REFERENCES

Bloomer, R. H., Word length and complexity variables in spelling difficulty. *J. Ed. Res.*, **49,** 531–555 (1956).

Filby, Y., Edwards, A. E., and Seacat, G. F., Word length, frequency and similarity in the discrimination behavior of aphasics. *J. Speech Hearing Res.*, **6,** 255–261 (1963).

Head, H., *Aphasia and Kindred Disorders of Speech.* Cambridge: Univ. Press (1926).

Howes, D., The intelligibility of spoken messages. *Amer. J. Psychol.*, **65,** 460–465 (1952).

——, On the relation between the intelligibility and frequency of occurrence of English words. *J. Acoust. Soc. Amer.*, **29,** 296–305 (1957).

——, and Geschwind, N., Statistical properties of aphasic language. *Nat. Inst. Hlth. Prog. Rep.*, Grant M 1802 (1962).

——, and Solomon, R. L., Visual duration threshold as a function of word-probability. *J. Exp. Psychol.*, **41,** 401–410 (1951).

Jastak, J., *Wide Range Achievement Spelling Test.* Wilmington, Delaware: C. L. Story Co. (1946).

Jones, L. V., and Wepman, J. M., Dimensions of language performance in aphasia. *J. Speech Hearing Res.*, **4,** 220–232 (1961).

King-Ellison, Patricia, and Jenkins, J. J., The duration threshold of visual recognition as a function of word-frequency. *Amer. J. Psychol.*, **67,** 700–703 (1954).

McGinnies, E., Comer, P. B., and Lacy, O. L.,

Visual-recognition threshold as a function of word length and word frequency. *J. Exp. Psychol.*, **44,** 65–69 (1952).

McNemar, Quinn, *Psychological Statistics (2nd. ed.)*, New York: Wiley (1955).

Postman, L., and Adis-Castro, G., Psychophysical methods in the study of word recognition. *Science*, **125,** 193–194 (1957).

——, and Rosenzweig, M. R., Practice and transfer in the visual and auditory recognition of words. *Amer. J. Psychol.*, **69,** 209–226 (1956).

——, ——, Perceptual recognition of words. *J. Speech Hearing Dis.*, **22,** 245–253 (1957).

Rosenzweig, M. R., and Postman, L., Intelligibility as a function of frequency of usage. *J. Exp. Psychol.*, **54,** 412–422 (1957).

——, ——, Frequency of usage and perception of words. *Science*, **127,** 263–266 (1958).

Schuell, Hildred, and Jenkins, J. J., The nature of language deficit in aphasia. *Psychol. Rev.*, **66,** 45–67 (1959).

——, ——, Reduction of vocabulary in aphasia. *Brain*, **84,** 243–261 (1961).

——, ——, and Carroll, J. B., A factor analysis of the Minnesota test for differential diagnosis of aphasia. *J. Speech Hearing Res.*, **5,** 349–369 (1962).

——, ——, and Landis, Lydia, Relationship between auditory comprehension and word frequency in aphasia. *J. Speech Hearing Res.*, **4,** 30–36 (1961).

Siegel, G. M., Dysphasic speech responses to visual word stimuli. *J. Speech Hearing Res.*, **2,** 152–160 (1959).

Solomon, R. L., and Postman, L., Frequency of usage as a determinant of recognition thresholds for words. *J. Exp. Psychol.*, **43,** 195–201 (1952).

Thorndike, W. L., and Lorge, I., *The Teacher's Word Book of 30,000 Words*, New York: Teach. Coll., Columbia Univ. (1944).

Weisenburg, T., and McBride, Katharine, *Aphasia, a Clinical and Psychological Study.* New York: Commonwealth Fund, and London: Milford, Oxford Univ. (1935).

Wepman, J. M., Bock, R. D., Jones, L. V., Van Pelt, Doris, Psycholinguistic study of aphasia: a revision of the concept of anomia. *J. Speech Hearing Dis.*, **21,** 468–477 (1956).

Zipf, G. K., *The Psycho-Biology of Language.* Boston: Houghton Mifflin (1935).

6

Phrase Length and the Type and Severity of Aphasia

HAROLD GOODGLASS
FRED A. QUADFASEL
WILLIAM H. TIMBERLAKE

HAROLD GOODGLASS, Ph.D., is director of psychology research at the Boston Veterans Administration Hospital.

FRED A. QUADFASEL, M.D., (retired) was with the division of neurology of the Washington, D.C., Veterans Administration Hospital.

WILLIAM H. TIMBERLAKE, M.D., is with the neurology service of the Lemuel Shattuck Hospital, Boston.

This work was supported in part by U.S.P.H.S. Grant MH04187 to Clark University.

General agreement on a consistent classification of aphasic disorders has been blocked by apparent discrepancies between traditional clinical categories and objective test results. This paper describes the findings of an experimental approach to classifying aphasia in which the measures developed reflect more faithfully the clinically significant variables. The practical and theoretical significance of these measures is discussed in the context of the general problem of classifying aphasia.

Careful analysis of the typology of aphasia from the classic writings of Broca and Wernicke to the present time reveals that the most significant difference between the major groups of patients resides in the character of their speech production and not, as commonly assumed, in the opposition between the functions of language intake and language output. Weisenburg and McBride (1935) give one of the most lucid discussions of the clinical distinction between "sensory" and "motor" aphasia, in the classical usage of these terms. They point out (p. 215) that both syndromes involve a disturbance of verbal expression, which may be as severe in sensory as in motor aphasia, although very different in quality. They further point out that the disturbance of auditory comprehension is a variable feature of "sensory" aphasia and may be virtually absent in some cases.

Most neurological authorities accept the localizing implications of the major dichotomy in types of aphasia; Broca's (motor) aphasia is associated with injury to the anterior portion of the speech area and Wernicke's (sensory) aphasia, with a more posterior injury, involving the temporal lobe. The third widely recognized type of aphasia—the amnesic variety (Head's "nominal aphasia") is also generally attributed to the posterior temporal or temporo-parietal region, a view supported even by Head, despite his marked theoretical antilocalizing bias. Amnesic aphasia is also known to arise under conditions of no localizing significance, such as fatigue, intoxication, or reduced level of consciousness.

It is an unfortunate paradox that Weisenburg and McBride, who so clearly described the classical forms of the motor and sensory aphasic syndromes, gave their support to the substitution of the terms "expressive" and "receptive"

From *Cortex* 1:133–53, 1964.

aphasia. These two words suggest that the contrast is exclusively between language intake and language output, creating the impression that this distinction also summed up the difference between "sensory aphasia" and "motor aphasia" as classically described. The notion of input and output as the major dimensions for classifying aphasic language disorders has naturally attracted experimental investigation by large scale analyses of test results.[1] Attention was directed away from the differences in the pattern of *productive speech defects* which may be the most significant differentiating clue among the several types of aphasia. For this reason, we have preferred to use the eponyms "Wernicke's" (rather than "sensory") aphasia and "Broca's" (rather than "motor") aphasia.

A review of the distinguishing features of the several classical syndromes makes it clear why conventional test procedures fail to represent these features in quantitative form. It is not surprising, then, that applications of quantitative test procedures, as by Schuell, Jenkins and Carroll (1962) and Bay (1962) have failed to distinguish the three classical syndromes and have left almost untouched the problem of accurately defining what elements determine the clinical impression created in each case.

Broca's aphasia is characterized by the following:

a) *Laborious articulation.* The articulation difficulty of the Broca's aphasic often involves merely awkwardness rather than phoneme-substitution, which would be more easily scored; moreover, even the awkwardness may disappear under conditions of repeating test words. On the other hand, the Wernicke or amnesic aphasic, whose spontaneous speech is fluently articulated, may show both awkwardness and phoneme substitution when he attempts to produce discrete responses on request. Consequently, the usual articulation test based on repitetion of test words, fails to distinguish between those patients, who in spontaneous speech have fluent articulation, in contrast to those whose articulation is awkward.

b) *Great reduction in the flow of speech.* This important symptom is not quantified in any published aphasia examination. It is obviously related to the severity of a Broca's aphasia and this relationship complicates its use as an isolated distinguishing feature. Moreover, certain severe Wernicke and amnesic aphasics also show a greatly reduced flow of speech when, instead of freely digressing to paraphasic or circumlocutory speech, they are inhibited by their word-finding difficulty.

c) *Loss of grammatical structure.* While the Broca's aphasic typically omits grammatical words and inflectional endings, no quantitative treatment of grammatical disturbances (agrammatism) is attempted as part of any published examination procedure. In fact, Goodglass and Mayer (1958), using repetition of standard test items, found that the aphasic who is not agrammatic in spontaneous speech has almost as many errors of omission and substitution as does the one who is agrammatic. No adequate formal test situation has yet been devised to assess the agrammatism of Broca's aphasia.

Wernicke's aphasia is distinguished in part by the following features, the first two of which are also distinctive of amnesic aphasia; the third belongs only to Wernicke's type:

a) *Naming difficulty.* This symptom is not adequately measured by an object-naming task, since severe aphasics of all types fail to name objects. Naming difficulty in Wernicke aphasics (as with amnesic aphasics) is disproportionately severe in relation to the fluent small talk of these patients. The fact that these patients may repeat the object name, when it is offered by the examiner, without recognizing it as correct, gives to their naming difficulty the peculiar character of an actual dissociation of sound from meaning. In any event, a specific naming difficulty can be measured only with reference to a measure of speech fluency as a denominator.

b) *Runs of rapid, fluently articulated speech.* The existence of such runs is ignored in conventional objective tests. It is not easy to establish a method of quantifying the feature of fluency, because the entire character of a speech pattern sometimes changes when a patient shifts from open ended conversation to answering specific informational questions.

c) *Uncorrected paraphasia in the form of sound transpositions and word substitutions.* Not all paraphasic errors are equally discriminating. Those which are most characteristic of the Wernicke aphasic occur in extended utterances, where they are not easily subject to quantitative treatment. Errors with individual words or short phrases as test responses

[1] The issue of pure, single-modality aphasic disorders has been inaccurately associated with that of the expressive-receptive dichotomy. Occasional cases of modality-pure aphasic disorders are well-documented, with supporting anatomical correlations. While such cases are of great importance, they are not immediately relevant for defining the major clinical types. Moreover the statistical analysis of data from large numbers of unselected cases is not effective in identifying the rare case.

are more readily scored, but are quite common with Broca's aphasics and mixed aphasics, especially as perseverations of earlier responses.

Since the chief distinguishing features of the classical types of aphasia are elusive to measurement in structured tests, we have turned, in this study, to the use of rating scales and the analysis of free conversation.

PROCEDURE

Selection of subjects

The position taken in this research is that the recognized clinical symptoms of aphasia represent the best available first approximation to the psychological lines of cleavage along which normal speech becomes disordered in aphasia. Consequently, a particular effort was made to include as many subjects as possible fitting the classical pictures of Broca's, Wernicke's, or amnesic aphasia, in preference to those with mixed symptoms. In fact, however, the supply of testable aphasic subjects was so limited that only those were excluded who were too impaired to cooperate or whose defects were too mild to contribute useful data. The aphasic sample included only a slightly greater proportion of "classical" types of aphasia than would be found in an unselected hospital population.

Other selective factors, however, operated to produce an uneven sampling of types of aphasia. Among these were the requirement that subjects be able to repeat short phrases and supply clearly comprehensible one-word responses, in order to participate in the principal portion of the research from which the present data is drawn. It was soon recognized that many severely impaired Broca's aphasics could meet the minimum requirements of the test battery, and were included as subjects. The severe Wernicke aphasics, in spite of their greater fluency in conversation, were rarely capable of responding to any specific test items because of their word-finding difficulty, combined with their ready flow of paraphasic speech, and sometimes because of poor comprehension. No count of excluded patients was kept during the collection of data. However, a survey of 49 successive patients treated in the Boston VAH aphasia unit since March 1963, showed seven (14%) severe Wernicke aphasics who would have been excluded from the sample. Another factor, however, lay outside of the scope of the experimenters' choice of subjects. This was the rarity of symptoms of Broca's aphasia at intermediate levels of severity. It appeared that most Broca's aphasics either remained grossly impaired or quickly attained a level of residual aphasia in which the classical features of agrammatism, telegraphic speech, and laborious articulation were no longer apparent. The imbalance in the distribution of types of aphasics necessitates careful interpretation of results, not only in this study, but in others which purport to take an unbiassed sampling of aphasics.

In all, 53 subjects from the aphasia programs of eight institutions in Boston and New York were included in this study. Age and sex were not considered in the selection of subjects. There were 39 men and 14 women, ranging in age from 26 to 79 years, with a mean age of 52.1. Non-aphasics with diagnosed cerebral disease were used as controls. They included seven men and three women, ranging from 37 to 70 years in age, with a mean of 54.1. No subject was examined until at least two months after the onset of the aphasia, so that testing carried out over a period of several days would not find the patient changing rapidly from day to day.

Test procedures

The raw data for this report consisted of the Conversational and Expository Speech subtest and the Auditory Comprehension subtests of the Boston VA Diagnostic Aphasia Test, which were included in the research battery. The Conversational and Expository subtest ordinarily consists of a structured conversation beginning with an exchange of greetings, requests for simple factual information and reminiscenses about work and the onset of the patient's illness, followed by the presentation of a picture-situation as a standard stimulus for expository speech. In the present study, the conversation preceding the picture presentation was extended to give a ten minute sample of free conversation with minimal guidance from the examiner.

The Auditory Comprehension section includes:

Word-discrimination. A multiple-choice picture identification test in which the stimulus is the spoken name of an object, color, letter, action, or geometric form. (Raw score from 0 to 72; converted score 0-6.)

Body parts. Twenty parts of the body are named, for the subject to identify by pointing. (Raw score 0 to 20; converted score 0-6.)

Commands. A set of five commands beginning with one informational element and progressing to five for a total of 15 scorable elements. (Converted score 0-6.)

Abstract material. A series of Yes-No discriminations of absurd and correct statements based either on common factual information (Will a stone sink in water? Will a board sink in water?) or on questions following an orally presented paragraph. Two Yes-No questions must be passed as a pair to earn each of 12 points. (Converted score 0-6.)

For the present study, a composite auditory comprehension score was obtained from the mean converted scores of the several subtests.

Severity rating

Differences in severity of aphasia may obscure the differences between types of aphasia. One of the central problems in classification is to distinguish variations based on severity from those based on type of aphasia. A patient with a severe, isolated anomia may fail badly on an object-naming task, yet converse fairly effectively by using circumlocutions, and show excellent comprehension during conversation. How is he to be compared to the Broca's aphasic who names almost every object, also has excellent auditory comprehension, but articulates words with such groping effort that most of his ideas remain unsaid? Since there appeared to be no valid way of combining objective subtest scores to give a meaningful composite rating, a six-step Severity Rating Scale (Table 6-1) was devised, based on functional efficiency in oral communication. The rating scale by itself includes no diagnostic criteria and its use in aphasia research assumes the exclusion of subjects with spuriously low ratings caused by peripheral defects or poor motivation.

In the present study, the tape recorded free conversation and oral picture description served as the basis for rating of severity by three independent judges. A reliability check, summarized in table 6-2, indicates that in 38 percent of cases the three judges showed full agreement; in 57 percent of instances two of the judges' ratings agreed, while the third differed from the others by one severity step. Only in 5 percent of cases were there still greater discrepancies of judgment.

Clinical classification

The first attempt at clinical classification consisted of a check list of speech characteristics on

TABLE 6-1. SEVERITY RATING FOR ORAL LANGUAGE DISTURBANCE IN APHASIA

0. No usable speech or auditory comprehension.
1. All communication is through fragmentary expression, with great need for inference, questioning, and guessing by the listener. The range of information which can be exchanged is limited, and the examiner carries the burden of communication.
2. Conversation about familiar subjects is possible with help from the listener. There are frequent failures to convey the idea but patient shares the burden of communication with the examiner.
3. The patient can discuss *almost all everyday problems* with little or no assistance. However, reduction of speech and/or comprehension makes conversation about certain material difficult or impossible.
4. Some obvious loss of fluency in speech or facility of comprehension, without significant limitation on ideas expressed, or form of expression.
5. Minimal discernable speech handicaps; patient may have subjective difficulties which are not apparent to listener.

TABLE 6–2. SUMMARY OF AGREEMENT AMONG THREE JUDGES IN SEVERITY RATINGS

Modal Rating	All Agree	1 point discrepancy; 2 ratings agree	More than 1 point spread
1	10	5	0
2	3	9	0
3	3	9	1
4	4	7	2
5	0	0	0
	20 (38%)	30 (57%)	3 (5%)

TABLE 6–3. DEFINITION OF SCALES AND CRITICAL POINTS FOR RATING OF THE CHARACTERISTICS OF APHASIC SPEECH AND COMPREHENSION

Scale designation	Minimum abnormality	Mid point	Maximum abnormality
Normal *melodic line*...	... connects all words within sentences or fragments of sentences	... restricted to short declarative constructions and stereotyped phrases	... is lacking between successive words
Maximum uninterrupted word group is ordinarily (excluding stereotyped expressions)	... seven or more words	... four words long	... one word long
Verbal agility in articulation	Sounds quite normal. (Literal paraphasic slips are permitted)	... is good only in stereotyped phrases and single words	... always sounds severely labored and distorted
Frames in *correct grammatical form*	Many kinds of constructions (even if sentences are incomplete)	Only simple declarative constructions; simple tenses	No groupings of words
Connected jargon speech (either neologistic or real words)	... never occurs	... sometimes occurs	... is included in every utterance
Auditory comprehension (based on converted score from objective test)	converted score of 7	converted score of 4	converted score of 1
Object-naming capacity is	better than conversational fluency	consistent with conversational fluency	much worse than conversational fluency
Inadvertent substitution of wrong individual words (*verbal paraphasia*)	... never occurs	.. occurs occasionally	... occurs in every utterance
Accidental sound transpositions (*literal paraphasic errors*)	... never occur	... occur occasionally	... occur in every utterance
Self-correction: Paraphasic errors in speech are	... always recognized (or never occur)	recognized about half the time	always ignored

the basis of which subjects were to be classified as having a Broca's (or motor) aphasia, a Wernicke's (or sensory) aphasia, an amnesic aphasia, or a mixed aphasia.

A set of six characteristic symptoms for each of the above four diagnostic categories was agreed on by the three authors. They then independently assigned each patient to one of the categories after having listened to the tape recorded Conversational and Expository Speech and inspected the auditory comprehension subtest scores. This method was abandoned when only 6 cases of agreement among the three raters were found in the first 28 cases classified.

A series of *rating scales* for all of the relevant speech characteristics was then substituted for the diagnostic check list. It was anticipated that the examiner's evaluations of individual speech characteristics would be more reliable than his forced decision on a single best fitting category. Table 6-3 defines the extremes and midpoint for each of 10 speech characteristics, which were presented as seven-step rating scales. These scales were completed by each judge while listening to the recorded speech sample of each subject. The Auditory Comprehension scale was the only one based on objective scores, as described above.

After the taped conversations had been rated, the average rating for each subject on each scaled variable was obtained and the average deviation of the three judges' ratings from their own mean was computed. By averaging these mean deviations across subjects, we obtained a measure of the reliability or consistency of the judgments on each scale. Seven of the scales had average deviations between .49 and .66. The three least reliable scales, having average deviations of .83 to .88, were eliminated. These were the scales for literal paraphasia, verbal paraphasia, and self-correction of errors. The remaining 7 scales, which continue in use, are seen in Fig. 6-1. This figure shows characteristic rating scale profiles for a Broca's, a Wernicke's, and an amnesic aphasic patient. These profiles are based upon the clinical features of each syndrome, as listed earlier in this paper.

Before accepting this profile as a criterion for clinical classification, a reliability test was conducted by having the profiles of all 53 subjects classified independently by one of the authors (H.G.) and by three psychologists who were unfamiliar with the subjects. By visual inspection, they assigned each profile to the category whose typical profile it most resembled. A category of "not classifiable" was included.

Table 6-4 summarizes the agreements and differences in classification in relation to the severity ratings of the patients. The four raters agreed in 38 (71%) of the cases. Excluding nine cases in which one or more raters withheld judgment by assigning the profile to the nonclassifiable group, there were seven disagreements (15%). Five of the seven involved a decision between the two varieties of posterior aphasia (i.e., Wernicke's vs. amnesic); in only two cases (4%) was there a disagreement in

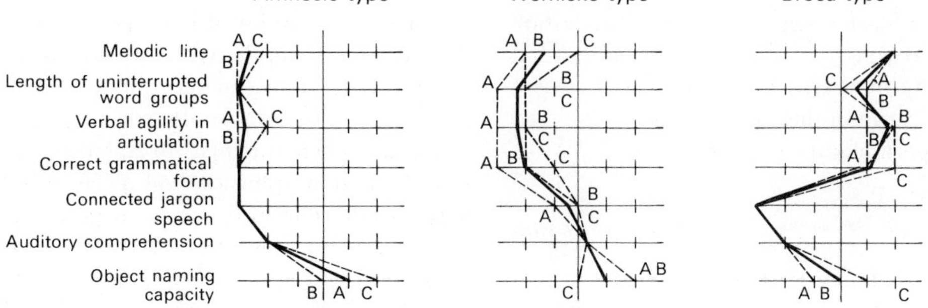

Fig. 6–1. Profiles of three judges' ratings (A, B and C) of speech characteristics of a representative case of each clinical type. Heavy line shows average profile.

TABLE 6-4. NUMBER OF CASES AT EACH SEVERITY LEVEL ASSIGNED TO EACH DIAGNOSTIC GROUP BY FOUR JUDGES, SHOWING DISTRIBUTION OF AGREEMENTS AND DISAGREEMENTS

	Combinations of diagnostic categories assigned						
Modal Severity Rating*	Amnesic Only	Amnesic and Wernicke	Wernicke Only	Wernicke or Amnesic with N.C.**	Broca's Only	Broca's with Wernicke or Amnesic	Broca's with N.C.
Level 1	0	0	0	0	8	2	6
Level 2	0	2	2	0	6	0	1
Level 3	1	2	7	1	3	0	0
Level 4	8	1	1	1	0	0	0
Level 5	2	0	0	0	0	0	0

* Level 1 = most severe; Level 5 = mildest
** N.C. refers to judgment "not classifiable"

judgment between Broca's aphasia and Wernicke's. The tabulation brings out the earlier observation that it is very difficult to distinguish among the speech patterns of residual aphasics of the various types. The profile of amnesic aphasia, as defined here, almost coincides with that of normal speech or of any mild aphasia. The one distinguishing feature of the amnesic type is the impairment of word-finding *relative to the level of conversational fluency*. Close examination of the eight cases classified as "amnesic" at Level 4 showed a considerable range in object-naming difficulty; the speech of the milder cases, particularly those at Level 5, can be distinguished from normal speech only by occasional lapses—if at all. We can only infer that mild cases of all types as well as true amnesic aphasics were placed in this category. While the absence of Broca's aphasics at the two mildest levels reflects the actual distribution of speech patterns, it is again emphasized that the sparsity of Wernicke aphasics at Levels 1 and 2 is a result of their inability to participate in the experimental program.

Phrase length ratio

The fluency of articulation to be found even in the severe Wernicke and amnesic aphasic proved so elusive to measurement with structured test items that a direct count from tape recorded conversations was decided upon. The count was designed to yield a frequency distribution of word groupings of different lengths to be found in the tape recorded Conversational and Expository speech sample.

Two listeners transcribed the tape independently, recording on a single line all the words spoken without pause or hesitation. A new line was started whenever the patient hesitated, whether this was appropriate to the grammatical sense or not. A new line was also started with the beginning of every new sentence. After differences between the two listeners were resolved, a tally was made of word-groups of each length from one-word to 5-or-more words. The ratio $\frac{\text{5-or-more-word groups}}{\text{1-word} + \text{2-word groups}}$ was determined for each sample, and called the "phrase length ratio."

Since the samples of conversation averaged 240 words in length, with one as short as 60 words, there is an obvious question about the stability of the phrase length ratio in short samples. When the first 40 aphasics and the first four non-aphasics had been tabulated, a split-half reliability test was performed on their phrase-counts by separating alternate phrases in each protocol into an odd half and an even half and recomputing the phrase-length ratio on each half of the sample. The reliability coefficient of .98 indicated considerable stability for the phrase length ratio, at least for speech elicited under fairly constant conditions of low constraint in choice of words. The samples of smallest size, in every case, came from severe "short-phrase dominant" aphasics who never show groupings more than two words in length.

RESULTS

Distribution of phrase length ratios

Inspection of Fig. 6-2 shows that there is a bimodal distribution of phrase length ratios in the aphasic population. Twenty-five subjects—the short-phrase dominant—had ratios of less than .15. No subjects fell in the interval between .16 and .30. The remaining 27 subjects—the long phrase dominant—had ratios of .31 or more. The fact that 75 percent of the aphasics were concentrated at ratios below .61 emphasizes the gap between the long-phrase dominant and short-phrase dominant groups. With 25 cases in the lowest interval and seven and eight cases respectively in the third and fourth intervals the chances of a fortuitous absence of cases in the second interval (.16 to .30) are very small (Chi square = 7.60; $p < .05$). Thus the dichotomy of aphasics into long-phrase dominant and short-phrase dominant types appears to represent the natural distribution of cases, rather than an arbitrary distinction. Inspection of Fig. 6-2 shows that non-aphasic controls overlap the entire range of phrase length ratios of the long-phrase dominant aphasics but that none extend into the short-phrase portion of the scale. It is noted, however, that more than half of the non-aphasic sample and only 22 percent of the long-phrase dominant aphasics had a ratio of 1.05 or more. It is likely that stylistic factors as well as impaired fluency may determine a patient's phrase length ratio—provided it is .31 or more.

Phrase length ratio and clinical classification

To what extent does the phrase length ratio predict the clinical classification, based on the profile of ratings of speech characteristics? That is, referring to the earlier listed characteristics of the several classical categories of aphasia, are the Broca's aphasics consistently short-phrase dominant while the Wernicke and amnesic aphasics are consistently long-phrase dominant? Table 6-4 is so set up that the groups for whom long-phrase dominance would be predicted are in the four left-hand columns, while those for whom short-phrase dominance is predicted are in the three right-hand columns.

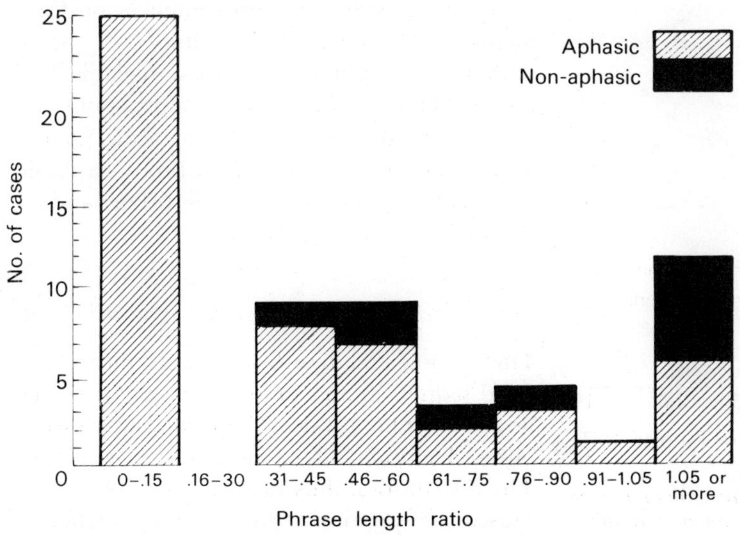

Fig. 6–2. Distribution of phrase length ratios of aphasics and non-aphasics.

In fact, only in two cases did the classification of the profiles turn out to violate this prediction. One was a Level 2 (moderately severe) patient classified as a Wernicke's aphasic by one rater (H.G.) and as an amnesic aphasic by the other three. Her severe word-finding difficulty and her many sentences which were aborted after a few words, resulted in an objective phrase count which differed from clinical impression. The other misclassified patient was a Level 4 (fairly mild) patient, unanimously categorized as amnesic on the basis of his profile. This man, a physician, spoke with a cautiously chosen, extremely high level vocabulary. Undoubtedly, his intonation, which seemed wholly appropriate to his over-deliberate style, influenced the judges' rating as to length of word groups, which placed him on the long-phrase dominant side, in opposition to his objective classification as short-phrase dominant.

One of the seven rating scales entering into the profile of speech characteristics, that of "maximum length of word groups," was designed to come as close as possible to duplicating the information of the objective phrase length ratio. Fig. 6-3 plots the distribution of 53 subjects' phrase length ratios against the judges' mean ratings of their maximum length of word-groups. Two patients of the 26 classified as short-phrase dominant by the objective ratio fell above 5.5 on the rating scale. One was the Level 2 amnesic aphasic already referred to. The other was a severe (Level 1) aphasic whose profile had been called unclassifiable by three and Broca's by the fourth judge. The one misclassified long-phrase dominant subject (out of 27) was the physician described in the preceding paragraph. Thus, the rating scale of "maximum length of word groups" proved to be a most efficient substitute for the tedious procedure involved in the determination of the objective phrase length ratio.

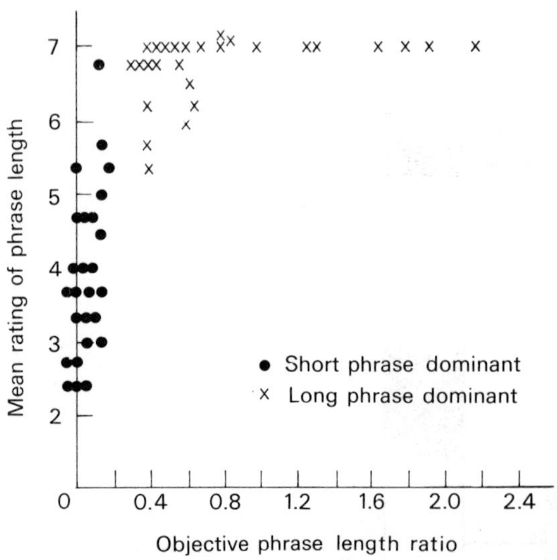

Fig. 6–3. Judges' mean ratings of maximum phrase length, plotted against objective phrase length ratio.

Other rating scales

While the rating scale for maximum length of word groups could be checked against an objective criterion, several of the other rating scales, taken by themselves, distinguished equally well between the Broca's aphasics and the Wernicke and amnesic aphasics. These were the scales for articulatory agility, for variety of grammatical forms, and for speech melody—all highly correlated with each other and with "phrase length." The speech melody scale, in fact, was the most perfect discriminator in the entire profile.

The point of minimum abnormality (scale score 7) was defined as, "Normal melodic line connects all words within sentences or fragments of sentences." The midpoint (scale score 4) was defined, "Normal melodic line restricted to short declarative constructions and stereotyped phrases." By taking scale point 5 as a cut-off, we found that no Broca's aphasic reached that point in the judges' ratings and no Wernicke or amnesic fell below it.

Phrase length ratio and severity

The obvious relationship between fluency in word sequences and mildness of aphasia could be expected to produce a high correlation when phrase length is judged against severity rating. The distribution illustrated in Fig. 6-4, in fact, caused the question to be posed as to whether

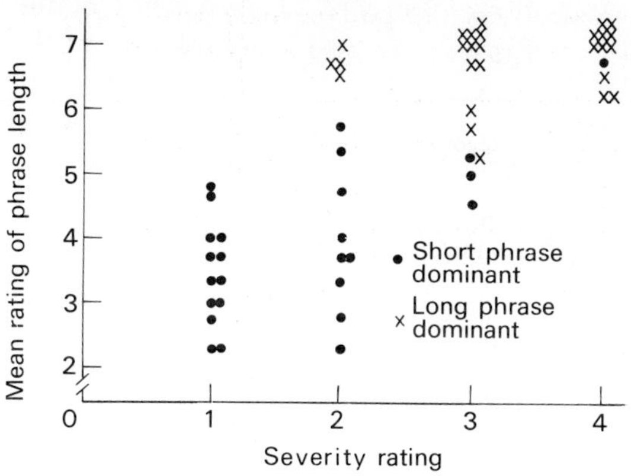

Fig. 6–4. Severity of aphasia, as rated by judges, plotted against mean rating of maximum phrase length.

we were dealing with any more than a severity measure.

In our sample, only three long-phrase dominant aphasics were rated at Level 2 (moderately severe), all of the remainder falling at the milder levels. The rating scale profiles for these three individuals showed the typical configuration of Wernicke's aphasia and were so classified by the judges. It is the severity of word-finding difficulty and the intrusion of uncorrected jargon which seemed to determine how much disability they had in oral communication. Three short-phrase dominant aphasics, assigned to severity Level 3, presented the typical rating scale profile, unanimously classified as Broca's aphasia. They differed from the more severe short-phrase dominant aphasics in the recovery of somewhat longer word groupings and of a few more grammatical constructions.

Clinical classification and locus of lesion

A number of physiological correlations have been cited supporting the interpretation of Broca's aphasia as indicating an anterior lesion, while Wernicke's and amnesic aphasia indicate a more posterior lesion. One of these is the observation that Broca's aphasia is more often accompanied by hemiplegia, since the lesion producing it impinges on the pre-Rolandic motor area, while the posterior temporal lesion of Wernicke's or amnesic aphasia can easily spare the entire motor area. In order to test the localizing predictions of the clinical classifications of our subjects, the medical summaries of the 24 aphasic patients from the Boston V.A. Hospital were reviewed to determine (1) the presence of hemiplegia (2) operative or other direct visual data as to the location of the causative lesion. In only six cases was there any direct visual data on localization—all were cases of space occupying lesions of the temporal lobe. Table 6-5 summarizes the distribution of hemiplegics (H) versus non-hemiplegics (h) and of verified temporal lobe cases (T), with respect to the diagnostic classification judgments made on the basis of the profiles of speech characteristics. Severity ratings are again represented in the table, since mildness of aphasia is inevitably correlated (in a group of cases) with mildness of other neurological symptoms, including hemiplegia.

Inspection of Table 6-5 reveals an overwhelming preponderance of hemiplegics, as predicted, in the three right hand columns. Basing comparisons only on cases in severity Levels 2 and 3, which happen to be equally represented on the Wernicke-amnesic side and on the Broca side of the table, the preponderance of hemiplegics on the right-hand side of the table is significantly greater by Fisher's exact test ($p = .025$). Here again is evidence that we cannot accept the facile conclusion that short-phrase dominance is merely a more severe degree of aphasia, on the evidence that most aphasics of this type are to be found at the more severe levels of impairment.

The six cases of established temporal lobe aphasia are all on the left-hand side of the table. If we were to disregard severity of aphasia, the chances are one in 64 that all six temporal lobe cases would be long-phrase dominant, without the operation of a causal link. Taking severity into consideration, we find that three of the six cases fall at severity Levels 2 and 3, where there are as many Broca's as Wernicke's aphasic cases. At these levels alone, the chance of an accidental one-sided distribution as predicted would be one in eight.

TABLE 6-5. INCIDENCE OF HEMIPLEGIA (H), ABSENCE OF HEMIPLEGIA (h) AND TEMPORAL LOBE LESION (T) TABULATED BY LEVEL OF SEVERITY OF APHASIA AND DIAGNOSTIC CLASSIFICATION ASSIGNED

	Combinations of diagnostic categories assigned						
Modal Severity Rating	Amnesic Only	Amnesic and Wernicke	Wernicke Only	Wernicke or Amnesic with N.C.*	Broca's Only	Broca's with Wernicke or Amnesic	Broca's with N.C.
Level 1					HH HH h	hh	
Level 2		h	TT hh		H h		H
Level 3			T h		HH		
Level 4	h hhh	h					
Level 5	T, H h						

*N.C. = "not classifiable"

DISCUSSION

This study reaffirms the pragmatic usefulness of the component symptoms classically ascribed to the syndromes of Broca's and Wernicke's aphasia. The difficulty of measuring objectively the critical variables was partly met by reducing them to rating scales. One of these variables—the phrase length ratio—was found, on objective measurement, to be the basis for a sharp dichotomy in the aphasic population. This variable is conceptualized as an indicator of the fluency of motor speech sequences. When defined, on a rating scale, in terms of the maximum number of words in uninterrupted runs, the bi-modal distribution of the objective count was reproduced fairly well by the judges' ratings. It thus appears that by defining more precisely what to listen for, we may have made some progress in identifying what is significant for the clinical classification of aphasia.

The conclusion that the phrase length ratio is significant for the typology of aphasia could have been ignored in favor of the obvious and trivial finding that it reflects the severity of aphasia. In our experience the actual distribution of aphasics in the neurological ward would tend further to obscure the independence of phrase length from severity of aphasia. There are several possible reasons for the fact that relatively few Broca's aphasics progress to moderate levels of recovery without losing the distinctive features of Broca's aphasia: labored, halting, grammatically simplified speech. This is the pattern which Wepman, in speaking of the motor type of aphasia with agrammatism, described as "having the statistical structure precisely the converse of the anomic type" (1956). We may conjecture that Broca's area contains critical structures which are so concentrated that a direct injury is likely to be permanently and severely damaging to speech, while injury closely adjacent to the critical area may result in early Broca's aphasia and subsidence of the worst symptoms as tissues peripheral to the injury recover their normal functions. Other, less anatomically oriented explanations are possible. Whatever the explanation, however, the Broca's aphasic who is able to recover seems to pass rapidly from the phase of severely interrupted speech to that of nearly fluent speech. Few individuals have a prolonged period during which they use halting, grammatically simplified sentences with a good vocabulary. More longitudinal case studies of recovering aphasics must be carried out in order to clarify this point.

Since all but six out of 53 cases conformed to the rule that Broca's aphasics are more severely impaired than Wernicke's, would it not be more economical to make the severity rating the only consideration in classification? There are two reasons why this procedure would not be acceptable, even from a purely quantitative viewpoint. First, the fact that 10 of the 14 cases at the two mildest levels were classified as "amnesic aphasia" on the basis of speech characteristics probably means that the profile alone does not produce a useful differentiation at the mildest levels, and that one must seek other data in order to make localizing decisions when speech is only minimally disturbed. Excluding these 14 cases, the proportion of exceptions to the correlation between severity and Broca's aphasia is changed to six in 39. As we have stressed previously, a significant number of severe, but fluent long-phrase dominant aphasics never found their way into this sample because they could not produce the one-word answers or perform the word and phrase repetitions required elsewhere in this project. It is estimated that if these patients were included, 30 percent of aphasics would be misclassified, if the principle were followed that the most severe aphasics were Broca's aphasics.

Schuell, Jenkins, and Carroll (1962) and Jones and Wepman (1961) report the results of factor analyses of aphasia test batteries to which one might turn for confirmation of the variables which have proved discriminating in this study. It is soon apparent that such confirmation was impossible from the onset because neither of the aforementioned test batteries included acceptable measures of the variables which were most critical in establishing the three-way clustering of aphasic symptoms discussed here. These variables include an adequate measure of continuity of word sequences, measure of melodic intonation, of articulatory agility, and of extended paraphasic intrusions in speech. We have discussed the difficulties involved in obtaining valid objective measures of these variables. Nevertheless, one cannot regard as comprehensive a study of factors in aphasia which does not incorporate these variables which are among the most prominent clinical features of aphasic speech.

SUMMARY

Three major syndromes of aphasia are repeatedly described in the neurological literature, characterized chiefly by the nature of changes in the speech pattern. The terms Wernicke's aphasia, Broca's aphasia, and amnesic aphasia are generally understood, but have slipped out of popularity. Terminology based on the distinction between language input and output has become popular, but actually does not correspond well to the syndromes and raises false issues concerning them. Moreover, the chief distinguishing characteristics of these syndromes are elusive to objective testing and have been ignored in factor analytic studies.

In this study, a series of rating scales was used in place of objective scores and each of the syndromes was defined by a profile of ratings. High reliability of diagnostic classification was obtained by this means, after impressionistic classification on the basis of a check list proved grossly unreliable.

An objective index of length of uninterrupted word-sequences was found to produce a sharp dichotomy in the aphasic population, separating Broca's aphasics from Wernicke and amnesic aphasics. This objective measure was reliably reproduced by several of the rating scales, including one which explicity required a judgment as to the longest number of uninterrupted words in nonstereotyped sequences. Physical signs of localization—i.e., presence of hemiplegia—and operative findings corresponded to the differences in the speech profiles.

Severity of aphasia must be taken into account, since the profile offers no differentiation among patients who have recovered to a level of mild or slight residual aphasia. Natural and artificial factors influencing the distribution of different types of aphasia must also be considered in interpreting test results from unselected aphasic groups. Such selective factors may produce artifactual correlations or else obscure fundamental relationships.

Acknowledgement. The authors are grateful to Dr. Norman Geschwind, Chief of Neurology at Boston V.A. Hospital, for his criticism. Thanks are also due to Mrs. Edith Kaplan, Miss Mary Hyde and Miss Celia Schulhoff for their participation in the collection and analysis of data. Appreciation is due to the staffs of the Massachusetts General Hospital Outpatient Language Clinic, Jewish Memorial Hospital (Boston), Holy Ghost Hospital (Cambridge), the Veterans Administration Hospitals in Manhattan and the Bronx New York, and the Bird S. Coler Hospital in New York for their courtesy in allowing us to test aphasic patients in their clinics or wards.

REFERENCES

Bay, E. (1962) *Aphasia and non-verbal disorders of language*, "Brain," **85,** 411–426.

Goodglass, H., and Mayer, J. (1958) *Agrammatism in aphasia*, "J. Sp. and Hear. Dis.," **23,** 99–111.

Head, H. (1926) *Aphasia and Kindred Disorders of Speech.* Macmillan, New York.

Jones, L. V., and Wepman, J. M. (1961) *Dimensions of language performance in aphasia*, "J. Speech Hearing Res.," **4,** 220–232.

Schuell, H., Jenkins, J. J., and Carroll, J. M. (1962) *Factor analysis of the Minnesota Test for Differential Diagnosis of Aphasia*, "J. Speech Hearing Res.," **5,** 349–369.

Weisenburg, T., and McBride, K. (1935) *Aphasia.* Commonwealth Fund, New York.

Wepman, J. M., Bock, R. D., Jones, L. V., and Van Pelt, D. (1956) *Psycholinguistic study of aphasia: a revision of the concept of anomia*, "J. Speech Hear. Dis.," **21,** 468–477.

7

Oral Responses of Aphasics under Different Syntactical Conditions

WALTER JEROME ROLLIN

WALTER J. ROLLIN, Ph.D., is with the department of special education of San Francisco State College.

This paper is based on a Master's Thesis completed in 1958 at the University of Pittsburgh under the direction of Dr. George Shames.

INTRODUCTION

This study was an attempt to test experimentally the effects of syntactical variations of question items upon the oral response ability of aphasic patients.

Although several writers (Eisenson, 1956 and 1957; Goldstein, 1948; Werner, 1956; Jacobson, 1955; Wepman, 1951), have referred to aphasia in terms of a linguistic involvement, little reference has been made in the literature to the work of modern linguistics and its possible value to the language testing and training of aphasics (Freud, 1953; Scargill, 1954).

Testing procedures for aphasics have often been criticized for their lack of standardization and objective scoring systems (Nash, 1955, Schotland, 1953; Yates, 1954). Current formal tests place much emphasis on the lexical meaning of question items requiring oral responses and fail to consider the grammatical functions of these test items (Eisenson, 1954; Halstead, 1949; Halstead and Wepman, 1949; Scargill, 1954; Schuell, 1957; Wells and Ruesch, 1945).

In testing for aphasia, the diagnostician will often vary the grammatical construction of a question in order to elicit a correct response from a patient. The patient unable to respond correctly to the question, "What is the color of a clear sky?" may respond correctly to the question when structured as follows: "Can you tell me the color of a clear sky?"

This re-wording of the question is of an arbitrary nature and has never been subjected to strict experimental test. Scargill (1954) suggests the construction of a test for aphasia, which would account for both the *lexical and grammatical* meanings of language, in order to be certain that the syntactical patterns do not confuse the patient. He believes that the patient's inability to respond to a particular question may be the result of his inability to recognize the structural pattern of the question as well as his inability to deal appropriately with the content of the question.

The hypothesis, stated in the null form, was as follows: There are no significant differences among responses given by a group of aphasic subjects to questions phrased in five different syntactical patterns.

PROCEDURE

Subjects

The thirty-two subjects for this study were brain injured patients obtained from Leech

From *Language and Speech* 7:167–75, 1964.

Farm Veterans Administration Hospital, Aspinwall Veteran Administration Hospital, University Drive Veterans Administration Hospital, and the Harmarville Rehabilitation Center, all in Pittsburgh, Pennsylvania; and Manhattan Veterans Administration Hospital, New York City, New York. All the subjects were diagnosed by physicians as having suffered brain injury. The presence or absence of aphasia was determined by clinical impressions and the use of formal diagnostic measuring instruments. The subjects ranged in age from 27 to 72 years with a mean age of 53.6 years.

Test Questions

Ten questions were selected for syntactical variation from the Auditory Verbal Comprehension sub-test of the Eisenson Test for Aphasia (Eisenson, 1954). Each item was changed so as to form five different syntactical patterns of speech. The term "syntactical" as used in this study was defined as a construction involving one of the four principal features of arrangements analysed by Block and Trager (1942).

The five patterns were developed with the condition that each pattern for a given item asks similar information depending on the item. Fries (1952) analyses the basic patterns of English sentences with regard to their structure and describes the patterns which ask for information. For the purpose of the present study the five syntactical conditions are identified by:

Pattern A	Interrogative Form
Pattern B	Interrogative Form
Pattern C	Imperative Form
Pattern D	Imperative Form
Pattern E	Declarative Form

An example of a test item showing the five syntactical patterns follows:

Pattern A	What do people wear on their heads?
Pattern B	Do you know what people wear on their heads?
Pattern C	Name what people wear on their heads.
Pattern D	Tell me what people wear on their heads.
Pattern E	On their heads people wear ——.

Because each item was represented by five patterns, the total number of questions asked of a subject equalled fifty. The fifty questions were randomized into five tests of ten questions each by a restricted method of randomization. This was done by originally randomizing the order of the ten test items and maintaining this item order throughout testing. Within each item the five patterns were also randomized. Finally, the presentation of the five tests to each of the subjects was then randomized in accordance with a systematic rotation of orders.

Testing Procedure

Each subject was given general instructions which were previously tape recorded. The instruction preceded each of the five tests. The testing session lasted no longer than a total of forty minutes. Each of the fifty items was asked twice with the requirement that the subject attempt to answer both times. The subject's responses were recorded as "correct" or "incorrect". For operational purposes, a correct response was defined as the oral response by the subject of the appropriate answer—the answer designated by the Eisenson Manual (1954). Misarticulation or synonym of the correct answer was considered "correct". An incorrect response was defined as the absence of any oral response of the correct answer by the subject. An interval of fifteen seconds between item presentation was the time allowed for an answer. The stimulus question items were presented by an examiner via a tape recording.

RESULTS

Analysis of Responses to the First Presentation of Items

A summary of the analysis of variance for evaluating variation among means of responses to the experimental conditions and for the evaluation of inter-subject variability, upon the initial presentation of the test items, is shown in Table 7-1. The value of F among methods (syntactical patterns) is 0.1. This value does not meet the requirements of significance for 4 and 124 degrees of freedom and thus indicates no significant difference among each of the five conditions.

TABLE 7–1. SUMMARIES OF ANALYSIS OF VARIANCE FOR EVALUATING ORAL RESPONSES UPON INITIAL PRESENTATION UNDER FIVE SYNTACTICAL CONDITIONS

Source of Variation	(df) Degrees of Freedom	(ms) Mean Square	F*
Conditions (C)	4	0.1	0.1
Subjects (S)	31	66.3	92.1**
Error (E)	124	0.7	
Total	159		

*F = msC/msE
= msS/msE
**Significant beyond 1% level

It can be seen, however, that the value of F among subjects is 92.13. This value is significant at the 0.01 level of confidence for 31 and 124 degrees of freedom and thus indicated wide variation of the individual subject means about the grand mean. It seemed, therefore, that any differences which may have been present among conditions could have been obscured by individual subject variability.

Analysis of Responses to the Second Presentation of Items

A summary of the analysis of variance for evaluating variation among means of responses to the experimental conditions and for the evaluation of inter-subject variability upon the second presentation of the test items is shown in Table 7-2. The value of F among methods (five syntactical patterns) is 0.9. This value does not meet the requirements of significance for 4 and 124 degrees of freedom and thus indicates no mean differences among the five conditions.

It can be seen, however, that the value of F

TABLE 7–2. SUMMARIES OF ANALYSIS OF VARIANCE FOR EVALUATING ORAL RESPONSES UPON SECOND PRESENTATION UNDER FIVE SYNTACTICAL CONDITIONS

Source of Variation	(df) Degrees of Freedom	(ms) Mean Square	F*
Conditions (C)	4	0.5	0.8
Subjects (S)	31	66.4	110.7**
Error (E)	124	0.6	
Total	159		

*F = msC/msE
= msS/msE
**Significant beyond 1% level

among subjects is 120.35. This value is significant for 31 and 124 degrees of freedom at beyond the 0.01 level of confidence, thus indicating wide differences among subject means. It seemed, therefore, that any differences which may have been present among conditions may have been obscured by the individual subject variability.

Analysis of Differences Between the Two Presentations

A summary of the analysis of variance for evaluating variation among means of responses to the presentations and for the evaluation of inter-subject variability upon both presentations is shown in Table 7-3. The value of F between orders (presentation 1 and 2) is

TABLE 7–3. SUMMARIES OF ANALYSIS OF VARIANCE FOR EVALUATING ORAL RESPONSES, UPON TWO PRESENTATIONS UNDER FIVE SYNTACTICAL CONDITIONS

Source of Variation	(df) Degrees of Freedom	(ms) Mean Square	F*
Presentations (P)	1	0.1	0.02
Subjects (S)	31	659.9	169.2**
Error (E)	31	3.9	
Total	63		

*F = msC/msE
= msS/msE
**Significant beyond 1% level

0.02. This value does not meet the requirement of significance for 1 and 31 degrees of freedom. These data, therefore, give no indication that the subjects responded to the second presentation of the items any differently than they did to the first presentation. The value of F among subjects is 166.43. This value is highly significant for 31 and 31 degrees of freedom at the 0.01 level of confidence and consistent with subject means differences seen in Tables 7-1 and 7-2. It seemed, therefore, that any difference which may have been present in presentations 1 and 2 could have been obscured by individual subject variability.

The Relationships of Responses Among the Five Syntactical Conditions

Coefficients of correlation (product moment *r*'s) among initial responses to each of the five experimental conditions were computed in order to investigate the degree to which each of the conditions elicited the same responses. As stated earlier, conditions A and B were in the Interrogative form; conditions C and D in the Imperative form; and condition E in Declarative form. These product-moment correlations ranged from 0.92 to 0.97 among the five syntactical patterns. These are shown in Table 7-4. Highly significant degrees of association between each of the conditions at beyond the 0.01 levels of confidence were revealed. The subjects seemed to respond similarly to each condition. They neither did better nor worse as a result of being asked the question in a different way.

TABLE 7-4. PRODUCT MOMENT INTERCORRELATIONS AMONG CONDITIONS A, B, C, D, E UPON INITIAL PRESENTATION

	A	B	C	D	E
A		0.94	0.96	0.95	0.95
B			0.94	0.97	0.92
C				0.95	0.95
D					0.94
E					

The Relationships Between First and Second Responses for Each of the Five Syntactical Patterns

Coefficients of correlation (product moment *r*'s), between first and second responses for each of the conditions were computed in order to investigate the degree to which the first presentation and response was associated with the second presentation and response under each syntactical condition. These product-moment correlations ranged from 0.92 to 0.98. As shown in Table 7-5, a highly significant degree of association between the first and second stimulus response situations for each of the conditions, beyond the 0.01 level of confidence was revealed. That is, the subjects seemed to respond to each presentation similarly for each of the conditions. They neither did better nor worse as a result of being asked the questions a second time.

TABLE 7-5. PRODUCT MOMENT CORRELATIONS AMONG PRESENTATIONS FOR EACH OF THE FIVE SYNTACTICAL PATTERNS A, B, C, D, E OF THE INITIAL PRESENTATION AND CONDITIONS A, B, C, D, E OF THE SECOND PRESENTATION

		FIRST PRESENTATION				
	Condition	A	B	C	D	E
	A	0.97				
SECOND	B		0.92			
PRESENTATION	C			0.97		
	D				0.98	
	E					0.98

DISCUSSION

The present study tends to support the hypothesis that oral responses given by a group of aphasic patients to question items do not differ significantly, at least quantitatively, under five syntactical conditions of presentation. It is important to note that a significantly high inter-subject variance was evident which would tend to obscure any differences found among experimental conditions. It seems, therefore, that a more homogeneous aphasic population would have been desirable for the purposes of this particular study. Such a selective procedure could, however, only be based upon the original medical diagnosis and subjective clinical judgments of each patient. The difficulty in utilizing these judgments as objective measuring instruments has been alluded to by Eisenson (1956) and Goldstein (1948) and therefore a selective sampling, in terms of type of aphasic problem, was not attempted here. For this particular study, subjects as made available at each of the particular hospitals were tested regardless of the extent of observable language dysfunction.

An analysis of variance performed on the second presentation of question items was consistent with the results obtained from the initial presentation of question items. As expected, inter-subject variance was again highly significant. The statistical results obtained in a between-presentation analysis seemed to indicate that, for this group, repetition of the question item did not help to elicit a better answer than was given upon the initial presentation. Quantitatively at least, the answers were interestingly consistent. A subject who answered a question *incorrectly* the first time would do so similarly the second time. In the same way, a subject who answered a question *correctly* the first time would do so similarly the second time. Also, since syntactical pattern had no observable effect upon oral responses, answers given by the subjects as a group remained quantitatively consistent throughout all conditions.

A statistical analysis of type of response was not performed in the present study so that consistency of qualitative response was not measured. However, an inspection of the verbatim responses revealed that answers given to each of the ten basic questions seemed to remain consistent under all syntactical conditions. That is, the words themselves, which the aphasics used in their responses, whether correct or incorrect, did not change. Several times subjects gave more than one response to an item, but these were not always consistent under all syntactical conditions. Not infrequently, subjects responded to questions asking for the warmest or coldest season of the year, by naming one or two of the summer or winter months. Such types of answers may suggest the concretism of response often found in aphasics (Wepman, 1953).

Several writers, among them Eisenson (1956), have suggested that inconsistency of response is one of the chief characteristic symptoms of aphasic patients. On the basis of the present study it would be difficult to explain the consistency effects other than in terms of possible perseverative behavior occurring with the immediate repetition of each item. Again this does not explain the consistency of response to the randomized syntactical patterns.

An analysis of the relationships among each of the syntactical conditions, utilising product-moment correlations, failed to indicate any differences among the effects of individual syntactical patterns. All correlations approached 1.00 to a highly significant degree. This further supports the results reported earlier in this discussion.

A descriptive item analysis supports Eisenson's statement concerning the varied complexity of the original items in his test for auditory aphasia (Eisenson, 1954). As a group, the subjects responded more correctly to items 8 and 10 than to the remaining items. The

TABLE 7–6. GROUP PERCENTAGES FOR THE TOTAL NUMBER OF SUBJECTS RESPONDING CORRECTLY TO EACH OF THE TEN ORIGINAL ITEMS UPON THE INITIAL PRESENTATION

Items	Total number of subjects responding correctly to the item	Percentage of subjects responding correctly
1	19	59
2	17	53
3	18	56
4	15	47
5	13	40
6	7	22
7	14	44
8	21	66
9	15	47
10	21	66

subjects' lowest scores occurred in response to item 6. Table 7-6 summarizes the number of subjects and the percentages of subjects who responded correctly to each of the items. These results further indicate the differences among subjects in terms of degree of impairment and point up the need for more rigid experimental controls and methodology in future research.

In summarizing, it can be concluded that no significant differences were revealed among responses given by a group of aphasic patients to question items presented under conditions of five different syntactical patterns. The study tends to question the efficacy of rearranging a question item syntactically, in a formal testing situation, in order to elicit an oral response from an aphasic patient. These data also suggest that the examiner may be doing something other than changing only the syntactical pattern when eliciting a different response with this procedure. A patient, unable to respond upon the initial presentation of the question, may receive certain clues through constant repetition of the question. It might be important to consider also the nature of other linguistic signs used by the examiner, namely those of inflection, intonation, and stress, and examine these variables experimentally. This study further demonstrates the difficulty in controlling the many variables inherent in an aphasic population, for the purposes of experimental research, and therefore suggests the need for standardized tests to be used as a basis for the establishment of distinct homogeneous groups.

REFERENCES

Bloch, B. and Trager, G. L. (1942). Outline of Linguistic Analysis (Baltimore).

Eisenson, J. (1954). Examining for Aphasia. A manual for the examination of related disturbances (New York).

——, and Berry, M. (1956). Speech Disorders (New York).

——, (1957). Aphasia in adults—classification and examination procedures in Handbook of Speech Pathology (ed., Travis, L. E.) (New York).

Freud, E. D. (1953). Recent trends in aphasia research. *Amer. J. Psychiatry*, **110,** 186.

Fries, C. C. (1952). The Structure of English (New York).

Goldstein, K. (1948). Language and Language Disturbances (New York).

Halstead, W. C. (1949). Manual for the Halstead-Wepman Aphasia Screening Test (Chicago).

—— and Wepman, J. M. (1949). The Halstead-Wepman Aphasia Test. *J. Sp. Hrng. Dis.*, **14,** 9.

Jakobson, R. (1955). Aphasia as a linguistic problem, in On Expressive Language (ed., Werner, H.) (Worcester).

Nash, J. (1955). The diagnosis of organic brain damage by psychological techniques: a review of the literature and present status. *Bull. Marit. Psychol. Assoc.*, **4,** 32.

Scargill, M. H. (1954). Modern linguistics and recovery from aphasia. *J. Sp. Hrng. Dis.*, **19,** 507.

Schotland, H. D. (1953). An evaluative study of two tests for aphasia. Unpublished Master's Thesis, University of Iowa.

Schuell, H. (1957). A short examination for aphasia. *Neurology*, **7,** 625.

Wells, F. F. and Ruesch, J. (1945). Mental Examiners' Handbook (New York).

Wepman, J. M. (1951). Recovery from Aphasia (New York).

—— (1953). A conceptual model for the processes involved in recovery from aphasia. *J. Sp. Hrng. Dis.*, **18,** 4.

Werner, H. (1956). Microgenesis and aphasia. *J. Abnorm. Soc. Psychol.*, **52,** 347.

Yates, A. J. (1954). The validity of some psychological tests of brain damage. *Psych. Bull.*, **51,** 359.

8

Agrammatism and Inflectional Morphology in English

HAROLD GOODGLASS
JEAN BERKO

HAROLD GOODGLASS, Ph.D., is director of psychology research at the Boston Veterans Administration Hospital.
JEAN BERKO (GLEASON), Ph.D., is a research associate at Clark University, Worcester.
This investigation was supported in part by fellowship MF9261, from the National Institute of Mental Health, Public Health Service, and in part by a grant from the Social Science Research Council.

Many aphasic patients, while beginning to recover a considerable speaking vocabulary, continue to omit articles, relational words, and inflectional endings from their speech. These patients, speaking in disconnected words rather than sentences, are said to exhibit "agrammatism" or "telegraphic speech." The phenomenon of agrammatism has been described by many clinicians in the classical literature on aphasia; it continues to be cited by Goldstein (*3*), Weisenburg and McBride (*12*), Brain (*2*), Wepman, Bock, Jones, and Van Pelt (*13*) as part of the syndrome of motor (or expressive) aphasia, as opposed to the speech pattern in the sensory and amnesic types of aphasia. Pick (*8*) undertook an analysis of grammatical disturbances in aphasia in 1913, but the problem then lay dormant for many years. Agrammatism and telegraphic speech have remained essentially subjective terms, based on clinical impression, in spite of their potential importance for clinical diagnosis and neuropsychological theory.

Recently, a series of contributions by Jakobson (*6*), Wepman, Bock, Jones, and Van Pelt (*13*), Goodglass and Mayer (*5*), and Luria (*7*) have applied psycholinguistic concepts and methods in the effort to define and make measurable the deficit which produces the symptoms of agrammatism. Jakobson applied the term "contiguity disorder" to this phenomenon and stated the symptoms in linguistic terms as follows: (a) reduction in the variety of sentences, (b) loss of syntactic rules, (c) dissolution of ties of grammatical coordination and subordination, (d) loss of words with purely grammatical function and loss of inflectional endings. Jakobson thus implicates inflections of grammar, which are obligatory in English, as well as syntactic arrangements, which are not so highly coded by the language. Contiguity disorder and agrammatism thus refer to language disturbances that more specifically fall under the linguist's headings of "morphology" and "syntax". Syntax here refers to the arrangement of words into sentences, and morphology includes the study of the rules for suffixes that are used to indicate grammatical relationships between words.

Goodglass and Mayer (*5*) selected five agrammatic and five nonagrammatic aphasics on the basis of clinical judgment. They found that these groups differed sharply with respect to errors with syntactic constructions (that is, positioning of words by grammatical function), and differed much less in their tendency to omit or confuse inflectional endings and the "small

From *Journal of Speech and Hearing Research* 3:257–67, 1960.

words" of grammar. These findings suggested that the morphological aspect of agrammatism might well be studied separately from the syntactical. Goodglass and Hunt (*4*) compared the ability of aphasics to answer questions correctly with words ending in a plural "-s" as opposed to a possessive "-s." They also required their subjects to judge the correctness of tape recorded sentences from which either a final plural "s" or a final possessive "-s" was omitted. The possessive was clearly more difficult than the plural, both in the expressive and the auditory-receptive parts of the experiment.

The present study is an investigation of the aphasic individual's ability to produce orally common English words with inflectional endings appropriate for the completion of English sentences. It affords some interesting comparisons with Berko's (*1*) study of this ability in preschool children. The principal questions to be answered by the data were conceived as follows:

a. Does there appear to be, in general, an order of difficulty for the English inflectional forms among aphasics and, if so, how does this order compare with the difficulty of these forms for children?

b. Is there any evidence from correlational data that a common factor governs the use of the various inflectional morphemes?

c. What relation can be discovered between impaired use of any of the inflectional morphemes and other, independently measured, aspects of aphasic disturbance?

The English inflectional items investigated were the regular forms of the plural and possessive of the noun, the simple past and the third person singular present indicative of the verb, and the comparative and superlative of the adjective, to make a total of 10 inflectional morphemes. These items include all of English inflection with the exception of the progressive "ing" form of the verb. All of these inflectional forms, except the comparative and superlative, occur in one of three differing forms, or allomorphs, depending on the last phoneme of the stem of the word; they are therefore said to be phonologically conditioned. These allomorphs are as follows:

a. The third person present singular indicative of the verb, the noun plural, and the possessive singular, phonologically identical and formed by [-əz], [-s], or [-z].

b. The past tense of the verb, formed by [-əd], [-t], or [-d].

c. The comparative and superlative of the adjective, formed by [-ər] and [-əst], respectively, endings which have no variants.

Ideally, a test aimed at the problem under consideration here uses nonsense words. That is, if a subject says that the plural of "watch" is "watches," it is always possible that he has no internalized rule for the formation of the plural, that his production represents a specific memorized form, and that he may be unable to form the plural of a word he has never before heard. Thus if the request is for the plural of a nonsense form like "gutch," these difficulties are overcome. The subject who produces "gutches" demonstrates the possession of an abstract rule. Berko (*1*) used such nonsense forms in her experiment with preschool children. In the present experiment with aphasic patients, real words were used because it was found that in the majority of instances the individual was unable or unwilling to complete a sentence containing nonsense words. Since inflections are obligatory in English, it was possible to construct sentences that necessitated their use, and the individual's deficits were readily measured.

PROCEDURE

Subjects

The subjects were 21 aphasic patients in the neurological wards of the Boston Veterans Administration Hospital and in the speech therapy program at Lemuel Shattuck Hospital.[1] They ranged in age from 24 to 65 years, with a mean of 48.1. Three were college graduates, including one physician; seven others had completed high school. The criterion for inclusion of a subject was that he have

[1] Testing of patients at Lemuel Shattuck Hospital was carried out by Miss Mary Hyde, Speech Therapist.

sufficient speech to complete the test sentences with scorable responses, but sufficient residual aphasia to make two or more errors. Two patients with minimal residual aphasia were excluded because they made no errors at all. One patient with a moderate anomic aphasia also was excluded because she made no errors in the experimental task.

Tests Used

A 60-item sentence completion test was composed to include six opportunities for the use of each of the ten inflectional morphemes chosen for study. The test was designed to be given in two equivalent sections of thirty items each. The 10 morphemes were plural [-z] or [-s]; plural [-əz]; past [-t] or [-d]; past [-əd]; present [-s] or [-z]; present [-əz]; possessive [-s] or [-z]; possessive [-əz]; comparative [-ər]; superlative [-əst]. An example of an item (simple past) follows: "It rains pretty often around here. It did rain last night. Last night, it ———."

Each sentence was read aloud by the experimenter with a natural or slightly exaggerated phrasing and intonation, in order to elicit the final word from the subject. The initial sound of the response word was supplied as a starting cue for subjects who needed this assistance, and the score of plus or minus depended solely on the correctness of the inflectional suffix. In some instances subjects misunderstood the item or gave a paraphrased answer and it was felt injudicious to press them to listen once more to the item. For this reason 18 (1%) of the responses could not be scored as right or wrong. These items were arbitrarily assigned plus or minus scores in alternation as they happened to fall on the data sheet. These ambiguous responses were evenly scattered; no test sentence elicited more than one unscorable response among the 21 subjects and no inflectional category (each involving 126 responses) had more than two. The error thus introduced is insignificant and random.

In the listing of test items it will be noted that final [-s] items are scored together with final [-z] items, and that final [-d] items are scored together with final [-t] items. The use of the unvoiced form in each of these cases does not depend on knowledge of the inflection, but is determined by prior phonological rules which are universal for English. That is, the final alveolar stop following [p, k, č, f, θ, s, š] is unvoiced and so is the final sibilant following [p, t, k, f, θ]. The assumption was made that the voiced and unvoiced forms were homogeneous in difficulty. A further assumption in the use of this test is that the six samples of each type of inflection are homogeneous in difficulty and that they reliably represent the level of difficulty of the entire class of inflections to which they belong. The basis for this assumption was that the task for the subject was phonologically and grammatically the same in all six samples of each type of inflectional ending. It was felt that differences in difficulty among the stems of the response words did not appreciably influence scores, since, with the help of a cue, if necessary, the subjects were capable of supplying the stem in every case. The validity of this assumption concerning homogeneity is examined statistically under *Results*.

As part of their examination routine, 15 of the subjects had had an aphasia examination which included objective ratings of effective "Functional Speech" and articulation. These subscores served as criteria of impairment in aspects of language performance apart from word endings. The Functional Speech score is obtained from a five-point rating, based on the Interjectional Speech and Spontaneous Expository Speech subtests of the Boston VA Hospital Diagnostic Aphasia Test.[2] This portion of the examination consists of a structured conversation, ranging from expletives and conversational automatisms to extended propositional utterances, including a narrative about a picture-situation. Subjects' performance was scored on a scale from *0* to *4* with *0* indicating no impairment and *4* indicating severe to total aphasia.

[2] The term "Functional Speech" applied to the rating of a structural conversation test and the principle of scoring several levels of speech productivity on a picture-situation were taken from the Minnesota Test for Differential Diagnosis of Aphasia by Schuell (*10*).

The rating scale was originally validated on 25 patients against the judgment of two clinicians who knew the patients well through testing and therapy. It has since been applied to more than 100 tested subjects with satisfaction that the objective scoring standard coincided with clinical judgment, based on extended observation, as to the patients' over-all verbal efficiency. Statistical evidence, though still scanty, supports the use of the Functional Speech rating as an index of the over-all severity of aphasic speech defect. In a study with 20 aphasic patients, rank order correlation coefficients obtained between Functional Speech and each of two subtests, Commands and Word Finding, were .71 and .72, respectively; intercorrelation of the two latter tests was only .49. The Functional Speech score is also based on performance closely similar in content to the two subtests (Giving Information and Picture Description) which Schuell and Jenkins (*11*) found to be tied for the second highest phi coefficient among 29 subtests which were tested for correlation with their full battery.

The articulation or Verbal Agility subtest required the rapid reiteration of a series of test words. Either one or two points per item could be earned, depending on the number of repetitions in a five-second span. Test words were presented both orally and visually, and timing of each word did not begin until the subject had succeeded in saying it, or clearly could not master its articulation. This task was designed as a wide range test of articulatory facility, as independent as possible of difficulties in auditory comprehension and in word-finding. It was included in the present experiment because of the impression gained during preliminary investigations that subjects who performed easily on the experimental task were facile in their articulation.

RESULTS AND DISCUSSION

Order of Difficulty of the Inflectional Endings for Aphasic Subjects

The difficulty of each type of inflectional ending for the aphasic subjects was measured by the number of errors on the six items representing each ending. Table 8-1 summarizes the data. From the column which gives the number of subjects failing each item it is possible to get a rough estimate of the uniformity of the difficulty of items within a class, as compared to the differences between classes. The Cochran Q test, as described by Siegel (*12*, pp. 161–166) was applied to each of the 10 sets of error scores. The null hypothesis in this test is that the items have equal probability of being passed. Rejection of the null hypothesis would indicate that the items in a set are clearly heterogeneous in difficulty. The null hypothesis could

TABLE 8-1. ERRORS MADE BY 21 APHASICS IN USE OF 10 INFLECTIONAL ENDINGS ON SENTENCE COMPLETION TEST IN WHICH EACH ENDING APPEARED SIX TIMES

Class of Inflection	*Number of Subjects Failing each Item*	*Total Errors*	*Mean Errors per Subject*
Plural [-s, -z]	4, 0, 6, 7, 5, 4	26	1.2
Plural [-əz]	7, 3, 5, 3, 5, 4	27	1.3
Past [-t, -d]	10, 9, 10, 10, 9, 6	54	2.6
Past [-əd]	13, 9, 13, 7, 5, 3	50	2.4
Present [-s, -z]	7, 9, 5, 4, 10, 11	46	2.2
Present [-əz]	10, 11, 11, 10, 9, 11	62	3.0
Possessive [-s, -z]	11, 10, 10, 6, 12, 9	58	2.8
Possessive [-əz]	12, 15, 10, 16, 14, 16	83	4.0
Comparative [-ər]	4, 8, 3, 6, 5, 4	30	1.4
Superlative [-əst]	10, 6, 7, 7, 6, 7	43	2.0
Total		479	22.8

not be rejected at the .05 probability level in any case except that of the past [-əd], where it could be rejected at the .01 level. Homogeneity of item difficulty thus may be assumed for all but one of the 10 sets.

Inspection of the several widely discrepant items suggests the possibility that some, but not all, of the easiest ones were more probable in English conversation than the others. On the whole, however, the assumption of homogeneity of difficulty within classes appears to have been justified. Consideration of the significance of differences between the error totals is therefore a legitimate next step.

Differences in error totals were tested for significance by means of the Wilcoxon signed ranks test, with results summarized in Table 8-2. It will be noted that the inflectional endings fall into at least three distinguishable groups with respect to difficulty, with the complex possessive by far the most difficult, the comparative and the two forms of the plural by far the easiest, and the remaining six occupying a middle range.

The decisive importance of grammatical function over phonological structure in determining the difficulty of an inflectional ending is illustrated by those items in which exact homonyms were used in different grammatical settings. For example, "horses" as a noun plural was failed by only three subjects in the item "The millionaire bought a new horse. He now has a whole stable full of ______." The possessive form "horse's" was failed by 15 subjects in the item "This blanket is for the horse. Whose blanket is it? It is the ______." "Watches" as a noun plural was failed by five subjects in the item "The doctor has a wrist watch and a pocket watch and a stop watch. He certainly has a lot of ______." The verb form "watches" was failed by 11 subjects in the item "John likes to watch while Tom draws pictures, so Tom draws and John ______."

The interpretation of the differences between the error scores may be limited by systematic differences in the probability structure of the incomplete sentences which were used to elicit the responses. That is, the order of difficulty of inflectional forms in free conversation is not necessarily the same as that obtained under the experimental conditions. It may be pointed out, for example, that the last word in the plural-demanding sentences is often preceded by a strong cue for a plural noun, such as "a lot of . . ." or the plural form of the verb. Yet, the item which had no such strong cue "My rose bush is in bloom. It is all covered with beautiful red ______." is just as easy, on the average, (five errors) as the other five items in its class.

A strong predominance in errors with the possessive was found also by Goodglass and Hunt (*4*). They used a stimulus structure that was apparently free of bias in the transitional probabilities of the words in the plural as compared to the possessive items. Their items were in the form: "The dog chewed up my

TABLE 8–2. SIGNIFICANCE LEVEL OF DIFFERENCES IN NUMBER OF ERRORS MADE, EACH INFLECTIONAL ENDING HAVING THE LARGER ERROR SCORE (LISTED FROM HIGHEST TO LOWEST) COMPARED TO EACH ENDING HAVING THE LESSER ERROR SCORE OF PAIR. FIGURES ARE BASED ON THE APPLICATION OF THE WILCOXON SIGNED RANKS TEST (TWO-TAILED) TO PAIRED ARRAYS OF ERROR SCORES OF THE 21 SUBJECTS.

Inflectional Ending (Larger Error Score)	*Inflectional Ending (Lesser Error Score of Pair)*								
	Present [-əz]	*Poss* [-s, -z]	*Past* [-t, -d]	*Past* [-əd]	*Present* [-s, -z]	*Superl* [-əst]	*Compar* [-ər]	*Plur* [-əz]	*Plur* [-s, -z]
Possessive [-əz]	.05	.01	.05	.01	.01	.01	.01	.01	01
Present [-əz]		ns*	ns	ns	ns	.05	.02	.01	.01
Possessive [-s, -z]			ns	ns	ns	ns	.05	.02	.01
Past [-t, -d]				ns	ns	ns	.05	.01	.01
Past [-əd]					ns	ns	.05	01	.01
Present [-s, -z]						ns	ns	ns	.01
Superlative [-ər]							ns	.05	.05
Comparative [-əst]								ns	ns
Plural [-əz]									ns

*Not significant

sister's gloves. (Read twice by examiner.) What did the dog chew up? Whose gloves were they?" It is therefore suggested that the differences in level of difficulty for the various inflectional endings, for aphasic subjects, cannot be dismissed as artifacts of the particular sentence structures chosen for the test items.

Comparison with Performance of Nonaphasic Subjects

The sentence completion tests used in the present study were given also to 15 brain-injured nonaphasic individuals who were neurological patients at the Boston Veterans Administration hospital. They were somewhat older than the aphasic subjects, ranging in age from 39 to 65 years with a mean age of 52.6. They closely resembled the aphasic subjects in educational attainment; two had graduated from college, four from high school. The two groups were not matched on performance IQs but the nonaphasic individuals appeared to have at least as much intellectual impairment as the aphasic subjects. The majority had right-sided brain damage or diffuse bilateral disease; two had been aphasic early in their illness.

Of the nonaphasic individuals, 10 performed with no errors at all, two made three errors, two made two errors, and one made one error. All five who made errors omitted the complex possessive [-əz]; this error occurred seven times. Three of the five omitted a simple possessive, as well, and one twice substituted a past tense for the third person present. None of these five had ever been considered aphasic. The most grossly deteriorated of these brain-injured individuals, who was confused, disorientated in time and place, and almost devoid of memory, performed without error under the conditions of the experiment. It is interesting to note that the items occasionally failed by the nonaphasics were also the most difficult for the aphasic subjects.

Comparison with Data on Children

According to Rapaport's (*9*, p. 186) summary, Ribot's rule holds that organic defects, such as aphasia, injure the latest learned patterns before they affect the earliest learning. One might therefore expect the aphasic's loss to mirror the pattern of the child's acquisition: that is, that the forms most difficult for the aphasic should be the ones acquired latest by the children. Data in the present study indicate that the pattern of aphasic deficit in English inflectional morphology only partially resembles the pattern of the child's learning, as found by Berko (*1*). For example, Berko found that children regularly have more difficulty with the phonologically complex[3] [-əz] and [-əd] than with the simpler [-s, -z] or [-t, -d] allomorphs in all the grammatical functions in which these endings are used. Percentages of correct responses of 80 children (four to seven years) to a sentence completion test, using nonsense words, are given in Table 8-3. For aphasics the corresponding difference in difficulty of the complex over the simple allomorph was found to a significant degree for the possessive; the difference between the simple and complex allomorphs of the third person singular tends in this direction; however, there is no difference, for aphasics, between the two forms of the plural or past tense endings. The errors of aphasics, as compared to children's, are much more influenced by morphemic differences than by phonological complexity. In some instances aphasics were unable to supply any of the allomorphs of a given inflectional morpheme, regardless of phonological simplicity. For example, three aphasics failed all of the possessive ending in the simple [-z] form. In the Berko study four-year-old children were consistently able to supply a simple possessive ending.

In making the comparison with children, it should be recalled that the aphasics were required to supply actual English forms; the children, on the other hand, had to demonstrate their generalization of the inflectional rules to nonsense words. Berko reports two instances in

[3] The expression "phonological complexity" here refers to the fact that the [-ez] and [-ed] forms apply to fewer cases and constitute exceptions to more general (hence "simpler") rules; it does not mean that these forms are harder to pronounce than their simple allomorphs.

TABLE 8–3. PERCENTAGE OF CORRECTLY INFLECTED NONSENSE WORDS SUPPLIED BY 80 CHILDREN, AGED FOUR TO SEVEN, AS REPORTED BY BERKO (1)

Inflectional Class	*Required Response*	*Percent Correct*
Plural [-z]	wugs	91
Plural [-əz]	tasses	36
	nizzes	28
Possessive [-z]	wug's	84
Possessive [-əz]	niz's	49
Present [-əz]*	loodges	56
	nazzes	48
Past [-d]	binged	77
Past [-əd]	motted	33

*The simple [-z] form of this inflectional morpheme was not sampled.

which real English words were to be supplied by the children. The past tense "melted" was supplied by 73% of her children as compared to 33% for the nonsense form "motted"; the plural "glasses" was supplied by 91% as compared to 36% for the nonsense form "nizzes."

Correlations among the Subscores

Rank order correlations were computed among the 10 arrays of error scores, with the results listed in Table 8-4. As a measure of the agreement between each of the subscores and their combined total, the rank order correlation was computed between each of the subscores and the total error scores of the 21 subjects. For this purpose the total error score was summed separately for each computation, omitting the score with which the total was being correlated. These correlations are also included in Table 8-3. Because of the small number of subjects, it would be rash to draw conclusions from any but the grossest differences between correlations. There appears to be a common factor contributing to the error scores of all the inflectional morphemes, with the possible exception of the simple past.

Relationship with Other Measures of Severity of Aphasia

The total error score on the experimental task was tested for correlation with the Functional Speech score and the Verbal Agility (articulation) score, which were described earlier. Unfortunately, these scores were available for only 15 of the 21 subjects. The obtained rho of .32 between Functional Speech and the total inflectional error score is well below the level

TABLE 8–4. INTERCORRELATIONS BETWEEN THE ERROR SCORES FOR THE 10 INFLECTIONAL ENDINGS. (WITH 21 SUBJECTS A CORRELATION COEFFICIENT OF .37 IS REQUIRED FOR SIGNIFICANCE AT THE .05 LEVEL)

	Plur [-əz]	*Past* [-t, -d]	*Past* [-əd]	*Pres* [-s, -z]	*Pres* [-əz]	*Poss* [-s, -z]	*Poss* [-əz]	*Compar* [-ər]	*Superl* [-əst]	*Combined Error Score*
Plural [-s, -z]	.45	.34	.50	.65	.63	.65	.33	.15	.53	.67
Plural [-əz]		.35	.72	.54	.65	.40	.46	.60	.53	.79
Past [-t, -d]			.32	.03	.16	-.18	-.02	.26	.21	.43
Past [-əd]				.42	.56	.40	.52	.43	.81	.70
Present [-s, -z]					.72	.62	.41	.03	.47	.63
Present [-z]						.62	.60	.19	.61	.74
Possessive [-s, -z]							.75	.18	.33	.60
Possessive [-əz]								.28	.35	.56
Comparative [-ər]									.21	.41
Superlative [-əst]										.51

required for statistical significance. This low correlation is illustrated clinically by the subject ranking fifth in the experimental task, who nevertheless had such a severe expressive aphasia that he could initiate practically no speech, although he could repeat words or short phrases. The patient ranking highest on the experimental task obtained a Functional Speech rating at the "moderately severe" level.

For the same group of fifteen subjects, a correlation of .69 was obtained between the Verbal Agility subtest and the total inflectional error score. This correlation accords with the clinical impression, gained in exploratory study, that patients who articulate individual words easily also have few omissions of inflectional endings.

Among the subjects who did well in the experimental task were some who had extreme word-finding difficulty and some whose speech was essentially limited to one-word sentences. That is, among the subjects who would be called clinically agrammatic because they speak in isolated words or short phrases, there are some—usually subjects having facile articulation—who are not much impaired in the test of grammatical morphology. It should be noted, however, that the correct syntactical context in each test sentence was already structured for the subject and was extremely important in determining the inflections supplied. This cue is absent in the normal speech of the patient who lacks a repertory of sentence patterns so that the correct inflections may be less in evidence under the conditions provided by their spontaneous speech. Under the present experimental conditions, at least, there appears to be a degree of independence between the morphological and syntactical aspects of agrammatism.

SIGNIFICANCE OF FINDINGS AND RESEARCH IMPLICATIONS

The present study has shown that aphasic subjects vary widely in their ability to supply inflectional endings under a particular experimental condition; that inflectional endings vary, according to their grammatical function, in their availability to aphasics. It further appears that if one eliminates the minimally aphasic and the totally aphasic, then the degree of aphasic handicap has little predictive value for the ability to supply inflectional endings. On the other hand, facility with articulation appears to be positively correlated with this ability. However, a considerably larger sample of aphasics should be tested before either of the two latter relationships can be claimed with any assurance.

As yet, there is no information on the relation between performance on the experimental task and use of inflections in a sample of free conversation; neither is the relation known between performance on the present test and facility with English syntactic forms, either in structured tests or in free conversation. A larger sample is necessary also before it can be determined whether any of the inflectional endings of the present test are differentially related to each other or to other diagnostic indicators. The present authors propose that continued application of linguistic categories to the design of experimental tasks offers the most promise for identifying agrammatism more precisely. As greater precision is gained in stating operationally *what* is meant by "agrammatism" it should be possible to suggest *how* or through what psychological process this defect operates.

From a comparison of the present experimental data with the performance of preschool children, it appears that no simple parallel can be drawn between the normal acquisition of inflectional forms and their loss through brain injury. However, the order of acquisition of regular inflectional endings by very young children is still not known. If they are acquired in a definite order, Berko's data suggest that this learning is nearly complete by the age of four when children are able to handle the more simple and regular forms of all English inflectional categories. In addition to information on the inflectional usage of three-year-olds, it would be useful to have a frequency count for the occurrence of the various English inflectional endings in normal adult speech.

SUMMARY

This study was concerned with the morphological, as distinct from the syntactical, aspects of grammatical disturbance in aphasia. Specifically, it investigated the ability of 21 aphasic subjects to supply, by means of a sentence completion test, correct inflectional endings for nouns, verbs, and adjectives. The results suggest the following tentative conclusions:

a. For aphasics, the difficulty of various inflectional endings follows a definite order which is based on grammatical function, not phonological similarity.

b. Phonological complexity is not as important for aphasics as for children in determining the difficulty of inflections.

c. A common factor appears to underlie adequate performance with all inflectional endings studied except the simple past.

d. The inflectional ending score is related to verbal agility in articulation, but it is not related to over-all adequacy of speech. It is suggested that, in some aphasics, the syntactic and the inflectional aspects of grammar may be impaired independently of each other.

REFERENCES

1. Berko, Jean, The child's learning of English morphology. *Word,* **14,** 1958, 150–177.
2. Brain, R., Aphasia, apraxia, and agnosia. In S. A. K. Wilson (Ed.), vol. 3, *Neurology* (2nd ed.). Baltimore: Williams and Wilkins, 1955.
3. Goldstein, K., *Language and Language Disturbances; Aphasic Symptom Complexes and Their Significance for Medicine and Theory of Language.* New York: Grune and Stratton, 1948.
4. Goodglass, H., and Hunt, J., Grammatical complexity and aphasic speech. *Word,* **14,** 1958, 197–207.
5. ——, and Mayer, J., Agrammatism in aphasia. *J. Speech Hearing Dis.,* **23,** 1958, 99–111.
6. Jakobson, R., Two aspects of language and two types of aphasic disturbances. In R. Jakobson and M. Halle, *Fundamentals of Language.* The Hague, Netherlands: Mouton, 1956.
7. Luria, A. R., Brain disorders and language analysis. *Lang. Speech,* **1,** 1958, 14–34.
8. Pick, A., *Die agrammatischen Sprachstorungen.* Berlin: 1913.
9. Rapaport, D., *Emotions and Memory.* New York: International Univ. Press, 1950.
10. Schuell, Hildred, *Minnesota Test for Differential Diagnosis of Aphasia.* Minneapolis: Univ. Minnesota Press, 1955.
11. ——, and Jenkins, J. J., The nature of language deficit in aphasia. *Psychol. Rev.,* **66,** 1959, 45–67.
12. Siegel, S., *Nonparametric Statistics for the Behavioral Sciences.* New York: McGraw-Hill, 1956.
13. Weisenburg, T., and McBride, Katharine E., *Aphasia.* New York: Commonwealth Fund, 1935.
14. Wepman, J. M., Bock, R. D., Jones, L. V., and Van Pelt, Doris, Psycholinguistic study of aphasia: a revision of the concept of anomia. *J. Speech Hearing Dis.* **21,** 1956, 468–477.

9

Meaning in Jargon Aphasia

EDWIN A. WEINSTEIN
OLGA G. LYERLY
MALVIN COLE
MARK N. OZER

EDWIN A. WEINSTEIN, M.D., is with the department of neurology of the Mount Sinai School of Medicine, New York City.

OLGA G. LYERLY, M.A., is with Psychological Assessment Associates, Washington, D.C.

MALVIN COLE, M.D., is with the division of neurology of the New Jersey College of Medicine, Newark.

MARK N. OZER, M.D., is director of the Learning Research Unit at The Children's Hospital, Washington, D.C.

Aided by a grant from the U.S. Army Medical Research and Development Command, Office of the Surgeon General.

The title of this paper may seem paradoxical since, in neurology, jargon is defined as utterances that have no meaning. In the literature the loss of meaning has generally been attributed to receptive defects and the breakdown of the phonetic, verbal and syntactical organization of language. However, Alajouanine (1956) has pointed out that jargon cannot be adequately defined only in terms of the intrinsic organization of speech. He states ". . . although not easily defined, it (jargon) is not difficult to recognize clinically, since it is an incomprehensible language, not because of abnormal utterance or defect of articulation but simply because it is completely lacking in meaning." Although word distortions and neologisms are common in jargon aphasia, they are not unique to it and occur commonly in the speech of other aphasics. On the other hand, well formed words used in proper grammatical sequence may constitute jargon under certain circumstances.

As Alajouanine stressed, the essential feature is the loss of meaning. This must be considered from the standpoint of communication between speaker and listener. Although the listener does not understand the speech of the jargon aphasic, the patient behaves as if neither he nor his auditor has any difficulty in understanding him. Patients with jargon are talkative and make no effort to determine whether or not they are being understood. While only a portion of the speech of patients with jargon aphasia is jargon, they do not indicate that they are aware of the change from normal to jargon speech. The patient not only behaves as if he is unaware of any speech disturbance but usually will deny that any exists when specifically questioned (Wyllie, 1894; Bastian, 1900; Weisenburg and McBride, 1935; Goldstein, 1948; de Ajuriaguerra and Hécaen, 1960; Brain, 1961; Allison, 1962; Alajouanine and Lhermitte, 1964). On the other hand, the aphasic patient without jargon is usually aware of his defect and may make a considerable effort to augment understanding by gesture, self-correction and reciprocal confirmation, much as an actor in a charade eventually brings comprehension to the other participants in the game. Even with an impoverished

From *Cortex* 2:165–87, 1966.

vocabulary much can be communicated.

The question of meaning arose in a recent study (Weinstein et al., 1964) of the relationship of anosognosia to aphasia in patients with right-sided sensorimotor defects. The series included two subjects with jargon aphasia who denied both their speech disturbance and motor and sensory loss. The approach was based on the idea that the manifestations of anosognosia are not a form of agnosia but are words and gestures in which the patient symbolically represents his disabilities. The predominance of anosognosia for the left side of the body over neglect and denial of right-sided sensorimotor deficits was explained on the basis of the aphasic patient's loss of metaphorical speech rather than in terms of minor versus major hemisphere localization per se. The anosognosic patient is not unaware of his disability in the sense of complete lack of knowledge of it. Rather, he is unaware of the way he is presenting his problem in his verbal language and his gesture. It was shown that patients commonly expressed knowledge of a disability in one form of language but not in another, and the jargon occurred predominantly in answer to questions about illness and disability. In this respect jargon had meaning in the way delusions about a paralyzed limb or selective silence in answer to questions about it may be felt by the examiner as meaningful. As in cases of anosognosia occurring with lesions of the non-dominant hemisphere (Weinstein and Cole, 1963), other alterations of language, including disorientation for place and/or time, confabulation and delusional reduplication (reduplicative paramnesia) were also present. These phenomena are classed as metaphorical in that personal experience are represented in terms of the physical environment; as events, places, objects and other people. In this formulation jargon is a mixture of aphasia and anosognosia in which the patient's attempt at metaphorical representation results in a highly personalized idiom, incomprehensible in the framework of referential speech.

The purpose of this paper is to determine the degree to which this formulation applies to jargon aphasia as a whole. Specifically, jargon will be considered in terms of:

1) the conditions of altered brain function,

2) the characteristics of jargon,

3) the association with other changes in language,

4) the comparison with non-jargon (standard) aphasics on a test of linguisitic skills.

METHOD

Eighteen patients with jargon aphasia were studied and compared with 26 standard aphasics, to be defined in a moment. Patients here considered as jargon aphasics were those who over a period of at least two weeks consistently produced speech which was incomprehensible to listeners but which seemed to be regarded as meaningful by the patients themselves. Standard aphasics were those commonly regarded as clinically aphasic, who did not use jargon speech or marked verbal stereotypy, and who were not markedly dysarthric. As jargon is seen less frequently, the 18 cases of jargon aphasia were collected over a longer period of time and included more civilians as compared to military (six civilians in the jargon group, two civilians among the standard aphasics). This was a factor in the age difference between the two groups; a mean of 42.9 years for the jargon and 31.4 years for the standard aphasics.

Patients were interviewed once or twice a week over periods up to several months. The interview was structured, kept its basic form through successive sessions and was transcribed verbatim. It included questions as to the patient's main symptoms, his reason for coming to the hospital and specific questions about particular disabilities such as the speech defect. Questions designed to elicit the presence of disorientation for place and time, confabulation and reduplicative delusions for place, time and person (reduplicative paramnesia) were also given. When these phenomena were marked and persisted through more than one interview, they were rated as + +. When they occurred in only a single session, they are scored as + (Table 9-1). Other, presumably less stressful, questions concerned the patient's home life and military history. A record was made of content, of rate and amount of speech

TABLE 9–1. CLINICAL PATHOLOGICAL FINDINGS IN JARGON APHASIA (CASES 1 TO 18) AND STANDARD APHASIA (CASES 19 TO 38)

Case	Sex	Age	Lesion	Neurological Findings	Disorientation Reduplication Confabulation
1	M	33	Aneurysm, junction of R. anterior cerebral, anterior communicating arteries	Transient R. hemiparesis after craniotomy	++
2	M	32	Closed head trauma, basilar skull fracture	Bilateral papilledema	++
3	M	34	Closed head trauma	None	++
4	M	43	L. frontal glioblastoma crossing midline to R. frontal lobe	Slight R. hemiparesis, bilateral extensor plantar responses	++
5	M	35	Meningioma involving L. sphenoid wing, middle fossa, clivus. Extension to posterior fossa	L. lateral rectus palsy. Left hemiparesis progressing to quadriparesis	++
6	M	22	Clcsed head trauma. Left parietal subdural hematoma	Bilateral papilledema. R. homonymous hemianopia.	++
7	M	24	Closed head trauma. Multiple skull fractures	Optic atrophy, blindness in O.S. Right temporal visual field defect	++
8	F	47	R. frontal glioblastoma extending deeply to midline	Bilateral papilledema. Ataxic gait	++
9	M	74	Senile Dementia (?)	Incoordination L.U.E. Extinction on D.S.S.	++
10	M	60	Metastasis to floor of anterior fossa of carcinoma of spheno-ethmoid sinus	Bilateral papilledema. Extinction on D.S.S.	++
11	M	41	Left parietal, occipital cystic astrocytoma	Anosmia, bilateral papilledema. Paralysis of R. lateral gaze, R. hemiparesis, hemisensory loss and R. homonymous hemianopia. L.-sided seizures	++
12	M	44	Bilateral aneurysms of Circle of Willis	Transient R. hemiparesis after craniotomy	++
13	M	59	Closed head trauma	Mild left hemiparesis	++
14	F	54	Multiple metastases from carcinoma of breast	Bilateral papilledema	++
15	M	47	Multiple metastases from carcinoma of lung	Bilateral papilledema	++
16	M	40	Closed head trauma. L. subdural hematoma	R. Babinski sign.	++
17	F	40	Left cerebral infarct, xanthochromic CSF, hypertension. Previous left hemiparesis	Incoordination L.U.E. Extinction on D.S.S.	?
18	M	52	Closed head injury	Slight R. hyperreflexia	+
19	M	19	L. temporal parietal astrocytoma	R. hemiparesis	+
20	F	41	L. sphenoid ridge meningioma	Sl. weakness R.U.E.	None
21	M	35	L. parietal temporal vascular malformation	R. hemiparesis and sensory loss	None

22	M	33	Aneurysm R. internal carotid artery	R. hemiplegia	None
23	F	28	Melanoma L. fronto-parietal area	R. hemiplegia	None
24	M	41	Meningioma, L. parietal occipital area	R. hemiplegia R. homonymous hemianopia	None
25	M	21	Closed head trauma	R. hemiplegia	++
26	M	32	? Occlusion L. middle cerebral artery	R. hyperreflexia	None
27	M	26	L. occipital A-V malformation (post excision)	R. homonymous hemianopia	None
28	M	49	L. cerebro vascular accident	R. hemiplegia and hemisensory loss	None
29	M	22	Laceration left fronto-parietal region	Marked R. hemiparesis and hemisensory loss	None
30	M	30	L. cerebral vascular occlusion	Marked R. hemiparesis	None
31	M	19	Aneurysms of R. internal carotid and bifurcation of L. anterior and middle cerebral arteries	R. hemiplegia and hemisensory loss	+
32	M	42	Metastatic liposarcoma L. parieto-occipital juncture	R. homonymous hemianopia; weakness of RUE	+
33	F	43	Ablation of anterior 6.5 cm of L. temporal lobe for seizures	R. superior quadrant visual field defect	None
34	M	21	Hematoma L. centrum semiovale extending beneath Broca's area to internal capsule	Marked R. hemiparesis and hemisensory loss	None
35	M	24	L. posterior parietal A-V malformation (post excision)	Mild weakness RUE Mild sensory loss RUE	None
36	M	48	L. parietal skull fracture	None	None
37	M	43	Metastatic lesion L. frontal lobe (post excision)	R. hemiplegia	None
38	M	18	Closed head injury	R. hemiplegia	None
39	M	24	L. parietal hematoma; ? vascular malformation	Mild R. hemiparesis	None
40	M	19	L. sided subdural hematoma particularly L. frontal	Mild R. hemiparesis	None
41	M	46	Metastatic tumor 1 cm below cortical surface beneath superior and upper middle frontal gyrus	Marked R. hemiparesis particularly RUE	None
42	M	24	L. parietal skull fracture and removal of L. epidural	Weakness R. face; R. hyperreflexia	+
43	M	51	? L.-sided vascular disease (no arteriogram)	Marked weakness R. face; mild weakness arm greater than leg	None
44	M	47	L.-sided vascular disease with multiple plaques on arteriography	Mild R. facial weakness, R. hyperreflexia	None

and of syllabic repetitions, hesitations and fillers such as "uh." Observations were also made of mood and gesture in the interview and notes were taken of casual, informal conversations with other patients, relatives and ward staff.

In addition to the procedures outlined above and the usual clinical neurological examination, subjects were tested on their ability to name 30 common objects and to interpret 15 common idiomatic expressions such as "getting the upper hand" and "looking through rose-colored glasses." The latter were scored not only for the number correct, but for the number of self-references used in the course of the interpretation. All of the 26 standard aphasics were given both tasks, while only ten of the jargon patients were tested on both object naming and idioms. This occurred because the jargon group was seen over a longer span of time and not all received the identical testing. These two tests are part of a longer *Language Test,* which involves ability to rhyme, give alliterations and use synonyms, antonyms, homonyms and acronyms, and perform calculations. Because of these discrepancies only the results of the two procedures described above will be reported in this paper.

OBSERVATIONS

Clinical pathological findings

These findings are summarized in Table 9-1 (see p. 94-95).

Of the 18 jargon cases, 7 patients had had acute head injuries, 3 had primary infiltrating tumors, 3 had metastatic lesions, 1 had a diffuse tumor of the base of the skull, 2 had had ruptures of aneurysms of the Circle of Willis, 1 was presumed to have senile dementia and 1 patient had had a cerebro-vascular accident.

In 14 of the cases the jargon came on acutely; after trauma, craniotomy or aneurysmal rupture. In all instances there was damage to the left (dominant) hemisphere with additional involvement of the other hemisphere. (All subjects were right-handed, except for one, Case 9, who was ambidextrous.) In Case 8 the tumor was mainly in the right frontal lobe even though the EEG abnormalities were mainly on the left side, while a patient (Case 11) with a left parieto-occipital astrocytoma had left-sided seizures. A patient (Case 17), whose jargon came on after a cerebral vascular accident associated with hypertension, had a history of a left hemiplegia three years previously. There was a paucity of unilateral right-sided sensori-motor loss. Only one patient had a marked or persisting right hemiparesis or hemisensory defect. Three had a right homonymous hemianopia.

The brain damage in the standard aphasics was more unilateral. The group included only 2 patients with closed head injury and only 1 with a primary infiltrating tumor. Clinically while 17 of the jargon group showed disorientation, confabulation and reduplication, only 5 of the standard aphasics did so. A striking difference lay in the incidence of hemiparesis and hemisensory loss, which occurred in 15 of the standard aphasics and only one of the jargon cases. Each group contained 3 subjects with right homonymous hemianopia.

Characteristics of jargon

The jargon consisted of phonetic distortions, of mispronounced words, of neologisms, of standard English words put together in meaningless sequence and of sentences seemingly irrelevant to the subject under discussion. Except in 2 cases (Cases 7 and 17), the phonetic structure was preserved in that the patients used phonetic combinations throughout that could be readily spelled and transcribed. In all cases, the rhythm and intonations of formal speech were preserved. All patients were clinically aphasic, but all but one (Case 17) could understand and cooperate in formal testing. Compared to standard aphasics, the jargon patients used very few "uh's," hesitations and syllabic repetitions and more unusual, "low frequency" words. They talked more than twice as much as the other aphasics but, although some were characterized as verbose, as a group, they did not talk more than paraplegics or patients with right brain lesions.

No patient used jargon exclusively and the

amount varied from a few jargon utterances to most of the total output. The degree of jargon depended in large part on what the patient was asked, how much he spoke and what he seemed to be trying to talk about. Some patients spoke well for a single sentence and jargon resulted when attempting to say more. Jargon occurred particularly when a patient seemed to be trying to explain, discuss or rationalize. Generally, the jargon was most severe in response to queries about disability and hospitalization, and in situations where the patient's capacities were being tested. Questions such as "what is your main trouble" yielded more jargon than those concerning the patient's family or when casual topics were discussed. The subject with the least jargon (Case 12) talked normally except when answering questions about his craniotomy. One patient (Case 7) was unintelligible only when referring to his accident. In another instance (Case 2) the patient gave a jargon distortion of a word when talking about his accident, but used the same word correctly in another context. In two instances, the nursing staff noticed no speech abnormalities in patients who used marked jargon in formal interviews and testing. Some patients would begin to speak normally, but would lapse into jargon when apparently trying to deal with themes of incapacity. Jargon was commonly elicited when a patient was pressed for an explanation of some error in speech. When one man (Case 1) was asked about a discrepancy in his location of the hospital, he explained that "each of these sections is divided percentagewise categorically across the country."

All subjects seemed unaware of their speech disturbance and talked and acted as if they were being understood. Of the 18 subjects 14 (Cases 1, 5, 6, 7, 8, 9, 11, 12, 13, 14, 15, 16, 17, 18) explicitly and consistently denied any difficulty in speaking and putting their thoughts into words when specifically asked. They also denied other disabilities such as motor weakness and visual defects. Even after speech had improved these patients seemed reluctant to admit that they had ever had any difficulty. Those patients who admitted some speech disturbance verbally were highly euphoric and, at times, paranoid. Three of them clowned and showed a bantering quality. One man (Case 6) boasted that he could speak four languages and went about accosting people in a kind of pseudo-Japanese. Another (Case 5) would hum and whistle in interviews, and would use such "French" expressions as "je ne scold pas" as when asked to give a synonym for the word "scold" on the *Language Test.* Patients with explicit verbal denial were not ludic, but serene and affable. They were particularly apt to use "officialese" involving professional, administrative and technical terms. The so-called catastrophic reaction was conspicuously absent in the jargon patients in contrast to the behavior of the standard aphasics, who frequently became upset over their errors. The only suggestion of a catastrophic reaction came in Case 17. While she would deny her speech deficit verbally, she occasionally was tearful. In one interview, in which she used marked jargon and slurring, she wept after making the clear utterance "I don't understand."

Associated changes in language

All jargon patients, with one possible exception, showed one or more of the following: confabulation, particularly about the onset of the illness or the reason for coming to the hospital; disorientation for place and time; and reduplicative delusions for place, time and person. The possible exception (Case 17) was the patient whose jargon was so severe that it was difficult to determine whether she was disoriented or confabulatory. At times it was difficult to differentiate disorientation for date from the aphasic defect itself, but such patients also had confabulations and reduplicative delusions. These occurred in the same interviews in which jargon appeared or came on after the jargon had improved. As with the jargon itself, the patients did not respond to correction or indicate in any fashion that they were aware of any inaccuracy in the way they designated events, places, people, things or units of time.

In 10 subjects the jargon cleared in the course of clinical improvement. In 9 of these some of the same questions that had yielded jargon now produced confabulations, reduplicative delusions or other forms of metaphorical or idiomatic speech. For example, in Case 1, the subject had originally answered the question of why he had come to the hospital with a jumble of officialese. Subsequently, he gave a number of confabulations including going into the bookbinding business and getting a janitorial job.

Jargon was also succeeded by, and associated with, euphemisms, colloquialisms, malapropisms, jokes, pedantic redundancies and other idiomatic and idiosyncratic expressions. A patient (Case 5) with a quadriparesis and history of sexual impotence referred to "weakness of the storage on my battery" and to being "sexually immune." In Case 1, after the patient no longer used jargon or confabulation, he stated that he had come to the hospital because "one facility was not working and they rectified that." Another man referred to the interviewer as "a leader of discovering injuries and illnesses." In Case 4, the patient attributed some scalp irritation after craniotomy to the "advent of some pills."

Another analog and sequel of jargon was the use of a term referring to some aspect of disability in another context or as a figure of speech. For example, in Case 2, after jargon had cleared, the patient complained of the "cussing" and "bad language" used by another soldier on the ward. Another patient, whose jargon followed the repair of an intracranial aneurysm, expressed worry about "going in debt over my head." Another man, who had been restrained for restlessness, when quizzed about his behavior, referred to a "confining job" and to a hospital whose functions were "confined" to certain conditions.

In some cases words literally referring to disability and military status were used repetitively, both in referring to the disability and in other contexts. Thus the patient with the quadriparesis (Case 5) repeated "grip" not only in reference to his weakness but in terms of a grasp of the situation. In Case 6, the patient was left with a visual field defect after his jargon cleared. Formerly, when asked about his accident, he had replied in jargon. Later, when questioned about it, he described it as follows: "I had a wreck, sir, an automobile accident (correct). I seem to don't remember. *See* I was going down the road . . . I was doing about 60 m.p.h. until I came to this place. It was foggy, so I slowed down to 40 or so I could *see*. I rolled my window down and put my head out of the window, so I could keep from *looking* out the shield and since I slowed down to 60, I wanted to *look* at this girl. I think it was awfully messy outside and I *looked* at her to ask her if she was in any sort of mind or mad at me for something or other and that is when the car hit the fence post." (Italics are ours).

These idioms, colloquialisms, stock phrases and other figures of speech are analogous to jargon in their selectivity and representation of problems of illness and disability. Just as the jargon patients appeared unaware of their speech disturbance, so did they seem unmindful of any malapropism or double meaning. Like jargon, these figures of speech served as an adaptation to the stresses of disability. The patients in whom these figures of speech occurred continued to be unperturbed and unworried about their residual deficits, even though some dysphasia remained. The only patient (Case 17), who showed a "catastrophic reaction" after the clearing of jargon, was the one in which jargon was not replaced by analogous figures of speech.

Language test

Results are given in Table 9-2.

There was no significant difference between the two groups in scores of object-naming or interpretation of idioms, so that in these respects the degree of aphasic impairment can be considered about equal.

Jargon patients differed, however, in their handling of the test. They did not acknowledge their errors or comment on wrong answers. They also differed from the standard aphasics in that "I don't know" and "I never heard that before" answers were not given. No "catastrophic reactions" were observed, while expressions of disappointment and frustration were common among the standard aphasics. As in formal interviews, jargon cases were wordier and used more pedantic, circumlocutory and flowery language. For example, the hands of a clock were called "indicators," and a plastic straw was designated by one patient as "a little apparatus called a sucking utensil."

TABLE 9–2.

	Jargon Aphasics	*Standard Aphasics*
Naming of Objects	$\bar{X} = 13.8$ (N = 16)	$\bar{X} = 16.7$ (N = 26)
	$S_{\bar{d}} = 3.05$, $t_{40} = 0.95$ NS	
Interpretation of Idioms	$\bar{X} = 4.0$ (N = 10)	$\bar{X} = 5.4$ (N = 26)
	$S_{\bar{d}} = 1.41$, $t_{34} = 1.01$ NS	
Number of Self-References	$\bar{X} = 3.9$ (N = 10)	$\bar{X} = 0.7$ (N = 26)
	$S_{\bar{d}} = 1.14$, $t_{34} = 3.83$ $p < .001$	

Jargon patients used misinterpretations of idioms to refer to personal matters, particularly those concerning illness, incapacity and professional status. The difference between the mean number of self-references for the two groups was highly significant ($p < .001$). Eight of the 10 jargon patients made such self-referential comments, while only 8 of the 26 standard aphasics did so. Of these standard aphasics who used self-references, the mean number used was 2.2 as compared to a mean of 4.8 self-references for the eight jargon aphasics. Thus, jargon aphasics not only used more self-references as a group but used them in greater number when they did appear. When the standard aphasics used self-reference, it was frequently not incorporated into the interpretation itself but was often a comment on failure, such as "I made a mess of that" or "back to school for you, Betty." There was no correlation between the number of errors and the number of self-references.

Even though jargon aphasics seemed completely unaware of any speech disturbance and would deny it vigorously when specifically questioned, there were references to speech in the idiom interpretation. Thus, one patient interpreted "butter-fingered" as "not articulating with your fingers." Long rambling references to work, couched in "officialese," were especially common.

The standard aphasics frequently simply repeated the idiom or gave a completely literal interpretation. When a jargon patient replied "concretely," he usually added a self-reference. Thus a patient with a left hemiparesis interpreted "caught flat-footed" as "caught—uh square-footed. Right foot even with the left foot"; or the interpretation might be a vehicle for humor as "I don't know who wants his foot in his mouth. I wouldn't want anyone's foot in my mouth."

Case reports

Case 2. A 32-year-old Army sergeant was in an automobile accident in Germany, sustaining fractures of his right humerus and left ankle. He was unconscious and hyperthermic for five days, and there was blood in the right external auditory canal, bilateral papilledema and bilateral extensor plantar reflexes. X-rays revealed a right parietal linear fracture and multiple long bone fractures. Cerebrospinal fluid was under an opening pressure of 320 mm of water; it was xanthochromic and contained 400 red blood cells and a total protein of 57 mg per 100 ml. Electroencephalographic examination showed "a basic patter of 10 cycles per second and suppression of activity in the left fronto-temporal areas." Three weeks after injury bilateral burr-holes revealed discoloration and contusion of the cortex, more marked on the left.

In the initial interview his right arm was still in a cast. He was euphoric throughout. The following is verbatim:

Doctor: Hello.
Patient: Hi, sir.
Doctor: What is your full name?
Patient: Edward Clarence Herzog. [Correct]
Doctor: Serial number?
Patient: RA 00000000. [Correct]
Doctor: What is your main trouble?
Patient: Just my arms and my one leg. It has been ripped open and it's getting pretty good now.
Doctor: How did it come about?
Patient: I think it was caused by a rood over in Koreeja. Corec reejus over in Koreeda.
Doctor: Why did you come to the hospital?
Patient: They sent me back, sir, on my one arm. I had one arm here in Koreejit and this one here on

for a corgent. They took part of that on the way back in [motioning to his cast] and my rove was renetted up and we got a crane secker that's where I got my injury in my head and my base. Both of my eyes were blacked and this lady that brought me back took it out. She was a captain, a nurse.

Doctor: Are you worried?

Patient: In a little way, I would like to go back on duty.

Doctor: What's today's date?

Patient: 22nd. of September. [24th.]

Doctor: Year?

Patient: 1953.

Doctor: What is the full name of this place?

Patient: Place they give you medicine.

Doctor: What is the name of it?

Patient: [No answer.]

Doctor: What kind of place is it?

Patient: It's an Army Hospital.

Doctor: You don't know the name?

Patient: They told me several times, sir, but things I got—sometimes I forget things. Hard in the last week to remember things.

Doctor: Why?

Patient: I don't know, sir. When my speaking . . . I get mixed up on words and times I different announce them over in Koreeda and canajit.

Doctor: Where is your home?

Patient: Georgia.

Doctor: Where in Georgia?

Patient: Farmville. [Correct]

Doctor: How far is that?

Patient: About 700 miles. [Correct]

Doctor: How long does it take to get there?

Patient: Almost a day, sir, because you have to go to Ohio and go to Cincinnati. That's close by.

Doctor: How do you sleep?

Patient: Pretty nice, sir. Last night I had a little trouble. The Major worked on my head yesterday. It got to hurting me.

Doctor: Did you have an accident?

Patient: Yes, sir.

Doctor: What kind?

Patient: Headquarters, M.P.

Doctor: What happened?

Patient: Over there? Well, sir, I was in Northern Korea and we had a place there, an outpost, and we guarded that. Got chased out of there and went down south and set up there to guard headquarters.

Doctor: But how did you get hurt this time?

Patient: This was through . . . I got hurt in the corbit was part of it too.

He named a pencil correctly, but gave "arptray" for ash tray; "keternic" for straw; "pridgit" for pitcher; "camel, rijit" (note perserveration) for cigarette; "ribitjav" for wheel chair; "canpaytrug" for crutch and "corat or ritjay" for cast.

In the next interview, five days later, his speech was improved in that he used fewer neologisms. Again, these appeared mainly when he was speaking about the accident as follows:

Doctor: What happened to you? What kind of an injury did you have?

Patient: I know, sir, I got through a marint with a truck and I know I got hurt in Korea, but I don't know whether it was incorpulate or whether I got shot.

Doctor: Anything the matter with your arms?

Patient: Yes, sir. I had this leg hurt. It was in pretty bad conshape.

There was repetitive use of the word "straighten."

Doctor: Are you worried about your condition?

Patient: Yes, sir. I try to figure out if I did things I can straighten out. Like I said, I hate to hurt the Arminy.

Doctor: If you had one wish, what would it be?

Patient: To get back on duty and try to straighten things out and see if I did anything wrong.

Doctor: Are you sleeping well?

Patient: Pretty good, sir.

Doctor: Have you had any dreams?

Patient: Sometimes, sir.

Doctor: About what?

Patient: Things my mind tries to straighten out, trying to figure out things.

Doctor: You think your speech is getting better?

Patient: Yes, sir. I am hoping I straighten it out O.K. because I like to stay in the Arminy.

Nevertheless, he showed no evidence throughout the interview that he was aware of speech errors. He showed reduplication for place, referring to a Walter Reed in New York. There was reduplication for the accident, the patient talking about a motor cycle wreck, an automobile accident with a woman and a tank wreck. He denied there was anything wrong with his arm and later said it had been fractured in Korea.

Two days later, however, he commented on his speech. He said that he had not realized other people could not understand him until he saw the puzzled looks on their faces. He used no jargon and made no errors in speech except "batoon" for "platoon." He did not use the word "straighten." He admitted having sustained his various fractures in a wreck in Germany and said his wife had told him. He was completely orientated and did not confabulate except to say he had been in an M.P. company in Germany (actually Ordnance). He expressed worry that he might be in trouble with the Army, both because of the accident and his financial accounts. He was also concerned that he had caused his wife so much worry.

The next interview was held two weeks later and the patient now used the word "straighten" only in reference to his speech. He began by referring to his speech therapy as "some of the girls come up here and try to straighten out my spelling." He recalled that "I couldn't say anything straight."

He continued to express worry about his status in the Army. He was also concerned about having talked in his sleep and what he might have said to his wife while he was disturbed. In his final interview he also expressed concern about the speech of fellow patients as follows:

> Like this boy in the next bed. He starts cussing and using bad language like I never heard before, and I've been in lots of Army Hospitals. That's strictly against regulations. I wouldn't even teach my own sons to speak that way. The Chaplain was up here and he cussed in front of him. I met a Chaplain at Fort Bliss, where my wife and kids were. I couldn't let this fellow cuss in front of him.

Comment. The case illustrates the selectivity of jargon and its association with other language patterns. It was of particular interest that he gave the neologism "Koreeja" when referring to his disability, but pronounced Korea correctly when talking about a military action.

Case 3. A 34-year-old Marine sergeant was first seen one week after sustaining a closed head injury in an automobile accident on his way home from a bar. On admission to another hospital he was found to have facial and scalp lacerations and ecchymoses. He was disoriented and unable to recall events of, and prior to, the accident. Apart from the mental status and disturbances in language, there were no abnormal neurological findings. The following are abstracted from the initial interview. The patient was pleasant and unruffled throughout.

Doctor: Now, how did your accident happen?

Patient: . . . I'm not sure. I think I just started getting trouble with colds and they found out I was tied up with some virus affair that the Army had and uh used me as a means to a cure that or . . . to put out a spread to it.

Doctor: And what's the name of the hospital?

Patient: Uh . . . patients or etimology, one of the two, I'm not sure, sir. I've been in part where you had the majority of them on the floor and some of them were not.

Doctor: Were you in an automobile accident?

Patient: Not to my knowledge I wasn't.

Doctor: I notice you have a couple of black eyes and a scar on your head. How did that happen?

Patient: Uh these, sir, I got through care of uh skin refractions uh some day while I was taking care of. I believe it was uh some areas that they were sending people into in Havana and all around they had some of these temperate discolorations and stuff like that . . .

Doctor: Do you have any trouble in putting your thoughts into words or figuring out what you mean?

Patient: No, I don't think I did. Uh I may have had at one time but it seems like I'm pretty much along the general lines of everyone else, [laughs] so I didn't do much straining to go in any particular way. My children are being raised . . . in their own country . . . thing started out.

Doctor: Do you have any trouble with your memory?

Patient: Uh . . . no, only . . . only possibly pertaining to child usage of any of the instruments, tools or anything like that.

There was less jargon when the patient was asked about events more removed from the accident.

Doctor: Where is your home? Where are you from?

Patient: Washington State. [Correct]

Doctor: Whereabouts?

Patient: Uh, Seattle, Washington. [Correct]

Doctor: Go to school out there?

Patient: Yes, sir.

Doctor: Where to?

Patient: I went to grade school in Fort Porter. I went to grade school in Seattle. I went through junior high school. Until I came into the service, then I came back in through the high school portion.

Doctor: How far did you go before the service?

Patient: Seventh or eighth grade.

On his *Language Test* he named 19 of the 30 test items. Six of 15 idioms and only one of the 18 synonyms and antonyms were solved correctly. He could give only one meaning for right. Calculation, spelling, and finger naming and placing were all done poorly.

In the next interview, three days later, jargon persisted and was mingled with confabulation. He explicitly denied any difficulty with his speech. When asked about the scars on his head, he replied:

> Uh, we were checking on mountain diseases for horses and hooves and such things as that and evidently what I have is a carry over from a foot disease of some kind, two horses that through my own usage and that as a result I'm stuck with them for the rest of my life, these scars and marks.

He continued to deny any speech difficulty. He stated that he was in San Diego and in his jargon referred to many other places where he had served as a Marine. He also mentioned children and family as:

> . . . and afterwards I was in service in Havana area somewhere around there. And as most people have, they've got families to keep records along with the local healths and mishealths and all that, and mine seems to follow pretty closely to the Cuban crisis down here, the population problem down here.

He later confabulated that his wife worked for the Red Cross and that he had four children (actually six) in Seattle.

During the period when he talked jargon in the interview situation most ward personnel had noticed nothing remarkable in his speech. Their conversation was in the nature of greetings and small talk and did not involve pressing for the details of the accident and disability.

The patient's wife was interviewed while he was in the hospital. She described him as the traditional Marine sergeant, devoted to his job and concerned about the "softness" of new recruits and policies. He was conscientious, stubborn and "married to the Marine Corps first and me second." He had never been ill and would not go to sick bay unless urged by his wife. She went into some serious problems in the marriage which had brought the couple to a consideration of divorce. The informant thought it might be partly her fault as she was frigid because of her fear of pregnancy. There had been six children, including two sets of twins and one retarded child, in the seven years of marriage. The wife believed that her husband was too demanding and arbitrary with the children and at the same time very jealous of her attention to them. Ten years previously, the patient's father had sustained a head injury in a quarrel with the patient over family matters. The episode was a near patricide as the father had been disabled and aphasic since.

Comment. The case illustrates explicit denial of the speech difficulty and the facts of the accident. It shows the degree to which the production of jargon may be influenced by the situation in which it is elicited. The formal interviews were held at the time of the Cuban crisis and there is a suggestion that the content of jargon may have been related to personal problems and spheres of identity. The patient certainly had a "population problem" at home.

DISCUSSION

The necessary conditions for jargon aphasia include a lesion of the dominant (left) hemisphere plus enough additional damage to give a disturbance of consciousness manifested by the association of jargon with confabulation, disorientation for place and time and reduplicative delusions. In all cases of jargon, bilateral brain involvement was indicated. In the only case in which a vascular lesion limited to one hemisphere appeared to have occurred, there was a history of a similar lesion involving the other hemisphere three years previously (Case 17). On the other hand, the brain disorder among the standard aphasics was more strictly unilateral and evidence of disturbance of consciousness was scant. It is not unusual, when there is an initial loss of consciousness, for a patient to present briefly first as a jargon and subsequently as a standard aphasic. These were not included in this paper for methodological reasons.

The paucity of right hemiplegia and hemisensory loss was conspicuous in the jargon group as compared to standard aphasics and this feature has been noted in the literature. Our explanation is that where there is sufficient brain damage to produce aphasia, hemiplegia and/or hemisensory loss and a disturbance of consciousness, the patient is apt to have too great a functional impairment for any substantial communication to be established. However, a relatively small temporal lobe lesion by reason of the greater connections of the temporal lobe with the limbic-reticular system may produce the necessary conditions of brain dysfunction with less diffuse damage than frontal or parietal lesions.

The study confirms Alajouanine's thesis that the explanation of jargon is not to be found in the breakdown of intrinsic speech structure. As a whole, jargon patients performed as well on language testing as did the standard aphasics and, with one exception, could understand instruction for formal testing. In the literature there has been much discussion as to the significance of receptive defects. Jargon has been attributed to the destruction of "auditory images" (Bastian, 1900; Weisenburg and McBride, 1935; Goldstein, 1948; Head, 1926; Kleist, 1962), and high level auditory discrimination defects have been held responsible for the production of jargon through a lack of auditory feedback and self-correction (Alajouanine and Lhermitte, 1964; Zangwill, 1960; Howes and Geschwind, 1964). In our series receptive difficulties were severe in only two cases and their jargon was not distinctive. It has also been noted that receptive difficulties are often mild in proportion to the degree of jargon and in some instances disappear while the jargon is still present (Wyllie, 1894; Dejerine, 1914). Also, Alajouanine has pointed out that the jargon patient can recognize the spoken jargon of others while he continues to use jargon himself. Further, what appears to be a receptive difficulty may itself be a manifestation of anosognosia. This is evidenced by the selectivity of much jargon which may appear suddenly in response to questions relating to disability after one or more fairly coherent answers of a relatively neutral nature.

Howes and Geschwind (1964) found that jargon and standard aphasics could be differentiated on the basis of word frequency studies. Standard aphasics showed higher mean frequencies, a greater number of immediate repetitions, lower rates of ad libitum word production, a lower proportion of interstitial or connective words in proportion to the above, and a higher frequency of pausal grunts and of incomplete or fragmented words. The jargon aphasics, on the other hand, showed only slight shifts in mean word frequencies, a normal or increased rate of speaking along with a normal proportion of immediate repetitions. In association tests, standard aphasics gave associations similar to those of normal subjects but with much higher latencies, while those jargon patients who could follow the instructions produced bizarre associations with relatively normal latencies. Intercorrelations among these variables are high only for standard aphasics, whereas profiles of deficit differed between mild and severe cases of the jargon type.

When these data are looked at within the context of meaning, they are applicable to the formulations of this paper. A careful perusal of the verbatim speech of standard aphasics will often show a tendency to lapse into odd words, neologisms, etc., but these are brief, typically one or two word utterances and are most often met with a reaction of frustration or annoyance on the part of the patient. His slower rate of speaking and the greater number of repetitions may represent the intensity of his efforts to cope with and convey meaning as indicated also by his essentially normal (except for latencies) responses on word association tests. This awareness may be the unifying factor that accounts for the observed intercorrelations.

The jargon patient feels that he is communicating satisfactorily and so does not show the halts, hesitations and corrections that mark standard aphasic speech. Much of what is said to him he interprets as concerning himself; hence the many rambling self-references and the pervading "officialese." Questions about illness and problems are likely to bring out the social idiom which constituted the patient's premorbid "problem solving language." The bizarre but unhesitating responses that are given in word association are attempts at self-referential usages in metaphorical, idiomatic or "humorous" speech. One subject, when asked to give a joke as part of the *Language Test*, rambled on in "joke language" of the "Pat sez to Mike" variety without ever coming to the point or conclusion—which had to be made by the exhausted examiner.

In jargon, one retains the structure if not the

substance of meaningful speech. Some sense of significance is felt even from nonsense rhymes or neologisms if they are put in a grammatical sequence. The demonstrated relationship between jargon and colloquialisms, stock phrases, clichés and officialese indicate that a sense of meaning is gotten from a particular style of speech and the anticipated response from the social environment that this language entails. The utterances of the jargon patient are bizarre to the listener who is trying to interpret them in the framework of referential speech. What is considered as jargon is to some extent variable in terms of the degree to which the listener is aware of the patient's problems and preferred social idiom.

SUMMARY

Jargon aphasia was studied as communication between speaker and listener rather than in terms of the intrinsic properties of speech. Eighteen cases were compared with 26 standard aphasics. Jargon subjects had bilateral brain involvement, showed other non-aphasic disturbances of language, denied speech difficulty and other deficits, and used jargon selectively, especially when attempting metaphorical representations of problems of disability. They did not show catastrophic reactions and, in the course of clinical improvement, the jargon was replaced by confabulations and forms of idiomatic speech such as clichés, puns and malapropisms. The greater the frequency of such verbalizations, the less was the degree of anxiety and overt concern.

On a formal test of linguistic skills the only significant difference was the marked tendency of the jargon group to interpret metaphors in a highly personalized idiom featuring themes of illness and occupation.

Jargon aphasia may be regarded as a mixture of aphasia and anosognosia in which a self-referential idiom is incomprehensible in the framework of referential speech.

REFERENCES

Ajuriaguerra, J. de, and Hécaen, H. (1960) *Le Cortex Cérébral.* Masson et Cie, Paris.

Alajouanine, T. (1956) *Verbal realization in aphasia,* "Brain," **79,** 1–28.

—— and Lhermitte, F. (1964) in *Disorders of Communication,* ed. by D. McK. Rioch and E. A. Weinstein. Williams and Wilkins, New York, Baltimore.

Allison, R. S. (1962) *The Senile Brain, A Clinical Study.* Edward Arnold Ltd., London.

Bastian, H. C. (1900) in *A System of Medicine,* ed. by T. C. Allbutt. Macmillan, London.

Brain, R. (1961) *Speech Disorders.* Butterworth, Inc., Washington.

Dejerine, J. (1914) *Sémiologie des Affections du Système Nerveux.* Masson et Cie, Paris.

Goldstein, K. (1948) *Language and Language Disturbances.* Grune and Stratton, New York.

Head, H. (1926) *Aphasia and Kindred Disorders of Speech.* Macmillan, New York.

Howes, D., and Geschwind, N. (1964) *Quantitative Studies of Aphasic Language* in Disorders of Communication, ed. by D. McK. Rioch and E. A. Weinstein. Williams and Wilkins, New York, Baltimore.

Kleist, K. (1962) *Sensory Aphasia and Amusia.* Pergamon Press, Oxford.

Weinstein, E. A., and Cole, M. (1963) *Concepts of Anosognosia,* in Dynamic Neurology, ed. by L. Halpern, Jerusalem Post Press, Jerusalem.

——, ——, Mitchell, M., and Lyerly, O. G. (1964) *Anosognosia and aphasia,* "Arch. Neurol.," **10,** 376–386.

Weisenburg, T., and McBride, K. E. (1935) *Aphasia.* The Commonwealth Fund, New York.

Wyllie, J. (1894) *The Disorders of Speech.* Oliver and Boyd, Edinburgh.

Zangwill, O. L. (1960) *Speech,* in Handbook of Physiology, Section 1, Neurophysiology, v. III. Waverly Press, Baltimore.

10

Disturbance of Gesture and Pantomime in Aphasia

HAROLD GOODGLASS
EDITH F. KAPLAN

HAROLD GOODGLASS, Ph.D., is director of psychology research at the Boston Veterans Administration Hospital.

EDITH F. KAPLAN, Ph.D., is with the department of psychology of the Boston Veterans Administration Hospital and Boston University. This work was supported in part by a grant from the Social Science Research Council and in part by Grant M-4187 from the National Institute of Mental Health.

INTRODUCTION

The literature on aphasia from the middle 1800's includes references to the ability of aphasic patients to indicate, by means of pantomime, their awareness of certain things which they cannot verbalize, as for example, how to use an object which they cannot name. However, in practice, we were impressed with the rarity with which such pantomiming is comprehensible, and the frequency with which it consists of aimless waving which leaves the examiner guessing and the patient frustrated. The present paper deals with an experimental investigation of gesture and pantomime in aphasia. The brief historical review which follows attempts to bring into focus the relevant issues.

In 1870 Finkelnburg (cited by Liepmann, 1905) introduced the concept of "asymbolia," a generalized disturbance in the capacity to express or comprehend symbols in any modality, including mimetic expression. Similarly, Jackson (1893) discussed pantomime in the context of "Words and Other Symbols." Subsequent workers including Brain (1961), Critchley (1939), Goldstein (1948) have treated the alterations in gesture and pantomime of aphasics as part of the aphasic communication disorder.

Thus Finkelnburg's concept of a central communication disorder is still implied in discussions where gestural disturbance is treated as a direct correlate of aphasia. If this idea is interpreted rigorously, it postulates a defect in representational or symbolic movements without a coexisting disturbance of movement *per se*. While treating defects in gesture and pantomime as a communication disorder in aphasia, many writers also discuss these defects in a quite different sense, in the context of ideokinetic apraxia: a disorder specific to movement. In ideokinetic apraxia as described by Liepmann (1905) there is a dissociation between the idea of the movement and its motor execution. On imitation some movements may be restored but on the whole performance is still defective. This definition includes difficulties in the purposeful manipulation of real objects as well as actions with pretended objects. While some writers, e.g. Nielsen (1951), make no distinction between these two forms of difficulty, Klein and Mayer-Gross (1957) consider difficulties in performing gestures and pretended movements a milder degree of apraxia than failures to handle actual objects correctly. Brain (1961) views

From *Brain* 86:703-720, 1963. Reprinted by permission of the editor of *Brain*.

testing for pretended actions outside of their normal context as "an exacting trial of praxis." Liepmann (1905) is the only one who unequivocally assigns all disorders of gesture and pantomime to the category of apraxia.

In an extensive study of 89 brain-injured patients Liepmann (1905) reported a high incidence of apraxic difficulty with the left hand in right hemiplegics with aphasia, a much lower incidence among right hemiplegics without aphasia, and no evidence of such a disturbance in the non-paralysed limb of left hemiplegics. He concluded that the control of all purposeful movements is in the left hemisphere; that supra-capsular lesions in the left hemisphere usually damage commissural fibres from the left brain to the right brain, which are necessary for normal performance with the left hand. For Liepmann, the significance of aphasia is that it serves as an indicator of a supra-capsular lesion as against a lesion of the internal capsule, which would produce a hemiplegia while sparing the fibres which cross to the minor hemisphere through the callosum.

In the light of these findings it is possible to clarify the issue of apraxia *v.* a central communication disorder. If we are dealing with an apractic disorder then (1) imitation as well as spontaneous production of gesture and pantomime should be disturbed; (2) this deficiency should be frequently encountered in association with aphasia, not through a causal relationship, but because of the contiguity of the pathways involved. Disturbance in gesture and pantomime should also be found, on occasion, in the absence of aphasia.

A third approach to gestural deficiency focuses on the role of non-specific intellectual damage, rather than on localizable disturbances either of movement or of communication. Goldstein (1948) believes that a general loss of abstract behavior may be manifested by the inability to execute pretended actions. Denny-Brown (1958) assigns a special use of the term "ideational apraxia" to a defect of purposeful movement which is limited to pretended actions. Denny-Brown and Goldstein both regard this defect as non-localizable. Critchley (1939) makes a single reference to the absence of gestural activity in cases of "total aphasia with gross mental deterioration." Bastian (1898) on the other hand attributes the entire gestural defect of aphasics to their "intellectual degradation." To date only one report has been found in which the relation of intellectual efficiency to gestural ability has been systematically studied. DeRenzi and Vignolo (1961) report finding expressive aphasics inferior to dements in expressive gesture.

The research reported here is based on the administration of an extensive test of gesture and pantomime to a group of 20 aphasic patients and a matched group of 19 non-aphasic brain-injured. The principal questions at issue are (1) whether with age and post-morbid intellectual level controlled, there is a difference between the aphasics and controls in ability to use gesture and pantomime, and (2) whether such a difference, if it is found, should be attributed to a central "communication disorder" in aphasia. Defining a defect in gesture as part of an aphasic communication disorder requires that it be correlated with the severity of aphasia. Furthermore, it should be distinguished from an apraxia by the absence of any related difficulty in purposeful movement *per se*, as in imitation of the examiner or in object manipulation. Secondary questions raised in the study relate to (1) specific difficulties which may exist for any definable class of gestural expression, and (2) an ordering of the difficulty of the various types of gestural movement.

Terminology

The term "gesture" is ambiguous in English. As an abstract noun, it subsumes the whole class of expressive and communicative movements, including pantomime. As a designation of a specific action, however, a "gesture" may be contrasted with a "pantomime," both of which may be considered types of gestural movements. The distinction is not a sharp one, but is based on the principle that "gestures," as used in the present study, are conventionalized movements which are generally embedded in a situation, where speech is also possible; pantomime is more improvised and ordinarily takes the place of speech when for some reason it is not possible or desirable to talk. This study excludes from consideration those gesticulations and expressive movements which may not be conventionalized, but are also properly referred to as "gestures." It may be mentioned in passing that the word signs of deaf mute sign language differ from gestures in that they are used like words in connected discourse. Their loss in aphasia may therefore be more akin to the loss of speech than to the loss of gestural ability in aphasics who are not deaf mutes.

Description of Tests

Gesture-pantomime test: Forty-six different items, divided among five types of gestural movement, were used in this test. The examination began with an introductory screening procedure in which the examiner gave the subject pantomimed instructions for manipulating some real objects. In one of the four tasks, for example, the examiner used pantomime to instruct the subject to draw an X on paper and then to erase it. None of the subjects had any difficulty in carrying out the required movements. The remainder of the examination was divided into two parts: the first half of items in each group constituted Form A; the second half constituted Form B. Half of the subjects were tested with Form A first in its entirety and then given Form B. The procedure was reversed with the remaining subjects. This counter-balancing was intended to compensate for the effects of fatigue and of practice during the test procedure. The five types of gestural movement under consideration were as follows:

(1) *Natural expressive gestures:* Commonly used, conventionalized communicative movements which give a direct action-picture of some crucial aspect of the message. Ten such items were elicited verbally, e.g. "Show me how you would hold your nose when you smell something terrible," ". . . how you would cover your ears to show it is too noisy."

(2) *Conventional gestures:* Commonly used, conventionalized communicative movements which are *not* obvious action-pictures of the message. These movements include some which have become so stylized that their original pictorial quality is no longer sufficient to identify them, e.g. saluting, showing "thumbs down." Ten items in this category were to be performed on verbal command. It was recognized that some of these gestures were lacking in universality, but in this community they were all well known.

(3) *Simple pantomime:* Improvised movements which are intended as direct representations of things, qualities or simple actions with objects. These movements may describe the physical properties of an object, such as the contour of a thumbtack, or some action imposed on the object, such as playing a piano.

(a) *Action with object.* The patient was required, on verbal command, to "Show how you would eat corn on the cob." ". . . how you would stir sugar in your coffee." Ten such items were presented.

(b) *Object description.* Three introductory buffer items consisting of pen drawings of a ring, a glass, and a banana were first demonstrated by the examiner. The patient was then required to use pantomime to convey to the examiner the idea of each of ten pictured presentations, e.g. a comb, a cigarette lighter.

Complex narrative pantomime: Improvised movements indicating sequences of actions or events, usually telescoping time and requiring inferences about causal relationships. Six pantomimed narratives of progressive complexity were given. The examiner first acted out the sequence, then verified the patient's comprehension through a multiple choice oral inquiry. For example, in the "Hot Soup" sequence the examiner pretended to pick up a spoon, place it in the soup, bring it to his mouth, startle and back away, blow twice over the pretended spoon, and then eat the soup. (This item was used for its expressiveness in spite of the poor etiquette it depicts.) The oral inquiry which followed consisted of the questions:

"Was I (a) eating soup?
(b) eating ice cream?
(c) whistling a tune?"
"Was the soup (a) too hot?
(b) too salty?"

Another more complex pantomime consisted of a "Hold-up" sequence in which the examiner first portrayed a bejewelled woman taking a walk, then a robber snatching her jewellery and running off, a call for help, and the arrival of a whistle-blowing policeman. After a set of three sequences had been demonstrated, the subject was asked to reproduce each as well as he could. The second set of three sequences was similarly administered.

To assess the patient's capacity for imitation of gestural movement, the examiner demonstrated some Natural and Conventional gestures, and Simple Pantomimes of Actions with Object. After performing the movement, the examiner first said "You know what I was doing, I was . . . (e.g. eating corn on the cob)," then repeated the movement and said, "Now you do it the way I did it."

In administering the examination, the examiner made descriptive notes, including a qualitative judgment sufficient to permit a fairly accurate reconstruction of the movement from the protocol. Subjects' difficulties in auditory comprehension were also noted. The basic scoring consisted of the assignment of the performance to one of three levels:

Adequate (Level 1): Within the expected range of intelligibility for a normal person, making allowance for awkwardness with a partially paralyzed or non-preferred limb.

Partially Adequate (Level 2): There is a discernible relation to the required movement but performance is more confused or incomplete than the patient's motor handicap could justify. Some examples of incomplete performance are pointing to the usual location of an object or indicating only the size of the object.

Totally Inadequate (Level 3): No recognizable relation to expected movement. Because it is often impossible to determine whether poor comprehension contributed to the inadequacy of performance, performances scored at Level 3 were deleted from all analyses in this study.

The basic scoring was further differentiated into a number of qualitative categories, of which the following were retained:

Gestural enhancement: Dramatizing or emphasizing a gestural movement by accompanying the required movement with additional expressive facial and/or bodily movements.

Pantomimed context: Pantomiming a situational setting in which the required movement is embedded.

Vocal overflow: In spite of instructions to refrain from verbalizing, the subject accompanies the gesture with an explanatory or exclamatory vocalization, as in saying "good-bye" while waving good-bye.

Body-part as object (BPO): Subject uses part of his body to serve as the object, as in hammering with a fist or stirring sugar with an index finger.

Scoring of gesture subtests. For Gestures and Simple Pantomime the score for each subject was a percentage, consisting of the ratio of Adequate responses, excluding *Body-part as Object*, to all Adequate plus Partially adequate responses. For Complex Pantomime the score consisted of the total number of identifiable elements produced by the subject for each sequence. No adjustment was made for the quality of performance, so long as the movement was recognizable.

Aphasia examination: A composite rank based on three separately scored sections of the Boston V. A. Hospital Diagnostic Aphasia Test served as the criterion for rating the severity of aphasia. These sections tested conversational and narrative speech, object naming and comprehension. All computations involving severity of aphasia were based on the mean rank of the aphasic subjects for these three subtests.

Wechsler Adult Intelligence Performance Scale: The Performance Scaled Score of the Wechsler Adult Intelligence Scale was used as a measure of intellectual efficiency[1] and, along with age, served as a matching criterion in the selection of the controls. The Scaled Score is the total of the weighted subtest scores and leads directly to the determination of the IQ through a table which introduces a compensation for age. In this situation it is preferable to deal with the direct measure of intellectual efficiency, which is the Performance Scaled Score, without adjustment for age.

Selection and Matching of Subjects

Twenty male aphasic patients from the Aphasia Unit of the Boston Veterans Administration Hospital were tested in this study. No restrictions were placed on age or on ætiology of the aphasia. Patients ranged in age from 24 to 74 years and consisted of mixed, predominantly expressive aphasics ranging from moderately severe to mild. Since much of the Gesture-Pantomime experiment involved oral instructions, it was necessary to eliminate severe receptive and global aphasics. It was decided that a control group of brain-injured but non-aphasic patients was essential if we were to duplicate the post-morbid intellectual efficiency of the aphasic subjects and yet have men with similar pre-morbid backgrounds. The 19 non-aphasics who constituted the control group also came from the neurological wards of this hospital. A twentieth control patient was tested but later discarded when his final diagnosis ruled out cortical damage. The remaining 19 control subjects, ranging in age from 22 to 70 years, had established diagnoses involving cerebral damage and all performed normally on aphasia screening tests of word-finding fluency and comprehension of commands. The ætiologies in both groups included cerebrovascular accidents, traumatic lesions, and post-operative brain tumours; Alzheimer's disease and post-encephalitic state were, in addition, represented in the control group. Neither group included any subjects whose onset of illness was more recent than three months prior to testing.

The experimental and control groups were closely matched in age and intellectual efficiency. Mean age for aphasics was 43.2 with a standard deviation of 12.9; for controls, 41.7 with a standard deviation of 14.0. Mean Performance Scaled Score for aphasics was 33.9 with a standard deviation of 10.7; for controls, 32.0 with a standard deviation of 10.2. These Scaled Scores correspond to mean Performance IQ's of 84 and 82 respectively.

The characteristics of the subject populations were further examined to see how closely age was related to intellectual deterioration within each group and to the severity of aphasia within the aphasic group.

[1] Digit Symbol subtest, which is disproportionately difficult for right hemiplegics was omitted and prorated in all cases.

Spearman rank order correlations were computed in each case.

It is apparent from Table 10-1 that the older aphasics were significantly more handicapped in speech than the younger ones. In the control group, the intellectual superiority of the younger patients is greater than can be attributed to chance. If the two groups had not been matched with respect to both age and intellectual efficiency it would have been impossible to distinguish the effects of the one from the other. The importance of matching for age and intelligence when dealing with brain-injured populations is underlined.

TABLE 10-1. SPEARMAN RANK ORDER INTERCORRELATIONS BETWEEN THE CRITERION VARIABLES (AGE, PERFORMANCE SCALED SCORE; SEVERITY OF APHASIA) FOR APHASIC AND CONTROL GROUPS

Correlated variables	Aphasics (N = 20)*	Controls (N = 19)*
Age × Scaled Score	−.32	−.57
Age × Severity of Aphasia	.42	—
Severity of Aphasia × Scaled Score	−.45	—

* Spearman rho of at least .39 is required for significance (p = .05) with 19 cases; a rho of .38 is required with 20 cases.

Reliability of Scoring

Our definitions of the levels of adequacy depend on a consensus as to the "normal range of intelligibility" of gestural movements. It is obvious that some movements are inherently more informative than others (e.g. "combing hair" *v.* "stirring sugar"). The rater's judgment was therefore based on how close the subject came to a "normal" attempt, rather than on the absolute intelligibility of the movement.

In order to test judge reliability, motion pictures with sound were made of three patients performing a total of 65 gestural movements taken from this experiment. These were observed and rated independently by five judges. Since the ratings must be converted to rank order scores it was decided to group the items into randomly grouped sets of five, as a means of avoiding an inordinate number of tied ranks. Inter-judge agreement as tested by Kendall's coefficient of concordance yielded a coefficient of .83, which is in the range of acceptability for individual clinical tests.

RESULTS

Intellectual Efficiency and Gestural Ability

The main body of data concerning the relation between post-morbid intellectual efficiency and capacity to use gesture and pantomime is summarized in Tables 10-2 and 10-3. Upon inspection of Table 10-2 it may be seen that the Gesture subtests are easier than the Pantomime subtests for both aphasics and controls. Further, there is a distinct progression in performance on both Simple Pantomime subtests as one moves from the groups with lowest to highest intellectual efficiency; this relationship is not apparent for the tests of Natural and Conventional Gestures, where there are comparatively few failures in either group. It may be that the distinction between Natural and Conventional Gestures is an artificial one. Most of the items in both subtests are highly over-learned and affectively charged. For the items used here, the pictorial quality of the Natural Gestures adds negligibly to the ease of performance.

The progression of score with intellectual level is particularly apparent in the Complex Pantomime subtest for both aphasics and controls. Inspection of the table of correlations (Table 10-3) computed for the foregoing data also reveals the significant influence of intellectual efficiency on both Simple and Complex Pantomime and its negligible influence on Gestures. While it is noted that the correlation coefficients in each instance are higher for the controls than for the aphasics, the size of our sample does not permit enough precision to evaluate the significance of these differences.

Returning to Table 10-2, it is at once apparent that the aphasic subjects were less adequate than the non-aphasic brain-injured in every type of gestural task. Moreover, while the order of difficulty for the types of performance is the same for both groups, the spread in scores between the easiest section (Natural Gestures) and the most difficult (Object Description) is considerably greater for the aphasics than for the controls.

The inferiority of the aphasics to their intellectual counterparts among the controls is found uniformly at all Scaled Score levels. In

TABLE 10–2. RELATION OF GESTURE AND PANTOMIME SCORES TO HIGH, INTERMEDIATE AND LOW PERFORMANCE SCALED SCORES, FOR APHASICS AND CONTROLS

	Mean percentage of fully adequate performance				Mean
	Natural gestures	Convent. gestures	Pantomime (object description)	Pantomime (action with object)	Score Complex pant.
APHASICS					
Scaled Score under 31 (N = 9)	83	74	20	25	16
Scaled Score 31 to 40 (N = 5)	77	74	23	41	24
Scaled Score over 41 (N = 6)	88	79	47	54	31
All Aphasics	83	76	29	38	24
CONTROLS					
Scaled Score under 31 (N = 9)	98	89	47	56	28
Scaled Score 31 to 40 (N = 5)	97	97	77	80	40
Scaled Score over 41 (N = 5)	95	98	70	73	42
All Controls	97	93	61	67	37

TABLE 10–3. RANK ORDER CORRELATIONS BETWEEN WAIS PERFORMANCE SCALED SCORES AND VARIOUS CATEGORIES OF GESTURAL MOVEMENT FOR APHASICS AND CONTROLS

	Gestures	Simple Pantomime	Complex Pantomime
Aphasics	.17	.48	.56
Controls	.28	.60	.85

fact, the average of the highest intellectual group of aphasics falls consistently lower than that of the most defective group of non-aphasic brain-injured.

The Mann-Whitney *U* test for significance of differences between independent groups, as described by Siegel (1956), was applied to the scores on each of the types of gesture and pantomime and the differences obtained between aphasics and controls were significant beyond the .01 level in each case.

Another approach to evaluating the influence of aphasia on gestural performance is through the correlation, within the aphasic group, between the severity of the aphasia and gestural proficiency. Table 10-4 reveals a significant correlation in the case of Complex Pantomime. The correlations for Gestures and Simple Pantomime are low enough to be considered fortuitous were they given out of context. From our limited sample, we cannot say with assurance whether the strength of the relation of Complex Pantomime to severity of aphasia is an accident of sampling or whether it represents a special feature of the Complex Pantomime task. In so far as Complex Pantomime leans considerably on the comprehension of verbal instructions, it is more likely that it would be linked to the

TABLE 10–4. RANK ORDER CORRELATIONS BETWEEN SEVERITY OF APHASIA AND GESTURAL PERFORMANCE

Types of gestural movement	Rho.
Gestures	–.26
Simple Pantomime	–.39
Composite Gestures and Pantomime	–.36
Complex Pantomime	–.66

severity of aphasia than would the other gestural subtests.

Tables 10-3 and 10-4 indicate that the Gesture and Simple Pantomime scores are related to intellectual efficiency to about the same degree as they are related to severity of aphasia. However, the fact that intellectual efficiency and severity of aphasia are also correlated raises the question as to which variable is carrying the burden of the correlation obtained with gestural proficiency. The strong relationship between Scaled Score and the Gesture-Pantomime scores for the control group (in the absence of aphasia) suggests that intellectual efficiency is the primary determinant and hence one may conclude that increasing *severity* of aphasia has little influence on gestural ability, beyond the effects of the accompanying drop in intellectual efficiency present in this sample.

Influence of Age on Gestural Ability

It was considered likely that the younger subjects would find it easier to adapt to a test of pretended actions than would the older. It is, therefore, of some interest to examine the relationship of age to gestural capacity.

Table 10-5 summarizes the correlations between age and scores on the several types of gestural movements. These correlations appear to be slightly higher than those between gesture and intellectual efficiency (although the difference is within the range of accidental variation).

TABLE 10-5. RANK ORDER CORRELATIONS BETWEEN AGE AND GESTURAL MOVEMENTS

	Gestures	Simple Pantomime	Complex Pantomime
Aphasics	−.40	−.72	−.32
Controls	−.05	−.65	−.45

Since, in the aphasic sample, age and Scaled Score are only slightly related, it is apparent that age would retain a significant relation with gestural skills, even if the effect of intelligence were statistically "partialed out." However, this inference does not necessarily hold for the control group, where age and intellectual efficiency are more strongly related.

Table 10-5 shows that Complex Pantomime correlates less with age than does Simple Pantomime. The one explanation that comes to mind is that the Simple Pantomime score is essentially a reflection of the qualitative adequacy of performance whereas the Complex Pantomime score is simply a count of the number of recognizable elements. Our figures may indicate that the quality of gestural movements deteriorates with age more consistently than does the number of movements attempted.

Body-Part as Object

Early in the experiment it was observed that aphasics frequently used their hands or fingers to represent an intended object, as in "hammer-

TABLE 10-6. PERCENTAGE OF BODY-PART AS OBJECT RESPONSES IN UPPER AND LOWER HALVES OF POPULATION FOR THREE CRITERION VARIABLES

	Composite Score on Gesture and Pantomime		WAIS Performance Scaled Score		Severity of Aphasia
	Aphasics	Controls	Aphasics	Controls	Aphasics
Upper half of distribution	14	6	21	7	19
Lower half of distribution	29	25	22	23	24
Sign.* of diff. between upper and lower halves	+	+	n.s.	+	n.s.

* Determined by Mann-Whitney *U* Test.
+ Represents significance at the .05 level or better.

ing" with the fist as the hammer, or "brushing teeth" with the index finger as the toothbrush. This phenomenon, termed *Body-Part as Object* (BPO) was also observed by one of the authors (E.K.) to predominate in children of preschool age.

Table 10-6 summarizes the distribution of BPO performances for the aphasic and control groups on the 20 items of Simple Pantomime. The results are given as percentages, since items which elicited total failure (21 percent for aphasics; 0.8 percent for controls) were omitted from the computations. The table divides the subjects into upper and lower halves with respect to the following variables: composite score on Gesture-Pantomime tests; intellectual level (WAIS Performance Scaled Score); severity of aphasia. The total number of BPO responses for aphasics was 77 or 22 percent; the number of controls was 56 or 15 percent. This difference, tested by the Mann-Whitney *U* test, was found to be significant at the .05 level of confidence. The differences between the aphasics and controls are confined to the upper halves of the distribution; the non-aphasics in the upper halves made very few BPO responses, while those in the lower halves performed like aphasics in this respect, with 23 to 25 percent BPO. Aphasics, whether high or low in the Performance Scaled Score and aphasia severity measures, produced the same proportion: about one in 4 or 5 responses.

We observed earlier that performance of Gestures and Simple Pantomime was clearly influenced by the *presence* of aphasia but only indifferently related to the *severity* of the aphasia. It is curious to note that BPO is also little influenced by the severity of aphasia. However, the aphasics who scored in the upper half of their group in *gestural* ability averaged only half as many BPO responses as did those who scored in the lower half.

Vocal Overflow

A common occurrence during the test performance was the emission of an exclamatory remark intended to supplement the gesture which was being portrayed: for example, exclaiming "Stop!" while demonstrating the movement of signalling someone to stop. It appeared to the authors that *vocal overflow* was a manifestation of the patient's inability to separate the representation or pretended action from his immediate involvement in the action. However, for the sake of scoring, no penalty was applied to movements which were otherwise adequate. Table 10-7 presents the distribution of *vocal overflow* responses for the aphasic and control groups on the 20 items of Natural and Conventional Gestures. *Vocal overflow* appears to be more characteristic of the total aphasic population. It occurs with no significant difference, in the upper and lower halves of the distribution on all the criteria (gestural ability, Scaled Score and severity of aphasia). The total incidence of *vocal overflow* for aphasics was 54 or 16 percent as contrasted with 17 or 4 percent for

TABLE 10–7. PERCENTAGE OF VOCAL OVERFLOW IN UPPER AND LOWER HALVES OF POPULATION FOR THREE CRITERION VARIABLES

	Composite on Gesture and Pantomime		WAIS Performance Scaled Score		Severity of Aphasia
	Aphasics	Controls	Aphasics	Controls	Aphasics
Upper half of distribution	11	1	15	4	14
Lower half of distribution	16	6	16	5	18
Sign.* of diff. between upper and lower halves	n.s.	+	n.s.	n.s.	n.s.

* Determined by Mann-Whitney *U* Test.
\+ Represents significance at the .05 level or better.

TABLE 10–8. PERCENTAGE OF GESTURAL ENHANCEMENT IN UPPER AND LOWER HALVES OF POPULATION FOR THREE CRITERION VARIABLES

	Composite Score on Gesture and Pantomime		WAIS Performance Scaled Score		Severity of Aphasia
	Aphasics	Controls	Aphasics	Controls	Aphasics
Upper half of distribution	14	13	11	13	14
Lower half of distribution	5	4	9	12	6
Sign.* of diff. between upper and lower halves	n.s.	+ +	n.s.	n.s.	n.s.

* Determined by Mann-Whitney *U* Test.
+ + Represents significance at the .01 level.

the controls. The difference, between aphasics and controls, was found to be significant at the .02 level of confidence, using the Mann-Whitney *U* test.

Gesture Enhancement and Pantomimed Context

The intensification of a gesture by means of supportive facial expressions or other accompanying bodily movements was termed *gesture enhancement.* For example, a response to the item "Show how you would hold your nose when you smell something terrible" might consist of grimacing strongly and turning the head away while holding the nose. Another form of embellishment—this one found in performances on the Simple Pantomime items—consists of leading up to the significant pantomime elements by means of a pantomimed situational context, e.g. for "stir sugar in your coffee," elaborately spooning the sugar from a sugar bowl and pouring cream before stirring.

Comparison of Tables 10-8 and 10-9 shows these forms of embellishment to characterize the more adequate performers equally in both the aphasic and control groups.

Imitation

The facilitating effect of having a model to imitate can best be determined by inspecting the performance on imitation for those items which had been inadequately executed on verbal request. Table 10-10 shows that Natural and Conventional Gestures improve much more readily on imitation than does Simple Pantomime, for both groups of patients. The non-aphasics have a much higher rate of improvement on imitation than do the aphasics. Thus, for the non-aphasics, 75 percent of the

TABLE 10–9. PERCENTAGE OF PANTOMIMED CONTEXT IN UPPER AND LOWER HALVES OF POPULATION FOR THREE CRITERION VARIABLES

	Composite Score on Gesture and Pantomime		WAIS Performance Scaled Score		Severity of Aphasia
	Aphasics	Controls	Aphasics	Controls	Aphasics
Upper half of distribution	18	19	18	18	17
Lower half of distribution	6	4	6	7	7
Sign.* of diff. between upper and lower halves	+ +	+	+	n.s.	+

* Determined by Mann-Whitney *U* Test.
+ + Represents significance at the .01 level or better.
+ Represents a level of significance at the .05 level or better.

TABLE 10-10. PERCENTAGE OF ADEQUATE AND INADEQUATE PERFORMANCES IN IMITATION FOR ITEMS INITIALLY POORLY EXECUTED

	Aphasics			Controls		
	Total Inad. Initial Perf. (No.)	Adequate Imit. (per cent)	Inad. Imit. (per cent)	Total Inad. Initial Perf. (No.)	Adequate Imit. (per cent)	Inad. Imit. (per cent)
Gestures	32	59	41	12	75	25
Simple Pant. (Action with Obj. only)	49	24	76	27	48	52
Total	81	39	61	39	59	41

originally failed Gestures are performed adequately on imitation, while only 59 percent are in the aphasic group. The difference between the two groups is more dramatic when the nonaphasics' 48 percent improvement rate for Simple Pantomime is compared to the aphasics' 24 percent. It is noteworthy that in each group, more than 80 percent of the inadequately imitated items were performed by subjects who had been classified as low in gestural ability.

DISCUSSION

Gestural Deficiency: Disorder of Communication or of Movement?

The proposition that gestural deficiency in aphasia is a consequence of a central communication disorder would have required the following evidence: (1) more severe gestural deficiency in the aphasic than in the control group, as well as (2) correlation of gestural deficiency with severity of aphasia and (3) disturbance in the formulation of movements without specific disturbance in the execution of movements (demonstrated by retained ability to imitate).

Our data verify only the first of these requirements: the inferiority of the aphasics is clearly established, and in this respect our results coincide with the recent report by DeRenzi and Vignolo (1961) as well as the earlier finding by Liepmann (1905). However, no clear relation exists between the severity of aphasia and the degree of gestural deficiency. Such a relationship was found only in that portion of the experiment (Complex Narrative Pantomime) which is not corrected for the effects of poor auditory comprehension.

The relative independence of *severity* of aphasia and gestural deficiency make the hypothesis of a common psychological factor hard to maintain. The occurrence of *Body-Part as Object*, discussed below, further exemplifies the independence of a specific kind of gestural disturbance from the *severity* of aphasia, although it is more characteristic of the aphasic group.

We must therefore join with Liepmann's interpretation that certain lesions in the left hemisphere, between the posterior frontal and parietal areas, have the effect of impairing gestural ability, regardless of the presence or severity of an accompanying aphasia.

There remains point (3), the issue of whether the difficulty experienced by the aphasics is specific to the spontaneous evocation of movements for communication or extends to the task of executing purposeful movements in general. Sparing of the ability to imitate was considered by the authors to be crucial for this distinction. In the present sample, only 1 out of 4 (24 percent) of the Simple Pantomimes originally failed was done adequately by the aphasics in imitation of the examiner. The improvement rate for this type of movement was 1 out of 2 (48 percent) in the control group. As one would expect, the more highly conventionalized Gestures are not only easier on initial request, but show a higher improvement rate on imitation. Here, too, however the aphasic group was inferior to the control group. It is necessary to conclude that the difficulty for the aphasics is indeed one of *reproducing* the movements. In this regard, too, our findings are in accord with those of Liepmann (1905), who concluded that the inability of his aphasics to improve on imitation was evidence of an apraxic disturbance.

The original focus on gestural deficiency as a communication disorder made freedom from aphasia the primary criterion in the selection of control subjects. The evidence that we are actually dealing with a movement disorder having its own implications for localization, makes it necessary to re-examine the lesions involved in the non-aphasic group. Of the 19 non-aphasics, *nine* had a clearly unilateral right cerebral lesion; *one* a unilateral left, and the remaining *nine* bilateral focal or diffuse damage. Of the *nine* right cerebral cases, *six* were in the upper half of the distribution (for the control population) of composite score for gestural ability; *two* were in the middle and only *one* was near the low end of the distribution. *Six* of the *nine* bilateral cases were in the lower half of the distribution, *one* in the middle rank, and only *two* in the upper half. The *one* left hemisphere case was *fifth* from the low end of the distribution.

Could the superiority of the right cerebral group have been due to a milder degree of intellectual impairment? Inspection shows that the right cerebral group was not spared intellectually any more than the bilateral group, since each group was split half and half between the high and low portions of the distribution for Performance Scaled Score.

Thus, re-examination of the data from our control group supports that portion of Liepmann's position which places the lesion responsible for gestural disturbance in the left hemisphere.

Both Liepmann's data and our own support the thesis that such a lesion need not always be accompanied by aphasia. Of Liepmann's 20 left hemisphere cases with apraxia, 14 were aphasic, but 6 were not. Among our 10 non-aphasics whose lesions involved the left hemisphere, 5 had 24 percent or more impaired performances. One patient, for example, who had 41 percent impaired performances demonstrated how he would eat corn on the cob by rubbing his right index finger across his lips, while smacking his lips. Another subject who was impaired on 27 percent of his performances demonstrated a spoon by holding his left fist to his mouth as though it were a glass, while opening and closing his lips. These 5 patients would be considered at least mildly apractic though not aphasic.

Intellectual Efficiency

Intellectual efficiency can no longer be ignored as a factor which contributes to the capacity to perform gesture and pantomime. Its effect has been demonstrated on the quality of gestural movements in both aphasic and control groups. In this respect we differ with Liepmann's report that his non-aphasics, however demented, were unimpaired in gesture and pantomime. This difference may be accounted for by the fact that, in this study, intellectual efficiency was controlled by an objective quantitative method and that each gestural performance was scored for quality and contributed to an objective total score. Experience with the intellectual assessment of aphasic and other brain-injured patients shows that impressionistic comparisons of patients often prove to be in error.

Auditory Comprehension as a Factor

Liepmann (1905) disagreed vigorously with the opinion of his contemporaries that the impaired gesture of aphasics was simply a reflection of their poor comprehension of instructions. He cited, as evidence of adequate comprehension, the fact that patients often demonstrated their understanding of material even more complex than the instructions for movements which they failed to carry out.

On the whole, our findings agree with Liepmann's belief that the gestural deficiency of aphasics is not entirely accounted for by poor comprehension. However, it is equally clear that he did not do justice to the role of reduced auditory comprehension as a contaminating factor in the evaluation of gestural ability. It is not sufficient, as Liepmann does, to cite the well-known fact that there are apraxic patients who cannot carry out simple movements for which they clearly understand the instructions. Even in the considerably smaller population from which our sample was drawn, there were severe aphasics (both receptive and mixed) whose comprehension was too impaired to permit their utilization as subjects. Liepmann does not acknowledge any such difficulties in selection and his argument seems designed to rationalize designating as "apraxic" all of the failures of the aphasics. In the present study it has already been noted that the only subtest score which was closely related to the severity of aphasia was that for Complex Pantomime, which was not corrected for auditory comprehension. Further studies of gestural ability should control or minimize the role of auditory comprehension, perhaps through the use of pictorial stimuli to elicit the required movements.

Body-Part as Object

The phenomenon of *Body-Part as Object* (BPO) is, at first glance, a quite novel and unpredicted by-product of the lessening of gestural ability. When one observes the impaired patient (or young child) in response to the instruction to carry out an action with a pretended object, there is frequently an effort to find some actual object to take the place of the absent one. With something actually in hand to manipulate, the task no longer involves a pretended object, but an actual one. The subject's own hands and fingers are always immediately present to serve this purpose. In a personal communication. Professor Heinz Werner suggested that the subject behaves as though he really had to "stir his coffee," "comb his hair," etc., and uses his fingers out of necessity.

Thus, BPO may permit the aphasics to evade the difficult task of reproducing a movement sequence outisde of the concrete context which ordinarily elicits it. It offers the "reality" of acting on an object and, one conjectures, permits a more vivid experience of the affective component of the pretended action. One observes the performer vigorously pounding the table with his fist as the hammer, raking his hair with his fingers as the comb, or rubbing his teeth with his index finger. One may say both of the child and of the brain-injured, dyspraxic patient that BPO permits them to avoid an impaired (or, for the children, undeveloped) function.

The incidence of *vocal overflow* in the aphasic group and its near absence in the control group suggests that the aphasic has difficulty in restraining his immediate emotional involvement in the reality of the act. This loss of distance may also be one of the prerequisites for the occurrence of BPO responses.

It follows from this reasoning that the patient who has difficulty in executing a pantomime can either approximate his intention with a "partially adequate" response or have recourse to BPO for which the movements may be quite adequately performed. However, BPO enters as a possible response only when an imaginary object is part of the representation—which is not the case in intransitive pantomimes (swimming, sleeping). Liepmann (1905) made a point of testing both transitive and intransitive movements but he makes no reference to differential response to the two types of request. In the present study the only intransitive movements required came under the heading of "Gestures," such as saluting, waving good-bye, applauding. It was assumed that the higher familiarity of the Gestures was sufficient to account for their being easier than the Simple Pantomime. However, it is also possible that the problem of dealing with a pretended object in all the Simple Pantomime items contributed to their difficulty. It is suggested that the relation between transitive and intransitive pantomime be examined in further studies of gestural behavior.

Gestural Deficiency as an Apraxic Defect

The disturbance of gestural ability now appears to be adequately subsumed under the heading of idiokinetic apraxia, as defined by Liepmann (1905) and used by Sittig (1931),

Schilder (1953), and Nielsen (1951). How does defective pantomime relate to an apraxia for the manipulation of actual objects? Klein and Mayer-Gross (1957) consider the disturbance of pretended action as a milder degree of the same defect. The fact that *none of the aphasic subjects in our sample had any difficulty* in handling real objects is not necessarily incompatible with the foregoing position; however, it suggests that there is a wide gap between these two levels of impairment, if indeed they are on a continuum. Within the sphere of gestural movements, it is clear that conventionalized or overlearned movements (i.e. gestures) are less difficult to execute than improvised ones (i.e. pantomime).

It would appear that we have supported the attribution of one more higher integrative function to the already overburdened left hemisphere. A comprehensive theory to account for the physiology of cerebral lateralization of functions is long overdue.

CONCLUSIONS

(1) Aphasics have a gestural deficiency which is best understood as an apraxic disorder consequent to a left hemisphere lesion; the concept of a general communication disorder is not supported. The bases for this conclusion are:

(*a*) Aphasics were inferior in gestural ability to their intellectual counterparts in a non-aphasic brain-injured control group at each level of intellectual efficiency.

(*b*) Aphasics were less able to profit from the opportunity to imitate than were non-aphasic controls.

(*c*) When the influence of auditory comprehension was controlled, gestural ability was not related to the severity of aphasia.

(*d*) In the absence of aphasia, left hemisphere lesions produced more impaired gestural movements than right hemisphere lesions.

(2) Gestural ability is impaired in direct relation to the loss of intellectual efficiency in brain-injured patients, whether aphasic or otherwise.

Acknowledgements. The authors are greatly indebted to Dr. Fred A. Quadfasel for his invaluable help and encouragement in carrying out this research. Thanks are also due to Dr. Norman Geschwind and Dr. Robert Efron who helped clarify the issues and assisted in refining the manuscript.

REFERENCES

Bastian, H. C. (1898) "A Treatise on Aphasia and Other Speech Defects." London.

Brain, W. R. (1961) "Speech Disorders." London.

Crtichley, M. (1939) "The Language of Gesture." London.

Denny-Brown, D. (1958) *J. nerv. ment. Dis.*, **126,** 9.

DeRenzi, E., and Vignolo, L. A. (1961) Abstract of paper presented at International Congress of Neurology, Rome. (Unpublished.)

Goldstein, K. (1948) "Language and Language Disturbances." New York.

Jackson, J. H. (1893) *Med. Pr.*, **107,** 205.

Klein, R., and Mayer-Gross, W. (1957) "The Clinical Examination of Patients with Organic Cerebral Disease." London.

Liepmann, H. (1905) *Münch. med. Wschr.*, **52,** 2322 and 2375.

Nielson, J. M. (1951) "A Textbook of Clinical Neurology." 3rd edition, New York.

Schilder, P. (1953) "Medical Psychology." New York.

Siegel, S. (1956) "Nonparametric Statistics for the Behavioral Sciences." New York.

Sittig, O. (1931) "Uber Apraxie." Berlin.

11

Impaired Recognition of Meaningful Sounds in Aphasia

HANS SPINNLER
LUIGI A. VIGNOLO

HANS SPINNLER, M.D., and LUIGI A. VIGNOLO, M.D., are with the Clinica delle Malattie Nervose e Mentali of the Università di Milano, Italy. This study was supported by a grant from the Centro Nazionale delle Ricerche.

Failure to recognize meaningful sounds or noises is often reported as the most convincing evidence of "auditory agnosia." The incidence and significance of such disorder in aphasia is, however, still imperfectly known, mainly because the descriptions of individual patients showing it as a prominent feature of their clinical picture tended to emphasize its purity with respect to the language disorders, rather than discussing their mutual relationships.

The purpose of this study was to investigate impaired recognition of meaningful sounds in terms of: 1. its frequency in aphasics, as compared to non-aphasic brain-damaged patients with focal lesions of the hemispheres; 2. its incidence in the different clinical forms of aphasia, and 3. its relationship with the disorders of auditory verbal comprehension.

MATERIALS AND METHODS

Patients

Thirty-five control patients without cerebral lesions and 96 patients with focal hemispheric damage were studied: of the latter, 29 had a right hemisphere lesion, 16 had a left hemisphere lesion without aphasia and 51 had a left hemisphere lesion with aphasia. Control patients had been hospitalized in our clinic because of psychoneurosis or neurological lesions below the level of the cervical spine. The side of the lesion in brain-damaged patients was determined on the basis of the clinical findings, usually supplemented by electroencephalographic and neuroradiological investigations. Assessment of aphasia in left brain-damaged patients was made by means of a standard aphasia examination, currently used in the aphasia unit of our clinic. Left brain-damaged patients, whose scores on the oral expression, repetition and auditory comprehension subtests were lower than the normal cut-off scores, were defined as "aphasics."

The characteristics of the four experimental groups are shown in Table 11-1. No significant difference among groups existed with respect to age and educational level. By contrast, aphasic patients were significantly different from non-aphasic patients with respect to etiology and length of illness. They showed a higher incidence of cerebrovascular accidents (as opposed to trauma and tumor) and were examined mostly after more than 3 months from the onset of illness. These characteristics of the aphasic group suggest that these patients suffered from long-standing and hence relatively stable lesions, without relevant side-effects.

Aphasic patients were divided into 6 broad clinical syndromes, according to the type of speech production and to the quantity of communication possible in two modalities of

From *Cortex* 2:337–48, 1966.

TABLE 11–1. CHARACTERISTICS OF PATIENTS IN THE 4 EXPERIMENTAL GROUPS

Variables		Examined patients (N = 131)				Significance of differences
		Control patients (N = 35)	Right brain-damaged patients (N=29)	Left brain-damaged patients: Non-aphasic patients (N=16)	Left brain-damaged patients: Aphasics (N=51)	
Age	≦ 40	13	10	5	13	
	41 - 59	16	13	9	23	Overall chi^2 = 3.406; $p<.80$
	≥ 60	6	6	2	15	
Years of schooling	≦ 5	17	17	11	23	Overall chi^2 = 3.751; $p<.40$
	> 5	18	12	5	28	
Etiology	vascular	—	16	10	45	Overall chi^2=12.695; $p<.005$
	non-vasc.	—	13	6	6	Aphasics vs. other brain-damaged pts.: chi^2 = 11.514; $p < .001$ Right vs. left non-aphasic brain-damaged pts.: chi^2 = 1.183; $p < .30$
Time elapsed from onset of illness	> 3 months	—	21	11	19	Overall chi^2=10.848; $p<.005$
	≦ 3 months	—	8	5	32	Aphasics vs. other brain-damaged pts.: chi^2 = 9.696; $p<.005$ Right vs. left non-aphasic brain-damaged pts.: chi^2 = 1.162; $p<.30$

TABLE 11–2. DEFINITION AND INCIDENCE OF APHASIC SYNDROMES

Syndrome	Type of Speech Production	Oral Expression score (mx score = 4)	Auditory Comprehension score (mx score = 4)
Global aphasia (N = 5)	*Laborious articulation* Speechlessness with recurring utterances; *or* "syndrome of phonetic disintegration"	0	0–2
Broca's aphasia, severe (N = 17)	*Laborious articulation* Speechlessness with recurring utterances; *or* "syndrome of phonetic disintegration"; *or* agrammatism	0–1	3–4
Broca's aphasia, moderate and mild (N = 3)	*Slight but obvious articulatory disorders* Phonemic paraphasias with anomia; agrammatism; disprosody	2–4	3–4
Wernicke's aphasia, severe (N = 9)	*Fluent speech, without articulatory disorders* Verbal and phonemic paraphasias, neologisms and/or anomia; *or* phonemic or verbal jargon	0–1	0–2
Wernicke's aphasia, moderate (N = 13)	*Fluent speech, without articulatory disorders* Verbal and phonemic paraphasias and anomia; *or* marked anomia	0–2	3–4
Wernicke's aphasia, mild (N = 3)	*Fluent speech, without articulatory disorders* Very few paraphasias and anomia	3–4	3–4

N.B. The results of the aphasia examination were lacking for one aphasic patient.

TABLE 11–3. THE SOUND RECOGNITION TEST (SRT)

Item no.	Sound played by tape-recorder	Pictures shown to the patient, corresponding to alternative responses			
		Correct response	"Acoustic" response	"Semantic" response	"Odd" response
Example[1]	The neighing of a horse	A neighing horse	A car braking hard	A braying donkey	A crying baby
1	The song of a canary	A singing canary	A man whistling	A crowing cock	A train in motion
2	Gun-shots	A huntsman shooting	Stones falling on a wooden floor	A sabre duel	A braying donkey
3	The crying of a baby	A crying baby	A cat mewing in the moonlight	Two dolls	An ambulance being driven
4	Storm-wind	Trees bent by the wind	Racing cars on a track	Thunder	A singing canary
5	The grunting of a pig	Pigs grunting	Capstan pulling the anchor	Some sheep bleating	A man whistling
6	Ambulance siren	An ambulance in action	Trees bent by the wind	Racing cars on a track	A cock crowing
7	The braying of a donkey	A braying donkey	Men using a saw	A neighing horse	A crying baby
8	The rumble of a train	A train in action	Some trotting horses	A bus	Some sheep bleating
9	The roaring of an aeroplane	A flying aeroplane	A flying hornet	A train in action	A neighing horse
10	The barking of a little dog	A barking dog	A pistol being fired	A cat mewing in the moonlight	Men using a saw

[1] This item was used as an example for the explanation of the task.

oral language, i.e., oral expression and auditory comprehension. The definition of the syndromes and their incidence in our series are summarized in Table 11-2.

The following types of patient were excluded from the study: those whose case history or clinical picture pointed to mental illness or to diffuse or obviously bilateral hemispheric damage; those who considered themselves left-handed or ambidextrous (or who were reported to be such by their relatives); those whose consciousness was impaired, who were confined to bed, or were absolutely unable to maintain the set necessary for carrying out the tasks. No other criterion of selection was applied.

No preliminary audiometric test was administered to any of our patients. However, since groups were balanced with respect to age, there is no reason to believe that hypoacusis specifically affected one experimental group more than any other.

Sound Recognition Test (SRT)

The test consists of 10 meaningful sounds or noises which are presented on a tape recorder. They were chosen out of a series of 60 meaningful sounds, by selecting those which were more easily recognized by 30 non-brain-damaged patients. All sounds in the test were both familiar and easily verbalizable. The subject was asked to listen to the sound played by the tape recorder and to indicate which of 4 pictures, which were shown to him, represented the natural source of the sound he had just heard. The list of the sound stimuli and of the corresponding pictorial alternatives is given in Table 11-3. It should be noted that, after hearing the sound (e.g., the song of a canary) the patient was required to choose one of 4 pictures, which represented respectively: 1. the correct natural source of the sound (e.g., a singing canary); 2. the natural source of a sound *acoustically* very similar to the presented sound (e.g., a man whistling); 3. a sound-producing event or object belonging to the same *semantic* category of the natural source of the presented sound, but producing a sound which is completely different from the presented one from an acoustic standpoint (e.g., a cock crowing); 4. a sound-producing event, animal or object which has no relationship with the presented sound from either the acoustic or the semantic aspect (e.g., a train in motion).

Thus, three types of error were possible: *acoustic* errors, when the patient indicated picture 2; *semantic* errors, when he indicated picture 3; *odd* errors, when he indicated picture 4. This was done in order to try to secure information about the quality of the recognition disorder. The distinction suggested by Feuchtwanger (1930) between *sound deafness* (disorder in precisely discriminating the sound Gestalt) and *sound agnosia* (disorder in associating the perceived sound Gestalt with its meaning) was adopted. It was assumed that *acoustic* errors reflect a discriminative disorder and *semantic* errors reflect an associative disorder, while *odd* errors have no distinct connotation in this respect.

An additional item was given to the subject as an example, before beginning the test. The multiple choice board with the four pictures was shown to him before each sound was produced, and the examiner made sure that the patient had no doubts as to the identification of the pictures, by asking him to name them or, if he was aphasic, by pointing to each picture and telling the patient its name. The 10 items of the test were presented to the patient in 2 subsequent rounds in the same order. Each response was scored as correct (1 point) or wrong (0 points); the overall score was the sum of the scores obtained in the 2 successive rounds (maximum score = 20). The type of error was also recorded.

RESULTS

Scores obtained by the 4 experimental groups on the test are shown in Table 11-4. The performance of the control group was used to determine to what extent an imperfect performance could still be considered to fall within normal limits. Performances which corresponded to a score inferior to that of all but the

TABLE 11-4. SCORES OBTAINED BY THE 4 EXPERIMENTAL GROUPS ON THE SOUND RECOGNITION TEST

SRT score	Control patients (N = 35)	Right brain-damaged patients (N = 29	Left brain-damaged patients	
			Non-aphasic patients (N = 16)	Aphasics (N = 51)
20	16	11	4	13
19	5	2	5	4
18	7	10	5	5
17	3	2		7
16	3	2	2	9
15		1		1
14	1			3
13		1		2
12				1
11				1
10				2
9				1
8				
7				1
6				1
5				
4				
3				
2				
1				

worst control patient (cut-off about 97%) were defined as *abnormal*. As Table 11-4 shows, the cut-off point was set at score 16. Thirteen aphasic patients scored below the cut-off point, while only 2 right brain-damaged patients and none of the non-aphasic left brain-damaged group fell below it.

Inspection of Table 11-4 shows that poor performance on the SRT was found only in the aphasic group, while both right and left non-aphasic patients behaved like normal controls. The number of aphasics falling below cut-off on the test was significantly greater than that of any other experimental group.

TABLE 11-5. SOUND RECOGNITION SCORES IN THE DIFFERENT APHASIC SYNDROMES

SRT score	Global (N=5)	Broca's		Wernicke's		
		severe (N=17)	mild (N=3)	severe (N=9)	moderate (N=13)	mild (N=3)
20		5	1	1	5	1
19	1	1		1	1	
18		3	1			1
17	1	3			2	1
16	2	3			3	
15			1		2	
14				1		
13		1		1		
12				1		
11				1		
10		1		1		
9				1		
8						
7				1		
6	1					
5						
4						
3						
2						
1						
0						

The incidence of sound recognition defects in the various aphasic syndromes is shown in Table 11-5, which discloses that such defects were very frequently associated with one particular syndrome, i.e., severe Wernicke's aphasia (7 patients out of 9). This finding suggests that the sound recognition defect is specifically associated with disorders of auditory verbal comprehension. The correlation between SRT scores and comprehension scores was found to be positive and significant (Spearman's $r_s = .56$, $p < .001$).

The performance of the aphasic group differed from that of the other groups also with respect to the type of errors. Figure 11-1 shows that, in aphasics, the mean number of semantic errors increased much more than that of acoustic and odd errors. The difference between the number of semantic errors in aphasics as compared to non-aphasic patients yields a $p = .00003$ (on the Mann-Whitney test), while the difference between acoustic errors yields a $p = .054$, which does not reach statistical significance. The figure also shows that aphasics were the only group which made more semantic than acoustic errors, while the opposite trend was consistently present in each of the remaining groups. In order to investigate this trend further, all subjects who did not reach the maximum score were divided into three classes: 1. those who made more semantic than acoustic errors; 2. those who made more acoustic than semantic errors; 3. those who made an equal number of semantic and acoustic errors. Odd errors were not considered. The distribution of the 3 classes in the 4 experimental groups is shown in Table 11-6. The significance of the qualitative differences between the groups was tested by putting together classes 2 and 3 and comparing aphasics with the non-aphasic group. Aphasics appeared to include a significantly larger number of patients with predominantly semantic errors than the entire non-aphasic brain-damaged sample ($chi^2 = 4.051$ with 1 D.F.; $p = <.05$).

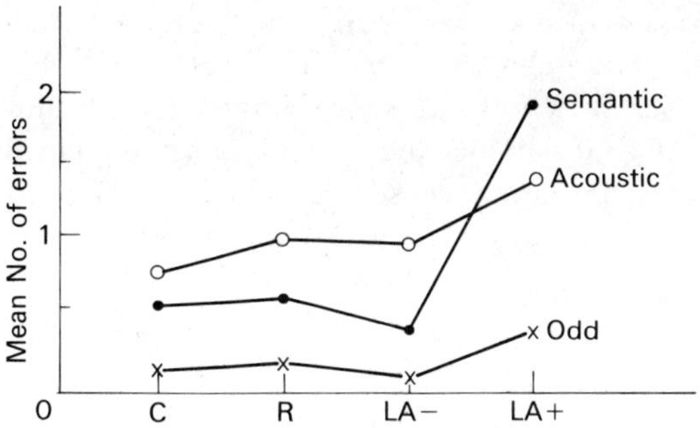

Fig. 11–1. Means of the different types of errors in the 4 experimental groups. C = control patients; R = right brain-damaged patients; LA− = non-aphasic left brain-damaged patients; LA+ = aphasic patients.

It should be noted also that, among aphasics, the proportion of semantic errors (as compared

TABLE 11–6. DISTRIBUTION OF PATIENTS ACCORDING TO PREDOMINANT TYPE OF ERROR IN THE EXPERIMENTAL GROUPS

	Control patients	Right brain-damaged patients	Left brain-damaged patients	
			Non-aphasic patients	Aphasics
S > A	6	4	3	18
S = A	1	6	2	6
S < A	12	8	7	14

S = "semantic" errors; A = "acoustic" errors.
S>A = patients who made more semantic than acoustic errors.
S<A = patients who made more acoustic than semantic errors.
S=A = patients who made the same number of semantic and acoustic errors.

N.B. Patients who made no errors are not represented in the table.

with acoustic) was greater in "agnosic" than in "non-agnosic" patients ($chi^2 = 4.982$, $p < .05$). On the other hand, the 2 right brain-damaged patients and the only normal control whose performances scored below cut-off point made more acoustic than semantic errors.

DISCUSSION

Our data indicate that, in an unselected sample of patients with focal hemispheric damage, defective sound recognition (as tested in this study) occurs frequently only in those who show aphasia and is specifically correlated with the auditory language comprehension defect. This correlation suggests that a common disorder underlies both verbal and non-verbal auditory impairment in aphasics. The nature of this disorder may be discussed. If only the quantitative scores were considered, one might be led to interpret it simply as a sound discrimination defect. Our findings would then appear to support the hypothesis that sound deafness is an essential determinant of the disorders of auditory verbal comprehension in aphasia—a concept which has been advanced by several authors (vide Kleist, 1934; Luria, 1958). However, the qualitative analysis of responses does not appear to confirm this view. Acoustic errors do not increase significantly in aphasics, as one would expect if these patients were suffering from a sound discrimination disorder. On the contrary, semantic errors are significantly increased, so as to become predominant with respect to acoustic errors. These findings strongly suggest that the aphasics' failure to recognize meaningful sounds is due not only to an acoustic-perceptual impairment as much as to the inability to associate the perceived sound with its correct meaning. If we were to define the aphasics' sound recognition defect in Feuchtwanger's terminology, we would be inclined to call it *sound agnosia* rather than *sound deafness*. In our opinion, this semantic-associative disorder, rather than an acoustic-discriminative one, is the more important determinant of the defects of both sound recognition and auditory language comprehension, which are found in an unselected group of aphasics. In support of this view, it may be recalled that semantic errors were reported to be predominant with respect to discriminative errors also in the auditory language comprehension defects of aphasics (Schuell, 1961; De Renzi and Vignolo, 1962). The disadvantage of the term *sound agnosia* is that it implies that the disorder is strictly specific to the acoustic sensory modality. On the contrary, we believe that it should be better conceived of as an intermodal associative defect, which is likely to manifest itself not only in the perception of acoustic material (verbal and non-verbal), but whenever the semantic decoding of a percept is required.

The SRT admittedly is not a very refined test of sound discrimination. In fact, the recognition of the sounds which make up the test is much more a matter of identifying them as meaningful wholes rather than a task involving subtle abilities to carry out fine discriminations in the acoustic field. Therefore, we are not in a position to state that acoustic discrimination defects do not contribute in an important way to impair sound recognition in aphasics. It may well be that such disorders play a greater role than we have been able to assess by our test. However, the fact remains that patients who made more acoustic than semantic errors were comparatively less frequent in the aphasic than in the non-aphasic group; while the 2 right brain damaged patients who scored below cut-off on the test both belonged to this category. In this connection, it is interesting to recall the data reported by Milner (1962), Shankweiler (1963) and Spreen, Benton and Fincham (1965). Both Milner and Shankweiler found that right brain-damaged patients performed defectively in tasks requiring acoustic discrimination and memory. Milner found that patients with right temporal lobectomy performed significantly more poorly on tasks for tonal memory, loudness discrimination and pitch discrimination, as compared to their pre-operative results. In Shankweiler's study, naming and repetition of well-known musical tunes were much more impaired in lesions of the right than of the left temporal lobe. Spreen, Benton and Fincham reported a remarkable case of isolated sound agnosia following right brain damage. Inspection of the published records of this patient discloses that his errors on a test of sound recognition (quite similar to ours) were acoustic rather than semantic. In our opinion, these findings suggest the tentative hypothesis that the sound recognition disorders which are found in aphasia, as a consequence of left hemisphere damage, are qualitatively different from those following right hemisphere lesions, in the sense that the former are associative rather than discriminative in nature, while the latter are discriminative rather than associative.

SUMMARY

Ninety-six right-handed patients with unilateral hemispheric damage (51 aphasics, 16 non-aphasic left brain-damaged and 29 right brain-damaged patients) and 35 control patients without cerebral lesions were given a sound recognition test requiring the identification of 10 meaningful sounds or noises. The patient was asked to listen to each sound and to indicate which of 4 pictures shown to him represented its natural source. The test allowed both a quantitative score (n° of correct responses) and a qualitative score (n° of *acoustic, semantic* or *odd* errors).

It was found that while non-aphasic left and right brain-damaged patients performed virtually like normal controls on the test, a significant proportion of aphasics (about 25%) fell below the normal cut-off score. The performances of patients with Wernicke's aphasia were particularly poor. In the entire aphasic sample, sound recognition scores appeared to correlate significantly with scores of auditory verbal comprehension ($r_s = .56$). When aphasics were compared to non-aphasic patients with respect to the quality of performance, aphasia was found to be associated more with semantic than with acoustic errors.

These findings seem to indicate that the impaired recognition of meaningful sounds, characteristic of aphasics, is due to a great extent to the inability to associate the perceived sound to its correct meaning, rather than to a merely acoustic-discriminative defect. The hypothesis is advanced that this semantic-associative disorder is the common factor underlying both the sound recognition and the auditory language comprehension defects, and that it may manifest itself also in other areas of the aphasic's behavior.

Acknowledgement. The Authors wish to thank Mr. M. Casadei of the RAI-TV of Milan for his aid in the realization of the Sound Recognition Test.

REFERENCES

De Renzi, E., and Vignolo, L. A. (1962) *Fattori verbali ed extraverbali della comprensione negli afasici,* in Atti del XIV Congresso Nazionale della Società Italiana di Neurologia, special volume of "Riv. Pat. Nerv. Ment.," 443-468.

Feuchtwanger, E. (1930) *Amusie.* Springer, Berlin.

Kleist, K. (1934) *Gehirnpathologie.* Barth, Leipzig.

Luria, A. R. (1958) *Brain disorders and Language analysis,* "Language and Speech," **1,** 14-34.

Milner, B. (1962) *Laterality effects in audition,* in Interhemispheric Relations and Cerebral Dominance, ed. by V. B. Mountcastle, John Hopkins Press, Baltimore.

Schuell, H., and Jenkins, J. J. (1961) *Reduction of vocabulary in aphasia,* "Brain," **84,** 243-261.

Shankweiler, D. P. (1963): quoted in Spreen, Benton and Fincham (1965).

Spreen, O., Benton, A. L., and Fingham, R. W. (1965) *Auditory agnosia without aphasia,* "Arch. Neurol.," **13,** 84-92.

12

An Experimental Approach to the Problem of Articulation in Aphasia

DONALD P. SHANKWEILER
KATHERINE S. HARRIS

DONALD P. SHANKWEILER, Ph.D., is with the department of linguistics of the University of Connecticut.

KATHERINE S. HARRIS, Ph.D., is a research psychologist with the Haskins Laboratories, New York City.

The work was supported in part by a Rehabilitation Research and Training Center Grant from the Vocational Rehabilitation Administration, U.S. Department of Health, Education and Welfare to the Institute of Physical Medicine and Rehabilitation, New York University Medical Center, and in part by a General Research Support Grant from the National Institutes of Health to Haskins Laboratories.

The purpose of this paper is to outline an experimental approach to an old problem: the nature of the articulatory disturbance which is often associated with so-called "motor" aphasia. It has long been known that in some cases of disturbance of expressive language, a breakdown of speech production occurs at the most molecular level; that is to say, the patient has major difficulties in producing the gestures words are made of. Patients who exhibit the syndrome Alajouanine has called "phonetic disintegration" articulate slowly, hesitantly, with extrinsic facial movements and with many substitutions of one phoneme for another. This condition, which is sometimes called "cortical dysarthria" (Bay, 1962) and "apraxic dysarthria" (Nathan, 1947), must be distinguished from dysarthric disorders arising from damage restricted to lower levels of the motor systems. In the latter, articulatory movements are impaired in a more stereotyped and regular fashion; the neural mechanisms responsible for organization of the gestures which convey the phonological units of speech are not involved.

Phonetic disintegration can occur in combination with widespread disorders of expression or, less frequently, in remarkably "pure" form. In the latter case, in spite of the difficulties in emitting speech sounds, expressive abilities (e.g., as shown in writing) may be well preserved, indicating continued access to vocabulary and continued adherence to the rules of syntax. Thus, speech may be selectively impaired at the phonetic level. Phonetic disintegration is most likely to occur as an isolated disturbance at a late stage in recovery from aphasia after remission of other expressive disabilities. It is easy to observe in these cases that the difficulties in articulation do not reflect a corresponding disturbance in speech recognition.

The phenomena of disordered articulation in aphasic patients have not received the study they deserve in view of the opportunities they provide to observe the breakdown of the processes of speech production. The reawakening of interest in the disorders of articulation

From *Cortex* 2:277–92, 1966.

associated with aphasia owes much to the work of Alajouanine and his colleagues. Alajouanine, Ombredane and Durand (1939) argue forcefully for the necessity of obtaining an adequate phonetic description of speech in cases with disturbed articulation, viewing this as an indispensable requirement for understanding the physiological bases of the syndrome of phonetic disintegration. Important suggestions are made about the ways speech production is linked to the various stages of recovery, ranging from the earliest stage in which only vowels can be produced to later ones in which virtually all segments of speech can be identified, though they are produced unreliably and in the wrong articulatory contexts. Unfortunately, the results of their phonetic studies are not presented in such a way that the reader can make his own evaluation of their findings. The work also suffers from failure to provide the necessary controls.

Fry (1958) has provided an illustration of a method for systematic analysis of the utterances of an aphasic patient with articulatory disorder. The problem was to develop an adequate test to enable an investigator to determine the relative difficulty of all the sounds of speech in their various articulatory contexts. Not only must the sample include all the words required for a complete survey, but it must include enough words of each type to provide adequate sampling. The problem was met by having the patient repeat a list of words chosen to meet these requirements. Phonetic analysis of the patient's tape-recorded utterances was carried out and a complete tabulation of all responses was made. This permitted a classification of all substituted phonemes according to place and manner of articulation. Fry's paper demonstrates the relevance to aphasia studies of a powerful method for discovering the dimensions of a phonological disturbance.

Mention must be made of another approach to the study of articulatory disorders. Lehiste (1965) has carried out meticulous spectrographic analyses of the utterances of a diverse group of patients suffering from a variety of neuromotor disorders, many of them due to damage to brain stem and cerebellar regions. We cannot compare her findings directly with our own because we did not use the technique of spectrographic analysis and because we confined our study to patients with presumably unilateral lesions of the left cerebral hemisphere.

The preliminary findings presented here are a part of a larger ongoing comparative study of articulatory function in cases of damage at different levels and sites in the sensorimotor system. In the present study we have tried to gain an accurate picture of the dimensions of phonemic error which occur in the syndrome of phonetic disintegration associated with "motor" aphasia. Information regarding the consistency and major directions of phonemic substitutions can then serve to guide more direct approaches to the defective speech gestures by means of electromyography, x-ray cinephotography and other techniques. Our program has these two interrelated aspects: first to obtain an adequate assessment of articulatory function in phonetic terms and secondly to study directly the gestures of speech in order to relate the phonetic description of the disordered speech output to the parameters of muscle movement. The present study is limited to the first aspect.

METHOD AND RESULTS

Subjects

Phonetic studies of speech were made in five patients with lesions of vascular origin involving but not necessarily restricted to the anterior portion of the dominant left cerebral hemisphere. All were patients of the Institute of Physical Medicine and Rehabilitation of New York University Medical Center. The group was composed of intelligent individuals with business and professional backgrounds, selected for their willingness to engage in intensive speech therapy. Each had suffered a stroke six months to seven years prior to the examination. The stroke in each case was followed by right hemiparesis and severe expressive aphasia with preservation of comprehension. At the time of testing, aphasic symptoms were greatly diminished, leaving a major residual deficit in articulation.

The patients' ages at the time of testing ranged from 39 to 61 years; three were under 50. None presented difficulties of chewing or swallowing. Some weakness of the right upper extremity was present in all patients, and in two the leg also was involved. Slight weakness of the right side of the face could be detected. All were able to perform movements of the lips, face and tongue on command, but with less than normal dexterity and speed. No cerebellar signs were present and there was no evidence of lower motor neuron paralysis. Audiometry revealed normal pure tone thresholds for frequencies below 2000 cps. In two cases the episode could be traced to occlusion of the left internal carotid artery. In a third case, angiography showed occlusion of the middle cerebral artery, and in two cases the origin of the lesion is not definitely known.

Although very different degrees of recovery of speech are to be found in the group, the sequence of events during recovery was similar for all. Writing was spontaneously adopted as the way around obstacles to oral communication. With the return of speech, the difficulties proved to be chiefly of an articulatory nature. All patients had reached a definite plateau in recovery at the time of testing. The residual level of articulatory impairment ranged from gross difficulty in producing all classes of speech sounds, with poor intelligibility, to mild impairment shown mainly in production of consonant clusters, with good preservation of intelligibility. None showed evidence of generalized intellectual deterioration.

Much interaction over a long period of time had convinced us on clinical grounds that the patients were nearly intact in comprehension of speech. A control, however, is needed in order to be reasonably certain that errors in articulation occur on the basis of impaired motor organization, rather than on the basis of perceptual impairment. A "rhyme" test was used to determine whether the acoustic cues which signal phonemic differences could be utilized normally by these patients.

Assessment of speech perception

Each patient listened to a taped recording of three 75 word lists of real word monosyllables. He was to encircle each word he heard in a set of five possible answers for that word printed on an answer sheet. For example, if the word spoken was *pat*, the answer sheet might offer the alternatives *pat*, *mat*, *slat*, *bat*, *cat*. In one-third of the list, the alternatives differed, as in the example given above, in initial sound; one third of the answer sets varied in terminal sound, and one third in vowel. Thus, we tested the patients for the ability to perceive initial, terminal and vowel sounds in words. We made

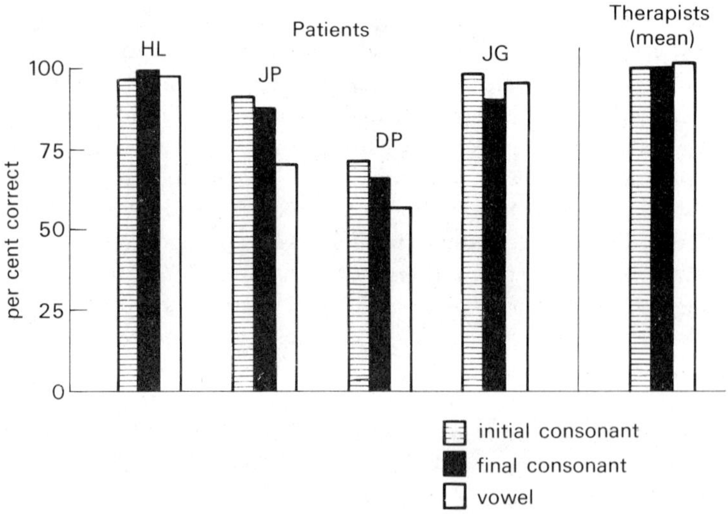

Fig. 12–1. Speech perception test: percent correct identification of initial consonants, terminal consonants, and vowels; shown individually for each of four patients and averaged for six therapists.

up the words for the vowel part of the test; the initial and terminal section lists were taken from a test described by House et al. (1965). As a further control, the same test was given to six speech therapists. The results for four patients (one left therapy before we could administer the test) and six therapists are shown in Figure 12-1.

Two patients performed virtually as well as the therapists. Moreover, one of these (JG) showed the greatest impairment of articulation of any member of the group (see Figure 12-3). This dissociation strongly confirms the impression that severe phonetic disintegration can occur independently of impaired recognition of speech sounds. Two patients performed less well for reasons which are not entirely clear. Some clues can be obtained from examining the pattern of errors. The error pattern in these cases contrasts strikingly to that in *producing* speech; i.e., the greatest incidence of error occurred on the vowel sounds in the rhyme test and on the consonant sounds in articulation. Special difficulty in perceiving vowels is not found in cases of perceptive disability due to sensorineural hearing loss. Errors in selecting the correct sounds from the multiple-choice sets do not, of course, necessarily reflect misperception. The difficulty may occur on some other basis. Analysis of the errors suggests that some can be attributed to reading impairment.

Assessment of articulation

Since the principal need was to study speech production at the phonological level, the investigation was limited to analysis of the productions of single words. A test consisting of 200 real word monosyllables was assembled. The distribution of phonemes in the word list was such as could be expected to bring into relief the difficulties in articulating the speech sounds of English. The list contains most singleton consonants, a sample of the most frequently occurring consonant clusters, and those vowels which in the regional dialect are not ordinarily characterized by glides. One respect in which this test differs from articulation tests designed for other purposes is in providing the same frequency of occurrence of all phonemes which occur in a given position in the words. Thus [z], a "rare" phoneme, has the same number of occurrences in initial position in the test as [d], a "common" phoneme. Even distribution of phonemes is highly desirable if one wishes to draw inferences about the relative difficulty of speech sounds. The test comprised 25 consonants and consonant clusters in initial position, each of which occurred eight times. Similarly, there were 25 sounds in terminal position, each occurring eight times, and there were eight vowel nuclei, each of which occurred approximately 25 times. The words were recorded on magnetic tape by a trained speaker and presented to the patient through earphones at a comfortable listening level. The patient's task was to repeat each word once. The responses were tape-recorded so as to be available for detailed analysis.

The results of articulation testing were treated in the following manner. The patient's recorded utterances were transcribed by a phonetically-trained listener. The transcription can best be described as broadly phonetic (IPA).[1] The intent was not to make the transcription reflect every phonetic nuance of speech production, for the practical reason that this would involve more categories than could be dealt with without obscuring the main features of the condition. A very broad transcription admittedly ignores features of speech which may have real importance for a physiological understanding of phonetic disintegration, but it has the virtue of allowing the gross features to stand in bold relief. Therefore, we have chosen to ignore narrowly phonetic features in this exploratory phase of our work.

The transcribed utterances for each patient were tabulated as confusion matrices; two such matrices appear as Figure 12-2. The matrix shows, with respect to each phoneme, the frequency with which it was "correctly" produced or replaced by another phoneme. Each row in the matrix refers to the phonemes

[1] In making the transcription, the listener was operating with reference to the normal allophonic ranges of the phonemic categories in the speech structure of English.

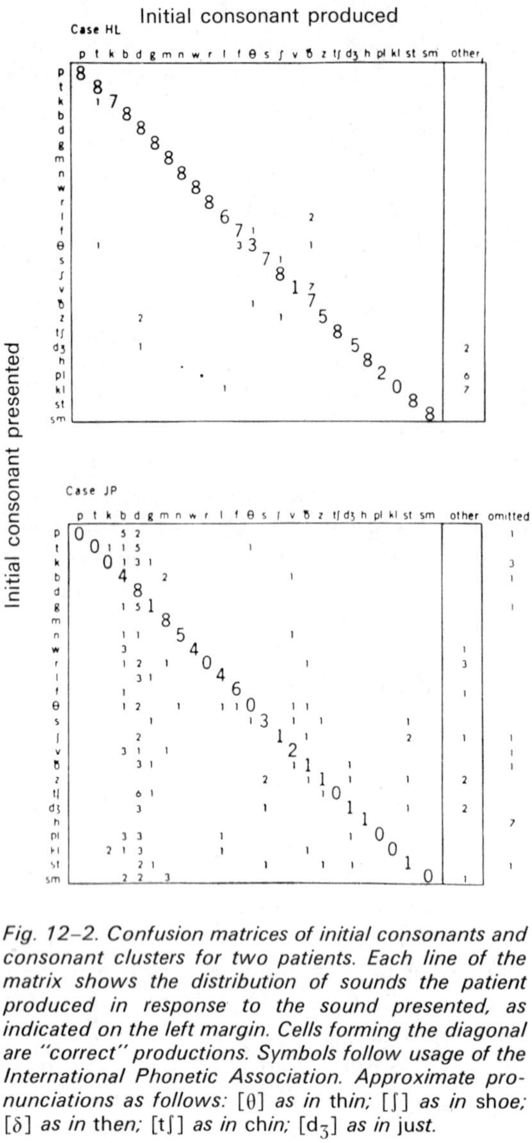

Fig. 12–2. Confusion matrices of initial consonants and consonant clusters for two patients. Each line of the matrix shows the distribution of sounds the patient produced in response to the sound presented, as indicated on the left margin. Cells forming the diagonal are "correct" productions. Symbols follow usage of the International Phonetic Association. Approximate pronunciations as follows: [θ] *as in* thin; [ʃ] *as in* shoe; [ð] *as in* then; [tʃ] *as in* chin; [dʒ] *as in* just.

occurring in the list, and each column refers to the sounds actually spoken by the patient. Since each initial consonant occurred eight times in the list, the figure *8* in the diagonal indicates that that phoneme was repeated "correctly" on every occasion it occurred. From the diagonal we can quickly discover the relative difficulty of the phonemes, and from the other cells in the matrix, we can discover the degree to which the phonemic substitutions fall into patterns.

Figure 12-2 gives the matrices of initial consonant substitutions of two patients who illustrate very different degrees of severity. Clinical judgment had placed HL as the least impaired in the group, and the data bear this out. Her errors in articulation were largely confined to a few consonant clusters and certain fricatives [θ, v, z, dʒ]. Clusters involving [l] were produced in a stereotyped manner by splitting the cluster and inserting a vowel in between, as [pəliz] (please) and [kəlin) (clean) thus producing disyllables. The patient lacked sufficient control to produce the cluster as a unitary gesture and had been taught this substitution by her therapist as a way of producing words in which these sounds occurred intelligibly if defectively. The lower matrix in the figure shows initial consonant distortions and substitutions of a severely impaired patient (JP). There is a striking tendency to substitute one of the three voiced stop consonants [b, d, g] for almost every other sound in the inventory.

Matrices of this type were made for each patient, one for initial consonants and clusters (e.g., the matrices shown in Figure 12-2), one for vowel nuclei and one for terminal consonants and clusters. These matrices, in turn, could be summarized by considering the overall percent correct for each matrix, shown in Figure 12-3.

It is apparent from Figure 12-3 that the errors in articulation are not evenly distributed throughout the word. This figure shows the tabulation of the total number of sounds "correctly" produced in each position in the word for every patient. Not surprisingly, consonant clusters are more difficult to produce adequately than singleton consonants. In every case consonant clusters in the initial portion of the word are the least accurately produced of all sounds. One patient (JG) failed to produce any of these sounds intelligibly. In four of the five cases, we can make the generalization that initial sounds are more difficult to produce than terminal sounds. The vocalic portion of the word is produced with greater accuracy than the nonvocalic portions. This is particularly striking in the case of JP.

Assessment of the production of vowels

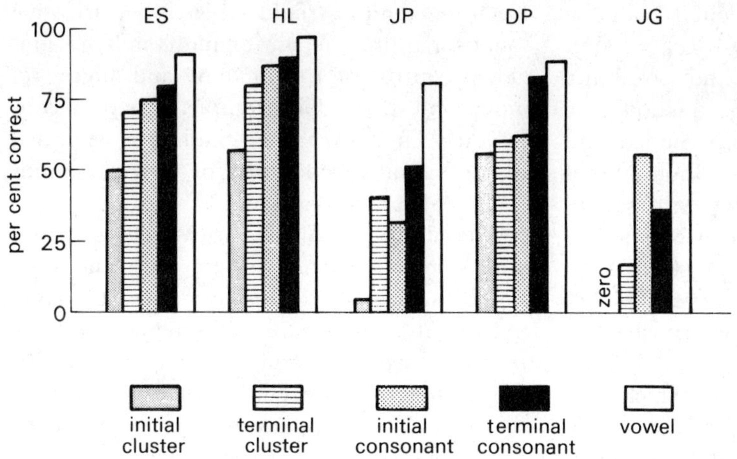

Fig. 12–3. Speech production test: percent correct for each indicated class of sounds for each patient.

introduces some special problems owing to the fact that differences in vowel quality are the main sources of phonetic variability between speakers of the same language. In view of this, the listener's assessments of the patient's vowels are more tentative than identification of other portions of the speech signal. In many instances there was uncertainty as to whether a certain feature should be attributed to pathology or to the fact that there may be several "correct" vowels for any given word. This ambiguity might sometimes be resolved by comparing each patient's productions against those of an appropriate control. This should be someone preferably of about the same age as the patient who has shared throughout life the geographic and social environment of the patient. In two cases we found available patients' siblings who met these requirements.

Patient-sibling comparisons were made (in cases HL and JP) by retabulating vowel production using the vowels of their siblings as targets. When this is done, HL's percentage accuracy rises from 97% to 99% and JP's figure changes from 81% to 88%. Although these changes are small, they are a further indication that the production of vowel sounds is very little affected by the disorder. Although the fifth patient, JG, has poor vowel production, we might expect some upward revision if an adequate control were available.

Considering the five cases as a group, there is a great deal of variability in the pattern of sound substitutions which occur, but some sounds were consistently misarticulated. Figure 12-4 shows the sounds which the group as a whole found difficult to produce.

It includes all phonemes in the inventory for which the wrong sound was produced on at least three of its eight occurrences by at least four of the five patients. The number to the right of each phoneme is the mean per cent error in producing it. It is noteworthy that the lists contain fewer sounds in final position than in initial, an additional indication that these patients have greater difficulty in producing initial sounds. The fricatives and affricates, together with certain consonant clusters, are the classes of speech sounds which are most consistently misarticulated.

The fricatives and affricates are also the most difficult sounds to perceive correctly.

INITIAL POSITION

Phoneme	%Error
θ	75
v	63
z	65
tʃ	55
dʒ	55
pl	82
kl	73
sm	65

FINAL POSITION

Phoneme	%Error
θ	62
ʃ	58
ð	55
lk	47
ps	65

Fig. 12–4. Speech sounds with highest error rates given as percentages of total opportunity for error.

Confusions are common, particularly among [f], [θ] and [v] (Miller and Nicely, 1955). Therefore we cannot ignore the possibility that some of these errors in production may reflect perceptual confusion, compounded with the likelihood that the transcription also is somewhat unreliable in dealing with sounds of this class. Both possibilities can be checked to some extent by retabulation. Consonant sounds may be classified in terms of the place in the oral cavity at which maximal constriction occurs in forming them (e.g., [b] is labial; [g] is velar), and the manner in which they are produced (e.g., [p] is plosive; [n] is nasal). The errors were classified according to whether the substituted sound differed from the target in place of articulation, manner of articulation, both place and manner, or whether the substituted sounds were unrelated to the target or omitted altogether. When the productions of stop consonants and fricatives were retabulated allowing manner errors, the error rate for fricatives was even greater than indicated by the original tabulation whereas that for stop consonants was less. Thus the fricatives remain the most impaired class of sounds when the tabulation allows as correct those substitutions which are likely to occur on a perceptual basis.

The results of the tabulations for all classes of speech sounds show a similar incidence of errors of place and manner with manner errors slightly predominating. The largest category of misarticulations, which accounted for one-third of all errors was the category of unrelated substitutions and omissions. Particularly common were the substitutions of consonant clusters for single consonants.

DISCUSSION

A feature of phonetic disintegration which is shared with many other disorders of articulation is the special difficulty in producing fricative and affricate sounds. Speech pathologists have observed that one fricative [s] is the most likely to be impaired in any type of pathological speech whatever the native language of the speaker (see, for example, Luchsinger and Arnold, 1965). The fricative sounds require the use of more muscles and closer control of the amount and timing of movement than, for example, the stop consonants. They are among the last to be added to the child's repertoire of speech sounds (Whetnall and Fry, 1964).

The finding that the fricatives, affricates and some consonant clusters are the only sounds which are consistently misarticulated by patients of our group points to the conclusion that no particular structure or region can be implicated to the exclusion of other parts of the articulatory apparatus. Sharply localized defects of specific muscles or muscle groups were not to be expected in a disorder of this kind. The possibility of dissociated defects of the lips and tongue has been raised (Denny-Brown, 1958), but we have found no evidence of differential involvement of these structures in any patient of our group. The preservation of vowel articulation, which was also observed by Nathan (1947), argues against any selective impairment of the tongue. So does the absence of general impairment of the lingual consonants. Thus, the particular difficulty with the fricatives and clusters, the frequent occurrence of errors of voicing and nasalization and the integrity of the vowels all point to a disturbance of coordinated sequencing of several articulators.

The hypothesis that the most rapid gestures of speech suffer most in phonetic disintegration was suggested by the fact that vowel production, which requires a relatively slow rate of movement, was least disturbed by the disorder. The implication of this hypothesis that production of the stop consonants (requiring the fastest movement) would be most impaired is contrary, however, to what was found.

To what extent do we generally find substitutions of "easy" sounds for "difficult" ones? This question has proved to be a stumbling block in considerations of the nature of phonetic disintegration. One reason is the ambiguity of what is meant by phonological difficulty. A relatively small proportion of the errors represent phonetic simplifications typical of young children (such as substitution of stop consonants for fricatives). A second class of errors must also be regarded as simplifications although they do not occur in children's speech (such as the breaking up of consonant clusters by insertion of a vowel between the normally linked pair of consonants). A third class of substitutions cannot be considered simplifications in any sense. On the contrary, the patients often emitted particularly difficult strings of consonant clusters which do not occur in English words and were nearly impossible to imitate.

Our findings, therefore, give little support to the idea (Jakobson, 1941; Alajouanine and Lhermitte, 1960) that speech in phonetic disintegration mirrors its development in the child. In this we are in agreement with Critchley (1952) and Fry (1958). It is true that our patients find difficult some of the same sounds the young child finds difficult (Morley, 1957), but there is little reason to assume that the difficulty has the same basis.

Phonetic disintegration differs from other disorders of articulation in a number of important ways. Children with developmental articulatory defects and adults with defects of the articulatory structures are predictable in the substitutions they make, whereas variability is one of the striking features of the speech of our group. The errors do not group systematically according to place of articulation. For example, there is no significant tendency for front consonants such as [p] to be better produced than middle or back consonants such as [t] or [k]. A number of errors occurred in the manner of articulation. Chief among these were errors of voicing, particularly the replacement of an unvoiced sound by a voiced one. This type of substitution rarely occurs in children's speech (Fry, 1958).

Many errors can be considered neither as poor approximations to the correct phoneme nor as clear-cut substitutions of related phonemes. The apparent unrelatedness of many of the substituted sounds to their targets, together with the marked lack of consistency of the substitutions, tells us much about the condition. To the extent that these features characterize a given patient's performance, the disorder must stem from disorganization of the process by which phonological units are encoded for production. It is almost inconceivable that residual spasticity or weakness could give rise to errors of this kind.

We have not attempted to describe all pathological features of speech in cases of phonetic disintegration. Certainly the patients have difficulties in producing connected speech which are not revealed by the method of analyzing monosyllables spoken in isolation. Syllabification, in particular, has been indicated as a problem in need of study. Lehiste (1965) and Tikofsky and his co-workers (1965) have shown that the intelligibility of utterances produced by their group of dysarthric patients varied with syllable content.

Even within the present restricted framework there are a number of questions which cannot be answered by studies of the acoustic speech output alone, whether by the trained listener or by spectrographic analysis. Neither can give direct information about the motor gestures of speech. New developments in the application of electromyography to speech research (Harris et al., 1964) make it possible to obtain a description of phonetic disintegration directly in terms of the disordered movements. An application of EMG to the study of a case of developmental dysarthria was illustrated by Rootes and MacNeilage (in press), and we are hopeful that this technique, used in conjunction with the method outlined here, can clarify a number of remaining questions. We would like to know, for example, whether the vowel gestures are as little affected by the disorder as the identification data would suggest.

It is of basic interest to learn whether or not all the normal components of each distinctive gestural unit of productive speech are present in the utterances of these patients, both when the target sound is acceptably produced and when another is substituted for it. If the gestures are intact in form, what errors of timing occur? What proportion of the errors are attributable specifically to problems of co-articulation? In the normal workings of speech all participant processes are so thoroughly fused in their integrated action that the relative contribution of each cannot be understood. We believe that careful examination of these questions in persons with localized interruption of a motor or sensory link in the speech chain can contribute new understanding to the processes of speech production.

observed less frequently than other errors which are not found in children's speech nor in the speech of adults with defects of the articulatory structures.

Systematic observation of speech in phonetic disintegration may well contribute new understanding of the fundamental processes of speech production.

SUMMARY

A phonetic analysis was made of speech production in five patients with major residual deficits in articulation following remission of more widespread disturbances of verbal expression. The findings demonstrate major disturbance of speech production at the most molecular level. Maximal difficulty in articulation occurred at the beginning portion of words. Consonant sounds were much more often misarticulated than vowel sounds. Fricative and affricate consonants and certain linked groups of consonants were the most often affected of all sounds of speech. Phonetic simplifications typical of young children were

Acknowledgements. We are indebted to Martha L. Taylor, Chief, Department of Speech and Hearing Therapy, Institute of Physical Medicine and Rehabilitation, New York University Medical Center, for providing the impetus for this study and for her considerable help and encouragement. Thanks are due to Ida Nathan for administering some of the tests and to Sheila Zelermyer for preparation of the confusion matrices.

The work was supported in part by a Rehabilitation Research and Training Center Grant from the Vocational Rehabilitation Administration, U.S. Department of Health, Education and Welfare to the Institute of Physical Medicine and Rehabilitation, New York University Medical Center, and in part by a General Research Support Grant from the National Institutes of Health to Haskins Laboratories.

REFERENCES

Alajouanine, T., Ombredane, A., and Durand, M. (1939) *Le syndrome de désintégration phonétique dans l'aphasie.* Masson, Paris.

——, and Lhermitte, F. (1960) *Les troubles des activités expressives du langage dans l'aphasie. Leur relations avec les apraxies*, "Rev. Neurol.," **102,** 604–633.

Bay, E. (1962) *Aphasia and non-verbal disorders of language*, "Brain," **85,** 412–426.

Critchley, M. (1952) *Articulatory defects in aphasia*, "J. Laryngol. Otol.," **66,** 1–17.

Denny-Brown, D. (1958) *The nature of apraxia*, "J. nerv. ment. Dis.," **126,** 9–32.

Fry, D. B. (1958) *Phonemic substitutions in an aphasic patient*, "Language and Speech," **1,** 52–61.

Harris, K. S., Rosov, R., Cooper, F. S., and Lysaught, G. F. (1964) *A multiple suction electrode system*, "J. EEG clin. Neurophysiol.," **17,** 698–700.

House, A. S., Williams, C. E., Hecker, M. H. L., and Kryter, K. D. (1965) *Articulation testing methods: consonantal differentiation with a closed-response set*, "J. acoust. Soc. Amer.," **37,** 158–166.

Jakobson, R. (1941) *Kindersprache, Aphasie und allgemeine Lautgesetze.* Almquist und Wiksell, Uppsala.

Lehiste, I. (1965) *Some acoustic characteristics of dysarthic speech*, "Bibliot. Phonet.," (Basel), Fasc. **2,** 1–124.

Luchsinger, R., and Arnold, G. E. (1965) *Voice-Speech-Language; Clinical Communicology: its Physiology and Pathology.* Wadsworth, Belmont, Calif.

Miller, G. A., and Nicely, P. E. (1955) *An analysis of perceptual confusions among some English consonants*, "J. acoust. Soc. Amer.," **27,** 338–352.

Morley, M. E. (1957) *The Development and Disorders of Speech in Childhood.* Williams and Wilkins, Baltimore.

Nathan, P. W. (1947) *Facial apraxia and apraxic dysarthria*, "Brain," **70,** 449–478.

Rootes, T. P., and MacNeilage, P. F. (1966) *Some speech perception and production tests of a patient with impairment in somesthetic perception and motor function*, in Symposium on Oral Sensation and Perception, ed. by Bosma, J. F. Thomas, Springfield, Ill. (in press).

Tikofsky, R. S. (1965) *Phonetic Characteristics of Dysarthria.* Office of Research Administration, University of Michigan, Ann Arbor.

Whetnall, E., and Fry, D. B. (1964) *The Deaf Child.* Heinemann, London.

13

Oral Apraxia and Aphasia

ENNIO DE RENZI
ALBERTO PIECZURO
LUIGI A. VIGNOLO

ENNIO DE RENZI, M.D., ALBERTO PIECZURO, M.D., and LUIGI A. VIGNOLO, M.D., are with the Clinica delle Malattie Nervose e Mentali of the Universitá di Milano, Italy.

Oral apraxia (O.A.) may be defined as the inability to perform voluntary movements with the muscles of the larynx, pharynx, tongue, lips and cheeks, although automatic movements of the same muscles are preserved. Jackson (1878) was the first to draw attention to the fact that some aphasic patients could not protrude the tongue on command, although they were perfectly able to move it when chewing or in response to a spontaneous stimulus, e.g. in licking the lips after drinking. Jackson explicitly connected this automatic-voluntary dissociation with that which is present in aphasic speech and suggested that such phenomena offered important cues to the understanding of the physiopathology of the entire aphasic process. These observations were more or less neglected for many years, even in the famous debate between Dejerine and Pierre Marie, which focused the attention of neurologists on the topic which is perhaps most closely related to oral apraxia, i.e., the nature of oral expressive disorders in so-called "motor" aphasia.

As is well known, some representatives of the classical school held that the speech disturbances of motor aphasics are due to loss of the motor images or engrams for words, i.e., to loss of the memory of the movements which are needed to articulate words. According to this conception, oral expressive disorders are entirely aphasic in nature; such images or engrams, in fact, strictly specialized as they are for word articulation, are constituent parts of the "notion du mot" (Dejerine, 1926) and therefore their loss also impairs inner language. This, in Dejerine's view, is the reason for disturbances of auditory comprehension, reading and writing in motor aphasia. In contrast, according to Pierre Marie, the expressive defect of these patients does not belong to aphasia, because it concerns merely the motor mechanism of articulation, thereby corresponding to dysarthria, or, in the severest cases, to anarthria. In his angry polemic against the representatives of the theory of images, Marie never precisely defined the nature of anarthria. He merely denied that it was due to paralysis of the oral muscles. Indeed, he did once define it as a "defect in the co-ordination of the movements of phonation" (1906a), and on another occasion (1908) he accepted Ballet's suggestion that it might be an apraxic disorder; nevertheless, he explicitly stated: "in my view the word 'anarthria' must be considered as free of any claim of physiological explanation; it merely describes a fact: loss or disturbance of articulated speech, with more or less complete preservation of inner speech" (1906b). For this reason he did not reply to Dejerine's objection (1908) that "while the anarthric patient (in the sense of the common dysarthric patient) also

From *Cortex* 2:50–73, 1966.

shows his motor defect in extra-articulatory movements, the patient with motor aphasia entirely preserves the functions of the bucco-pharyngo-laryngeal apparatus in all movements other than speech movements." Marie's failure to reply is perplexing, especially when one considers that his disciple, Moutier, had just written in his book, *L'Aphasie de Broca* (1908): "Let us ask an anarthric patient to stick out his tongue; the patient opens his mouth, makes some desperate efforts, shows with his gesture that he has perfectly understood our command. Yet his tongue lies still in his mouth, or it barely moves. This is not present in all anarthric patients, nor in all Broca's aphasics, particularly those at an advanced stage of their evolution; nevertheless, it may frequently be observed, and we have already seen it ourselves in about ten patients."

It appears as if the authors of this period did not grasp all the implications connected with the presence of disturbances involving even non-verbal oral movements in "motor" aphasics. The association between speech disorders and O.A. in Broca's aphasia was also generally ignored or overlooked in later studies, even though the hypothesis that the majority or all of the expressive deficits in Broca's aphasia were apraxic in nature had already been advanced by Liepmann (1900) and Ballet (1908), and was to be revived by Foix (1928), Nielsen (1946) and others. Thus, whether the speech disorders in these patients should be defined as "aphasic" or "apraxic" was merely a terminological question.

The significance of this association has been grasped only recently by some investigators who have continued along the path opened by Pierre Marie. These authors maintained that it is possible to demonstrate, in a number of aphasics, some articulatory disturbances ("anarthria," "cortical dysarthria," "syndrome of phonetic disintegration," etc.), which are extraneous to the specific language disorders and which, at least in the initial stages of the syndrome, are associated with disorders of nonverbal movements of the oral muscles.

De Morsier (1949) called attention to swallowing difficulties in two cases of motor aphasia, and Nathan (1947) described six cases of motor aphasia with facial apraxia. Alajouanine and co-workers (1939, 1960, 1961) and Bay (1957) made major contributions in this direction. The use of recording devices (Rousselot's cylinder, cathode-ray oscillograph, Rey's glossograph) complemented clinical observation in their studies. According to Bay (1957), O.A. is constantly present in aphasic patients with anarthria (or, as he calls it, "cortical dysarthria") and its course coincides with the evolution of the articulatory disorders; certain features, such as obvious effort, explosiveness and spasms of the oral movements, are common to both disturbances. Alajouanine and Lhermitte (1960, 1961) also believe that O.A. is a very common finding in Broca's aphasia, but point out that the association is often limited to the first stages of the illness, because non-verbal oral movements, being less complex than articulatory movements may recover more rapidly. Moreover, while according to Bay O.A. appears only in Broca's aphasia, Alajounine and Lhermitte maintain that it may be found not exceptionally in Wernicke's aphasia. In such a case, however, the disorder of oral movements is associated with a particular clinical picture: oral language is worse than written language, paraphasic perseverations are frequent, repetition is particularly impaired, and oral expression of one word is not facilitated by reading the word aloud.

Geschwind (1965) has recently called attention to the common occurrence of facial apraxia in patients with conduction aphasia, i.e., aphasic patients whose spontaneous speech is usually copious, but grossly paraphasic, and whose repetition is severely impaired, while comprehension is good. This clinical picture is ascribed to a lesion in the arcuate fasciculus connecting Wernicke's with Broca's area. O.A. in these patients does not seem to reflect a causal relationship between verbal and extraverbal symptoms; on the contrary, it seems to be due to the common anatomical background subserving both oral performances. In fact, disruption of the arcuate fasciculus would prevent verbal commands from reaching the motor association cortex, which is responsible for both kinds of oral movements. When oral praxic movements are performed on visual command (e.g., on visual imitation) presence of O.A. in conduction aphasics would indicate that the lesion involves the supramarginal gyrus, where the arcuate fasciculus runs close to the occipito-frontal fibers.

In contrast to the above-mentioned writers, the vast majority of English-speaking authors seem to pay very little attention to the phenomenon of oral apraxia and to its possible physiological implications. Few of them seem to agree with Nathan's (1947) opinion, that "as facial apraxia is a common accompaniment of aphasia, it should be considered as a possible cause of the dysarthria, whenever the aphasia is of the type known as Broca's aphasia (aphasia and dysarthria)." This discrepancy is probably due to the fact that O.A. has been described up to now in a limited number of patients who showed it to a very conspicuous degree. A systematic investigation involving a large sample of brain damaged subjects, in order to assess the frequency of occurrence of O.A. and its association with different aphasic disorders, is still lacking. The purpose of the present study is to fill this gap.

In undertaking this research, we have been faced with a number of difficulties, which deserve discussion in order to clarify the method which has been adopted to classify aphasic patients in this study. If one needs to classify a large number of patients according to the type of aphasia, one is faced with the difficulty of defining aphasic syndromes according to objective criteria which could be applied in each particular case. The most currently accepted clinical pictures of aphasia (such as Broca's aphasia and Wernicke's aphasia) have never been defined on the basis of rigorous criteria which could be immediately applied to a great number of unselected aphasics. While general agreement is easily reached with respect to the most severe cases belonging to the most classical forms, the classification of a not inconsiderable number of aphasics whose symptoms are either mild or not quite typical is open to question. This fact entails considerable difficulties whenever one wishes to evaluate the actual incidence of O.A. in the various forms of aphasia in which it has been previously reported.

A different approach, which allows us to overcome these drawbacks, consists of limiting the investigation to assessing whether or not the severity of O.A. is correlated with the severity of anarthric disorders of expression, deliberately ignoring the overall classification of aphasic syndromes. Unfortunately, anarthria too has always been defined by reference to its most severe forms (e.g., total blocking, recurring utterances, etc.). When the milder symptoms of anarthria are considered, it is easily realized that they have many features in common with disturbances of inner speech involving the *phonemic level of language expression.* We mean by this term all disorders which intervene in the expression of phonemes at a pre-articulatory stage of word formation, i.e., at the level of the mechanisms through which phonemes to be uttered are chosen among the repertory of phonemes afforded by the spoken language. Disruption of such mechanisms reverberates on written as well as oral expression and does not *per se* imply poor articulation.

As Table 13-1 shows, the most severe articulatory defects in aphasia (e.g., total blocking, explosive speech, etc.) can be clearly distinguished from the most severe phonemic disorders (e.g., phonemic jargon); the milder forms of the two orders of phenomena, however, may bear too close a resemblance to be easily differentiated. For example, it is hard to decide if the substitution of voiced consonantal sounds (e.g., b, v, g) by the corresponding voiceless consonants (p, f, and k respectively) is due to wrong choice of phonemes (perhaps as a consequence of auditory discrimination defects, as postulated by Luria, 1958) or to lack of synergy of the vocal chords with the muscles of articulation (as in the "syndrome of phonetic disintegration" described by Alajouanine, Ombrédane and Durand in 1939). Moreover, phonemic errors, while often uttered with great fluency, as in a typical Wernicke's aphasia with anosognosia, may sometimes be ejaculated with uncertainties, sudden stops and partial repetitions; a good example of this is what the French

TABLE 13-1. SCHEMATIC ILLUSTRATION OF DIFFICULTIES IN THE DIFFERENTIAL DIAGNOSIS BETWEEN ARTICULATORY AND PHONEMIC DISORDERS IN APHASIA

Overall clinical severity of observed symptom	Observable symptom in spontaneous aphasic speech	Possible nature of underlying defect	
		Articulatory	Phonemic
more severe	total blocking	+	
	explosive speech	+	
	slurred speech	+	
	scansion	+	
less severe	rare pauses within words	+	+
	phonemic paraphasias	+	+
	"conduites d'approche"	+	+
	neologisms		+
more severe	phonemic jargon		+

authors call "conduites d'approche," i.e., sets of consecutively uttered phonemic paraphasias which are phonemic variations of the same word. In such cases it is difficult to say whether this jerky speech betrays a concomitant disorder of articulation or whether it mirrors the patient's attempts at self-correction.

We do not deny that, in a number of patients, one may overcome these diagnostic uncertainties by relying on one's clinical intuition. However, we have not been able to set up *objective* differential criteria which could be applied to all aphasic subjects. Therefore we decided to consider phonemic and articulatory disorders as equivalent for the purposes of the present research and to subsume them under the comprehensive concept of *"phonemic-articulatory disorders."* This way of dealing with the problem, while justifiable from a practical standpoint, entails as a consequence that aphasics whose disorders are traditionally considered as belonging to different types of aphasia fall in the same category. For example, both anarthric patients—who are usually labelled as Broca's aphasics—and patients with phonemic jargon—who are usually labelled as Wernicke's aphasics—would be considered as belonging to the "severe phonemic-articulatory disorders" group.

On the basis of the above considerations, it seemed advisable to approach the problem of the relationships between O.A. and aphasic disturbances of oral expression by determining:
1. the correlation between O.A. and the severity of phonemic-articulatory disorders;
2. the incidence of O.A. in the different clinical syndromes of aphasia, focussing one's attention, in particular, on the forms in which a concomitant presence of O.A. has been reported in the literature.

The present study was designed to answer the following questions:

1) Does O.A. appear in patients with lesions of the left hemisphere, or is it associated also with lesions of the right hemisphere?

2) In left brain damaged patients, is O.A. constantly accompanied by aphasia?

3) Is there any correlation between presence and severity of O.A. and presence and severity of the phonemic-articulatory disorder? What is the incidence of O.A. in the different clinical syndromes of aphasia?

4) What is the relationship between O.A. and limb apraxia (L.A.)? This question is justified by the possibility that O.A. may occur in subjects who show no phonemic-articulatory disturbance; in such cases, is O.A. merely a part of a more general apraxic disorder, i.e. is it always accompanied by L.A.?

MATERIALS AND METHODS

Subjects

Forty control subjects without cerebral lesions, 40 patients with focal lesions of the right hemisphere and 134 patients with focal lesions of the left hemisphere were studied.

Control patients had been hospitalized either in our clinic for psychoneurosis or for neurological lesions below the level of the cervical spine, or in general medical wards for internal diseases. The side of the lesion in brain damaged subjects was determined on the basis of clinical findings, usually supplemented by electroencephalographic and neuroradiological investigations. Patients who had an obvious involvement of both hemispheres were excluded from the study. All subjects who considered themselves left-handed or ambidextrous (or were reported to be such by their relatives) were also excluded. Since the gestural tasks of our apraxia tests were very elementary in nature (vide infra), no attempt was made to match the groups with respect to cultural level. In contrast, age was considered, the mean age being 48.2 years for the normal group, 53.1 years for the right brain damaged group, and 51.5 years for the left brain damaged group. No significant difference with respect to age was found among the three groups ($F=1.56$; $p>.05$).

Assessment of aphasia

All left brain damaged patients were administered a standard aphasia examination, currently used in the aphasia unit of our clinic, in order to (1) separate aphasics from non-aphasic patients, and (2) classify aphasic subjects according to the presence and severity of phonemic-articulatory disorders in oral expression and according to the type of aphasia. The examination allows an accurate recording of qualitative phenomena of oral expression and a quantitative assessment of the following performances: oral expression, auditory comprehension, repetition, spontaneous writing, reading comprehension, writing to dictation, reading aloud and copying. For each section there is available a cut-off score, i.e., a score exceeded by 100% of normals, obtained from the administration of the examination to control subjects.

The separation between aphasics and non-aphasic patients was made on the basis of the oral language sub-tests only, since the specific disturbance which we wished to correlate with aphasia might be expected to show some affinity merely with disorders of oral language. Reading and writing were not considered. Thus, left brain damaged patients, whose scores on the oral expression, repetition and auditory comprehension sub-tests were lower than the normal cut-off scores, were defined as "aphasics," while left brain damaged patients whose disturbances were limited to written language (i.e., "pure" alexic and/or agraphic patients) were considered "non-aphasics."

Twenty-nine left brain damaged patients turned out to be non-aphasic, and 105 to be aphasic. As mentioned, the aphasic patients were considered from two points of view: 1. the presence and severity of phonemic articulatory defects, and 2. the overall clinical picture to which they belonged.

With respect to the presence of phonemic-articulatory defects, aphasic patients were classified as having severe, mild, or no phonemic-articulatory disturbances by an independent observer (who did not know their score on the apraxia tests) on the basis of the quality of speech disorder recorded on two sub-tests: a) description: men were asked to describe accurately what they did when shaving and women were asked to describe accurately what they did when cooking spaghetti; b) naming of 20 pictures representing common objects, such as a table, an umbrella, etc. Repetition was not used to assess phonemic-articulatory disorders of speech because it is not necessarily a more sensitive indicator of articulatory defects than spontaneous speech (Goodglass, Quadfasel and Timberlake, 1964) and because the performance of it may be impaired by disturbances which are extraneous to oral expression, such as lack or instability of set and auditory receptive defects.

The following criteria were used:

1) A patient was classified as having *severe* phonemic-articulatory disorders if he showed:

a) *speechlessness with recurring utterances;*

b) *the "syndrome of phonetic disintegration"* of French authors (Alajouanine, Ombrédane and Durand, 1939) and similar syndromes. Speech in these patients is characterized by a conspicuous laboriousness of articulation: articulatory movements are difficult to initiate and to maintain; the beginning of each utterance, preceded by a latency period, is often explosive, and speech goes on with a chopped up, syllabic cadence. Phonemic paraphasias are constantly present: phoneme substitutions (voiceless consonants instead of voiced consonants, occlusives instead of fricatives), assimilations (e.g. *l*ailor for *t*ailor), metatheses (e.g. sig*an*ture for sig*na*ture) or elisions (e.g. nessary for ne*ce*ssary) are commonly found. One aphasic patient who showed severe and unusual pseudo-stuttering, i.e. uncontrolled rythmical repetition of some syllables, was also included in this group.

c) *phonemic or syllabic jargon;* i.e. meaningless syllables, articulated in quick succession and with an apparently normal prosody or "melody of speech." Patients with this type of jargon were included in this group even when the phonemic disorder was not accompanied by slurred articulation, as may sometimes occur.

Forty-five patients were included in the group with severe phonemic-articulatory disorders.

2) A patient was classified as having *mild* phonemic-articulatory disorders if his speech showed at least 4 neologisms or phonemic paraphasias *plus* some sudden interruptions breaking a word into two or more parts (and therefore not explainable merely in terms of word-finding difficulties). All aphasics who showed the so-called "conduites d'approche" belonged to this group. Subjects whose disturbances were limited to a few phonemic paraphasias plus an obviously altered melody of speech ("dysprosody") were also included. Twenty-six patients belonged to this group with mild phonemic-articulatory disorders.

3) A patient was classified as having *no* phonemic-articulatory disorders if none of the preceding phenomena were present in his speech production. A few patients who showed some neologisms within a picture of many verbal paraphasias (i.e., word substitutions) were also included in this group. We believe, in fact, that whenever other phonemic-articulatory disorders are missing, a few neologisms may be uttered as a by-product of severe disturbances in the choice of words. Thirty-four patients turned out to have no phonemic-articulatory disorders.

It is important to point out that the designations "severe," "mild" and "no" phonemic-articulatory disorders refer solely to the qualitative aspects of speech, and do not imply any judgment as to its quantitative aspect, i.e., as to the degree of the impairment of the patient's ability to communicate through speech. Actually, 21 out of 26 (81%) patients with *mild* phonemic-articulatory disturbances were suffering from *severe* impairment of their verbal communication, for reasons other than their phonemic-articulatory defect (e.g. anomia, verbal paraphasias, extreme speech reduction, etc.). Of course, all patients with *severe* phonemic-articulatory disorders were totally unable to communicate.

From the clinical standpoint the following discrete types of aphasia may be singled out with sufficient certainty among the 105 patients in our series:

a) *Broca's aphasia.* Of the patients with severe phonemic-articulatory defect those with severe anarthria were included in this category. There were 26 speechless patients with recurring utterances, and 12 patients with the syndrome of phonetic disintegration. Moreover, 3 patients who showed mild phonemic-articulatory disorders (1 patient with agrammatism and 2 with dysprosody and rare phonemic paraphasias) were also included in this group. It should be pointed out that Broca's aphasia is defined here according to Pierre Marie's conception: the severity of the receptive defect was not taken into consideration.

b) *Phonemic jargon aphasia.* This syndrome was present in 6 patients with "severe phonemic-articulatory defects." Its position among the main forms of aphasia is a matter of controversy. Delay and Lhermitte (1963) tend to consider it as a particular type of Wernicke's aphasia. Actually 5 out of 6 of our patients showed a severe impairment of oral comprehension on our standard examination for aphasia, which may justify labelling them "Wernicke's aphasia." At any rate, this sub-group should be kept separate from the more common forms of Wernicke's aphasia, on account of the type of the speech defect, which is exclusively phonemic in character.

c) *Conduction aphasia.* This form was defined in conformity with Geschwind's (1956) clinical description: 1. quality of speech production: spontaneous speech is fluent, but grossly paraphasic; 2. a striking discrepancy between auditory comprehension (preserved) and repetition (impaired). Our standard aphasia examination provides us with scores for expression (description plus naming), auditory comprehension (sentences and isolated words) and repetition (sentences and isolated words). Scores for each modality range from 0 to 4 and are weighted so that manipulation of whole sentences is given more weight than manipulation of isolated words in each language modality. Subjects whose comprehension score was 3 or 4 and whose repetition score was at least 2 points lower than their comprehension score were included in the "conduction" group. Nine patients belonging to the "mild" phonemic-articulatory disorders group met these requirements and were therefore classified as "conduction aphasics." It should be noted that 8 out of these 9 patients were severely impaired in oral communication, i.e. they scored 2 or less in the expressive section of our aphasia examination.

d) *Wernicke's aphasia.* All of the 34 patients with no phonemic-articulatory disturbances may be considered as suffering from Wernicke's aphasia. The degree of their expressive defect ranged from semantic jargon with anosognosia to moderate verbal paraphasias and to rare word-finding difficulties. Their comprehension defect was also very variable, but there was never a discrepancy between comprehension and repetition.

e) *Unclassifiable aphasics.* As we pointed out, we were not able to discriminate, in patients with milder forms of phonemic-articulatory symptoms, between articulatory defects (connoting Broca's aphasia) and purely phonemic defects. As mentioned before, the presence of agrammatism and dysprosody permitted us to identify 3 such patients as cases of Broca's aphasia, while 9 cases met the requirements of conduction aphasia, as previously defined. The remaining 14 cases could not be included in any of the preceding categories and were therefore considered as "unclassifiable" aphasics.

Assessment of O.A. and L.A.

Oral apraxia (O.A.) was assessed in all experimental groups by means of a 10-item test in which subjects were asked to perform oral gestures following verbal command and, if necessary, on imitation. The following gestures were requested:

1) Stick out your tongue
2) Whistle
3) Yawn
4) Try to touch the tip of your nose with your tongue
5) Give a "Bronx cheer" or "raspberry"
6) Show how you would kiss someone
7) Show how your teeth chatter when you are cold
8) Click your tongue, imitating the sound of a horse galloping
9) Puff or blow
10) Clear your throat.

The verbal command was given first. If the patient performed perfectly, he was given a perfect score. If this was not the case, the gesture itself was shown to him by the examiner, and only the patient's performance on imitation was scored. In so doing, we wished to avoid possible confusion between praxic errors and errors due to lack of verbal comprehension. This could also mean that we may, to a small extent, have under-estimated the number of apraxic errors. The patient's behavior was rated on a 3-point scale (0, 1, 2). Maximum score on the whole test was 20. Possible re-

TABLE 13–2. POSSIBLE RESPONSES AND SCORES ON THE ORAL APRAXIA TEST

Definition of response	Observed behavior	Score
Correct	a) accurate performance immediately follows oral command (or demonstration).	2
	b) accurate performance is preceded by protracted pauses, during which unsuccessful movements may be present.	1
Raw	overall pattern of gesture is acceptable though movements are defective in terms of amplitude, accuracy, force and/or speed.	1
Partial	some important part of gesture is lacking, though the rest is performed correctly.	0
Perseveration	gestures elicited by preceding items are performed.	0
Irrelevant	some other incorrect oral performance (including speech sounds) is produced.	0
Nil	no oral performance is produced.	0

TABLE 13–3. SCORES OBTAINED BY THE DIFFERENT EXPERIMENTAL GROUPS ON THE ORAL APRAXIA TEST

				Left Brain Damaged Patients			
	Oral Apraxia Scores	Control Patients (N = 40)	Right Brain Damaged Patients (N = 40)	Non-aphasic Patients (N = 29)	Aphasics		
					No Phon-art. (N = 34)	Mild Phon-art. (N = 26)	Severe Phon-art. (N = 45)
none	20	28	30	18	15	5	
	19	5	2	2	4	3	1
	18	3	3	3	6	3	1
	17	4	3	3	2		1
	16		2		5	3	1
mild	15				1		1
	14			1	1	6	3
	13					2	3
	12						1
	11					2	2
severe	10			1			6
	9					2	4
	8						2
	7						3
	6						2
	5						3
	4						2
	3						4
	2			1			3
	1						
	0						2

sponses and their corresponding scores are shown in Table 13-2.

Assessment of limb apraxia for intransitive movements[1] (L.A.) was also made in all patients by means of a 10-item test (maximum score = 20) in which subjects were asked to perform gestures with the upper limb homolateral to the side of the lesion. Both the administration and the scoring system were similar to those of the O.A. test. The following gestures were requested:

1) Make the sign of the cross
2) Salute
3) Wave goodbye
4) Threaten somebody with your hand
5) Show that you are hungry
6) Thumb your nose
7) Snap your fingers
8) Make the sign of the horns to designate a cuckold
9) Indicate that someone is crazy
10) Make the letter O with your fingers.

Although some of these gestures are not generally used in other countries, all of them are common it Italy.

RESULTS

Oral apraxia versus phonemic-articulatory disorders and limb apraxia

Table 13-3 shows the scores obtained on the O.A. test by the 6 experimental groups. The lowest score obtained by any of the control subjects was 17. Right brain damaged subjects showed a similar performance, their lowest score being 16, i.e., only one point below that of the worst normal subject. Sixteen was chosen as the cut-off point, i.e., patients with scores of 15 or less were classified as orally apraxic. This was done on the assumption that certain non-specific factors, which may exert a negative influence on oral performance, such as paresis of oral and facial muscles and overall awkwardness due to cerebral damage, are present in right brain damaged subjects as well as in left brain damaged subjects.

Three non-aphasic left brain damaged patients, 2 aphasics without phonemic-articulatory disorders, 12 aphasics with mild phonemic-articulatory disorders, and 41 aphasics with severe phonemic-articulatory disorders had a score lower than the cut-off point. These patients may be defined as "oral apraxic" subjects. A further distinction was made between *mild* O.A. and *severe* O.A., the cut-off point being arbitrarily set at 11, i.e., patients with a score of 10 or less were considered to be severely affected.

The aphasic group was partitioned into a 3 × 3 contingency table, according to presence and degree of severity of both phonemic-articulatory and O.A. disorders, as shown in Table 13-4.

TABLE 13-4. PARTITIONING OF APHASIC PATIENTS ACCORDING TO PRESENCE AND SEVERITY OF PHONEMIC-ARTICULATORY AND ORAL APRAXIC DISORDERS

		Phonemic-articulatory Disorders		
		S	M	N
Oral Apraxia (O.A.)	S	31	2	0
	M	10	10	2
	N	4	14	32

chi² = 72.660
p < .001
C = .640

(S = severe; M = mild; N = none)

The chi^2 of this table is highly significant ($p < .001$). The value of the corresponding contingency coefficient ($C = .640$) is close to the maximum obtainable value ($C\,max = .816$). This indicates that the severity of phonemic-articulatory disturbances is highly correlated with severity of O.A.

The lowest score obtained by control subjects on the L.A. test was 18, while the lowest score obtained by right brain damaged patients was 17. In analogy with the criterion used for O.A., the latter score was chosen as the cut-off point

[1] The term "intransitive" movements was used by Liepmann (1905) to designate movements which are always made without the handling of an object. This class of limb movements was chosen because our oral apraxia test also included only intransitive movements.

to discriminate L.A. patients from non-L.A. patients, while the cut-off point between *mild* and *severe* L.A. patients was set at 11. All left brain damaged patients (non-aphasics as well as aphasics) were classified according to presence and severity of O.A. and L.A. in Table 13-5.

TABLE 13–5. PARTITIONING OF LEFT BRAIN DAMAGED PATIENTS ACCORDING TO PRESENCE AND SEVERITY OF ORAL APRAXIA AND LIMB APRAXIA

		Limb Apraxia (L.A.) S	M	N
Oral Apraxia (O.A.)	S	11	10	14
	M	1	6	16
	N	2	6	68

$chi^2 = 36.448$
$p < .001$
$C = .461$

(S = severe; M = mild; N = none)

The chi^2 of this table yields a $p<.001$ and a contingency coefficient $C=.461$ (to be compared with a maximum value of .816). This indicates that O.A. and L.A. also tend to appear together with a frequency which is far greater than chance. However, in the entire left brain damaged group, this correlation is significantly lower than the correlation between O.A. and phonemic-articulatory disorders of speech, as shown by the comparison carried out by Goodman's method (1964) in Table 13-6.

Among the patients with severe O.A. some had mild or no phonemic-articulatory defects. The presence of L.A. in these patients was investigated. Out of 3 patients without aphasia, but with severe O.A., none had L.A. Two aphasics without phonemic-articulatory disorders had O.A.: of these one did not have L.A. Finally, 2 aphasics with mild phonemic-articulatory disorders had severe O.A.: only one of these had L.A. It is evident, therefore, that when O.A. appears in the presence of mild or absent phonemic-articulatory disorders, one cannot argue that it is part of a general apraxic disturbance.

Oral apraxia and aphasic syndromes

Table 13-7 shows the scores obtained on the O.A. test by the patients suffering from the different syndromes. Ninety percent of Broca's aphasics and 83% of phonemic jargon aphasics showed O.A. No significant difference was found between these 2 types of aphasia with respect to severity of O.A. ($p=.37$ on the Mann Whitney U test).

O.A. was present in 33% of cases with conduction aphasia. The incidence of O.A. in this group was nearly similar to the incidence of O.A. in the non-classifiable group, in which there was no discrepancy between comprehension and repetition.

Finally, only 2 out of 34 Wernicke's aphasic patients (i.e., less than 6%) showed mild O.A.

Relative difficulty of oral praxic performances

Table 13-8 shows the relative difficulty of the different items of the O.A. test, expressed as the

TABLE 13–6. COMPARISON BETWEEN O.A. VS. PHONEMIC-ARTICULATORY DISORDERS AND O.A. VS. L.A. IN THE ENTIRE LEFT BRAIN DAMAGED GROUP

		Phonemic-articulatory Disorders +	−
Oral Apraxia (O.A.)	+	53	5
	−	18	58

		Limb Apraxia (L.A.) +	−
Oral Apraxia (O.A.)	+	28	30
	−	8	68

$y^2 = 4.246 \quad p < .05$

N.B. Sign + indicates presence of the disorder (either severe or mild); sign — indicates absence of the disorder. Both the aphasic patients with no phonemic-articulatory disturbances and the brain damaged patients with no aphasia are classified as "phonemic-articulatory disorders —" in the table.

TABLE 13–7. ORAL APRAXIA IN DIFFERENT APHASIC SYNDROMES

Oral Apraxia Scores	Broca's Aphasia (N=42)	Phonemic Jargon (N=6)	Conduction Aphasia (N=9)	Non Classifiable (N=14)	Wernicke's Aphasia (N=34)
20			3	2	15
19	1	1		2	4
18	1		2	1	6
17	1				2
16	1		1	2	5
15	1				1
14	2	1	1	5	1
13	4		1		
12	1				
11	1	1		2	
10	7				
9	2	2			
8	2				
7	3				
6	2				
5	3				
4	2				
3	4				
2	2	1	1		
1					
0	2				

mean score obtained on each item by the entire group of aphasics.

It is noteworthy that the performance, failure of which was stressed by Jackson in his original description, i.e., protrusion of the tongue, was the easiest of the entire test and was, in fact, impaired only in subjects with the most severe oral apraxia.

DISCUSSION

The lesions responsible for O.A. were found only within the left hemisphere in our series. However, the possibility of finding O.A. in a right brain damaged patient cannot be excluded, since such an association has occasionally been reported in the literature (see Nathan, 1947). In any case, O.A. with right hemisphere lesions must certainly be uncommon, especially when we consider the high incidence (43%) of O.A. in lesions of the left hemisphere. In this series, the incidence of O.A. was greater than that of L.A. (27%).

Within the left brain damaged group, O.A. and phonemic-articulatory disorders appear together very often, and this is a fact which,

TABLE 13–8. RELATIVE DIFFICULTY OF ORAL PRAXIC PERFORMANCES IN APHASIC PATIENTS

Item	Mean score	Rank
1. Stick out your tongue	1.82	1
9. Puff or blow	1.58	2
10. Clear your throat	1.52	3
3. Yawn	1.38	4
6. Show how you would kiss someone	1.35	5
2. Whistle	1.33	6
4. Try to touch the tip of your nose with your tongue	1.29	7
7. Show how your teeth chatter when you are cold	1.27	8
5. Give a "Bronx cheer" or "raspberry"	1.00	9
8. Click your tongue, imitating a horse galloping	.79	10

N.B. 1) The scoring scale ranges from 0 to 2 for each item.
2) Performances are ranked from easiest to most difficult.

whatever its possible interpretations, cannot be ignored. As Table 13-6 shows, the association between O.A. and phonemic-articulatory disturbances of speech is significantly stronger than that between O.A. and L.A. Oral apraxia characterizes patients whose speech productions may be very different from one another, and therefore their inclusion by us in the same group might seem arbitrary. Yet no difference can be found between the mean severity of O.A. in anarthric patients, who have either severely reduced or absent speech, and in phonemic jargon aphasics, whose speech is fluent though meaningless. Thus, it looks as if phonemic jargon is closer to classic anarthria than to verbal jargon—at least with respect to O.A. This finding is interesting when one considers that phonemic and verbal jargon aphasics, because of their fluent speech production, are traditionally subsumed under the same category of "jargon aphasia" which is usually distinguished from the group labelled "anarthria."

As a rule, the severity of O.A. is also directly proportional to the severity of phonemic-articulatory disorders. Exceptions are represented mainly by those subjects (N=28) in whom the verbal disturbance is more severe than the non-verbal one. In the majority of these cases (24 out of 28) the discrepancy was small (from severe to mild or from mild to none): this is concordant with the view expressed by Alajouanine and Lhermitte (1960) that articulation is more severely impaired and slower in recovery than non-verbal movements because of its greater complexity and differentiation. This interpretation is, however, unsatisfactory in cases in which the discrepancy between the two symptoms is great, i.e. when severe phonemic-articulatory disorders appear in a setting of virtually normal oral praxis. Four such cases were found in our series. Their clinical features may be summarized as in Table 13-9.

It should be noted that these patients differed from each other with respect both to type of speech production and to time elapsed from the onset of illness.

Even rarer were patients showing the opposite dissociation, i.e. whose O.A. was more severe than their phonemic-articulatory disorder. There were 7 such subjects in all: 4 aphasics plus 3 non-aphasic left brain damaged subjects. As shown in Table 13-3, the discrepancy between the 2 symptoms was small in 5 of these patients. The discrepancy was striking in 2 non-aphasic left brain damaged subjects.

TABLE 13-9.

Patient No.	Sex	Age	Etiology	Time elapsed from onset of illness	Type of speech disorder	Score on O.A. test
1	F	42	Cerebrovascular accident	26 days	Phonemic jargon	19
2	F	35	Cerebrovascular accident	35 days	Syndrome of phonetic disintegration	18
3	M	33	Cerebrovascular accident	More than six months	Syndrome of phonetic disintegration	17
4	M	53	Cerebrovascular accident	More than two years	Recurring utterances	16

One of these was a 57-year-old male patient who had suffered from a CVA with right hemiparesis and dysphasia 2 months and 20 days before testing. When seen in our aphasia unit, he showed mild central paresis of the right facial nerve and no aphasic defect on our standard aphasia examination. He scored 10 on the O.A. test and 20 on the L.A. test. The second patient, a 55-year-old male patient, had a long history of vascular insufficiency of the left hemisphere. Angiography showed a left internal carotid thrombosis at the bifurcation, with clear collateral circulation through the ophthalmic artery. At the time of testing the patient showed right hemiparesis with greater involvement of the lower limb and of the proximal part of the upper limb. He complained of some slight difficulty in oral language during conversation, not detectable on our standard examination of aphasia. By contrast, he showed marked dysgraphia and dyslexia, mild constructive apraxia and some difficulties with color recognition (green-blue). He scored 3 on the O.A. test and 18 on the L.A. test.

Let us now consider the possible implications of our findings with reference to the clinico-anatomical aspects of aphasia. The behavioral level on which the present research was carried out does not allow us to make reliable inferences concerning the anatomical and functional relationships which exist between O.A. and speech disorders. Nevertheless, on account of the interest of the problem, some hypotheses may be advanced. O.A. is present in the great majority of patients with severe Broca's aphasia. This might be due to the concomitant impairment of two discrete but independent associative areas: the area where engrams for words are stored and the area which is responsible for the integration of non-verbal oral movements. An alternative hypothesis is that oral movements, both verbal and non-verbal, are subserved by one single associative motor area, a lesion of which would manifest itself through both phonemic-articulatory and oral apraxic disorders. In this case the phonemic-articulatory disturbance of Broca's aphasia could be considered apraxic in nature, not merely in analogy with O.A., but also because lesions of motor associative areas always tend to manifest themselves with apraxia (Geschwind, 1965). The absence of O.A. in 3 severe Broca's patients seems to support the former hypothesis: the possibility that the two functions be independently impaired would demonstrate that they have discrete cortical representation. On the other hand, the second hypothesis appears to be more probable when one considers that, from the point of view of the economy of the C.N.S., it would be strange if the same muscles depended upon two different cortical areas, according to the type of movement which was required from them. It is likely that the cortical representation of "la faculté de coordonner les mouvements propres du langage" (to quote the expression originally used by Broca when discussing aphemia in 1861) is not different from that of the ability to co-ordinate extra-verbal oral movements. Therefore, the disturbance in the 4 patients (out of a sample of 38 patients) whose phonemic articulatory impairment of speech was not accompanied by oral apraxia, could be explained in terms of earlier recovery of non-verbal movements, because of their lesser complexity and differentiation.

Personally, we would favor the latter hypothesis, i.e. that all intentional oral movements, both verbal and non-verbal, are controlled by a single key-board, derangement of which produces both phonemic-articulatory disorders and O.A. Commands impinging upon this keyboard might come, in the case of verbal movements, from the posterior language centers, via the arcuate fasciculus (Geschwind, 1965) and, in the case of non-verbal movements performed on imitation, from the visual-kinesthetic area, possibly via the occipito-frontal fasciculus. A lesion involving both pathways may produce speech and oral apraxic disorders at the same time, and thus explain the presence of O.A. in patients other than Broca's aphasics. The most common site of such a lesion seems to be the parieto-temporal region. Our knowledge of the morbid anatomy of phonemic jargon aphasia is still too scarce to enable us to say whether or not this form—where O.A. and speech disturbances coexist—fits the proposed locus of lesion. As far as other cases are concerned, two considerations are relevant: 1) O.A. is found in a certain number (33%) of patients with conduction aphasia, even if not so frequently as suggested by Geschwind (1965); according to this author, these cases should correspond to a lesion of the supramarginal gyrus region. 2) At least one of the two left brain damaged patients who presented severe O.A. without aphasia showed additional symptoms (e.g., constructive apraxia, dyslexia, dysgraphia, color dysgnosia, etc.) which suggested an inferior parietal lesion. This case seems to demonstrate that a lesion in the inferior parietal lobe may impair the fiber tracts which subserve oral praxic mechanisms, without involving the anatomical structures for either limb praxis or oral verbal movements.

SUMMARY

This study was undertaken in order to assess the frequency and to explore the role of oral apraxia in expressive disturbances of speech. Forty right brain damaged patients, 134 left brain damaged patients and 40 control patients were given an oral apraxia test and a limb apraxia test for intransitive movements. In the left hemispheric group the presence and quality of aphasia was assessed by means of a standard aphasia examination. On the oral apraxia test, the performance of the right hemispheric group was similar to that of the control group. All the left brain damaged patients who scored below the lowest score obtained by any of the right brain damaged patients were considered oral apraxic. A strong association was found between oral apraxia and phonemic-articulatory disorders of speech, the exceptions being mainly in the sense of a poorer verbal than praxic performance. However, severe oral apraxia was found in two non-aphasic left brain damaged patients. When considered with respect to the clinical syndromes of aphasia, it was found that oral apraxia was a very common accompaniment of Broca's aphasia and of phonemic jargon aphasia, it was present in one third of conduction aphasics and it was usually absent in Wernicke's aphasia. Oral apraxia was not uncommonly found to be independent of limb apraxia. Moreover, the majority of patients with severe oral apraxia and mild or no phonemic-articulatory disturbances did not show limb apraxia: therefore, one cannot argue that, in these cases, oral apraxia was part of a general praxic disturbance.

Acknowledgement. The authors wish to thank Dr. Norman Geschwind for his valuable advice on the manuscript.

REFERENCES

Alajouanine, T., Ombredane, A., and Durand, M. (1939) *Le Syndrome de Désintégration Phonétique dans l'Aphasie*, Masson, Paris.

——, and Lhermitte, F. (1960) *Les troubles des activités expressives du langage dans l'aphasie. Leur relations avec les apraxies*, "Rev. Neurol.," **102,** 604-633.

——, ——, (1961) *Les désorganizations des activités expressives du langage dans l'aphasie* in Reports at the VII International Congress of Neurology, Edition for the Congress, Roma.

Bay, E. (1957) *Die corticale Dysarthrie und ihre Beziehungen zur sogenannten motorischen Aphasie*, "Deutsch. Zeitschr. f. Nervenheilk.," **176,** 553-594.

Ballet, G. (1908) *Apraxie faciale (impossibilité de souffler) associée à de l'aphasie complexe (aphasie motrice et aphasie sensorielle). Apraxie et aphémie*, "Rev. Neurol.," 445-447.

Dejerine, J. (1908) in *Discussion sur l'aphasie*, "Rev. Neurol.," 626.

—— (1926) *Sémiologie des Affections du Système Nerveux*. Masson, Paris.

Delay, J., and Lhermitte, F. (1963) *Aphasie* in Encyclopédie Médico-Chirurgicale, Neurologie, vol. 1, Paris.

De Morsier, G. (1949) *Les troubles de la déglutition et des mouvements de la langue dans l'anarthrie (aphasie motrice)*, "Pract. otorinto-laryng.," **11,** 124-133.

Foix, C. (1928) *Aphasies* in Nouveau Traité de Médicine, vol. 18, Masson, Paris.

Geschwind, N. (1965) *Disconnection syndromes in animals and man*, "Brain," **88,** 237–294, 585–644.

Goodglass, H., Quadfasel, F. A., and Timberlake, W. H. (1964) *Phrase length and the type and severity of aphasia*, "Cortex," **1,** 133–153.

Goodman, L. A. (1964) *Simple methods for analyzing three-factor interaction in contingency tables*, "J. Am. Statist. Assoc.," **59,** 319–352.

Jackson, J. H. (1878) *Remarks on non-protrusion of the tongue in some cases of aphasia* in Selected Writings, vol. 2, 153–154, Hodder and Stoughton, London, 1932.

Liepmann, H. (1900) *Das Krankheitsbild der Apraxie ("motorischen Asymbolie")* "Monatschr. Psych. Neurol.," **8,** 15–44, 102–132, 182–197.

—— (1905) *Uber Störungen des Handelns bei Gehirnkranken*, Karger, Berlin.

Luria, A. R. (1958) *Brain disorders and language analysis*, "Language and Speech," **1,** 14–34.

Marie, P. (1906a) *Que faut-il penser des aphasies sous-corticales?* in Travaux et Mémoires, Masson, Paris, 1926.

—— (1906b) *Un cas d'anarthrie transitoire par lésion de la zone lenticulaire* in Travaux et Mémoires. Masson, Paris, 1926.

—— (1908) Discussion on Ballet's communication, "Rev. Neurol.," 447.

Moutier, F. (1908) *L'Aphasie de Broca*, Stenheil, Paris.

Nathan, P. W. (1947) *Facial apraxia and apraxic dysarthria*, "Brain," **70,** 449–478.

Nielson, J. M. (1946) *Agnosia, Apraxia, Aphasia*, Hoeber, New York.

Siegel, S. (1956) *Non Parametric Statistics for the Behavioral Sciences*, McGraw Hill, New York.

14

Prosodic Factors in Grammar—Evidence from Aphasia

HAROLD GOODGLASS
IRIS G. FODOR
CELIA L. SCHULHOFF

HAROLD GOODGLASS, Ph.D., is director of psychology research at the Boston Veterans Administration Hospital.
IRIS G. FODOR, Ph.D., is with Northeastern University, Boston.
CELIA L. SCHULHOFF, Ph.D., is with the Lexington, Massachusetts, School department.
This investigation was supported in part by Public Health Service Research Grants No. MH 04187 from the National Institute of Mental Health to Clark University, and NB 06209 from the National Institute of Neurological Diseases and Blindness to Boston University.

The pathology of grammar, as seen in aphasia, has aroused much speculation but little systematic investigation on the part of the psycholinguistic community. The dissociation, through pathology, of the component processes of grammar complements the study of the acquisition of grammar in children—a field which is receiving a great deal of study. Each is a testing ground for principles derived from the other area and both are challenges to a comprehensive psychology of language.

In this study, we were principally concerned with the conditions under which the function words of grammar are omitted or confused in aphasic speech. The loss of function words, which gives rise to the clinical symptom of telegraphic speech, is usually considered to be the central feature of motor agrammatism as seen in Broca's aphasia. However, omission of nonessential words is characteristic of many abnormalities of speech, and confusion in the use of grammatical words is heard in the speech of many types of aphasics. Among the questions at issue, then, is whether the motor agrammatic indeed has some objectifiable, distinctive difficulty with function words, and if so, whether this is a difference in degree only, from the misuse of function words in other varieties of aphasia.

It is important to bear in mind that the function words constitute the most commonly used words in English. They are easy to pronounce and, while chiefly monosyllabic, are phonetically distinct from each other. They constitute a closed class in that their limited number is sufficient for all usages in the language and has remained very stable down through the history of the language. Thus, their selective disturbance in aphasia would seem to contradict the familiar psychological principle of frequency of use.

Previous considerations of the psychological attributes of function words have emphasized the lack of meaningfulness of these words, which have no conceptual referent, and which come into use only to indicate relationships between lexical words. For example, Goldstein (1948) assumes that their lack of a referent makes them abstract and therefore diminishes their availability to patients who have lost the capacity for an "abstract attitude." Braine (1963) proposes an argument

From *Journal of Speech and Hearing Research* 10:5-20, 1967.

for the positional learning of function words, from which it follows that a major component of the meaning of these words may be a rather tenuous position association dependent on the contiguity of a lexical word. Howes and Geschwind[1] point out that the exclusive use of function words to relate other words to each other makes their occurrence unlikely in speech made up of one-word utterances. Glanzer (1962), on the basis of Braine's theory, reasoned that function words might be better retained as paired associates when learned in contiguity with other words—even nonsense syllables—than when learned as isolated responses; and he found this to be the case. Brown and Fraser (1963) consider the function of stress in early versus late acquisition of various grammatical function words.

In an earlier discussion, Goodglass (1962) attempted to account for the most prominent symptoms of Broca's (or motor) aphasia in terms of two postulates: (1) that the principal defect in this form of aphasia can be understood as an increased threshold for initiating and maintaining the flow of speech; and (2) that we can hypothesize a variable of "psychological salience" which characterizes the points in a message at which the Broca's aphasic can break through his raised speech threshold. After each such breakthrough, speech may continue for a number of syllables, after which the patient requires a new start with another salient word. It was suggested that salience depends interchangeably upon the informativeness, the intonational or amplitudinal stress, the phonological prominence, or even the affective quality, of a word or part of a word. This pair of postulates seemed sufficient to account for: (1) the existing indications that unstressed initial function words were omitted from the motor aphasic's speech; and (2) the sharply dichotomized distribution of aphasics when classified as to number of words per uninterrupted run of speech.

In the ensuing presentation we shall make use of the earlier reported finding by Goodglass, Quadfasel, and Timberlake (1964) that this dichotomy corresponds to a split between Broca's aphasia on one hand and Wernicke's (sensory) and amnesic aphasia on the other. We refer to the two latter as *fluent aphasia* with the reservation that the diagnostic distinction between fluent aphasia and Broca's aphasia breaks down at the milder levels. In general, the speech of fluent aphasics is characterized by frequent runs of five or more words and by well-preserved intonational patterns, while their major deficiencies lie in word finding, in errors of word and sound transposition, and in impaired comprehension. The Broca's aphasics initiate speech with effort, and speak in short word groupings with poor intonational patterns.

[1]Howes, D., and Geschwind, N., *Statistical Properties of Aphasic Speech*. Unpublished progress report on NIMH grant (1962).

EXPERIMENT 1

The first of our observations that agrammatic errors might hinge chiefly on prosodic variables was based on the frequent omissions of unstressed words (subject pronouns, conjunctions, articles, auxiliary verbs) when they occurred as the first word of a sentence in a Sentence Repetition Test.

On the basis of judges' ratings, the 50 aphasic subjects in this study were placed into the two major diagnostic groups, fluent aphasics and Broca's aphasics. The procedure for these judges' ratings is detailed by Goodglass, Quadfasel, and Timberlake (1964). It is based on ratings of the following seven speech characteristics: melody, articulatory agility, length of uninterrupted word-runs, grammatical variety, presence of paraphasia in running speech, auditory comprehension, and word-naming. A profile of the ratings made from each patient's tape recorded speech is assigned to a diagnostic category by reference to a standard profile for each diagnostic group.

While the fluent aphasics in this sample were consistently rated as milder in severity than the Broca's aphasics, the two groups were, in fact, closely matched on a Word-Span Repetition Test. This test contained a total of 15 groups of 3-word sets, of which one third were nouns (book, candle, light), one third function words (of, from, but), and one third mixed words suggesting a sentence (bottle, close, drink). Each set was pronounced twice immediately prior to the subject's attempt to repeat it, and was scored with one point for each word included in the patient's repetition, plus an extra point for any word group reproduced correctly as a unit. The distribution of scores of the two groups is reproduced in Figure 14-1, where it can be seen that the over-all scores did not distinguish between the groups. Further examination of these data showed that the two groups did not differ in their ability to repeat grammatical function words, as contrasted with nouns. For both groups, repetition of noun sets was superior to repetition of function words by a statistically insignificant margin. In view of the disparity in severity of the two groups, we may state that the fluent aphasics are at a disadvantage in their span for repetition of word-lists, when compared to Broca's aphasics of equal severity.

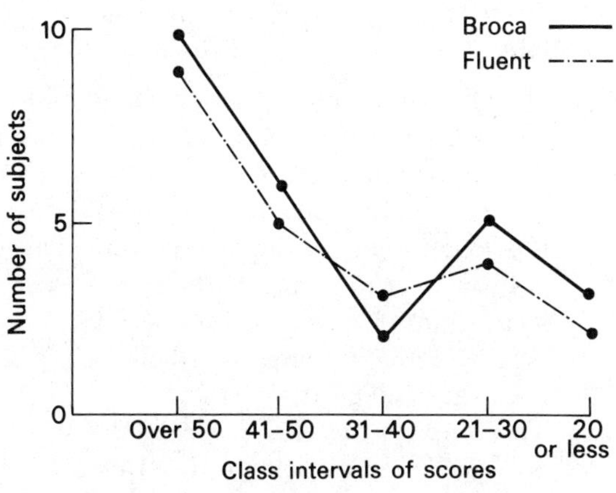

Fig. 14–1. Distribution of scores of Broca's and fluent aphasics on three-word repetition span.

The Sentence Repetition Test consisted of a series of 40 four- and five-word sentences of eight grammatical types. Fifteen of the test sentences began with subject pronouns (e.g. "*He* is staying home"), five with the word *if* ("*If* he wakes, call me"), five with the interrogative auxiliary *do* or *does* ("*Does* he feel better?") and five consisted of *the* plus a noun, with a modifying clause ("*The* man who won"). The remaining 10 sentences began with a stressed word (five imperatives and five interrogative adverbs). In contrast with the presentation of the Word Span Test, where grammatically unrelated words were spoken with equal stress, these sentences were pronounced by the examiner with normal conversational intonation, although care was taken to articulate distinctly. Under these conditions, the initial unstressed word was omitted with much greater relative frequency than the initial stressed words. Moreover, this type of omission was not distributed evenly between the groups, but was much more frequent in the Broca's aphasics than in the fluent aphasics. The distribution of omissions of initial unstressed words is compared for both groups in Figure 14-2. The difference between the two distributions was tested for statistical significance by splitting both groups into those subjects having more than two and those with fewer than two omissions. A chi-square test computed on this basis was significant beyond $p = 0.01$. It was found that omission of initial words is grossly unrelated to severity of aphasia in the group of fluent aphasics, and not significantly related to severity within the Broca's group, although

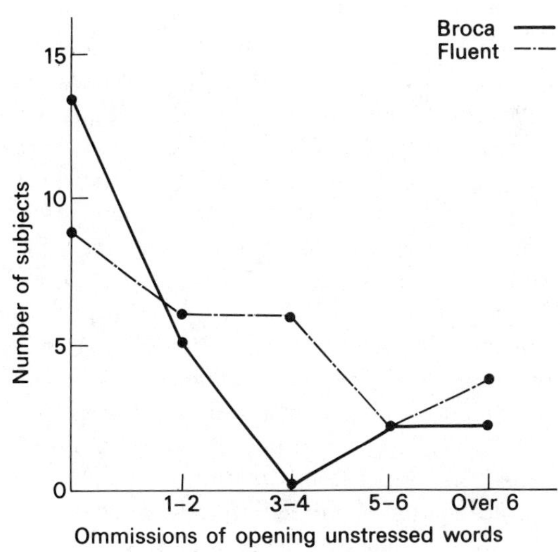

Fig. 14–2. Comparison of 27 Broca's aphasics and 23 fluent aphasics with respect to omission of opening unstressed words in sentence repetition.

a loose relationship in the latter group appeared to exist.

While this finding demonstrates a difference in type of words omitted by the two types of aphasics, it leaves open the question as to whether the same parts of speech in any other position would be treated differently. The Sentence Repetition Test provided too few instances of function words following an initial stressed word to constitute a test of this issue.

EXPERIMENT 2

Case Description

Patient S. L. was a 52-year old former chief cook for a large state institution, who had gradually developed aphasia over a period of four years, during which he had also developed tingling of his right hand and had one episode of unconsciousness. He had given up work only two months before this examination because he could no longer communicate adequately for the demands of the job. He had no hemiplegia and his language pattern was overwhelmingly that of Broca's aphasia, except for some difficulty in understanding complex spoken or written material. His aphasia was sufficiently severe that he did not initiate speech without stimulation by questions or pictures. When stimulated by conversation with an interviewer he produced brief answers consisting mainly of content words. His word finding was difficult, but beyond this partially spared ability to produce isolated ideas, there was no flow of speech. His verbs were generally uninflected, showing no tenses. His articulation was occasionally labored, but he had no consistent dysarthria. He demonstrated to a remarkable degree the tendency to repeat back model sentences in agrammatic form, with small words and inflectional endings omitted. Thus, his repetition—in spite of having a correct sentence immediately in memory as a model—duplicated the defects which characterized his efforts to formulate speech on his own. In addition to his expressive agrammatism, this patient acknowledged that he was unable to distinguish between the meanings of the various prepositions and auxiliary words.

Experimental Procedure

A series of three-word groups was constructed, consisting chiefly of sentences, but including some phrases as well, in which the patient's handling of the function word in the first or second position was the principal feature to be observed.

The major comparisons undertaken were:

(1) Comparing the ability to use function words in the following positions and stress patterns.

Position of Test Word	*Stress Pattern*	*Examples*
Initial	˘ ˘ ´	(a) "in the house"
		(b) "Is he home?"
Initial	˘ ´ ´	(a) "Can Jim come?"
		(b) "We all went."
Medial	´ ˘ ´	(a) "Close the door."
		(b) "So can you."
Medial	˘ ˘ ´	(a) "Is he home?"

(2) Given a particular position in a stress pattern, to compare the influence of the type of grammatical construction on the patient's ability to include the word in his repetition; for example, in the stress pattern ˘ ´ ´, to compare the initial word in a group of questions such as "Is John here?" with the initial word in a simple declarative like "It worked fine."

(3) To compare the effect of prosodic stress on an initial function word ("Doesn't he smoke?" versus "Does he smoke?") in competition with the effect of grammatical complexity, as introduced by the negative construction. Complexity might be expected to make the negative interrogative more difficult than the simple interrogative, while stress is expected to act as a facilitating influence.

(4) To compare the survival of several specific grammatical function words (*my, the, a, do, can, are*) under various prosodic and grammatical conditions.

Each test sentence was presented with normal conversational rate and intonation, with care taken to articulate even unstressed words carefully. The contrast between stressed and unstressed words was maintained as uniformly as possible through the several types of sentences.

In order to avoid fatigue and boredom, the testing was broken up into six sessions. Responses were taken down verbatim and checked against a tape recording, which was made concurrently. The first response which included the stem of one or more of the words in the test phrase was scored. Second attempts, whether they constituted self-corrections or contaminations were omitted in this tabulation, as were responses given after a repetition of the stimulus by the examiner.

For purposes of quantitative analysis, the following categories were established—all referring to the first function word in the sentence.

Scoring Category	*Definition*
Correct	Test word is produced in correct temporal relationship to one of the other words. Initial function word produced by itself is also accepted.
Substitution	Another function word is substituted.
Grunt	An inappropriate syllable occupying the rhythmic position of the test word (e.g., "Da Jack here?").
Omit only	Test word is omitted, but the other two words are correct.
Omit plus other error	Omission of test word plus a second word; also, interrogative in which an initial *is* or *are* was omitted from its proper position and placed after the subject.

S.L. was able to supply a scorable response falling into one of the above categories, for every test sentence.

Results From Testing Patient S. L.

The data summarized in Tables 14-1 and 14-2 reveal significantly higher omission rates for unstressed function words in the first position (49 omissions in 70 items or 70%) than for unstressed function words between two stressed words (6 omissions in 44 items, or 15%). Chi square $= 31$; $p < 0.01$.

Test phrases beginning with an unstressed function word were further subdivided into syntactic subcategories which appear to fare differently in this patient's speech. For example, in 3-word prepositional phrases (e.g., "In the house") the opening unstressed preposition was reproduced correctly in five of seven items, represented by a "grunt" once, and only once completely omitted. The anapestic rhythmic pattern of two unstressed words followed by a stressed word (items E through H of Table 14-1) was compared with the pattern of an unstressed word followed by two stressed words (items A through D). The difference favoring the anapestic pattern over the other is well short of statistical significance.

Looking more closely at differences between syntactic constructions having the same rhythm, we observe that in 22 simple declaratives beginning with an unstressed initial personal pronoun or possessive pronoun, the first word was omitted 18 times. In 16 interrogatives beginning with an unstressed auxiliary verb (*do*, *does*, or *can*) the first word was omitted 12 times—demonstrating essentially the same rate for the interrogative as for the declarative construction.

No significant differences are observed in percentage correct among the six types of construction using the rhythm ´ ˘ ´. We do note that the conditional construction using the unstressed word *if* medially ("Close, *if* open"), was correctly produced 4 out of 9 times, while the *if* degenerated to *iss* 4 times and was scored as a "grunt." There was only 1 total omission for the medial *if* as compared to 16 omissions in 22 phrases beginning with *if*. The difference between the initial and medial *if* is significant beyond $p = 0.01$ (chi square is 7.6). Here is some indication that the "grunt" is an intermediate phase in the mastery of grammatical morphemes. Similar use of a vague syllable as a primitive function word is described for children's speech by Braine (1962).

TABLE 14–1. REPETITION BY S. L. OF INITIAL UNSTRESSED FUNCTION WORDS

		Response Category				
Paradigm of Sentence Type	*Number of this Type*	+	*Subst. in Class*	*Grunt*	*Omits Test Word Only*	*Omission Plus Other Error*
A. His egg broke.	4	0	0	0	2	2
B. He feels good.	5	0	0	0	5	0
C. The wrong time	3	0	1	0	2	0
D. Can birds fly?	5	2	0	0	3	0
Subtotal (A thru D)	(17)	(2)	(1)	(0)	(12)	(2)
E. If he moves.	22	5	1	0	4	12
F. Can he dance?	11	1	1	0	0	9
G. He can dance.	13	4	0	0	1	8
H. In the house.	7	5	0	1	0	1
Subtotal (E thru G)	(53)	(15)	(2)	(1)	(5)	(30)
Total (A thru G)	(70)	(17)	(3)	(1)	(17)	(32)

TABLE 14–2. REPETITION BY S. L. OF MEDIAL UNSTRESSED FUNCTION WORDS

		Response Category				
Paradigm of Sentence Type	*Number of this Type*	+	*Subst. in Class*	*Grunt*	*Omits Test Word Only*	*Omission Plus Other Error*
I. Here they come!	4	4	0	0	0	0
J. Throw him out!	10	9	0	1	0	0
K. Wells are deep.	5	4	0	1	0	0
L. Where is Jack?	5	5	0	0	0	0
M. Close, if open.	9	4	0	4	0	1
N. Can't he dance?	11	6	0	0	0	5
Subtotal (I thru N)	(44)	(32)	(0)	(6)	(0)	(6)

It is notable that 9 of 16 stressed initial auxiliaries in the negative interrogative were reproduced correctly (e.g., "*Can't* he dance") as compared to 1 out of 11 unstressed auxiliaries in simple interrogatives of the class: "Can he dance?" Here the facilitating role of stress overrides the complexity of the syntactic structure, if we assume that the negative interrogative is a more complex syntactic form than the simple interrogative.

Since we could not use each unstressed word an equal number of times in each type of rhythmic pattern, the question arises as to whether the medial unstressed words, which were retained, are easier (because of frequency) than the unstressed openers which were dropped. Table 14-3 shows how each function word in a test sentence was handled by the patient when it occurred (a) as an unstressed initial word, (b) between two stressed words, or (c) as a stressed opening word. *The, it, if, is* have enough repeated use to demonstrate that the influence of the stress pattern applies, even when the same word is used in the various position with respect to stress.

EXPERIMENT 3

In order to test the generality, among Broca's aphasics, of the speech behavior of patient S. L., we assembled a set of 48 sentences for repetition—12 in each of four different stress-syntax patterns. The performance to be scored was the correct production of a function word in one of the following positions:

TABLE 14–3. TREATMENT OF IF, THE, IT, IS, CAN, DO(N'T) IN THREE DIFFERENT STRESS-POSITION COMBINATIONS

	Opening Unstressed				Medial Unstressed				Opening Stressed	
Word	+	Subs.	Grunt	Omit	+	Subs.	Grunt	Omit	+	Omit
if	5	1	0	16	4	—	4	1	4	—
is	0	0	0	4	3	0	0	0	1	3
the	0	1	0	4	5	0	0	0	—	—
can	—	—	—	4	2	0	1	0	3	1
it	1	0	0	3	6	0	0	0	0	0
do(n't)	1	—	3	—	—	—	—	—	3	1

Position of Function Word	*Grammatical Role*	*Paradigm*
Initial unstressed	Auxiliary in simple interrogative, followed by noun and verb.	Dŏ bírds flý?
Initial, stressed	Auxiliary in negative interrogative, followed by noun and verb.	Dón't bírds flý?
Initial, stressed	Auxiliary in negative interrogative, followed by pronoun and verb.	Dón't thĕy flý?
Medial unstressed	Copulative or modal verb between two stressed words.	Dógs căn bárk.

Subjects were 12 fluent aphasics and 10 Broca's aphasics who had been clinically classified by judges on the basis of their recorded speech as described by Goodglass, Quadfasel, and Timberlake (1964). The same response categories which were developed for patient S. L. were used to analyze these data.

From Figures 14-3 and 14-4 it can be seen that the initial unstressed function word was the least often correctly reproduced by the Broca's patients, but was within one point of the easiest sentence type for the fluent aphasics.

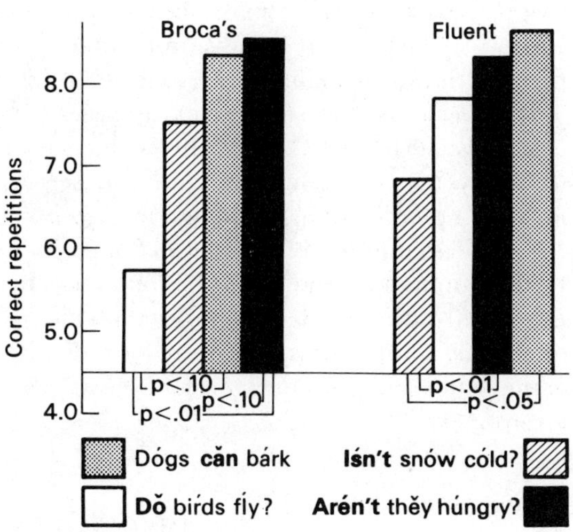

Fig. 14–3. Mean number of correct repetitions by Broca's and fluent aphasics of function words in four conditions of stress and position. (Test words in heavy print in key. Significance tests indicated are Wilcoxon two-tailed tests).

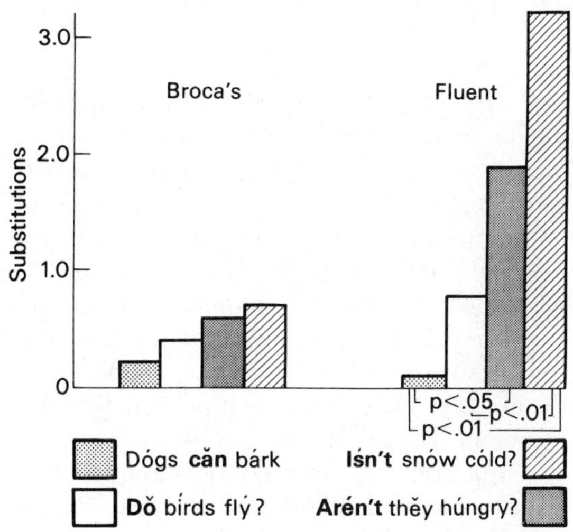

Fig. 14–4. Mean number of substitutions made by Broca's and fluent aphasics for function-words in four conditions of stress and position. (Words tested are in heavy print in the key. Significance tests indicated are Wilcoxon two-tailed tests).

In contrast, the stressed-opening of the type "Don't birds fly?" produced more than 3 (25%) substitution responses from the average fluent aphasic and was more correctly reproduced by the Broca's aphasics. These substitutions consisted chiefly of using the unstressed simple interrogative in place of the stressed negative interrogative. The same contrasting incidence of substitution errors can be seen, to a lesser degree, with the sentences of the type "Aren't they hungry?"

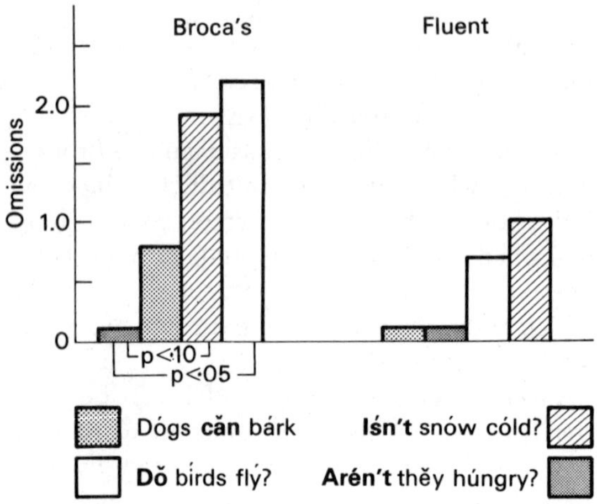

Fig. 14-5. Mean number of omissions of function words (heavy print in key) embedded in four different conditions of stress and position.

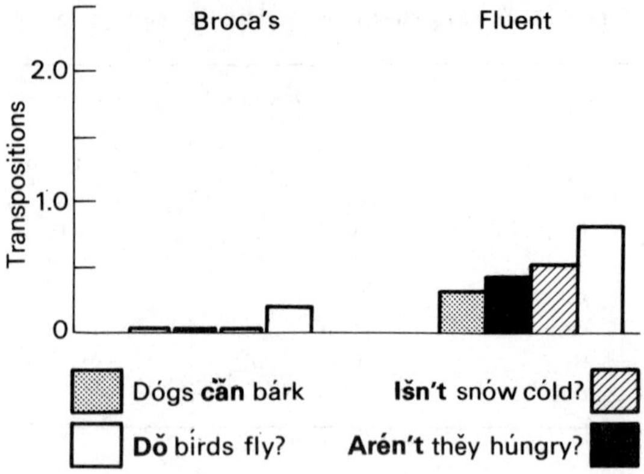

Figure 14-6. Mean number of transpositions of function words embedded in four different conditions of stress and position, as indicated by words in heavy print in key.

Figure 14-5 shows that the Broca's aphasics had more omissions in three of the four sentence types than did the other group and that the unstressed opening function word of the type "Do birds fly?" was the most vulnerable, although the stressed form "Isn't snow white?" was a close second. The number of transpositions, on the other hand, was uniformly greater on the part of the fluent aphasics (Figure 14-6). Six of the 12 fluent aphasics produced 23 transpositions, while only 2 of the 10 Broca's aphasics produced one transposition apiece. This type of error was significantly related to the severity of the disorder in the fluent aphasics.

In Table 14-4, we compare the relative difficulty of the four stress-syntax patterns, pair by pair. It is predicted that the pattern "Do dogs bark?" is more difficult for Broca's aphasics than any of the other three stress patterns with which it is matched, but no directional predictions appear justified among the remaining pairs. This pattern proved also to be the second most difficult for the fluent aphasics—their most difficult being the pattern of "Isn't snow white?" Thus, in comparison A, we find a significant reversal in order of difficulty experienced by Broca's and by fluent aphasics, in accord with experimental expectations. The negative interrogative, using three stressed words is almost always easier for Broca's aphasics than is the simple interrogative, with an opening unstressed auxiliary. The reverse is true for fluent aphasics. In comparisons B and C, the same sequence of difficulty between sentence types is observed for both aphasic groups, although in each case, the greatest number of instances of opposition to the dominant trend are to be found among the fluent aphasics. It is notable that in five of the six comparisons, the order of difficulty of the sentence types is the same for both aphasic groups.

DISCUSSION

Our data indicate that the position of a function word in the immediately surrounding stress-pattern helps to determine whether the word is retained or dropped in an aphasic's

TABLE 14-4. COMPARISON OF SUCCESS RATES FOR REPETITION OF FUNCTION WORDS, WITH RESPECT TO STRESS AND POSITION OF WORD IN SENTENCE. PRESENTED AS A SERIES OF PAIRED COMPARISONS OF CONTRASTING STRESS-POSITION CONTEXTS

Paradigm Test Sentences (Test Word is Italicized)	*Number of Patients Scoring Higher* Broca's a>b	b>a	a=b	Fluent a>b	b>a	a=b
a. *Isn't* snow white? versus b. *Do* birds fly?	8	2	0	2	10	0*
a. *Aren't* they hungry? versus b. *Do* birds fly?	9	0	1	6	1	5
a. Dogs *can* bark. versus b. *Do* birds fly?	8	2	0	7	4	1
a. Dogs *can* bark. versus b. *Aren't* they hungry?	4	5	1	4	7	1
a. Dogs *can* bark. versus b. *Isn't* snow white?	6	3	1	8	2	2
a. *Aren't* they hungry? versus b. *Isn't* snow white?	5	2	3	10	0	2

* Difference between groups significant at p 0.025 by Mann-Whitney U Test.

speech. In some cases, this factor was found to override considerations of grammatical complexity and of frequency of usage. In particular, the omission of the initial unstressed function word characterized the Broca's aphasic, in contrast to the fluent aphasic, and appears to account for at least one component of the agrammatism of these patients.

The term *agrammatism* is used also by Brown and Fraser (1963) in relation to the speech of young children who, like Broca's aphasics, speak in lexical words, while their function words are omitted or misused. Thus, one may reasonably ask whether the opening unstressed position is also the most vulnerable spot for function words in children's language, as it is for Broca's aphasics. A survey of the children's utterances cited by Brown and Fraser (1963) and Brown and Bellugi (1964) suggests that, in repetitions of short sentences and phrases, such omissions occur as frequently immediately after the first lexical word as before it. However, the inspection of such a small sample does not provide an adequate answer to the question about the possible parallel between the agrammatism of children and that of aphasics.

We have discussed earlier the proposal that the defect underlying the agrammatism of Broca's aphasics is a reduced capacity to initiate or maintain the production of sequences of speech sounds. Loss of certain function words would then be a defect that requires linguistic definition, but which may be nonlinguistic in origin. There is, in fact, no reason to expect the difficulties of children to follow the pattern resulting from this defect.

While accounting for one factor contributing to the ill-defined cluster of defects called agrammatism, we have left other symptoms unaccounted for. One of these symptoms is the inability to discriminate between the meanings of function words and inflectional endings, on hearing them or reading them, or to choose correctly among them in speech or writing. This difficulty, which we may call conceptual agrammatism is not universally present in our Broca's aphasics. The full distribution of conceptual agrammatism in relation to other aphasic symptoms is not known.

Thus, the concept of a unitary deficit underlying all grammatical difficulties in aphasia is not consistent with the results of analytic study. For example, Jakobson's (1956) "contiguity disorder" as an explanatory principle is too inclusive, since it requires the coexistence in agrammatic subjects of certain component symptoms which are not demonstrable, in nature, to cluster in any patient.

Two clinical types of aphasics were found to have contrasting responses to variations of stress pattern in word repetition and sentence repetition tests. In particular, the responses of Broca's aphasics appeared to account for certain agrammatic features of their speech. The ability of these tests to discriminate between our two clinical groups supports the meaningfulness of our categorization into Broca's aphasics on one hand and fluent aphasics on the other, the latter being composed of the standard clinical types Wernicke's and Amnesic aphasia, treated as a single group. Specific findings were:

1. When required to repeat short word sets as uniformly stressed lists, grammatically fluent aphasics were at a disadvantage compared to the equally severe Broca's aphasics.
2. All of the aphasics repeated three-word lists of nouns as easily as lists of function words, despite the greater frequency of the latter in English. Differences in grammatical fluency between the aphasic groups did not affect their ability to repeat functions words in three-word lists.
3. Broca's aphasics preserved initial stressed function words on sentence-repetition more successfully than did fluent aphasics, while fluent aphasics were more likely to substitute an unstressed for a stressed initial form.
4. For all aphasics, the stress pattern: ´˘´ was easier than any of the other three-word patterns tried, when reproducing a function word accurately in the first or second position. The facilitating effect of this stress pattern appeared to override variations in the actual grammatical construction of the three-word sentences. Thus, the negative interrogative in the form "Can't you swim?" is easier to say than the grammatically simpler form "Can you swim?"

The foregoing findings are consistent with the suggestion that Broca's aphasics depend upon the stressed features of an intended utterance in order to initiate and then maintain the flow of speech. This fact, in turn, can account for certain features of their agrammatism—particularly the omission of initial function words and the predominance of short bursts of speech. This explanation does not account for all aspects of grammatical difficulty in aphasia.

REFERENCES

Braine, M. D. S., On learning the grammatical order of words. *Psychol. Rev.*, **70,** 323–348 (1963).

Brown, R., and Bellugi, U., Three processes in the child's acquisition of syntax. *Harvard Educ. Rev.*, **34,** 133–151 (1964).

——, and Fraser, C., The acquisition of syntax. In C. N. Cofer (Ed.), *Verbal Learning and Verbal Behavior.* New York: McGraw-Hill (1963).

Glanzer, M., Towards a psychology of language structure. *J Speech Hearing Res.*, **5,** 303–314 (1962).

Goldstein, K., *Language and Language Disturbances.* New York: Grune & Stratton (1948).

Goodglass, H., Redefining the concept of agrammatism. Proc. XIIth Congr. Int. Assn. Logopedics and Phoniatrics, Padua (1962).

——, Quadfasel, F. A., and Timberlake, W. H.,

Phrase-length and the type and severity of aphasia, *Cortex*, **1,** 133–153 (1964).
Jakobson, R., Two aspects of language and two types of aphasic distrubances. In R. Jakobson and M. Halle, *Fundamentals of Language.* The Hague: Mouton (1956).

15

Acalculia

F. GREWEL

F. GREWEL, M.D., is with the department of ortho-education of the Universiteit van Amsterdam, The Netherlands.

In 1900 attention was first paid to disorders of calculation developing in patients who hitherto had shown no disturbance of their arithmetical faculties. Acalculia was systematically described and named by Henschen (1919) after a thorough survey of the material available. Henschen found that difficulties in the identification and in the naming of printed or written figures and numbers may occur without accompanying disorders of calculation. As on the other hand cipher- or number-blindness may be seen in many cases of acalculia without word-blindness, Henschen assumed that a visual factor, bound up with the occipital cortex, plays a part in calculation. Acalculia was observed in occipital, frontal, parietal and temporal lesions including atrophies, in the absence of aphasia. Henschen, therefore, concluded that the integrity of several areas of the cortex is essential for calculation and that a separate system, independent of the apparatus for the use of language and of music, exists in the human brain. Yet it remains remarkable that as a rule acalculia is associated with "acopia," or the incapacity to copy a text, notwithstanding an ability to read which is impaired but slightly, if at all.

Other neurologists, such as Peritz and Sittig, found acoustic, visual and ideational defects in cases of acalculia. Acalculia naturally implies a disturbance of modern computation, or Western arithmetic. Calculation was formerly regarded as a particular ability of the merchant. Not until the eighteenth century, when children learned tables by heart at school, did arithmetic become a common ability. We visualize the tables memorized in the first school years, when they were learned visually as well as motoro-acoustically. They were recited aloud and with most of us they still resound in our mental ear when we come to use them. Thus calculation is not a primary or biological human capacity, but one which bears in its practical realization the stamp of our cultural configuration.

This means that we are compelled to study the psychology of modern arithmetic before facing the problems pertaining to acalculia. Primitive people, as well as children, do not count, but work with sets of objects, with groups—aggregates or manifolds, as they are called in mathematics; they distinguish the relations "bigger and smaller," "more or less" and "part or whole," with the insight that the whole is more than a part. Piaget (1941) observed that children at this stage have not yet the notion of, nor the insight into, quantity, and that the above-mentioned aspects are still qualities. These fundamental qualities are the foundations of calculation, addition and subtraction, and so on.

The conception of number as a cardinal, that is as something belonging to a group as a whole,

From *Brain* 75:397–407, 1952. Reprinted by permission of the Editor of *Brain*.

has, as a prerequisite, the idea of a whole consisting of its parts. A group is counted, the insight being necessary that only one number is the "image" of a given group. Mathematically speaking only one number (that is, one place in the numerical series) represents a given aggregate or set. The irrevocability or unambiguity of the result of counting is its cardinal principle, even of calculation. The mathematician is fully aware of what he is doing in calculation in that he works with aggregates as well as with numerical quantities, and therefore with the symbols used for number-notation. The representation of numeral quantities by words is called numeration; the representation by written signs is called notation. The systems adopted for numeration and for notation do not always agree (or fully correspond) with one another, as for instance in France where eighty is called "quatre-vingts" or "four-twenties."

We use the Hindu system for the notation of numbers, which proceeds by ones, tens, tens of tens, etc. Essential features of this system are:

(1) the limitation of the number of different symbols to ten, however large the number in question;
(2) the use of the zero to indicate the absence of a power;
(3) the principle of local value, by which the value of a digit changes according to its position within a number-notation.

In our notation of natural numbers we thus not only make use of the denary scale but we represent the first nine natural numbers by different symbols, namely, the digits. The ingenious symbol for the zero, the "nought" (0), was devised as late as the seventh century in India; in the Middle Ages it came to Western Europe by way of the Arabs. The zero is no natural number[1] and its symbol therefore does not represent a number, but in arithmetic it is treated like a figure—a fact of the utmost importance. The conception of the zero and the introduction of its symbol made arithmetic as easy as it is nowadays.

Upon the symbols for the first nine numbers and the 0, a logical system is erected for the notation of the higher numbers, beginning with the ten (10). This plural cipher notation proceeds from right to left, and the local value of a digit within a number notation is counted from the right, its place corresponding to the power at the base. The absence of a power within a number-notation is indicated by a 0, which may be called a "place filler."

A number has its place in the set of number names. Man's ingenuity has developed a logical symbolism in the form of sets of symbols, visible numerical signs, that enable him to judge immediately whether the number it represents is lesser or greater than another number, represented by another plural cipher notation, provided that he knows the ten fundamental symbols and the numerical value they represent, as well as the rules governing plural cipher notation. The basic principle underlying this is the isomorphism of the numerals as visible numerical signs with the numbers.

Such a system of symbols manipulated according to certain conventions is called a semantic (or semiotic) system.[2] To handle such a system one must know the elements and the rules of their combination. It is evident that ideational as well as visual factors play a part here.

A patient who does not know the ten basic symbols any longer may suffer from dementia, from visual agnosia or from asymbolia. Inability to handle the plural cipher notation, the patient still recognizing the digits, may be due to visual agnosia or to the loss of insight into the composition of these notations, dementia, or asemasia. Some patients no longer regard a numeral as an entity, for example 286 may be regarded as 2, 8 and 6 or as 2 and 86. The succession or the place-value may have lost its meaning; 26 may be identified as sixty-two; 10 may be one-nought, or 1 or 0.

Our arithmetical procedures are based on the semantic system of number-notation using

[1] From a philosophical point of view "one" is not a number either (Husserl).

[2] Other semantic systems include languages, maps, morse and braille signs—such games as cards and chess; signal systems like semaphores, flags, etc.

the Hindu symbols and their arrangement. Clearly in written arithmetic we are not handling numerical quantities, numbers proper, but their symbols—this according to the principle of the isomorphism of both series. Arithmetical operations are free from ambiguity. If we bring the parts of plural cipher notations in relation to each other in the more or less complicated ways we have been taught, we rightly assume that the ensuing symbol is indeed the symbolic notation of the answer, that is, the number wanted or sought. Those skilled in arithmetical operations no longer wonder about the technicalities, and forget the painful steps taken in learning the procedures of calculation, as well as the training necessary to handle them fluently.

The process of thought in additions like $378 + 497$ is complicated indeed. One must remember that units are added only to units, tens to tens, etc., and hence it is convenient to write units of the same denomination under one another in the same column. The ciphers in each of these columns must be "brought in relation" to each other. Every 10 units of one denomination (like the 10 of 15 in our example) must be "carried" as a unit to the next column, in this case to that of the tens, the same as we "borrow" in subtractions from the cipher at the left side in the minimend if this is necessary. The main arithmetical fact is that we *regroup* the numerical quantities represented by the numbers; e.g. in our example $8 + 7$ not as $9 + 6$, but as $10 + 5$. This is self-evident no doubt, but it is none the less an ingenious procedure.

In the case of multiplication there are further complexities. The digit of the units in the multiplier is consecutively brought in relation to the digits for the units, the tens, etc., of the multiplicand. If one puts every cipher exactly in the right column the result of the computation by figures is a notation representing the product.

It is useful to realize the intricacy of this method of calculation, which took centuries to develop to its present level. By this method one can work with numbers and solve calculations which without this complicated semantic system would have been impossible.

The sources of difficulty within this method are manifold, as are the procedures which must be learned. For some children, the difficulties, especially of subtraction and division, prove unsurmountable. Without constant training many tricks (especially of division) are forgotten soon after the school years.

Obviously there are many sources of failure in calculation in the case of mental disturbance due to cortical lesions. However, these failures always bear the stamp of *our* method of calculation and of *our* notation system, that is of the difficulties and intricacies inherent to this peculiar system. No doubt there still existed other difficulties and disorders in the case of finger calculation, the use of the abacus, or with Roman numerals, and probably even greater when one thinks of such a problem as CLXXIV × XCVII.

The disturbances we can deduce theoretically from the semantics of calculation are repeatedly seen in patients with acalculia. Unawareness of the necessity to rearrange the groups; inability to arrange units, etc., in columns; failure to bring the digits of one number in relation with the corresponding digits of others in an addition or with all the figures of the multiplicand in a multiplication, are frequent errors with such patients. The procedures of "carrying over" and "borrowing" may be forgotten; or the patient may no longer remember how to proceed. He may write down the 1 of 15 in the wrong place, e.g. under the 5 or in the column of the tens. He may have a vague memory of what he is expected to do but be at a loss to realize it. Horizontal and perpendicular directions may be confused; the fact that 12×17 is identical with $\begin{smallmatrix}17\\ 12\\ \overline{\times}\end{smallmatrix}$ may prove bewildering.

In short, the numerous failures in calculation which these patients show are understandable as soon as we start from the semantic system of number-notation and the ensuing semantic (or better syntactic) system of calculation—calculation being taken as computation by means of our system of figures.

Following Berger (1926), we distinguish between primary and secondary acalculia. Many mental affections such as dementia, memory and retention disorders, perseveration and aphasia, may cause difficulties in calculation. The partial sum or product may be forgotten before it can be utilized, e.g. in mental arithmetic. The tables may be lost. Or there may be a disturbing perseveration of a cipher, e.g. $7 \times 7 = 47$, or $9 + 13 = 13$; or of a sum, e.g. $6+6=12$, $6+8=12$, etc. Inability to formulate the answer because of aphasia may prevent its notation.

Cipher agnosia and apraxia generally result in acalculia. A visual factor plays a part in calculation; but it has been shown experimentally that there is no parallelism, even no manifest relation between mental arithmetic and visualization or "Gestalting" ability; nor between ability in calculation and visual or acoustic powers.

In cases of primary acalculia, calculation itself is affected; though on deeper analysis one finds that calculation is a complicated psychological procedure that may be disturbed or hampered in many ways. As a rule mental arithmetic suffers more than calculation on paper.

Henschen (1926) already stressed the fact that every calculation, even the most simple one, is a mental process, and one which confronts us with a problem requiring a series of thinking tasks. Ranschburg showed experimentally with well-taught children of the higher classes in a primary school that even simple sums always demand a certain effort. Berger (1926) thought that disturbances of logical thinking are always accompanied by acalculia; this is not true, though arithmetic does presuppose a more or less intact intelligence.

The occipital type of primary acalculia is the result of gross lesions of that part of the brain. It can be explained only in part by difficulties in the handling of cipher symbols and by impaired visual retention and visualization.

Cases of frontal acalculia are said to show more severe disturbances in dealing with abstract than with concrete numbers. My experience does not confirm this assertion. Though psychologically the concrete precedes the abstract, the latter being based on the former, in patients with acalculia there is a deterioration in computation and there is no reason why this should be expressed more in abstract computation. Moreover, while addition and subtraction may in the first instance be limited to numerical quantities, multiplication and division necessarily introduce the idea of pure number. Practical calculation on the other hand makes use of a well-learned conventional technique, and at any rate in a multiplication only one of the numbers can be concrete. Finally it remains an open question whether any number is ever really abstract. We may conclude from these remarks that the idea of abstract and concrete numbers in frontal acalculia is superficial. The intensity of acalculia in frontal lesions shows a certain parallelism with the general lowering of the level of productive thinking and of initiative in these cases.

Hitherto, from a psychological point of view, parietal acalculia formed the most interesting type of primary acalculia. Henschen (1919, 1920) and Peritz (1918) already emphasized that in lesions of part of the left angular gyrus typical acalculia might ensue. It is well known that small lesions in and around this area may cause several symptoms: disorders in thinking and in language, disturbances of left-right orientation and of the body scheme. In Gerstmann's syndrome, finger-agnosia, acalculia and sometimes agraphia—another symptom of this region—are combined.

Such patients often show that type of apraxia described by Kleist (1936) and his pupil Strauss as "constructive apraxia." It is a disorder of spatial handling and modelling, though there is neither paralysis nor apraxia, and the awareness and the planning of the task to be fulfilled is unimpaired. This disturbance can best be demonstrated by drawing, and in constructions with blocks or sticks. One realizes that these patients are incapable of forming spatial relations though well aware of this defect.

Krapf (1937) showed that such patients often cannot write down a plural cipher notation. In written sums they cannot combine ciphers and numbers correctly; horizontal and perpendicular directions are interchanged. The same occurs in drawing. According to Krapf, the fundamental disturbance in these cases of parietal acalculia is an inability to manipulate spatially parts of number notations and the parts of numbers (notations) in relation to each other. One might perhaps call this "constructive acalculia." Few cases of acalculia have been adequately studied along these lines; in my own cases the picture was always much more complicated.

Several problems remain. For example, why does counting become more difficult beyond the figure 10; why is one operation still possible while another, apparently an easier one, is not? From a psychological standpoint there are often paradoxical features in these cases, as, for example, when a patient cannot subtract 9—6, but nevertheless gives the unexpected answer to 9+6 as 3. Or a patient may not be able to add 1+8+3, but afterwards asked to make a number containing a 1, 8 and 3 he answers 12. It has been said that automatization and spontaneity have suffered in these cases or that tasks are carried out passively which they cannot solve actively. Singer and Low (1933) remarked that this is a translation rather than an explanation. In my opinion the cause of this phenomenon lies in an impairment of the so-called "distributive attention," as seen in frontal and parietal lesions.

The rare and laborious follow-up studies of cases of progressive acalculia give a deeper understanding of the psychology of acalculia, provided that one looks upon calculation as a highly complicated symbolic-semantic system and upon its disturbances as a series of highly diverse disturbances of the manipulation of this system. With this in view, one notices that in various types and grades of acalculia different faculties and different parts of the procedure of calculation have suffered. In the most severe defects the notion of aggregate and/or of quantity may have been lost, or the insight into the conception of part and whole has disappeared. The relation of bigger and smaller may have lost its meaning, though seldom if ever is it found that a patient who still has a vague idea of what subtraction means, will try to subtract the bigger number from the smaller one.

Counting may be impossible. The unambiguous correspondence between a number, viz. a numerical quantity, and the manifold it represents may no longer be clear to the patient. The so-called transitive rule in arithmetic may no longer be evident. These are all intellectual and ideational disturbances.

Moreover a patient may show asymbolia not only for the ciphers but also for the operational symbols (+, −, =, etc.), that is for the whole of the so-called pasigraphic system. In these cases the relation between the language symbols of numerical quantity, that is the name of the numbers, and the ideographic notation system of ciphers and signs used in number and calculation notation, is disturbed. In this connexion it is necessary to point to the remarkable fact that for the notation of ciphers, numbers and operational symbols we make use of an international ideographic system, not only independent of the system of language notation, but also of linguistic formulation. Thus "3" is "three," "trois," "drei," "tre," "drie," and so on; 3 is the symbol for the idea three, or for the fact ///, or for the numerical quantity three; 3 is a notation symbol; but 3 is *not* a rendering or reproduction of the *word* three. This fact explains that asymbolia and agraphia for letters and words and those for ciphers and numbers do not always concur; the one and the other represent different systems of symbolization of different semantic systems. In parentheses we may add that the semantic system used in musical notation is independent of the others and therefore each of the three systems may be affected independently of the other two. Often each one is impaired, but with very different degrees of intensity.

Since the various disturbances of computation, calculation and of notation, as well as the constructivo-apraxic defects, often go together, sometimes being combined with language disorders and dementia, it will be obvious that the study of acalculia offers many difficulties.

One point to be remembered is the fact that our language denomination of numbers generally follows a certain rule; e.g. 3456 is three thousand, four hundred, fifty, six. But this parallelism does not obtain in every case. In many languages the denomination of the teens follows another rule of succession; e.g. 14 is four-teen and not ten, four. This divergency exists in different languages for different numbers; it therefore is a source of different agnosic-apraxic troubles in these languages according to their linguistic peculiarities.

It is not our intention to go further into the special problems of the different types of acalculia. One example may suffice to show that the study of acalculia may afford a deeper psychological insight into the problems of arithmetic itself. It has been maintained that arithmetic must be looked upon, and therefore studied and taught, from a Gestaltist point of view. One of Wertheimer's (1912) earliest studies dealt with calculation in primitive peoples from the Gestaltist angle; in his opinion a holistic approach to the problems of arithmetic was necessary. Fettweis (1927) was able to show that in reality primitive peoples usually have some notion of number.

In our experience cases where the conception of aggregate, of quantity *per se*, has suffered, are very rare. Most patients with acalculia have retained the notions of whole and part, of bigger and smaller; but they still cannot calculate. In the first mentioned rare cases, Wertheimer's Gestalt considerations have their value. However, in most cases of acalculia as our analysis has shown, it is not the configuration of groups, but the command over the symbolic-semantic system which has suffered; this aspect of calculation is relevant in the disorder. This is the place to point out that the regrouping in computation, e.g. $8+7=10+5$ is not a regrouping of Gestalts but the manipulation of counted elements, viz.:

$8 + 7 = 8 + (2 + 5) = (8 + 2) + 5 = 10 + 5$; or
1, 2, 3, 4, 5, 6, 7, 8, ...
. . . . .1, 2, 3, 4, 5, 6, 7,
1, 2, 3, 4, 5, 6, 7, 8, 9, 10, 11, 12, 13, 14, 15.

The Gestaltist point of view does not hold good in the study of modern arithmetic and its advocates (e.g. in the school) get no support from the study of acalculia.

As already shown, a differentiation between asymbolic and asemantic acalculia is fruitful.

The asemantic types of acalculia remind us of Head's (1926) semantic aphasia. In these cases the patients do not grasp and do not realize the full implication, the wider meaning of what has been said. These patients moreover no longer understand games, cards or caricatures. If one refers to the case-histories in Volume II of Head's book one finds that every one of these patients showed a manifest acalculia. Moreover, all of them had outspoken constructional disturbances. It is well known that Head localized their cortical lesions to the supramarginal and angular convolutions, but it is often forgotten that Head described these symptoms even before Kleist and Straus.

The fundamental common factor of many of these disturbances is an asemasia, revealing itself in different semantic systems.

Certain considerations require discussion: In the first place arithmetic appears to be such a complicated process that a simple cortical (and functional) "localization" is out of question. Its study confronts us with the rapidly developing branch of neurology, namely, neurological psychology or neuropsychology. This study requires an adequate knowledge of modern psychology and our study may demonstrate that when we are dealing with "new" problems semantic analysis of the functions studied is necessary as well.

Secondly, we realize that with the study of aphasia, agraphia, and acalculia, a special domain is opend to neurology. In these syndromes it is not a biological function which has deteriorated, as in the case of a hemiparesis, but it is the patient's participation in cultural acquisitions, in acquired cultural patterns which is disturbed, viz. his sharing of a language system, of a graphic notation system, of a calculation system. This offers an opportunity for a more intimate co-operation between neurology, social psychology and cultural anthropology.

Thirdly, the result of our analysis sets us speculating about the possible intimate relations between our mental make-up and our bodily constitution. The combination of finger-agnosia with acalculia is all the more remarkable, because our counting probably had its origin in pointing (that, and that, and that) or/and in counting on the fingers. The use of the denary scale in notation is due to its use in numeration and this again springs from the primitive use of the fingers for counting, as exemplified in English by the use of the word "digit." Is not acalculia than an unavoidable accompaniment of the loss of the knowledge of one's fingers?

Further speculation is tempting. Considering acalculia in its relation to difficulties with spatial manipulation, i.e. with the control of one's space (body and action space, or near and distant space), and even with the concept of time (as was the case in Head's patients), one may attach a great value to Descartes' happy idea of attaching numerical value to vectors. Herewith analytical geometry was founded, geometry came within the scope of measure and number, and algebraic formulas could be depicted. This means that counting and the scheme of three-dimensional space were brought into intimate relation. Is it not then remarkable to see that anatomical lesions causing disorders of calculation are so often accompanied by impairment in the control or command over space? Can it be then that anatomical proximity within one convolution is the real basis of Descartes' intellectual combination?

One must beware of the lure of such speculations. We know that acalculia, agraphia and many subtle disturbances are seen with lesions of the parieto-temporo-occipital borderland, but that spatial disturbances, in part at any rate, are due to gross subcortical interruption of pathways correlating the "praxis" of the hand with the visual field, i.e. with the "guiding eye." On the other hand the three-dimensional space of geometry is not our "real" biological space, but merely a useful schema; and as such it is itself part of yet another semantic system. We are not permitted to use these schemata as if they were realities, so committing what Whitehead has called the "fallacy of misplaced concreteness." This means that Man's creative thinking permits him to lay connexions between a certain space scheme and his arithmetical system, but that there is not the least "real" connexion between both. Man's specifically human analytic-synthetic power (i.e. Spearman's "correlative" power); his ability to create as it were connexions, relations and correlations; his gift to fix these relations in symbols and his faculty to handle them abstractly lie at the foundation of the correlating of different schemes such as Descartes did.

Many of the psychological disturbances treated in this study may be explained by a shortage of these faculties of relating, correlating, and symbolizing, as well as of the semantic faculty. When these highest intellectual faculties of Man are impaired we are confronted, amongst other things, with asymbolic and asemantic disturbances.

This insight is a more realistic basis for science than speculations and esthetic pseudo-scientific pursuits. As for the new field of neuropsychology, illustrated in this article by the example of acalculia, it must be founded on a sound combination of neurological and psychological exact research.

REFERENCES

Berger, H. (1926) *Archiv. Psychiat. Nervenkr.*, **78,** 238.

Conrad, K. (1932/33) *Mschr. Psychiat. Neurol.*, **84,** 28.

Fettweis, E. (1927) Das Rechnen der Naturvölker. Berlin.

Gerstmann, J. (1927) *Z. ges. Neurol. Psychiat.*, **108,** 152.

Grewel, F. (1948) *Nederl. Tijdschr. v. Geneesk.*, **92,** 767.

—— (1950) *Nederl. Tijdschr. v. Psychol.*, **5,** (with literature).

Head, H. (1926) Aphasia and Kindred Disorders of Speech. London.

Henschen, S. E. (1919) *Z. ges. Neurol. Psychiat.*, **52,** 273.

—— (1920) Klinische u. anatom. Beitrage z. Pathologie des Gehirns, V, Stockholm.
—— (1926) *Z. ges. Neurol. Psychiat.*, **100,** 1.
Kleist, K. (1936) Gehirnpathologie. Leipzig.
Krapf, E. (1937) *Schweiz. Arch. Neurol. Psychiat.*, **39,** 330.
——, and Courtis, B. (1937) *Rev. Neurol. de Buenos Aires*, **1,** 280.
Lewandowsky, M., and Stadelmann, E. (1908) *J. Psychol. Neurol.*, **11,** 289.
Nielson, J. M. (1938) *Arch. Neurol. Psychiat.*, **39,** 536.
—— (1947) Agnosia, Apraxia, Aphasia. 2nd Ed., New York.
Peritz, G. (1918) *Dtsch. Z. Nervenheilk.*, **61,** 234.
Piaget, J., and Szeminska, A. (1941) La génèse du nombre chez l'enfant. Paris.
Singer, H. D., and Low, A. A. (1933) *Arch. Neurol. Psychiat.*, **29,** 162.
Sittig, O. (1919) *Z. f. Pathopsychol.*, **3,** 39 and 298.
—— (1921) *Mschr. Psychiat.*, **49,** 299.
Wertheimer, M. (1912) *Z. f. Psychol.*, **60,** 321.
—— (1952) Drei Abhandlungen zur Gestalttheorie.

16

The Fiction of the "Gerstmann Syndrome"

ARTHUR L. BENTON

ARTHUR L. BENTON, Ph.D., is with the department of neurology of the University Hospital, University of Iowa.

This investigation was supported by a grant (B-616) from the National Institute of Neurological Diseases and Blindness, U.S. Public Health Service.

The problem with which this study is concerned can be stated as follows. A patient with parieto-occipital disease may show one or more of a relatively large number of diverse behavioral deficits. When he presents with two, three, or more of these symptoms, the latter may be viewed by the clinical observer as forming a naturally occurring combination of deficits and given the status of a syndrome, this status implying that the concurrence of deficits is not a chance one, that there is an underlying factor responsible for it, and that it possesses a distinctive neuropathological significance. Once such a special combination or syndrome is established, not only is it used in the observation and description of subsequent cases but it may also determine which aspects of a patient's behavior are selected for study and which are not. The "Gerstmann syndrome" represents such a combination of behavioral deficits. The study to be reported examines the question of whether, as is usually assumed, this "assembly of unlikely and unexpected symptoms" (Critchley, 1953) is a naturally occurring combination or whether it is only one of a very large number of more or less fortuitous combinations of behavioral deficits which may be encountered in patients with cerebral disease.

Reproduced from *Journal of Neurology, Neurosurgery and Psychiatry* 24:176–181, 1961, by permission of the editor and author.

The history of the Gerstmann syndrome has been recounted in detail elsewhere (cf. Critchley, 1953; Benton, 1959); only a few major points need be mentioned to introduce the present investigation. Before the end of the nineteenth century, the four behavioral deficits comprising the syndrome—right-left disorientation, acalculia, agraphia, and finger agnosia—had been described as occurring in patients with cerebral disease. The first three were well-known symptoms but the description of finger agnosia in 1888 by Jules Badal had escaped the attention of neurologists, a fact which is not altogether surprising in view of the circumstances that the Bordeaux eye specialist published in an ophthalmological journal, and the finger agnosia which he quite clearly described was only one of a large number of deficits shown by his patient. In 1924, Gerstmann once again described finger agnosia, designating it as "a circumscribed disorder of orientation to one's own body". In 1927, he advanced the idea that finger agnosia and agraphia formed "a new syndrome". However, in 1930 he enlarged the syndrome to include right-left disorientation and acalculia and proposed that it had a highly specific neuropathological significance. At the same time, he discussed the question of the *Grundstörung* responsible for this presumably "natural" concurrence of behavioral deficits.

Clinical experience appeared to confirm the real existence of the syndrome; case reports of patients manifesting it appeared in the literature and speculations regarding the basic impairment underlying its occurrence were offered. However, it was certainly not rare to encounter patients who showed one, two, or three deficits but not the full syndrome. While such observations were often interpreted as simply representing *formes frustres* of the syndrome, they did indicate at least that the four symptoms did not necessarily occur together in every case and they did have implications regarding the cogency of those theoretical formulations which had been advanced to account for an obligatory concurrence of the deficits. On the other hand, a wide variety of other deficits were also observed to occur in connexion with any or all of the four symptoms. These were given a subordinate status as accompanying symptoms which might or might not be manifested. Among them were general mental impairment, aphasic disorders, colour agnosia, visual disorientation, dyslexia, and constructional apraxia. Indeed, the last-named deficit, constructional apraxia, has been observed so often to accompany one or more of the four deficits that some authors have come to consider it, explicitly or implicitly, as part of the syndrome. For example, Ajuriaguerra and Hécaen (1960), discussing the interrelations of the elements of the syndrome and the connexions with other symptoms, remark that "the most frequent and most important association is that between finger agnosia and constructional apraxia. We have seen that such an association cannot be considered to be simply fortuitous or anatomically conditioned".

If the "Gerstmann syndrome" is a naturally occurring combination of interrelated deficits, all of which are expressions of a single basic impairment, and not merely the product of selective attention and observation, the four behavioral deficits which comprise it should show stronger "associative bonds", so to speak, among themselves than they do with symptoms which are considered to be outside of the syndrome. If unbiased analysis should show this to be the case, the findings could be reasonably interpreted as evidence for a special coherence of the four symptoms and both the designation of the combination as a syndrome and a search for the common factor responsible for the coherence are justified. On the other hand, if such analysis should disclose that this is not the case, the findings could be reasonably interpreted as indicating that this particular combination of deficits is no more or less likely to occur in patients with cerebral disease than a great many similar combinations and that, unless it can be shown to have a distinctive neuropathological significance, neither its designation as a syndrome nor the postulation of a common psychoneurological factor to account for it (as distinguished from other combinations) is justified.

It might be thought that a comprehensive survey of the pertinent clinical literature would provide the answer to this question of the phenomenological reality of the Gerstmann syndrome. However, the literature proves to be virtually without value in this respect. The methods and criteria utilized for making clinical judgments regarding the presence or absence of defect in the performances investigated are so diverse that the findings from one case to another are not comparable. Not infrequently the criteria employed in making judgments of deficit are not mentioned and notations such as "slight finger agnosia", "questionable right-left disorientation", or "no noteworthy constructional apraxia" are made. Moreover, the majority of case reports fail to mention the presence or absence of one or more pertinent accompanying deficits and hence must be excluded from a systematic analysis. Finally, the factor of selective attention and observation when one is dealing with an already established entity, such as the Gerstmann syndrome, may introduce a bias in the original observations for which the reviewer cannot correct.

It seems evident that the question of the status of the Gerstmann syndrome as a behavioral phenomenon can be answered only by an investigation which has been deliberately designed to answer it and which employs explicitly described procedures for assessment and criteria for judgment. The present paper reports such an investigation.

CASE MATERIAL AND METHODS

The case material consisted of 100 non-psychotic patients with unequivocal diagnoses of disease or injury involving the cerebral hemispheres who had been seen in the neurological and neurosurgical services of the University Hospitals and Veterans Administration Hospital, Iowa City. Any patient who was suffering from acute illness, whose behavior raised the question of psychosis, who had a history of treatment in hospital for a psychiatric disorder, or whose history was suggestive of a state of mental defect dating back to childhood, was excluded from the study. All the patients were between the ages of 16 and 64 years and were clearly capable of understanding directions, co-operating in the test procedures and undergoing one to two hours of examination without discomfort. The mean age of the group was 42 years. The mean educational level was 10 years (range: 5 to 16 years). A variety of cerebral conditions, focal and diffuse, was represented in the group. The performances of 12 right-handed patients with focal disease involving the left parietal lobe were analyzed separately, in addition to the main analyses of the total group of 100 patients of which they formed a part.

A control group of 100 non-psychotic patients from the neurological, neurosurgical, and medical services who showed no evidence or history of cerebral disease or injury were also examined, their performances being utilized to establish objective normative standards on the basis of which the presence or absence of impairment could be defined. The mean age of this group was 41 years (range: 16 to 65 years) and mean educational level was 10 years (range: 5 to 14 years).

All the patients were given a battery of seven tests designed to provide objective and comprehensive assessments of the following capacities: (1) right-left orientation; (2) finger localization; (3) arithmetic calculation; (4) writing; (5) constructional praxis; (6) reading; (7) visual memory. The testing procedures were as follows:

Right-left Orientation. This test battery (32 items) required the patient to execute localizing movements to oral command and assessed the following aspects of right-left orientation: (A) with the aid of vision, identification of single lateral body parts on one's own body; (B) with the aid of vision, execution of double uncrossed and crossed commands with respect to lateral body parts on one's own body, *e.g.*, left hand on right eye; (C) without the aid of vision, identification of single lateral body parts; (D) without the aid of vision, execution of double commands; (E) identification of single lateral body parts on a front-view representation of a man; (F) execution of double commands involving identification of lateral body parts of both the patient and the representation, *e.g.*, patient's right hand on a man's right eye. The details of this test battery may be found in a paper by Benton and Kemble (1960). Level of performance was defined as the number of correct localizations made by the patient.

Finger Localization. This test battery (80 items) assessed the following aspects of finger identification: (A) with the aid of vision, presentation of single fingers on oral command; (B) identification of single fingers on schematic drawings of the hands; (C) with the aid of vision, identification of single fingers which had been touched; (D) without the aid of vision, identification of single fingers which had been touched; (E) without the aid of vision, identification of pairs of fingers subjected to simultaneous tactile stimulation. (For details regarding the arrangements for tactile stimulation of the fingers, see Benton, 1959.) Level of performance was defined as the number of correct localizations made by the patient.

Arithmetic Calculation. This untimed 16-item written test consisted of simple problems in addition, subtraction, multiplication, and division involving one- and two-digit numbers. Level of performance was defined as the number of correct solutions.

Writing. The patient was asked to write his name, copy two simple sentences, write two simple sentences to dictation, and write down anything that came into his mind. Unlined $5\frac{1}{2} \times 8$ in. paper was used. Each specimen of writing was independently rated by two examiners on the basis of the following factors: alignment of lines; elisions and omissions; formation of letters; spelling; substitutions and additions. Each of these factors was rated from 0 (poor) to 2 (within normal limits). Level of performance was defined in terms of an overall rating consisting of the sum of the two examiners' ratings on each of these factors. However, in the case of patients with sensorimotor deficits of the preferred hand, the "formation of letters" factor was excluded from consideration, and a weighted sum of the examiners' ratings on the other factors was computed.

Constructional Praxis. Both two-dimensional and three-dimensional praxis was assessed. The two-dimensional task consisted in having the patient copy six "stick" designs presented by the examiner while the three-dimensional task consisted in having him copy four models made of rectangular blocks of various sizes and dimensions. The patient was allowed to use only one hand in arranging the sticks or blocks. Level of performance was defined as the number of sticks and blocks correctly placed.

Reading. The patient read four short paragraphs and, with the paragraphs in view, answered questions which assessed his understanding of them. Level of performance was defined as the number of questions correctly answered. No time limit was enforced.

Visual Memory. Multiple choice form G of the visual retention test (Benton, 1953) consisting of 15 designs was used. Each design was presented to the patient for 5 sec., after which he was required to identify the design on a card containing it and three similar designs. Level of performance was defined as the number of correct choices made by the patient.

Distributions of the scores of the 100 control patients on each of the seven tests were made and inspected. For each distribution, a score which was equalled or exceeded by 91 to 94% of the patient's was selected as a "cutting score" and scores below this level were considered to indicate significantly defective performance. Natural "breaks" which occurred in the lower ends of some of the distributions were utilized in establishing these cutting scores, a circumstance which accounts for the slight variation in the percentage values of the various scores.

THE INVESTIGATION

Relationships among performances

The inter-correlations among the seven performances for the total group of 100 brain-damaged patients are shown in Table 16-1. These are "second-order" correlation coefficients, from which the effects of variation in age and educational level on performance have been eliminated. Inspection of this matrix suggests that the correlations among the elements of the syndrome are neither higher nor lower than those between these elements and the performances which presumably do not belong to the syndrome. Thus, while the highest correlation coefficient in the matrix (0.62) is between two syndrome performances (right-left orientation vs. finger localization), it will be seen that the lowest correlation coefficient (0.35) is also between two syndrome performances (finger localization vs. calculation). The mean correlation coefficient of the performances within the syndrome (derived from averaging the six relevant correlation coefficients) is 0.48. This may be compared with the mean correlation coefficient between the syndrome performances and those performances which are outside of the syndrome. This statistic (derived from averaging the 12 relevant correlation coefficients) is 0.52, indicating that the syndrome performances show no closer relationship among themselves than they do with performances outside of the syndrome.

TABLE 16-1. SECOND-ORDER CORRELATION COEFFICIENTS (AGE AND EDUCATION "PARTIALLED OUT") IN 100 BRAIN-DAMAGED PATIENTS

	Finger Localization	Writing	Calculation	Constructional Praxis	Reading	Visual Memory
Right-left	0.62	0.48	0.46	0.51	0.48	0.57
Finger localization		0.52	0.35	0.60	0.42	0.50
Writing			0.46	0.44	0.57	0.52
Calculation				0.51	0.60	0.58
Constructional praxis					0.42	0.47
Reading						0.56

A more detailed analysis of the strength of the relationships existing among elements of the syndrome as compared with that existing between them and the other performances is presented in Table 16-2, which shows the mean correlation coefficient of each syndrome performance with the other three syndrome performances and of each extra-syndrome performance with the four syndrome performances. The findings indicate quite clearly that constructional praxis, reading, and visual memory are as closely related to the elements of the syndrome as the latter are among themselves, *i.e.*, that the elements of the syndrome do not show particularly close associative bonds.

Cohesiveness of syndromes

As has already been noted, the mean intercorrelation among the elements of the syndrome is 0.48, which may be interpreted as an index of its "cohesiveness", *i.e.*, of the tendency of elements to vary concurrently. Thirty-five combinations of four performances each can be formed from the seven "parietal" performances investigated in this study. Each combination will include one or more elements of the syndrome, one of them being the syndrome. If there is a special tendency for the elements of the syndrome to vary concurrently, its observed mean intercorrelation of 0.48 should be higher than those derived from combinations consisting of mixtures of syndrome and non-syndrome elements. The mean correlation coefficient (derived from the six relevant correlation coefficients) of each of the 34 mixed combinations was computed. They ranged in size from 0.48 to 0.54. Two coefficients were as high as 0.54 and four were as low as 0.48. It is clear from these findings that all 35 combinations of elements show about the same degree of cohesiveness and that the syndrome is not at all distinctive in this respect.

The incidence of significant deficit in performance (as defined above, *i.e.*, performances which fell within the lowest 6 to 9% of the scores of the control group) was computed for each patient. Twenty-nine showed no significant deficits and 23 showed only one deficit. The remaining 48 patients showed two to seven deficits, 10 of them showing four deficits. Examination of these 10 sets of four deficits disclosed that all involved combinations of syndrome and non-syndrome performances. The pure Gerstmann syndrome did not appear. The combination of deficits in finger localization, writing, reading, and constructional praxis appeared twice. Eight other combinations appeared once. Again the findings indicate no particularly strong tendency for the symptoms of the Gerstmann syndrome to appear concurrently.

Performances of Patients with Left Parietal Lesions

It might be argued that assumptions about the essential unity of the elements of the Gerstmann syndrome hold only for patients with parieto-occipital disease of the dominant hemisphere and that a study involving patients with various types of lesion cannot provide cogent evidence about these assumptions. This contention is quite debatable. The explanations which have been advanced to account for the supposedly obligatory concurrence of the symptoms have

TABLE 16-2. MEAN CORRELATION COEFFICIENTS BETWEEN INDIVIDUAL PERFORMANCES AND THE SYNDROME IN 100 BRAIN-DAMAGED PATIENTS

	r
Right-left vs. finger localization—writing—calculation	0.52
Finger localization vs. right-left—writing—calculation	0.51
Writing vs. right-left—finger localization—calculation	0.49
Calculation vs. right-left—finger localization—writing	0.42
Constructional praxis vs. right-left—finger localization—writing—calculation	0.52
Reading vs. right-left—finger localization—writing—calculation	0.52
Visual memory vs. right-left—finger localization—writing—calculation	0.54

TABLE 16-3. MEAN CORRELATIONS BETWEEN INDIVIDUAL PERFORMANCES AND THE SYNDROME IN 12 PATIENTS WITH LEFT PARIETAL LOBE DISEASE

Right-left vs. finger localization—writing—calculation	0.53
Finger localization vs. right-left—writing—calculation	0.38
Writing vs. right-left—finger localization—calculation	0.21
Calculation vs. right-left—finger localization—writing	0.51
Constructional praxis vs. right-left—finger localization—writing—calculation	0.53
Reading vs. right-left—finger localization—writing—calculation	0.61
Visual memory vs. right-left—finger localization—writing—calculation	0.44

been of a broad psychological or psychoneurological nature and have no necessary reference to a specific locus of the responsible lesion. Thus such concepts as the importance of intact finger gnosis for writing and calculation, of intact right-left orientation for calculation, or of intact spatial thinking for all the performances have been applied to all situations in which the deficits appear, *e.g.*, developmental deficit, and are not dependent upon the presence of a specified lesion. Nevertheless, it seemed worthwhile to make a separate analysis of the performances of the 12 right-handed patients in the group who had disease of the left parietal lobe to determine the nature of the relationships of the syndrome performances among themselves and with the other performances.

The mean correlation coefficient of each of the syndrome performances with the other three syndrome performances and of each extra-syndrome performance with the four syndrome performances is shown in Table 16-3.

It is evident from inspection of this table that constructional praxis, reading, and visual memory are as closely related to the elements of the syndrome as the latter are to each other. Thus in this group of patients with focal disease of the left parietal lobe there is also no evidence that the elements of the syndrome show any noteworthy strength of association.

The significant deficits in performance shown by these 12 patients are shown in detail in Table 16-4. It will be seen that no patient showed the full Gerstmann syndrome. Four patients (E.H., R.K., A.P., D.T.) presented with three Gerstmann symptoms but in each case these appeared in association with other deficits.

DISCUSSION

This investigation represents an attempt to determine whether the four behavioral deficits

TABLE 16-4. INCIDENCE OF DEFICITS IN PATIENTS WITH LEFT PARIETAL LOBE DISEASE

No.	Patient	Right-left	Finger Localization	Writing	Calculation	Constructional Praxis	Reading	Visual Memory
1	N.F.	o	o	o	o	+	o	+
2	E.H.	+	+	o	+	+	o	+
3	V.H.	o	o	o	o	o	o	o
4	R.K.	+	+	o	+	+	+	+
5	E.K.	o	o	o	o	+	o	o
6	A.P.	+	+	o	+	+	+	o
7	D.T.	+	o	+	+	o	+	o
8	E.H.	o	o	o	o	o	o	o
9	R.M.	o	o	o	o	o	o	o
10	E.M.	o	o	o	o	o	o	o
11	J.C.	+	+	o	o	+	o	o
12	J.D.	o	o	o	o	o	o	o

(+ = Deficit; o = no deficit)

comprising the so-called "Gerstmann syndrome" form a distinctive constellation. A variety of analyses, which provided evidence concerning the strength of the relationships existing among these elements and that existing between the elements and performances which do not belong to the syndrome, were done. These analyses, made both on a large group of patients with diverse types of cerebral disease and a smaller group of right-handed patients with focal disease of the left parietal lobe, consistently indicated that the particular combination of behavioral deficits which form the syndrome show no stronger internal associative bonds than do a score of other combinations of behavioral deficits. A large number of combinations of four behavioral deficits may be presented by patients with cerebral disease. The analyses of the present study suggest that there is about an equal probability of occurrence for any one of them, including the combination known as the Gerstmann syndrome.

These results provide a reasonable explanation of the frequent reports in the clinical literature of so-called incomplete forms of the syndrome as well as the even more frequent reports of symptoms which are observed to "accompany" it. Such behavioral pictures are simply other combinations of deficits which tend not to be accepted in their own right because of the predilection of clinical observers to look first for elements of the Gerstmann combination and to use these elements as an anchoring point to which accompanying symptoms may be attached. The findings also indicate that theoretical speculations concerning the basic impairment which must underlie the so-called Gerstmann syndrome are hardly warranted. There is no obligatory concurrence of deficits to account for and, in any case, if it is necessary to explain this particular combination of deficits, it is equally necessary to explain the existence of a score of other combinations of behavioral deficits.

A tenable conclusion from these results is that, judged from the standpoint of behavioral analysis, the Gerstmann syndrome is a fiction; it is simply an artifact of defective and biased observations. Objective, unbiased observation discloses a large number of combinations of parietal deficits. Since all these combinations appear to be about equally strong with respect to their internal associative bonds and frequency of occurrence, either all or none should be designated as syndromes.

This study has not been concerned directly with the question of the possible neuropathological significance of the combination of deficits known as the Gerstmann syndrome. Despite the fact that this combination of deficits does not seem to be any different from many other combinations of parietal symptoms, there is the possibility that when it is manifested in pure form it does possess the highly specific focal diagnostic significance which has been claimed for it, namely, a lesion of "that nodal area which corresponds to the angular gyrus in its transition to the second occipital convolution" (Gerstmann, 1957). However, Critchley (1953), reviewing the clinical literature, was inclined to conclude that the syndrome was more reasonably interpreted as a sign of parietal disease in general rather than specifically indicating a lesion of the angular gyrus. Similarly, Heimberger, DeMyer, and Reitan (1957) found that when patients manifested the full syndrome, the responsible lesion, even when restricted to the dominant hemisphere, was invariably an extensive one. Finally, there are case reports, such as the recent one by Brusa, Rossi, and Tartarini (1960), of the occurrence of the syndrome in patients with lesions apparently restricted to the frontal lobes. Thus those analyses of the question as have been done throw considerable doubt on the assertion that the syndrome has a highly specific focal diagnostic import. If it does possess such a significance, it might be expected that the other 34 of the 35 syndromes investigated in this study would also have a similarly specific significance. But the weight of clinicopathological evidence gathered over the last 60 years makes it extremely unlikely that such "punctate" localization of functions or deficits exists.

In directing the attention of neurologists both to certain disorders of the body schema and to the unusual variety of combinations of behavioral deficits which a brain-damaged patient may show, the Gerstmann syndrome has perhaps been a useful fiction during the past 30 years. Now that these purposes have been accomplished, adherence to the fiction may well operate to retard further advances in the understanding of the patterns of behavioral deficit which may occur as a consequence of cerebral disease, for it tends to prejudice clinical observation and to produce a distorted picture of the organization of abilities and disabilities in brain-damaged patients.

SUMMARY

Systematic, objective analysis of the performances of patients with cerebral disease on seven "parietal" tasks (right-left orientation, finger localization, writing, calculation, constructional praxis, reading, visual memory) indicates that many combinations of deficits, including that known as the "Gerstmann syndrome", may be observed. The syndrome appears to be no different from the other combinations in respect to either the strength of the mutual interrelationships among its elements or the strength of the relationships between its elements and performances not belonging to it. These results hold both for patients with diverse cerebral conditions and for those with focal lesions of the dominant parietal lobe.

The findings are interpreted as indicating that the Gerstmann syndrome is an artifact of defective and biased observation. Further, a review of the pertinent clinical literature offers little support for its alleged focal diagnostic significance. The general conclusion is that the syndrome is a fiction which has perhaps served a useful purpose in the past in certain respects, but which now carries the hazard of retarding advances in the understanding of the organization of abilities and disabilities in patients with cerebral disease.

REFERENCES

Ajuriaguerra, J. de, and Hécaen, H. (1960). *Le Cortex Cérébral.* Masson, Paris.

Badal, J. (1888). *Arch. Ophtal. (Paris)*, **8,** 97.

Benton, A. L. (1953). *Manuel pour l'Application clinique du Test de Rétention Visuelle.* Editions du Centre de Psychologie Appliquée, Paris.

—— (1959). *Right-Left Discrimination and Finger Localization: Development and Pathology.* Hoeber, New York.

——, and Kemble, J. D. (1960). *Psychiat. et Neurol. (Basel)*, **139,** 49.

Brusa, A., Rossi, R., and Tartarini, E. (1960). *Encéphale*, **49,** 319.

Critchley, M. (1953). *The Parietal Lobes.* Arnold, London.

Gerstmann, J. (1924). *Wien klin. Wschr.*, **37,** 1010.

—— (1927). *Z. ges. Neurol. Psychiat.*, **108,** 152.

—— (1930). *Nervenarzt.*, **3,** 692.

—— (1957). *Neurology (Minneap.)*, **7,** 866.

Heimberger, R. F. DeMyer, W., and Retain, R. M. (1957). Paper read at the American Academy of Neurology, Boston.

17

Language After Section of the Cerebral Commissures[1]

MICHAEL S. GAZZANIGA
ROGER W. SPERRY

MICHAEL S. GAZZANIGA, Ph.D., is with the department of psychology of New York University.
ROGER W. SPERRY, Ph.D., is with the division of biology of the California Institute of Technology, Pasadena.
Aided by U.S. Public Health Service grant MH 3372 and the Frank P. Hixon Fund of the California Institute of Technology.

INTRODUCTION

Some of the functional effects that appear in man following surgical separation of the hemispheres produced by complete transection of the corpus callosum plus the anterior and hippocampal commissures, with separation of the massa intermedia have been described in earlier reports (Gazzaniga, *et al.*, 1962, 1963, 1965). The observations were based on two patients operated on by Drs. Philip Vogel and Joseph Bogen of the California College of Medicine at the White Memorial Medical Center in Los Angeles for relief of intractable seizures. In general the post-surgical studies indicate a striking functional independence of the gnostic activities of the two hemispheres. Perceptual, cognitive, mnemonic, learned and volitional activities persist in each hemisphere, but can proceed separately in each case outside the realm of awareness of the other hemisphere. The subjective experience of each hemisphere is known to the other only indirectly through lower level and peripheral effects.

This disruption of interhemispheric integration produces remarkably little disturbance in ordinary behavior, temperament, or intellect. The functional deficits tend to be compensated by the development of bilateral motor control from each hemisphere, also by bilaterality in some of the sensory projection pathways and by a variety of other unifying factors that we deliberately avoid or exclude so far as possible in the testing procedures. Ordinarily there would seem to be a large common denominator of similar and closely related background activity in right and left hemispheres.

This paper describes some of the further findings obtained to date with reference specifically to language functions. As might be expected, it is in activities involving language and especially speech, that the effects of sectioning the cerebral commissures become most conspicuous. It is the severing of connexions that link the minor hemisphere to the speech centers in the major hemisphere that is directly responsible for many of the more pronounced functional disturbances.

General Background

Three patients from a total of six who have undergone the surgery are included in the

From *Brain* 90:131–148, 1967. Reprinted by permission of the Editor of *Brain*.

[1]All subjects examined were patients of Drs. Philip Vogel of the California College of Medicine and Joseph Bogen of the Ross Loos Medical Group, Los Angeles. We are also grateful to Dr. Joseph Bogen for his continuing interest and cooperation in carrying out the language studies.

present study. All three have been virtually free of seizures since their surgery for four, two-and-a-half and one years respectively to date. Three others have had various complications and have shown little or no improvement over the pre-operative condition. The medical case histories of two of those included here have already been described (Bogen and Vogel, 1962; Bogen *et al.*, 1965). Both these persons have continued to give full co-operation in functional testing. A third case (L.B.) from the same series who, like the others, had undergone a similar disconnexion of the hemispheres for the same reason, is included here. The surgeons were confident in this case that both fornices and all main cortical veins draining into the sagittal sinus had been spared. This third patient, a right-handed 12-year-old boy, had no history of traumatic brain injury. He was a bright, affable and generally happy individual with a pre-operative I.Q. of 115 (WISC)[2] scored under anti-convulsant sedation. Pre-operative testing of the visual fields, somatic sensibility and motor co-ordination disclosed no significant abnormalities.

The language capacity of the minor hemisphere in Case 1 proved to be almost negligible and was decidedly inferior to that of the other two subjects. Also, Case 1, unlike the others, had sustained considerable brain damage, especially in the minor hemisphere, prior to surgery. For these reasons it was assumed that findings in Cases 2 and 3 could be relied upon to reflect more accurately the typical effects of cerebral disconnexion *per se*, whereas Case 1 is more representative of the kinds of disconnexion syndrome seen in cases of brain tumor, vascular accidents, or other cerebral pathology.

OBSERVATIONS

Early Recovery

The most rapid recovery was seen in the third and youngest patient. During the first twenty-four hours after surgery this boy was conversing with the hospital staff with good comprehension, made quips about having a "splitting headache," and was able to recite "Peter Piper picked a peck of pickled peppers," etc. rapidly with no apparent difficulty. From his comments and his general attitude in the intensive care unit, it seemed evident that the same humor, mannerisms and general personality that characterized this person pre-operatively were already present from the first day after surgery.

By the second day he was feeding himself, consuming normal portions of solid food. He was walking around the hospital at the end of the first week, and earlier mobility would probably have been possible, had it been permitted. At this time he also displayed only a little of the apraxic difficulty in making voluntary movements with the left hand to verbal command that had been so marked for months in Case 1 and for weeks in Case 2. What little inability he had in this regard involved the individual control of the left fingers. Shoulder, elbow and wrist movements all could be made at will or to verbal command, and he was able upon request to make a closed fist moving all fingers together. The left fingers could be controlled individually at this stage if the verbal command was accompanied with an overt "do this" type of demonstration. Case 3 was discharged three weeks following surgery. During the next two months general somatosensory and visual testing showed a course of recovery almost identical to that described for Case 2 (Gazzaniga *et al.*, 1965) with the time scale somewhat advanced by almost two months.

A short period of mutism followed the surgery in the other two cases lasting for approximately thirty days in Case 1 and one to two days in the second patient. Case 2, a 30-year-old housewife and mother, was talking over the telephone on Day 3 and was walking with assistance and feeding herself at the end of the first week. During the first two weeks after surgery she displayed an erratic emotional lability in her conversation. At one moment, for example, she would be conversing in a normal manner. Suddenly and for no apparent reason, she would be on the verge of tears while, however,

[2] Administered by Mrs. E. Gunther, Hacker Clinic, Los Angeles.

keeping the main train of thought. Then just as abruptly she would resume talking in a normal manner. During the same two week period she was also prone to confabulate a good deal during interviews—especially with the onset of fatigue. It was considered highly probable that part or all of her right fornix had been divided in the surgery.

During this period Case 2 displayed good memory for many of her pre-operative experiences up to and including her hospitalization for the surgery. On Day 4 she acknowledged and appeared to recognize from among a group of strangers someone whom she had seen only briefly on the second day before surgery. She was able, during the first week after surgery, to hum with good tonal quality several of her old favorite tunes. Complaints that her memory was poor were received from the family, however, for about four months following the surgery.

In Case 1, a 48-year-old right-handed male payroll clerk, speech reappeared after one month and had returned to approximately normal so far as ordinary conversation was concerned by about the eighth week. At this time there appeared to be no change in gross temperament or intellect in this person, and he repeatedly remarked that he hadn't felt better in years—probably attributable in part to the reduction in medication that proved to be possible after the surgery.

After these persons were well recovered from surgery and had again settled into their routines at home, more detailed lateralized tests were started including those described below aimed at determining among other things the extent to which speech and language had been preserved in each of the disconnected cerebral hemispheres. The positive findings reported below were evident starting from about the fourth month for Case 2 and the second month for Case 3. Prior to this function seemed to be depressed below the normal level presumably from disruption of the tonic influence of the corpus callosum and other diaschistic effects.

In the following tests and their interpretation we take for granted some of the basic findings already reported, such as the absence of any interchange of cognitive experience or any transfer of learning or memory from one hemisphere to the other (Gazzaniga *et al.*, 1962, 1963, 1965). In view of the evidence for independent mental function in the two disconnected hemispheres, it makes for confusion to try to describe the behavior and cerebral symptoms with reference to the individual person in the ordinary way. Accordingly we continue the practice of referring specifically to the perceptual, cognitive and other mental functions of each hemisphere independently. We also take the position for reasons reviewed elsewhere (Sperry, 1964, 1966; Sperry and Gazzaniga, 1965) that conscious awareness is commonly present in the minor as well as in the major hemisphere and that the two separate spheres of conscious experience may proceed concurrently as well as in alternation.

LANGUAGE EXPRESSION

Speech

In tests aimed to determine the capacity to speak with reference to information specifically lateralized to one or the other hemisphere, very different results were obtained for the right and left sides. Whereas spoken descriptions of stimulus material and other verbal responses obtained from the left hemisphere showed from the beginning little or no impairment, the right hemisphere appeared in similar testing to be totally incapable of speech. For example, visual stimuli such as numbers, letters, words and pictorial material presented tachistoscopically in the right visual half field at one-tenth second as described elsewhere (Gazzaniga *et al.*, 1965) were reported correctly and described normally.

The same was true for stimuli presented to the right hand with vision excluded. A familiar item placed in the subject's right hand, like a spoon, knife, comb, toothbrush, block letters, or any of a series of simple geometric shapes were readily recognized, named and described by both subjects. Speech was also used with normal facility in making various somatosensory discriminations involving weight, pattern, and temperature applied anywhere on the right half of the body. This was true as well for the left side of the face and head, and we have assumed this to be correlated with the presence of an ipsilateral component in the afferent projections of these areas to the left hemisphere. In short, any sensory information entering the left hemisphere, or the results of the central processing of that information, could be reported through speech in much the usual manner.

Conversely, both subjects were totally unable to give accurate spoken reports for even the simplest kind of sensory information projected to the right hemisphere. Test material presented to the left hand or to the left half of the visual field evoked in each case only irrelevant confabulatory spoken responses or none at all. For example, a pencil placed in the left hand might go unnoticed and elicit no verbal comment whatever, or more typically, its presence would be recognized but it would be called a "can opener" or a "cigarette lighter," etc. Such guesses came presumably from the left dominant hemisphere and were based on whatever indirect cues happened to be available to that hemisphere. All visual stimuli flashed to the left half field similarly went undescribed or were reported vocally, as just a "flash" or a "white flash." Whereas Case 1 had been unable to localize verbally points of stimulation on the left side of the body below the neck, Cases 2 and 3 had little trouble in reporting verbally the correct localization of cutaneous stimuli applied to the left side of the entire body, excepting only the hands and feet. This again seems best attributed to bilateral cerebral projection of sensory cues for cutaneous and deep local sign including an ipsilateral component to the major hemisphere, that is particularly strong in the case of the face and head.

Writing

The right hand with its main motor control centered in the left hemisphere along with speech was always capable of writing correctly the names and descriptions of visual or tactile stimuli presented to the left hemisphere with no special difficulty evident. When the same stimulus material was presented to the right hemisphere, however, none of the stimuli could be described or named in writing by any of the patients using either hand. For example, when a spoon or a knife was placed in the left hand, or a picture flashed to the left visual field, any written responses seemed to represent mere guesswork by the major hemisphere. Writing to dictation posed no problem for these persons when they were using the right hand.

Some simple writing to dictation was possible with the left hand also after the seventh month in Case 2 and after the first month in Case 3, but not at all in Case 1. This performance with the left hand seems best ascribed to the bilaterality in motor control. This ability of each hemisphere to govern movement of the ipsilateral as well as the contralateral limb showed definite improvement in all cases during the post-surgical observation period. That the writing with the left hand was directed from the major and not the minor hemisphere is shown by the above-mentioned inability to write when the stimulus is strictly lateralized to the right hemisphere. Further, the name of an object flashed to the left hemisphere could be written with the left hand in the absence of audible or other intermediary cues. The left arm writing was guided more easily from the proximal joints than from the fingers.

Drawing

Although not language, expression of understanding by drawing is closely related to some of the foregoing and is included here for comparison. None of the patients had a highly developed talent for drawing pictures prior to surgery, although Case 3 at 12 years had some favorite caricature sketches that he did moderately well and he was able to repeat the same sketch upon request. This capacity to sketch his favorite caricature with free hand use was severely impaired during the first several months following surgery, but then improved with the right hand to almost its former level. The drawing capacity of the two older patients after surgery was decidedly poor even with the preferred right hand suggesting that cerebral interaction through the commissures may have some particular importance for artistic drawing in the normal brain.

Within their reduced artistic limits, each patient was able to reproduce by drawing with the right hand various geometric figures like triangles, parallelograms, trapezoids, stars and other line drawings presented to the right visual half field. They could do the same for familiar objects like a comb, fork and alphabet letters presented out of sight for palpation and stereognostic exploration by the right hand. And they could draw with the right hand simple objects and patterns named vocally by the experimenter. When stimulus material was presented to the right hemisphere via the left hand or in the left half visual field, Cases 2 and 3 were both able to make recognizable reproductions of very simple material using the left hand. For example, flat wooden cut-outs including a circle, square, triangle, toy alphabet letters and other simple shapes could be drawn after having been explored by the left hand. This contralateral performance, controlled from the minor hemisphere, however, was generally inferior to that of the right hand in response to stimuli presented exclusively to the left hemisphere.

When the subjects were shown three-dimensional forms like the Necker cube, a house, or other objects involving more complex spatial relations and asked to reproduce them, their performance with the left hand was consistently superior to that with the right so far as getting correct spatial representation was concerned, as described earlier (Gazzaniga *et al.*, 1965; Bogen and Gazzaniga, 1965).

Ideation in the Absence of Linguistic Expression

With regard to the major hemisphere there was little reason to question the preservation of thought, imagination, reason, judgment and other cognitive functions since these were amply demonstrated in conversation and behavior generally as well as in the testing situation. Scores on the WISC I.Q. tests at two to three months after surgery were not significantly lower than those obtained before surgery when one omitted test items requiring use of the left hand. That the surgery has produced at least subtle impairments in some of these higher cognitive functions, however, can neither be asserted nor denied at this time without more refined and specific testing of these factors than we have attempted to date.

In regard to the minor hemisphere, on the other hand, even the approximate level and quality of cognition remained highly obscure from the beginning. The inability of this hemisphere to express itself in speech or writing, and the apparently low, but uncertain, level of comprehension for verbal material, as indicated below, made any assessment of the mental capacity of the minor hemisphere difficult and devious. With respect to the total picture of the functional effects of the surgery, the cognitive properties of the speechless and agraphic minor hemisphere has always posed the outstanding and most challenging unknown. Accordingly our main testing efforts were directed at this problem. A variety of related questions are involved here that concern possible interrelations between the development of language and cognition.

When stimulus material was presented to the minor hemisphere, under conditions in which its comprehension could be indicated by purely non-verbal responses, it became evident that the mute minor hemisphere was quite capable of perceptual understanding and of forming ideas or concepts that went well beyond a mere image of the stimulus. Not uncommonly these test performances seemed to involve some abstraction, generalization and mental association. This was demonstrated, for example, in tests that combined the presentation of visual pictures to the right hemisphere followed by the retrieval of a matching object with the left hand using the sense of touch. The subjects were able on the first exposure to match such disparate stimuli as a crude ink drawing of a skeleton key presented visually with a very differently shaped car key selected by touch. Similarly when a picture of a wooden match was presented, they retrieved correctly a book of paper matches and so forth. Both visual and tactile stimulation had to be in the same hemisphere; cross-integration of these inter-modal tasks failed consistently. Similar performances were described in connexion with tests for vision (Gazzaniga, *et al.*, 1965) and many others are given below in tests for symbol comprehension.

Other examples of ideation in the absence of linguistic expression were obtained within the somatosensory sphere in which recognition and retrieval tests were performed with the left hand, vision and audible speech being excluded. Following presentation of a sample object to the left hand for stereognostic recognition, the left hand might then search for a considerable time, up to a half-minute or more, among a series of other objects before coming to and selecting the correct one. Some of the incorrect objects, especially those most resembling the correct item, might be lifted and explored at length before being rejected. When additional delay periods were imposed as part of the task in this situation, rememberance of the stimulus object could be held for periods of time exceeding one minute. This was true for Case 3 even when distractions were introduced during the delay, such as irrelevant conversation, and asking the patient to walk out of the room, down the hall, and back. After picking out the correct item at the end of such a delay period, the verbal response of the subjects, when questioned, indicated that the major hemisphere had no idea what the object was that had been perceived and remembered by the right hemisphere. The proficiency of Cases 2 and 3 on these tasks far exceeds that described earlier in Case 1 in which the minor hemisphere had sustained extensive damage ten years prior to the surgery. The upper limit of such delayed-reaction capacities has yet to be determined.

LANGUAGE COMPREHENSION

The findings throughout the foregoing are consistent with the inference that language functions had survived with little, if any, impairment in the left, major hemisphere. Conversely, the same tests suggest the possibility of complete absence of any language development in the minor hemisphere, in that correct responses were unobtainable for the simplest of words, numbers, or even single letters when these were presented solely to the right hemisphere. In tests like the foregoing the minor hemisphere appears to be alexic, word blind, word deaf, agraphic and astereognostic (for review, *see* Geschwind, 1962, 1965). The question of the extent to which language is represented in the subordinate hemisphere has long been a matter of controversy with authoritative proponents supporting both sides of this issue (*see* Zangwill, 1962). The tests that have been described thus far in the present study required in addition to perception and comprehension of non-verbal stimulus material only an ability to use language at most for the expression and communication of this understanding. It thus remained possible that the minor hemisphere was capable of some recognition and comprehension of language and other symbolic information but that this comprehension had not been evident for lack of any means for expression.

To investigate the possibility of this we applied tests that were designed to separate the comprehension of language from its expression. The motor activity in these tests was non-verbal and depended in most instances upon pointing with the left hand to a correct answer presented as one item among an array of incorrect items. Even these tests failed to reveal any significant language comprehension in the damaged right hemisphere of Case 1. In the other two cases, however, in which prior brain damage had been absent or minimal, it was possible to demonstrate comprehension of verbal and other symbolic material presented visually, audibly or tactually as outlined in the following.

Visual Comprehension

Both Cases 2 and 3 proved to be capable of reading letters, numbers and short words in the left visual field. For example, when the names of familiar objects were flashed at one-tenth second to the left field, the subject though unable, as described above, to give a correct verbal response, was nevertheless able to retrieve the matching item from among a series of 10 objects laid out in open view in front of him. If words such as *cup, knife, pen, orange,* etc., were tachistoscopically presented in the left visual field, in the set-up illustrated in Fig. 17-1, the patient could also readily point out the correct one from among 10 items arrayed in free view before him. Similarly, if a picture, for example, of a ship, were flashed into the left visual field, these subjects would verbally deny having seen anything. When urged to let the left hand try, however, they would then proceed to pick up the card with "ship" written on it from a series of 10 laid out in open view in front of them. It was difficult to determine the upper limits of such comprehension under these conditions because the choice of stimulus material was restricted to what could be read in the brief exposure time required to avoid eye movement.

The same sort of result was obtained in tasks that required intermodal integration going from vision to touch and vice versa. When a sample word such as pencil, tack, knife, sock, comb, etc., was presented in the left visual half field, the left hand, *but not the right,* could be used to search out the described correct matching object by touch from among an array of others, all shielded from vision. In such instances, when the stimulus and the matching answer were both presented exclusively to the right hemisphere, the subjects remained completely unaware of the given stimulus and response selection in their dominant conversant hemisphere. After making a correct manual response through the mute hemisphere they would commonly describe the selected object as some totally unrelated item that was obviously a pure guess. Where the objects for choice were laid out where both hemispheres could see them, the speech hemisphere would routinely confabulate after the fact, and state that a particular word had been seen to fit the object to which the left hand already had pointed. Under the latter conditions they would guess correctly the word that had been pro-

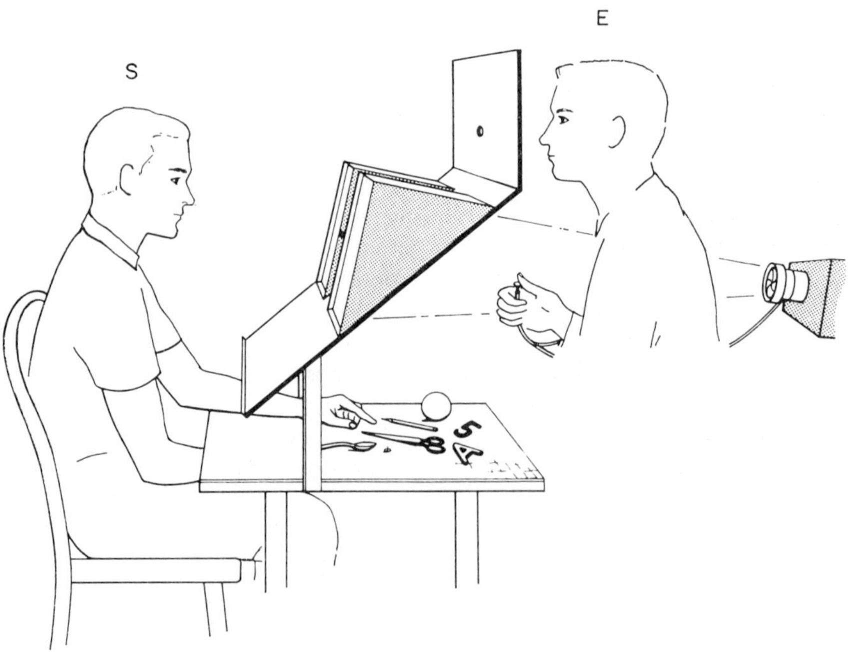

Fig. 17–1. Testing apparatus: Slanting shield on table prevents subject from seeing test items on table, his hands, or the examiner. It contains ground glass viewing screen for back projection of 2×2 slides, and also serves to hold cards or other test items set before subject in free view. Examiner flashes slides when subject's gaze is seen to be properly centred on designated fixation point. A second examiner beside subject records trials and subject's reactions.

jected to the minor hemisphere but often the guesswork in the dominant hemisphere was revealed in the subject's use of a synonym that did not have even remote resemblance in spelling.

Comprehension of Spoken Words

Because of the bilaterality of auditory afferent projection, tests for the comprehension of words presented audibly to the right hemisphere were run, not by trying to lateralize the original input, but by limiting the available answers exclusively to the right hemisphere. In one test situation the patients were required to push a response button held in the left hand, when they saw that one of a series of five nouns projected in serial succession to the left visual field, matched the test word spoken previously. They were able to do this and also to pick out the correct word from among a series presented to the left half field that fitted a descriptive phrase read aloud by the examiner. For example, the examiner would read, "Used to tell time," and would then flash five choice words in succession to the left visual field. In this instance the patients made a correct manual signal to the word "clock." When one of them was asked in passing what word he had seen, the reply (from the major hemisphere) was "watch." Here again was another demonstration of what we constantly encounter in testing these persons, namely, complete agnosia in one hemisphere for cognitive experiences that have just transpired in the other hemisphere.

Comprehension of the spoken word by the minor hemisphere was further shown by the patients' ability to retrieve by blind palpation with the left hand an audibly named object from among an array of objects presented to the left hand. The patients for example had no problem retrieving a safety pin when it was presented along with: *ring, coin, sock, tack, marble, pencil, pen, flashlight bulb*, and *spoon*. This was true also for a group of geometric solids as well as other series of objects all made of the same material and all of approximately the same weight to exclude any possible cues such as sound or weight, etc.

Comprehension Through Stereognosis

For the detection of latent linguistic and other symbolic mental functions in the aphonic noncommunicative hemisphere, tests based on tactile input from the left hand were found to have certain advantages. There was no need, for example, to limit the presentation of the test material to a brief exposure of a fraction of a second as with vision. The subject could take time to explore the stimuli and the complexity of the test material could be increased accordingly. Also, competitive function in the other hemisphere could be reduced more effectively by elimination of non-specific visual and auditory distractions which is more difficult to achieve with visual and auditory testing. As with visual and unlike auditory material the perceptual process in the case of stereognosis can be confined to a single hemisphere.

The tests involving stereognosis were carried out in the general testing apparatus illustrated in Fig. 17-1. The slanting screen served to exclude vision of the hand and arm and the test objects. The eyes were closed for difficult tasks to aid concentration on the performance with the left hand. Also, the table was covered with acoustic soundproofing material to exclude auditory cues in manipulation of the objects which the subjects' major hemisphere was very quick to use to facilitate guessing the correct response. Preliminary testing of Case 3 confirmed the findings in the earlier cases with respect to the more generalized features of stereognosis following forebrain commissurotomy. Stereognosis was approximately normal for each hand in Case 3 so long as the motor response was through the same hand, i.e. by motor demonstration of how the test object is used, by retrieval through touch of the same item from among others, or by pointing to matching pictures, etc. Cross-matching or cross-comparison of stereognostic discriminations from one to the other hand failed consistently in all cases. All three subjects have always been unable to describe verbally or in writing any stereognostic discriminations made through the left hand. Only the presence of a stimulus and very gross differences of localization and in the direction of movement of a stylus across the left hand were detectable by the speaking hemisphere. In short, practically all stereognostic discriminations made with the left hand were processed entirely by the right hemisphere and vice versa.

Tasks that depended upon stereognosis in the left hand could, therefore, be used to investigate the perceptive capacity of the minor hemisphere. For example, the ability to use the left hand to search out by touch an object described by spoken or written words could be taken to mean that there must have been comprehension of those words within the minor hemisphere. This presumes the exclusion of indirect sophisticated strategies of various sorts that seemed to be ruled out under our present testing conditions. Conversely, after a test object had been perceived solely by the left hand, the ability to select a correct audible or written name for that object could also be taken as evidence of comprehension of those words in the minor hemisphere. A large battery of tests designed along these lines was applied to subjects 2 and 3 with results in both cases that further confirmed the conclusion that there is considerable comprehension of language present in the minor hemisphere despite the incapacity of this hemisphere for motor expression.

A series of 10 objects was placed one at a time in the subject's left hand out of sight behind a screen and a printed list of the 13 names of the test objects was set up on a card in front of the subject for free visual inspection. Both subjects, after having felt each of the 10 items in scrambled order, were able then to point correctly to the name of the given item in the printed list. A large variety of everyday items were correctly identified under these conditions. Typically the subjects would spontaneously offer the correct name by saying it aloud, but only after the left hand had first pointed correctly, never before. If asked to point to the name of an object with the right hand while feeling it with the left hand, they sometimes could do so especially if the names were individually placed 6 to 12 inches or more apart. However, apraxia in the form of hesitancy, false moves, and outright errors of response were not uncommonly seen under these conditions. Frequently, after an error had been made with the right hand, the left hand would then jerk up spontaneously from under the screen to point to the correct answer. Confusion in the right hand control was potentiated under these conditions by conversation with the subject, presumably by bringing in the left hemisphere.

Under similar testing conditions the subject was asked to signal the correct name of the test object held in the left hand by raising the hand at the proper time when a list of names was read aloud by the experimenter. Comprehension of spoken words similar to that shown for written words above was clearly demonstrated. These two types of tests were extended from simple nouns into verbs, adjectives and phrases of different categories. There is almost no limit to the variety and refinement that could be introduced into such tests more thoroughly to analyze in detail the language capacity of the speechless hemisphere. Samples of some of the more complicated test words for which some recognition and understanding seemed to be present in the right hemisphere are listed as follows:

rough, smooth, round, cone, rectangle, cylinder, square, pyramid, flashlight bulb, tweezers, safety pin, measuring instrument, door latch, clown, Indian, etc.

In other tests a definition was first read aloud by the examiner after which the subject then explored blindly a series of objects with the left hand feeling for an item that would satisfy the examiner's definition. By careful selection of words of increasing difficulty in the spoken definition, this type of test also was extremely informative and could be extended over a wide range even though the test objects themselves remained fairly simple. Under the same conditions, the definitions, names, descriptive words, phrases and adjectives could be written out for free visual, instead of auditory, presentation.

In similar tests, the linguistic cues for comprehension and retrieval by stereognosis were flashed tachistoscopically to the left half visual field. Only simple short, usually single, words could be used with this form of presentation. On the other hand, this procedure gave the greatest assurance that the left hemisphere was not contributing to the performance. The words were printed vertically in some cases as well as horizontally and presented near the vertical mid-line on the left side in order to utilize central vision as much as possible. When words like *coin, ball, apple, comb,* etc. were flashed to the right hemisphere the subjects were able to search out the item named by palpating blindly with the left hand. They were asked what the item was on occasional trials after a correct selection had been made and while the item was still in the left hand but out of sight behind a screen. If the item were named correctly, as happened very rarely, the trial was thrown out on the supposition that the eyes had probably moved from the fixation point at the time of exposure and had allowed the test word to be projected to the left hemisphere. With these rare exceptions it was clear from the verbal responses that the left hemisphere was only guessing and that knowledge of the correct answer had been confined to the right hemisphere.

Spelling

Tests were run to find out to what degree the right hemisphere might have the ability to order and arrange individual letters into words. Alphabet letters about four inches high cut from heavy cardboard were presented out of vision to the left hand for manual palpation and arrangement. Thus the patients had only to feel and recognize the individual letters and then place them in correct spatial order from left to right. Case 2 failed to perform convincingly, but the significance of this was questionable in view of the left-handed hypesthesia. Only Case 3 was able to spell consistently with the subordinate hemisphere as indicated in results like the following: The subject was told to spell a word like "dog" after which the examiner placed the appropriate three letters, one at a time in random order, into the subject's left hand for placement on the table. Very simple familiar words like *the, how, what, pie, hat,* were spelled correctly under these conditions but only slowly and with considerable effort. When an occasional mistake was made in letter order, the examiner would suggest that the subject check the word, and usually the error was found and corrected on the first such check. During this particular test wherein the left hemisphere also heard, the subject would often talk in a confabulatory way. Thus while holding the "O" for "dog" in his left hand the subject would say, "That's the 'D'." Nevertheless the left hand would continue to spell correctly, demonstrating the ability of the minor hemisphere to maintain its own reasoning, will and intent in the presence of competitive ideas and other distracting influences from the major hemisphere.

In further tests, a group of three or four letters was presented out of vision to the left hand and the subjects were instructed to "spell a word." The word to be spelled was not stated and it remained for the right hemisphere to recognize the individual letters and to arrange them into a meaningful order. Case 3 again proved able to do this and spelled such words as *cup, not, cake, love* and *what.*

Calculation

With stimuli presented tactually to the minor hemisphere through the left hand, Cases 2 and 3 demonstrated a limited ability to add correctly the numbers one or two to numbers under ten. They were unable, however, to subtract or multiply at this level. In this test, a set of from one to four wooden pegs (2.5 × .8 cm.) implanted upright in two inch wooden blocks were presented to the patient's left hand, out of view and in random order. Initially it was shown that the patients, upon command, could readily pick out blocks 1, 2 or 3, etc. With a card with printed numbers from 1–8 placed in open view in front of the patients, two blocks were serially presented to the left hand and the patients were required to point with the left hand to the number representing the sum. They usually succeeded with these numbers under five but were unable to subtract the number of pegs in one block from those in another or to double or triple the number of pegs.

All of the above tasks, of course, were performed easily with the other hand. In addition, much more complicated problems and general experience with the use of mathematics, changing money, estimating food quantities, etc. all made it questionable that calculations carried out with the major hemisphere were at all impaired. Case 3 had some difficulty during the fourth and fifth months after surgery in carrying out written mathematical calculations. This proved to be a problem not so much in the ability to calculate *per se*, but in taking care to scan far enough to the left so that all numbers fell in the right half field.

DISCUSSION AND CONCLUSIONS

Some of the main points that emerge here regarding the cerebral organization of language and the cerebral disconnexion syndrome generally, may be summarized briefly as follows. Information perceived exclusively or generated exclusively in the minor (right) hemisphere could be communicated neither in speech nor in writing; it had to be expressed entirely through non-verbal responses. By contrast, there was no noticeable impairment of speech and writing with reference to information processed in the major (left) hemisphere. Linguistic expression seemed, thus, to be organized almost exclusively in the left hemisphere. The possibility that a few simple emotional, tonal, or extremely familiar words might be expressed through the minor hemisphere in these cases, however, cannot be completely ruled out from the present data.

In tasks involving calculation the separated minor hemisphere was unable to multiply or divide even small numbers or items by two or by three, and subtraction of two or more from numbers below ten failed. Mathematical computations by the major hemisphere, on the other hand, were not markedly below preoperative standards under optimal conditions where distractions were minimized and careful concern reinforced. Like speech and writing, calculation in these patients seems thus to be confined almost exclusively to the major hemisphere. This same hemisphere also, of course, was shown to process all visual functions for the right half of the visual field and the stereognostic functions for the right hand.

In contrast to the highly lateralized organization of verbal expression, the comprehension of language, both spoken and written, was found to be represented in the minor as well as in the major hemisphere. Present evidence indicates that the minor hemisphere is less proficient than the major in this respect, although the upper limits of language comprehension, ideation, and related activities in the minor hemisphere have yet to be determined. The minor, like the major hemisphere, was able to perform intermodal tasks such as the matching of tactually-perceived words and vice versa. Performances with the right hemisphere involving word and object association, sorting, retrieval and related tasks showed evidence of ideation, emotion, mental concentration and other high order mental capacities.

The observed ability to write with the left hand legible and meaningful material, though with rather poor penmanship, can be explained in terms of the bilateral motor control of both hands from the major hemisphere. Therefore it is not a contradiction of the above conclusion that writing is organized only in the major hemisphere. The bilaterality in motor control applies to a lesser degree to the control of the right hand from the minor hemisphere. This latter combination is clearly inferior to the above, in part because the dominant hemisphere tends to interfere more by imposing its own control on the right hand.

The foregoing applies also to the drawing of simple objects and geometric shapes perceived either visually or stereognostically. After presentation to the major hemisphere either hand could draw the object, but the performance was clearly superior with the right hand. Following such presentation to the minor right hemisphere, the left hand drew moderately recognizable reproductions. Drawing with the right hand, however, was highly erratic under these conditions and was commonly disrupted by interfering functions in the major hemisphere.

The general picture of the cerebral disconnexion syndrome that emerges from the present two cases would seem to stand somewhere well between the extremes arrived at by Akelaitis (1941; 1943; 1944) on the one hand and that outlined more recently by Geschwind (1962; 1965*a*, *b*). Whereas the results in our initial case conformed fairly well with the Liepmann-Geschwind interpretation, these more recent findings require a significant shift on a number of the important features of the disconnexion syndrome well over in the Akelaitis direction.

Though based on only two cases and clearly at variance with many reports in a literature filled with contradictions, there nevertheless are reasons at this time for thinking that the general picture as seen in these two individuals may represent, by and large, a common and perhaps the typical situation.

With respect to apraxia our present observations coincide rather closely with those of the Akelaitis series, and also with our own observations in subhuman primates. They favor the view that each hemisphere is able to direct the motor control of the ipsilateral, as well as the contralateral hand under normal conditions and also after pure commissural lesions. The appearance of apraxia or dyspraxia in connexion with long standing callosal lesions suggests, as concluded by Akelaitis, the presence of associated cerebral brain damage. The implication we would emphasize here, however, is not that the associated cortical damage itself is responsible, but rather that it is in most cases the combination of lesions that is critical. From recent evidence it appears that the ipsilateral control system in each cortex is delicate and easily deranged by minor damage that leaves the more robust contralateral system with little detectable impairment (Gazzaniga and Sperry, 1966).

The ipsilateral elements in the control system are not confined to the precentral region but are more diffuse. Also, good ipsilateral control is dependent on the functional integrity of the contralateral control system. And further, target references once established in an ipsilateral cortex are frequently bilateralized automatically or indirectly, thus allowing much of the final details of the motor patterning of coordination to be handled from the contralateral side (Gazzaniga, 1966). This complex of factors provides an interpretational scheme that seems to account for most of the data and conflicting observations in the experimental and clinical studies on apraxia following cortical and callosal lesions.

Our evidence that the disconnected minor hemisphere perceives and comprehends both the written and spoken word, as described earlier (Sperry, 1964; Gazzaniga, 1965; Sperry and Gazzaniga, 1965; Gazzaniga and Sperry, 1965) contrasts with previous reports of "word blindness" and "word deafness" following callosal lesions (Geschwind, 1962). Since the present two patients also appeared alexic and "word blind" in tests that involved verbal communication, one wonders if the application of appropriate non-verbal testing methods might not have demonstrated the presence of comprehension in the minor hemisphere in the earlier studies as well. Also the earlier cases of word blindness and deafness involved extensive cortical lesions in the dominant hemisphere. It becomes increasingly evident that the functional capacity of a unilateral cortical area with its contralateral counterpart intact may appear to be quite different from that seen in the presence of contralateral lesions. Allowing for considerable individual variation in the cerebral organization of language, the general picture as outlined in the present two cases could well prove to be more typical than exceptional so far as we can tell from the evidence now available.

REFERENCES

Akelaitis, A. J. (1941) *Arch. Neurol. Psychiat., Chicago*, **45,** 788.

—— (1943) *J. Neuropath. exp. Neurol.*, **2,** 226.

—— (1944) *J. Neurosurg.*, **1,** 94.

Bogen, J. E., Fisher, E. D., and Vogel, P. J. (1965) *J. Amer. med. Ass.*, **194,** 1328.

——, and Gazzaniga, M. S. (1966) *J. Neurosurg.*, **23,** 394.

——, and Vogel, P. J. (1962) *Bull. Los Angeles neurol. Soc.*, **27,** 169.

Gazzaniga, M. S. (1965) *Science*, **150,** 372.

—— (1966) *Exp. Neurol*, **16,** 289.

——, Bogen, J. E., and Sperry, R. W. (1962) *Proc. nat. Acad. Sci.*, **48,** 1765.

——, ——, —— (1963) *Neuropsychologia*, **3,** 1.

——, ——, —— (1965) *Brain*, **88,** 221.

——, and Sperry, R. W. (1965) *Fed. Proc.*, **24,** 522.

——, ——(1966) *Fed. Proc.*, **25,** 396.

Geschwind, N. (1962) *In* "Reading Disability," edited by J. Money, Baltimore.

—— (1965*a*) *Brain*, **88,** 237.

—— (1965*b*) *Brain*, **88,** 585.

——, and Kaplan, E. (1962) *Neurology, Minneap.*, **12,** 675.

Sperry, R. W. (1964) James Arthur Lecture, New York, American Museum of Natural History.

—— (1966) *In* "Brain and Conscious Experience," edited by J. C. Eccles. Heidelberg (In press).

——, and Gazzaniga, M. S. (1965) *In* "Brain Mechanisms Underlying Speech and Language," edited by F. L. Darly. Grune and Stratton (In press).

Zangwill, O. (1964) *Res. Publ. Ass. nerv. ment. Dis.*, **42,** 103.

18

Psycholinguistic Aspects of Aphasia

OTFRIED SPREEN

OTFRIED SPREEN, Ph.D., is with the department of psychology of the University of Victoria, British Columbia, Canada.

Psycholinguistics in the area of aphasia is often very loosely defined. In a sense, of course, aphasia itself is a psycholinguistic phenomenon in that it refers to language as produced by an individual. However, for this review only studies which deal with aphasic speech as a linguistic phenomenon are included. Consequently, studies with psychometric tests of performance only are omitted. For example, the review does not include tests measuring name-finding performance in general, but includes studies of naming in relation to what is being named. Studies with diagnostic applications of aphasia tests are omitted, but studies which investigate the grammatical structure of responses in such tests are included. Even with this restriction, it is impossible to cover all pertinent studies in this area.

The topic can be organized in many ways, for example, by linguistic units, by types of impairment, or by the theoretical models employed. For this review a few basic theories of language impairment seem to provide a useful guide for the organization of the material.

REGRESSION

The first such theory is the concept of regression in aphasic language, which is becoming popular again in some recent studies. This concept was very much a part of the *Zeitgeist* around 1880. It originated from Herbert Spencer's work and was first used in connection with aphasia by Kussmaul (1877). In 1879 Hughlings-Jackson referred to it as the law of evolution and dissolution of nervous system functions. It is used extensively in Ribot's book on memory disorders (1883) and applied to polyglot aphasia by Pitres in 1895. Freud, of course, has stimulated the use of the concept of regression in his interpretation of neurotic development, but he first used the concept in his monograph on aphasia (1891). Arnold Pick (1913) comments upon what he calls "Ribot's law" in his book on the psycholinguistics of agrammatism —perhaps the first truly psycholinguistic treatment of aphasia. He discussed the regression concept later when he described some apparent exceptions in 1921. He also made the specification that this principle does not apply directly to the acute symptomatology but rather to the chronic sequelae of the lesion (Pick, 1931, p. 1443).

Jakobson (1962) refers to regression in the disintegration and reacquisition of sound patterns which "mirror the child's acquisition of speech sounds," and proposes a regression towards early infantile stages on a level of larger linguistic units in his concept of "contiguity disorders."

More recent studies have presented experimental investigations of regression. Lambert and Fillenbaum (1959) tested Ribot's law in

From *Journal of Speech and Hearing Research* 11:467–480, 1968.

bilinguals and concluded that this law can be tentatively confirmed for patients with coordinate bilingualism, i.e., that languages acquired later in life tend to be more severely affected by aphasia. However, in compound bilingualism with continual and concurrent use of two languages (for example, in Montreal and certain areas of southern France) such selective loss tends to follow more strength of habit, preference, and emotional factors.

Rochford and Williams (1962, 1963) investigated the breakdown of the use of names in aphasia. They tested adult aphasics as well as children ranging in age from 2 to 12 with the task of naming three objects and four of their parts. The authors found a close parallel between degree of difficulty in naming and age of acquisition. They were able to demonstrate that the same phenomenon can be produced in normal speakers under stress, distraction, or confusion after electroconvulsive treatment (ECT); here again they found the same regression pattern when compared to word acquisition in children. A final paper by these authors showed that reacquisition of names tends to follow the same rule.

Spreen and Benton (1967) confirmed this finding. The errors made by aphasic patients in naming 40 common objects were correlated with age of acquisition in children between the ages of 2 and 13. The rank correlation coefficient was found to be 0.86 for the toal sample; after blocking across ties the correlation increased to 0.92.

The regression principle applied to phonetic patterns (phonetic disintegration), on the other hand, has not fared as well in experimental studies (Fry, 1958; Shankweiler and Harris, 1966). Attempts to demonstrate Ribot's law for difficulties of forming inflectional endings (Goodglass and Berko, 1960) have remained inconclusive. Goodglass and Berko obtained difficulty levels for various types of inflectional endings in aphasics with agrammatical disturbance. Unfortunately, their comparison group was too old to show developmental types of errors in this study. However, they demonstrated that the order of difficulty appeared to be the same for aphasics and nonaphasic brain-damaged patients even though the latter group made very few errors.

With the exception of phonetic regression it appears to be well established that aphasic patients do not show a highly peculiar pathological deficit, but that they tend to follow normal rules of acquisition and tend to make errors on those items which also prove to be the most difficult for the normal speaker.

However, the problem is more complex than this. Schuell, Jenkins, and Landis (1961) investigated the auditory comprehension of words in the Ammons Picture Vocabulary Test in aphasics and found that difficulty of comprehension of a word was inversely related to frequency of occurrence of that word in the English language (estimated on the basis of the Thorndike-Lorge word count). Newcomb, Oldfield, and Wingfield (1965) reported the same finding; these authors used latencies—the time it takes to name an object—as a measure of difficulty. Correlations between frequency and latency ranged between -0.80 and -0.87. They were also able to demonstrate the same relationship in normals and for errors in name finding itself rather than for latency (Oldfield and Wingfield, 1964).

It would seem that after both age of acquisition and frequency of usage have been found to be related to naming difficulties, acquisition age and frequency themselves should be strongly related; for example, in general, words learned earlier in life are most frequently used in the English language.

These studies and theories seem to establish some general rule of language acquisition and of the degree of difficulty in language usage which holds for both normal and aphasic speakers. Does it also alter our concept of aphasic disturbances? Wepman, Bock, Jones, and Van Pelt (1956) argued that students of aphasia tend to isolate "anomia" as a specific aphasic deficit, implying that it is the use of nouns which is most severely impaired. Examining the normal frequency of occurrence of various parts of speech, these authors observed that nouns are relatively infrequent in normal speech and that other parts of speech tend to have the highest frequencies of occurrence. If, therefore, nouns are the most difficult words for aphasics, this would merely follow general frequency rules. Words with the highest frequency (non-nouns) are retained better than low frequency words (nouns). The analysis of actual speech samples from aphasic and normal speakers tends to confirm the impression that "anomia" is not a very meaningful concept if defined as a predominant loss of nouns. Rather, all types of words are lost in aphasia, with nouns showing the most impressive loss because of their relatively low frequency of occurrence. This is confirmed by a study by Sefer and Henrikson (1966). They investigated word-association difficulties of aphasics in relation to parts-of-speech classification and found the same general pattern of variance as in normal speakers. Siegel (1959) obtained a similar finding for word classes.

MICROGENETIC REGRESSION

So far, some rules regarding what is lost in aphasia have been shown to exist. Another question in this context is the "how" of loss of speech; for example, the type of distortions, substitutions, and the possibility of relating the erroneous productions to the process of speech generation.

Many theories have been advanced in the past as to how the aphasic patient makes an error. Arnold Pick's monograph in 1913 centers around this major question. He suggested a process of speech generation which proceeds from the nonverbal content through the thought schema to a language schema. He suggested that certain determinating tendencies would be present immediately in this process; for example, a bilingual Czech-German patient would not pick a German grammatical construction or a German word if the situation and his general "set" called for speaking Czech. He would generate a grammatical sentence schema with the appropriate syntax. Pick expounded the principle of the primate of the sentence and deduced that the choice of words for making the utterance itself would be only the final step in producing language. He indicated that this was why word-finding difficulties appear to be the most frequent language difficulties found in patients as well as in normal speakers and the ones most likely to persist when the aphasic recovers. Thus the theory asserts that most patients know fairly well what they are going to say and how they are going to say it. Most errors occur at the last stage of language production. These are not likely to be random, but are rather errors which are closely related to the intended words, often caused by a lack of inhibition or a lack of resistance towards incorrect choices.

This theory of microgenesis or of language generation can be subjected to experimentation. Following Pick's suggestions and the work of Sander in 1928, Werner (1965) and Conrad (1947, 1950) developed the concept of a "pre-gestalt" arrest of language in the aphasic. According to this view, the process of generating language—whether it takes fractions of a second or minutes—is interrupted, arrested, or left incomplete for other reasons before it reaches the final gestalt. In his early experiments Werner presented single words and two- and three-word combinations tachistoscopically at 1/50 sec and after each exposure had normal subjects report what the words were. He reported that many subjects experienced "spheres of meaning," a global "microgenetically early" impression of the words, which frequently was very close to the actual meaning itself. Werner (p. 351) quotes many examples which seem to indicate that aphasic patients may produce "atmospheric" impressions—in terms of formal stylistic properties of a sentence—which "precede the specific, correct articulation of the text." Thus if a patient sees the word *green* and says, "red, no, blue, no, yellow, no, green," he indicates that he already has grasped the concept of color; that is, he has a very definite general idea of the content of the word without being able to reach the final gestalt. Conrad quotes similar errors. For example, a patient is asked to read the word "earth" and says "something (makes a circular movement with his hands) like a ball." Another patient may make statements like, "He was to sail by train to the south," or, "He spoke the violin." (Weisenburg and McBride, 1935.)

Schuell and Jenkins (1961) asked aphasic patients to choose the response to a test word from four multiple-choice pictures, one of which was the object referred to, one an object with a rhyming name, one an object closely associated, and one an unrelated object. For example, *chair* matched with *stair* (rhyme), *table* (association), and *apple* (unrelated). Their findings indicated that the types or errors made by aphasics were highly similar whether the word was heard, named, read, or written. The errors appeared to be predominantly associative. Errors of the rhyming type were much less frequent and unrelated errors were extremely rare. The study seems to confirm that errors made by aphasic patients are not made at random. Most errors appear to be substitutions of closely associated words for the word intended by the patient.

Even in jargon speech, although it is regressed more deeply and possibly constitutes a language deficit which is complicated by other deficits, sentence melody, rhythm, intonation, and sometimes even grammatical structure are preserved (Weinstein et al., 1966). Such evidence seems to support Pick's view of a disturbance predominantly at the final stage of language generation, not at microgenetically earlier levels. Weinstein et al. follow Alajouanine's (1956) interpretation of jargon in a similar fashion. An additional feature of jargon may be the phenomenon of disinhibition referred to later on.

ABSTRACTNESS AND OTHER WORD PARAMETERS

The microgenetic regression hypothesis predicts that words with high associative meaning tend to be more easily substituted than others. Another approach to this question goes back to Kurt Goldstein (1948), who advanced the hypothesis of an impairment in abstract behavior in the brain-damaged person. He extended this to aphasia, indicating that the use of abstract words tends to be more impaired than the use of concrete ones. This principle survived in spite of many futile attempts at empirical research and, until recently, has not been tested experimentally in its application to aphasic speech. Howes (1964) refers to it in his paper on frequency distributions and offers an ingeniously simple explanation. He points out that even in the normal speaker abstract usages are less frequent than concrete ones. This assumption can easily be sustained by a look at the frequencies of abstract and concrete words in the Thorndike-Lorge count. Considering the finding that aphasics use rare words less frequently and familiar words more frequently, abstract words should be more affected than concrete words since they are found in different positions on the frequency distribution curve.

In some studies by Spreen and his associates, a new approach to this question was used with a technique borrowed from verbal learning research. In order to vary abstractness independently from frequency of usage, words with the same frequency level were used. Spreen and Schulz (1966) selected all A-frequency nouns from the Thorndike-Lorge list for this purpose and scaled them for abstractness in a rating experiment. Since even within the A-frequency word category the actual frequencies vary from 50 to 100 per 100,000 words, the abstraction ratings were correlated with the actual numerical frequency. The correlation between frequency and abstractness rating was 0.001.

This material was used in studies of perception and immediate memory (Borkowski, Spreen, and Stutz, 1965; Spreen, Borkowski, and Benton, 1967; Spreen, Borkowski, and Gordon, 1966). If abstractness is strictly a function of frequency, then the ratings obtained would have to be considered an artifact of the forced ratings, and consistencies of perceptual behavior in relation to abstractness should not be observable. In these studies, however, words rated as concrete were perceived and reported or recalled significantly better than words rated as abstract. This held consistently in six different experimental groups with three different word lists presented under superimposed noise and also in the dichotic listening situation.

The tentative conclusion is that the abstract-concrete dimension overlaps heavily with frequency, but if frequency is eliminated as a variable, abstractness shows an effect all its own.

The foregoing findings were made with normal subjects. Two experiments with mental retardates (Jones and Spreen, 1967a, b) showed a somewhat stronger correlation between recognition of words and abstractness although significance for this difference between normals and retardates was not demonstrated. It seems possible that pathological groups would follow the trend predicted by Goldstein's theory, i.e., that abstract words are more difficult for the retardate than for the normal person. Unfortunately, results with aphasics are not available as yet. Previous studies with aphasics by Siegel (1959) and Greenberg (1963) remained inconclusive since word frequency was not adequately controlled in these studies.

Abstractness is not a very clearly defined concept. Roger Brown (1958) uses the term strictly as superordinate-subordinate, for example, *dime* vs. *money*. Another possible definition is the lack of sense experience with the item designated by the word, e.g., *faith* as abstract, *goat* as concrete. In the study cited above (Spreen and Schulz, 1966), ratings were made separately for each of these two definitions. They overlapped significantly so that in subsequent experiments the sum of both ratings was used.

Abstractness is not the only important variable which should be considered in the search for characteristics of words which make them difficult for the aphasic, A recent review of the area of stuttering by I. K. Taylor (1966a, b) shows how much more work can be done in aphasia. Taylor reviews the many studies investigating articulatory complexity, difficulty of initial phoneme, position of word in the sentence, grammatical function of the stuttered word, etc. An experimental approach would also allow a check into such parameters as pronunciability as a measure of articulatory difficulty; difficulty of initial, medial, or final phonemes; and associative strength in terms of Noble's *m*. The words in the Spreen and Schulz list have been scaled for *m* and PR, but so far no studies with these parameters have been done in aphasics. One would predict that in the normal speaker most of these variables would have an effect similar to abstractness and that all of these effects would likely be more severe in the aphasic.

MATHEMATICAL LINGUISTICS

The preceding studies show that words with low association strength, low frequency of occurrence, and late acquisition in life tend to be the words most easily impaired in aphasia. From this finding it is only a small step to more comprehensive investigations of the relationship between frequency of occurrence of a word in the English language—or, for that matter, in any language—in relation to the impairment of its use by the aphasic. The basic inventory of the English language for this type of study still remains the word count of Thorndike and Lorge (1944). It is based on written English in books and magazines 40 and more years old and is therefore not the ideal material, but so far the only one available in such comprehensiveness.[1] The frequency (*f*) of occurrence of any given word in such a sample can be plotted against the cumulative proportion of the total sample (omega) or its rank on a logarithmic scale. Thus in a sample of 5000 words, the word occurring most frequently is assigned to omega 1 and the word with the lowest frequency has the omega value of 5000. It has been shown, first by Zipf (1935) and in more appropriate terms by Howes (1964), that the Thorndike-Lorge count plotted in this fashion follows a well-known normal function ($\text{rank} \times \text{frequency} = c$): it cuts more or less diagonally across a diagram of this sort as a straight-line function (lognormal function). The same function has been shown to exist for word counts in other languages, such as

[1] A word count in normal speakers published recently by Howes (1967) now provides the material for studies of oral frequencies although it is based on a sample which is smaller than the Thorndike-Lorge count and, perhaps, still biased by regional and situational word preferences.

German. Other statistical models developed by Mandelbrot (1961) ("Canonical Law" $Pr=P(r+s)^{-B}$),[2] Simon, and others have been used to obtain an approximation of the lognormal distribution. It may suffice here to say that this lognormal distribution holds for most long texts whether derived from written material, formal speeches, or interview transcripts.

Some valid criticism has been made of the meaningfulness of such investigations (Plath, 1961; Simon, 1955; Herdan, 1960, 1966). As both Plath and Herdan point out, the more meaningful question is whether a particular individual or group of individuals (for example, aphasics) follow the same rules or not; that is, whether this model may be used as a basis for the measurement of significant deviations in linguistic behavior. Howes and Geschwind (1964) have shown that individual normal speakers producing 5000 words do follow the same lognormal distribution in their word usage. Howes (1964) investigated the question whether aphasic speech samples show significant deviations from the lognormal function. At first glance, his data on 60 patients apparently follow exactly the same curve as described for normal speakers, that is, a straight line gradient. Looking at specific parameters of these samples, however, Howes noted that the mean log frequency and/or the standard deviation of log frequency show a definite shift in most aphasic patients. A shift of the first of these parameters indicates that the word-frequency distribution is shifted towards the right side at the median of the sample; that is, the words at any rank tend to occur less frequently than in normal speech. The second parameter indicates a counterclockwise rotation of the curve within the graph, indicating that rare words are even more rarely used by aphasics.

For our understanding of the aphasic patient, the shift in the two parameters would indicate that the least frequent words are the ones most easily lost, illustrating a regression in vocabulary as discussed in the first section of this paper. A similar regression has also been demonstrated on a much smaller scale for spelling difficulties in aphasics (Thurston, 1954). However, Howes calls attention to the fact that the lognormal shape of the distribution is preserved in aphasics. This is an important qualification of the regression hypothesis. It would mean that although rare words are used less frequently, they are not completely absent in aphasic speech. As Howes points out, there is no true loss of vocabulary in the aphasic patient, but rather a reduction in the use of low-frequency words. Failure to examine for a complex relationship between frequency and discrimination difficulties probably accounts for the non-significant results obtained by Filby, Edwards, and Seacat (1963).

TYPES OF APHASIA BASED ON LINGUISTIC EVIDENCE

One further step in the free-speech analysis of Howes and Geschwind is the attempt to isolate types of aphasics. They do this partly on the basis of the mathematical formulas derived from their speech samples. As an additional measure, Howes used rate of speech, that is, number of words per minute. He found a large variation on this measure, and concluded that rate of speech neatly reflects the severity of the aphasia as rated by the clinical examiner. However, the distribution was bipolar, with the normal rate of speech as a reference point. That is, with increasing severity some aphasics produced fewer words per minute, but another part of the aphasic group tended to produce more words per minute as severity increased, moving towards the opposite end of the scale. Patients with lowered rates of speech also tended to have more immediate repetitions of words. This was rare in patients with increased rates of speech. Patients with lowered rates of speech also tended to show less shift in the previously described parameter; they used more rare words, whereas the rapid talker tended to have fewer rare words in his sample. Thus Type A, with decreased rate of speech, more repetitions, and more rare words, can be distinguished from Type B, with increased rate

[2] Pr = frequency, P, s, B = constants, r = rank.

of speech, more frequent words, and a normal number of repetitions. Howes also found that perceptual thresholds for words presented under superimposed noise conditions show more variability in Type B and that controlled association experiments with this type are almost impossible, or bizarre in their results. Type A, on the other hand, shows long latencies on word association, but normal types of associations and little increase in perceptual threshold. In conventional terms, Howes appears to be describing an expressive-amnestic type of aphasia and a second type which is less consistent, characterized by jargon and paraphasias. Evidence from the neurological examinations suggested also that Type A shows more deficit in the anterior cortical areas, whereas lesions for Type B tended to be found predominantly in the posterior region. The increased rate of speech in Type B, incidentally, fits in with Pick's (1931) explanation of paraphasia, jargon, and logorrhea on the basis of a "disinhibition principle" (in contrast to Wernicke's interpretation of it as a pure T_1 area phenomenon). The patient lacks the normal inhibition in his choice of words or parts of words from the many incorrect ones, and ends up with a paraphasic jargon response. Pick draws the parallel with normal states of disinhibition caused by exhaustion and stress, which tend to produce similar lapses of speech. Related to this evidence is Weinstein's observation of associated tendencies towards euphemisms, malapropisms, jokes, etc. in the "jargon aphasic" (Weinstein et al., 1966). In a grand design for a principle of disinhibition, Pick (1931) hypothesized a hierarchy of disturbances beginning with the literal paraphasic, continuing through verbal paraphasia and logorrhea to the most severe form of echolalia. This hierarchy is viewed as a progressive disinhibition at different levels of speech generation. The most severe disturbance occurs with disinhibition at the thinking level, a different level of disinhibition produces deficits of grammatical structure, but disinhibition can also occur at the level of word choice. Even if the word is found, the completion of the word may be defective since the speaker lacks the inhibition to reject defective forms.

Research of the mathematical linguistic type so far has shown that some of the salient features of well known clinical types can be demonstrated with this technique and described in more efficient terms. Some of the evidence seems to modify our concept of Wernicke's aphasia in that it stresses the factor of disinhibition in combination with an explanation in terms of a pure receptive defect.

Several linguistic studies attempting to differentiate types of aphasia have been published by Jones, Wepman, and associates. In this context their classifications based on testing of speech functions, and the contrasting results obtained by Schuell and her collaborators, are not reviewed here. However, their findings based on free speech samples are pertinent. Fillenbaum, Jones, and Wepman (1961) used a sample of 12 aphasic and 12 matched control subjects and obtained a free speech sample based on the patients' stories in response to the Thematic Apperception Test cards (TAT). This type of material, used throughout the studies of these authors, tends to limit generalizations of a linguistic nature since the frequency of many of the words used in TAT stories is dependent on the stimulus cards. It also presents some difficulties of analysis because of the sharply varying length of individual responses. In the earlier study (1961), the authors used a dictionary type of classification of parts of speech which was later replaced by a more logical one (Jones, Goodman, and Wepman, 1963). They found that aphasic speech differed from normal speech in 9 out of 12 cases. It is somewhat difficult to assess from the report what actual differences were found since there was great variability from one subject to another. Basically, differences were in the use of grammatical form classes, sequential dependencies in form-class usage, and in stereotypy of vocabulary. However, the investigators felt that there were some consistencies within subgroups of aphasics which suggested that they could be subdivided into three groups—semantic, syntactic, and pragmatic aphasics—as well as admixtures of these three. This was based on a linguist's classification of the speech samples into three types without reference to the calculated variables. The semantic type was mainly characterized by word-finding difficulties, the syntactic type by grammatical errors, whereas the third type, the pragmatic type, was characterized by lack of meaningful speech. In Jakobson's terms the first two types correspond roughly to his similarity disorder (i.e., loss of ability to nominate symbols) and to his contiguity or arrangement disorder. In general clinical terms, the three types converge with the amnestic, expressive-agrammatical and what Alajouanine and Lhermitte (1964) call the semantic jargon type of aphasia.

TAT productions of 50 aphasic speakers were empirically classified into six categories in a study by Siegel, Jones, and Wepman (1965). The six categories were based on a classification into distinct subgroups by linguists without further instruction. The authors showed that by two discriminant functions performed on the Language Modalities Test for these groups a discrimination on a dimension of "intelligibility" and a second one on a dimension of "grammatical correctness" could be established. Thus again we find the types of "jargon" and of "agrammatical-expressive" aphasia emerging from linguistic analysis.

Wepman and Jones (1964) have expounded their three-type classification of syntactic, semantic, and pragmatic aphasia in further detail but without further linguistic data. In their 1964 paper and in other contexts they have added two further types, the phonetic jargon and the global aphasic. In a theoretical outline they draw a parallel between the five types of aphasia and five stages of language development in children. Thus we find, once again, the regression concept invoked in a somewhat different context, the classification of aphasia. Since the regression hypothesis of this type implies a gradual continuity between successive types, Wepman and Jones conclude that recovery from aphasia should follow these stages too. This exciting hypothesis is illustrated by individual cases, but so far remains without substantiating evidence. It will not be hard to investigate this hypothesis in longitudinal studies, since, if it is true, recovery should never jump from type 1 to 4 or reverse from 3 to 2, but follow a predictable course. It also implies interesting modifications in our thinking about aphasia as a multidimensional or unidimensional phenomenon.

Goodglass, Klein, Carey, and Jones (1966) examined the expressive and receptive difficulties aphasic patients had with semantically different kinds of words. They found that name finding for objects was hardest, followed by numbers, colors, actions, and letter names, in that order. They found a different order of difficulty among these categories for the understanding of words. Since frequency of usage was not taken into account, these overall results are somewhat difficult to interpret. The authors proceeded with a discriminant function analysis with patient groups defined clinically as Broca, Wernicke, and amnestic aphasia. Differences in naming and understanding of the different categories of words utilized in two separate discriminant function analyses allowed a 75% prediction rate of group membership on the basis of these parameters.

RESUME AND OUTLOOK

As this survey of psycholinguistic studies of aphasia shows, the approach has considerable promise. It tries to capture the elusive features of "speaking style" and express them in terms which can be subjected to statistical treatment, as any other research data. The clinician observing an aphasic patient often regrets that traditional testing methods limit his approach to the statement of loss and an expression of "how much." He senses that the patient's speech is "impoverished," simplified, or distorted in its grammar, or deviant in the choice of words, but these characteristics cannot be readily expressed and compared in the clinical examination. The psycholinguistic study provides the opportunity to analyze these features and to supply new evidence for research in aphasia.

The surveyed studies have added new

information about the regression concept, both on an ontogenetic and a microgenetic level. The basic studies preliminary to an investigation of "abstract" vs. "concrete" use of language have been completed. Mathematical linguistics has attacked the possibility of shift in the frequency of word usage. The question of types of aphasia—of prime importance to the clinically oriented researcher—has been approached with linguistic data.

One disappointing aspect of these studies is that none of them so far has used an extensive, strictly linguistic type of approach to defining aphasia. Most authors use a loose classification into types by "a linguist" either with or without the use of a preselected classification schema, and then hasten to relate these types to test data, traditional clinical types, or theoretical types proposed by linguists like Jakobson. A discriminant function analysis of linguistic data between traditionally defined clinical groups is not likely to come up with new ideas for the classification of aphasia nor is it likely to supply independent evidence for the validity of the old ones.

One would wish to see a complete departure from older concepts and a fresh look at the patients and aphasia on the basis of purely empirical linguistic data. The main reason this has not been done seems to lie in the limited scope of the linguistic measures used in most studies and their inherent difficulties. Jones' and Wepman's list of measures is the most comprehensive so far.

A look at the statistical analysis of literature samples shows how much more can be done (Leed, 1966; Seboek and Zeps, 1960; Wachal, 1966). These studies often deal with authorship problems and employ no fewer than 20 and as many as 600 different parameters in the definition of the writing "style" of an author. These measures include frequency counts (of the number of words of a particular grammatical class, of word and phrase length, etc.) as well as complex measures of ratios (such as adjective-verb ratio, type-token ratio, derivational suffixes per word). We might borrow a useful new approach from this neighbor discipline.

In addition to these descriptive linguistic measures, the advance of transformational linguistics offers new approaches to the study of aphasia. Studies of the particular difficulties of aphasics in the generation and understanding of transforms, as suggested by Goodglass and Hunt (1958), may be of great promise. So far, no studies of this type are available. The main obstacles to research of this kind lie in the problem of obtaining truly "free" speech samples and in transcription, but they are not insurmountable. Another problem is the phonetic distortions and confusions made by the speaker. These defects are of interest by themselves, but tend to confound the problem of analyzing the structure of speech. Again, little has been done to tackle this problem.

It would seem that we are just at the beginning of psycholinguistic research in aphasia.

REFERENCES

Alajouanine, T., Verbal realization in aphasia. *Brain*, **79,** 1-28 (1956).

——, and Lhermitte, F., Aphasia and physiology of speech. In D. M. Rioch and E. A. Weinstein (Eds.), *Disorders of Communication.* Baltimore: Williams and Wilkins, 204-219 (1964).

Borkowski, J. G., Spreen, O., and Stutz, J. Z., Ear preference and abstractness in dichotic listening. *Psychon. Sci.*, **3,** 547-548 (1965).

Brown, R. W., How shall a thing be called? *Psychol. Rev.* **65,** 14-21 (1958).

Conrad, C., Ueber den Begriff der Vorgestalt. *Nervenarzt*, **21,** 58-63 (1950).

——, Ueber den Begriff der Vorgestalt und seine Bedeutung fuer die Hirnpathologie. *Nervenarzt*, **18,** 289-298 (1947).

Filby, Y., Edwards, A., and Seacat, G., Word length frequency and similarity in the discrimination behavior of aphasics. *J. Speech Hearing Res.*, **6,** 255–261 (1963).

Fillenbaum, S., Jones, L. V., and Wepman, J. M., Some linguistic features of speech from aphasic patients. *Lang. Speech,* **4,** 91–108 (1961).

Freud, S., *On Aphasia, a Critical Study* (1891). New York: Intern. Univ. Press (1953).

Fry, D. B., Phonemic substitutions in an aphasic patient. *Lang. Speech,* **1,** 52–61 (1958).

Goldstein, K., *Language and Language Disturbance.* New York: Grune and Stratton (1948).

Goodglass, H., and Berko, J., Agrammatism and English inflection. *J. Speech Hearing Res.* **3,** 257–267 (1960).

——, and Hunt, J., Grammatical complexity and aphasic speech. *Word,* **14,** 197–207 (1958).

——, Klein, B., Carey, P., and Jones, K., Specific semantic word categories in aphasia. *Cortex,* **2,** 74–89 (1966).

Greenberg, F. R., An investigation of paired associate learning in adult dysphasic subjects. Doctoral dissertation, Univ. of Iowa (1963).

Herdan, G., *The Advanced Theory of Language as Choice and Chance.* New York: Springer (1966).

——, *Type-token Mathematics: A Textbook of Mathematical Linguistics.* The Hague: Mouton (1960).

Howes, D., Application of the word-frequency concept to aphasia. In A. V. S. de Reuck and M. O'Connor (Eds.), *Disorders of Language.* Boston: Little, Brown, 47–78 (1964).

——, A word count of spoken English. *J. verb. Learn. verb. Behav.,* **5,** 572–606 (1966).

——, and Geschwind, N., Quantitative studies of aphasic language. In D. M. Rioch and E. A. Weinstein (Eds.), *Disorders of Communication.* Baltimore: Williams and Wilkins (1964), pp. 229–244.

Jackson, H., On affection of speech from disease of the brain. *Brain.* (1879). Reprinted *Brain,* **38,** 107–174 (1915).

Jakobson, R., Kindersprache, Aphasie und allgemeine Lautgesetze. In *Selected Writings,* Vol. I. S'Gravenhage: Mouton (1962).

Jones, D., and Spreen, O., Dichotic listening by retarded children. The effects of ear order and abstractness. *Child Developm.,* **38,** 101–105 (1967a).

Jones, E., and Spreen, O., The effects of meaningfulness and abstractness on word recognition in educable retarded children. *Amer. J. ment. Defic.,* **71,** 987–989 (1967b).

Jones, L. V., Goodman, M. F., and Wepman, J. M., The classification of parts of speech for the characterization of aphasia. *Lang. Speech,* **6,** 94–107 (1963).

——, and Wepman, J. M., Grammatical indicants of speaking style in normal and aphasic speakers. In K. Salzinger and S. Salzinger (Eds.), *Research in Verbal Behaviour and Some Neuro-Psychological Implications.* New York: Academic Press (1967) pp. 169–180.

Kussmaul, A., Die Stoerungen der Sprache. Versuch einer Pathologie der Sprache. In H. von Ziemssen (Ed.), *Handbuch der speziellen Pathologie und Therapie,* Vol. 12. Leipzig: F. C. W. Vogel (1877).

Lambert, W. E., and Fillenbaum, S., A pilot study of aphasia among bilinguals. *Can. J. Psychol.,* **13,** 28–34 (1959).

Leed, J., *The Computer and Literary Style.* Kent, Ohio: Kent State Univ. Press (1966).

Mandelbrot, B., On the theory of word frequencies and on related Markovian models of discourse. *Proc. Sympos. Appl. Math.,* **12,** 190–219 (1961).

Newcomb, F. B., Oldfield, R. C., and Wingfield, A., Object-naming by dysphasic patients. *Nature,* **207,** 1217–1218 (1965).

Oldfield, R. C., and Wingfield, A., The time it takes to name an object. *Nature,* **202,** 1031 (1964).

Pick, A., Aphasie. In A. Bethe et al. (Eds.), *Handbuch der normalen and pathologischen Physiologie,* **15,** Part 2, Berlin: Springer (1931), pp. 1416–1524.

——, Die agrammatischen Sprachstoerungen. Studien zur psychologischen Grundlegung der Aphasielehre.I.Teil. *Monogr. a. d. Gesamtgeb. d. Neurol. u. Psychiat.,* Heft 7, Berlin: Springer (1913).

——, Die neurologische Forschungsrichtung in der Psychopathologie und andere Aufsaetze V. Zur Erklaerung gewisser Ausnahmen von der sogenannten Ribotschen Regel. *Monatsschr. Psychiat. Neurol.,* Beiheft **13,** 1–247 (1921).

Pitres, A., Etude sur l'aphasie chez les polyglottes. *Rev. Medic.,* **15,** 873–899 (1895).

Plath, W., Mathematical linguistics. In C. Mohrmann, A. Sommerfelt, and J. Whatmoughs (Eds.), *Trends in European and American Linguistics, 1930–1960.* Utrecht: Spectrum (1961).

Ribot, T. A., *Les maladies de la memoire,* 2nd ed. Paris: Libraire Germer Bailliere (1883).

Rochford, G., and Williams, M., Studies in the development and breakdown of the use of names. I. The relationship between nominal dysphasia and the acquisition of vocabulary in childhood. *J. Neurol. Neurosurg. Psychiat.,* **25,** 222–233 (1962).

——, ——, Studies in the development and breakdown of the use of names. III. Recovery from nominal dysphasia. *J. Neurol. Neurosurg. Psychiat.,* **26,** 377–381 (1963).

Sander, F., Experimentelle Ergebnisse der Gestalt-psychologie. In *Bericht ueber den X.Kongress fuer experimentelle Psychologie*. Berlin: Springer (1928).

Schuell, H., and Jenkins, J. J., Reduction of vocabulary in aphasia. *Brain*, **84,** 243–261 (1961).

——, ——, and Landis, L., Relationship between auditory comprehension and word frequency in aphasia. *J. Speech Hearing Res.*, **4,** 30–36 (1961).

Seboek, T. A. and Zeps, V. J., Computer research in psycholinguistics: towards an analysis of poetic language. *Behav. Sci.*, **6,** 365–368 (1960).

Sefer, J. W. and Henrikson, E. H., The relationship between word association and grammatical classes in aphasia. *J. Speech Hearing Res.*, **9,** 529–541 (1966).

Shankweiler, D., and Harris, K. S., An experimental approach to the problem of articulation in aphasia. *Cortex*, **2,** 277–292 (1966).

Siegel, D. K. Jones, L. V., and Wepman, J. M., Test responses as predictors of free-speech characteristics in aphasic patients. *J. Speech Hearing Res.*, **8,** 349–362 (1965).

Siegel, G. M., Dysphasic speech responses to visual word stimuli. *J. Speech Hearing Res.*, **2,** 152–167 (1959).

Simon, H. A., On a class of skew distribution functions. *Biometrica*, **42,** 425–40 (1955).

Spreen, O., and Benton, A. L., Age of acquisition for names and selective loss of names in aphasia. Unpublished manuscript (1967).

——, Borkowski, J. G., and Benton, A. L., Auditory word recognition as a function of meaningfulness, abstractness and phonetic structure. *J. verb. Learn. verb. Behav.*, **6,** 101–104 (1967).

——, ——, and Gordon, A. M., Effects of abstractness, meaningfulness and phonetic structure on auditory recognition of nouns. *J. Speech Hearing Res.*, **9,** 619–625 (1966).

——, and Schulz, R. W., Parameters of abstraction, meaningfulness, and pronunciability for 329 nouns. *J. verb. Learn. verb. Behav.*, **5,** 459–468 (1966).

Taylor, I. K., The properties of stuttered words. *J. verb. Learn. verb. Behav.*, **5,** 112–118 (1966).

——, What words are stuttered? *Psychiat. Bulletin*, **65,** 233–242 (1966).

Thorndike, E. L., and Lorge, T., *The Teacher's Book of 30,000 Words*. New York: Columbia Univ. (1944).

Thurston, J. R., An empirical investigation of the loss of spelling ability in dysphasics. *J. Speech Hearing Res.*, **19,** 344–349 (1954).

Wachal, R. S., Linguistic evidence, statistical inference and disputed authorship, Doctoral dissertation, Univ. of Wisconsin (1966).

Weinstein, E. A., Lyerly, O. G., Cole, M., and Ozer, M. N., Meaning in jargon aphasia. *Cortex*, **2,** 165–187 (1966).

Weisenburg, T., and McBride, K. E., *Aphasia, a Clinical and Psychological Study*. New York: Commonwealth (1935).

Wepman, J. M., Bock, R. D., Jones, L. V., and Van Pelt, D., Psycholinguistic study of aphasia: a revision of the concept of anomia. *J. Speech Hearing Dis.*, **21,** 468–477 (1956).

——, and Jones, L. V., Five aphasias: A commentary on aphasia as a regressive linguistic phenomenon. In D. M. Rioch and E. A. Weinstein, (Eds.), *Disorders of Communication*. Baltimore: Williams and Wilkins, 190–203 (1964).

Werner, H., Microgenesis and aphasia. *J. abn. soc. Psychol.*, **52,** 347–353 (1965).

Zipf, G. K., *The Psycho-Biology of Language*. Boston: Houghton-Mifflin (1935).

19

Temporal Perception, Aphasia and Déjà Vu

ROBERT EFRON

ROBERT EFRON, M.D., is chief of the Neurophysiology-Biophysics Research Laboratories of the Martinez, California, Veterans Administration Hospital.

Moreover, something is or seems
That touches me with mystic gleams
Like glimpses of forgotten dreams—
Of something felt, like something here;
Of something done, I know not where;
Such as no language may declare.
(*Tennyson*)

"Yossarian shook his head and explained that déjà vu was just a momentary infinitesimal lag in the operation of two coactive sensory nerve centers that commonly functioned simultaneously."
—*Heller* (1961)

In order to deal appropriately with the events in its environment, an animal must perform at least two essential actions. It must be able to identify or characterize an event, and it must also be able to determine when the particular event occurred in relation to other events. Without the capacity to accurately identify both the nature as well as the time of occurrence of an event, effective action would be impossible.

The capacity to perform these functions is necessary to all information-processing systems whether they are conscious or not. The necessity for the identification of the event itself is obvious. An illustration of the need to identify the time of occurrence is, perhaps, most familiarly illustrated in a ship's log. This is a *bound* book in which is kept a chronological account of the events which have occurred. Each event carries with it a "time-label." From such a log it is possible to reconstruct the complete history of the ship. If the record had been kept on loose sheets of paper which were not filed in order, it would be more difficult to reconstruct the history. If the loose record had no time or date "labels," it would be virtually impossible to reconstruct more than fragmentary parts of the history, and finally, if each word were on a separate card and they had been randomly mixed, reconstruction would be theoretically impossible. "Meaning" requires that the unitary bits of information be kept in a proper sequence.

A word is a sequence of auditory events (phonemes). Each word of a language is a unique sequence (except for rare homonyms such as "here"—"hear") of the small number of phonemes which serve as the base of a particular language. Let us suppose that an individual loses the capacity for identifying the

From *Brain* 86:403–424, 1963. Reprinted by permission of the Editor of *Brain*.

correct order of phonemes. The word "electrician" "i lek′ tris′ an" might as easily be interpreted as "tris′ lek′ an i" or as "an i tris′ lek." The unique coding having been lost, words will be either meaningless or incorrect (such as, "stop"—"pots" which happen to have the same phonemes). An occasional word might be correctly identified by chance, but the vast majority would be erroneously identified.

As languages are highly redundant, and as certain phoneme-sequences do not occur in particular languages, the jumbled phonemes might on occasion be sorted out by applying the rules of the language deductively. This would be a slow process analogous to cryptogram solving and would almost certainly be insufficient to understand normal English speech which contains 120–150 words per minute and an average of 5 phonemes per word. This is a rate of roughly 80 milliseconds per phoneme. Any reduction in the capacity to "time-label" or "sequence" phonemes from 80 milliseconds to 100 or 200 milliseconds should, by our reasoning, have some effect upon comprehension of speech. What is the importance of this function in aphasic disorders? A similar defect in the efficiency of producing a proper phoneme or word sequence might result in jargon, neologisms and "word-salad"—more symptoms of aphasia. Lashley (1951) has discussed the logical necessity of proper sequence in verbal output but did not analyze the similar necessity of input sequence discrimination. Brain (1950) has discussed the necessity for input sequence analysis.

Previous studies (Efron, 1963*a*, *b*, *c*) have been concerned with the physiological basis for the judgments of simultaneity and of sequence of two sensory events. The data of these experiments lent considerable support to the hypothesis that certain information (relative to the time of occurrence) is transferred from nondominant to dominant hemisphere before temporal discrimination of simultaneity and order can be performed. It is in this sense only that we may say that the function of temporal perception of sequence is "located in" or "performed by" the hemisphere which is dominant for speech. This hypothesis was tested quantitatively in several experiments and was found to be consistent with the results.

The hypothesis did not specify which part(s) of the dominant hemisphere was concerned with this function. However, if the hypothesis is correct, it should be possible to detect a defect in sequencing activities in patients with lesions in the "dominant" hemisphere, and by analysis of the results, it may be further possible to localize the region performing this activity even more precisely. Thus, the detection of any sequencing defect in dominant hemisphere lesions (as contrasted with nondominant hemisphere lesions) will strongly support the hypothesis previously formulated.

It is the purpose of this paper to present the evidence which suggests that the regions in the left hemisphere concerned with temporal discrimination lie in the temporal lobe and extend posteriorly at least as far as Wernicke's area and the angular gyrus. In addition, evidence will be presented which indicates that some differentiation of various functions of temporal analysis can be detected within this region.

The implications of these findings as they may apply to a general theory of hemisphere dominance and to some of the specific symptoms of aphasia, and déjà vu will be discussed.

METHODS

Visual stimuli consisted of 5 millisecond "square" pulses of light. The characteristics of the light source and the means of controlling its duration were described previously (Efron, 1963*a*). Two independent light sources were projected (by means of a half-silvered mirror) upon a Ramsden eye piece. A red filter was placed before one light and a green filter was placed before the other light. The subject, looking into the eyepiece monocularly, perceived a round homogenous flash of light subtending approximately 30 degrees. The subject was allowed to use either eye. No attempt was made to correct for the difference of intensity of the two flashes of different color. The two colored flashes were separated by various intervals of time from 0 to

600 milliseconds, and the pair of flashes was repeated every four seconds. The subject was required to indicate whether the red or green light appeared first.

Auditory stimuli consisted of tones of 10 milliseconds' duration. The tones were produced by feeding a small earphone with a train of pulses from a gated Tektronix wave form generator, Type 162. Two pulse frequencies were used—2500pps and 250pps—thus giving rise to a high-pitched "bleep" and to a low-pitched, somewhat rasping "bop." There was no attempt to make these sounds of equal energy, or of equal apparent loudness. They were both suprathreshold. Again, the subject merely had to report which sound was first when the pair of sounds was repeated every four seconds.

Subjects were selected from the in-patients on the neurology wards. Twelve subjects were obtained with unequivocal lesions of the left hemisphere of whom 11 had some degree of aphasia. Four subjects were obtained who had unequivocal lesions of the right hemisphere in the same general areas. The 5 subjects without aphasia constituted the control group and were matched as closely as possible for age and general alertness. Patients with diffuse cerebral disease were excluded, as well as those with clinically obvious dementia. Patients with such a profound aphasia that they could not be instructed in the task were regretfully excluded. Some of the aphasic patients gave their responses by hand signals. They were instructed to point upward for high-pitched sound first, downward for low-pitched sound first, and to slap their thighs when the stimuli were considered "together" or "simultaneous" or "don't know." Similarly, they pointed to a red or green piece of filter to indicate which light flashed first. Considerable patience was necessary, and in a few subjects a large number of practice trials, before they understood the instructions.

EXPERIMENTAL PROTOCOL

The subjects were first introduced to one stimulus—the high tone, for example, and this was identified and the appropriate expression evolved. Then the low tone was introduced alone and identified. Finally, the two signals were introduced with a one-second interval between them, and they were instructed to indicate by pointing (or by speech if this was possible) which tone or colored light appeared first. A three-choice answer was permitted—the third choice being "don't know" or "together."

The experiment consisted of 130 determinations of which 10 were made when the stimuli were simultaneous, 60 in which the high tone or red light was first and 60 in which the low tone or green light was earliest. Thirteen selected intervals (no interval counting as one) were given randomly but ensuring that 10 determinations were made at each of the thirteen intervals. The subject was permitted to observe as many pairs of flashes as he wished before he gave his reply. It was possible, during the instruction period to determine the overall range which would be covered and select the thirteen intervals so that a 100 percent correct response would be given on the first and thirteenth intervals. Occasional errors were made in this selection so that some subjects did not quite get a perfect score on the first and thirteenth intervals and others had perfect scores for the first and last two or three interval periods. It will be seen that these methodological errors do not lead to any confusion or to significant statistical problems. They occurred only because of the necessity to keep the number of determinations to a small number to prevent fatigue.

Half the subjects were first instructed and tested with visual stimuli, the other half were first tested with auditory stimuli. Every subject was tested for both visual as well as auditory tasks. Only one subject (SU) failed to recognize that the two tests were essentially similar and he therefore required equally detailed instructions for the second test. The others immediately recognized the similarity of the instructions as to signalling their answer. There were obviously no such problems for the control subjects whose speech was normal.

RESULTS

The two most striking facts which emerge from the results are (1) that the lesions which produce disturbances in the discrimination of temporal sequence are all in the hemisphere which is dominant for speech functions and (2) that every subject with a dominant hemisphere lesion who had difficulty with temporal analysis also had some degree of aphasia.

The experimental subjects were divided into two major groups—those with or without aphasia. Table 19-1 lists the results of the performance in all sixteen subjects for both auditory and visual tests. In this table, the numerical value used is the interval (expressed in msec.) at which the subject correctly identified the sequence in each of ten trials (100 percent correct). As some difference frequently occurred in the two thresholds (red first vs. green first), each value is listed and the mean of these two figures has been calculated. It is immediately apparent that the nonaphasic patients gave 100 percent correct discriminations at shorter intervals than the aphasic patients. That this finding was true for all other criteria of performance of less than 100 percent is seen in figs. 19-1 and 19-2 for auditory and visual tasks. In these figures, the "simultaneous" or "don't know" replies were equally divided between the other two choices. These two figures also show that the auditory sequence analysis was more severely affected than the visual analysis.

Examination of the results obtained on the control group reveals that the accuracy in the determination of correct sequence is similar for both visual and auditory stimuli. The 75 percent threshold values (Table 19-2) were 80 and 75 milliseconds respectively in the control group. This confirms the observations of Hirsh

TABLE 19-1. 100 PERCENT CORRECT THRESHOLD BY SUBJECT

		Visual			Auditory		
Subject	Age	Green first	Red first	Mean	Low tone first	High tone first	Mean
Non-aphasic							
CH	37	100	150	125	150	150	150
BE	31	150	100	125	150	200	175
MO	64	100	100	100	75	50	62.5
ZW	49	150	150	150	150	175	162.5
CU	53	75	75	75	100	100	100
Aphasic							
BU	43	125	100	112.5	700	600	650
AN	55	125	150	138	600	500	550
A. MAS	43	200	300	250	700	700	700
GAR	31	200	200	200	700	600	650
EL	44	150	150	150	700	700	700
AR	61	250	150	200	150	400	275
CL	55	300	300	300	350	250	300
B. GAL	63	300	300	300	200	250	225
MAN	44	250	300	275	200	300	250
HA	51	350	350	350	175	150	162.5
C. SU	51	650	550	600	600	600	600
BRE (LH) Word-blind	45	400	500	450	>700	>700	

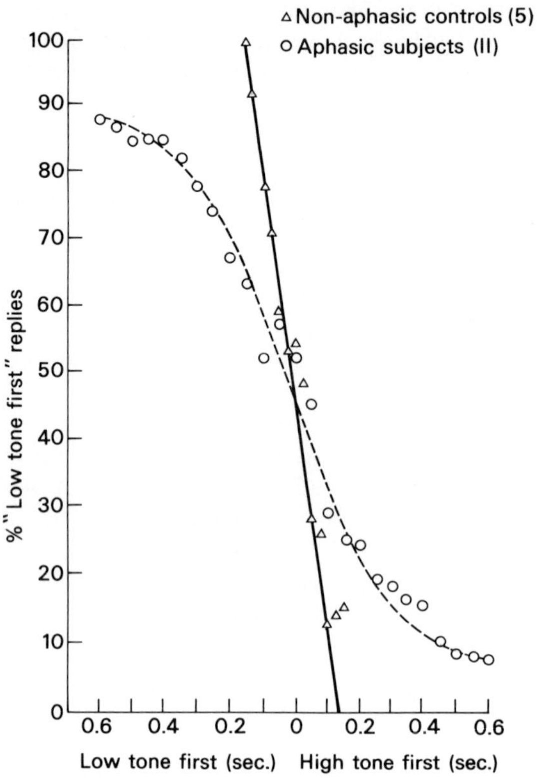

Fig. 19–1. *Auditory sequence discrimination.*

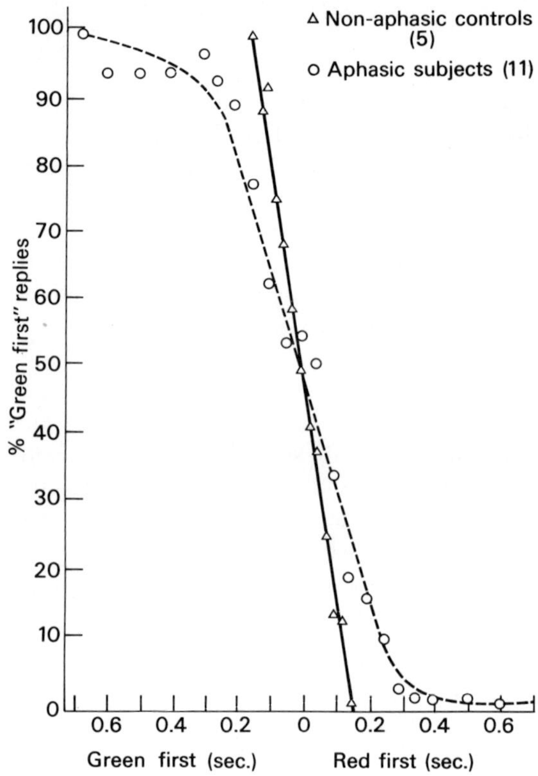

Fig. 19–2. Visual sequence discrimination.

and Sherrick (1961) who found that the interval required for 75 percent correct discrimination of sequence was the same for visual,

TABLE 19–2. 75 PERCENT CORRECT RESPONSE THRESHOLD (MSEC.)*

	Visual	Auditory
Control subjects	80	75
Expressive aphasics	100	400
Receptive aphasics	160	140

* Interpolated value derived from Figs. 19-3 and 19-4.

auditory, and tactile stimuli. The value obtained by Hirsh and Sherrick, using normal subjects, was 20 milliseconds which is appreciably smaller than that obtained by our hospitalized patients. The poor performance on tasks of sensory discrimination by hospitalized patients is well known and could account for the elevated threshold in our control group.

The aphasic subjects listed in Table 19-1 were further divided into two groups. Group A consisted of those subjects who could be classified as having a predominantly "expressive" aphasia, by the criteria of markedly reduced verbal output, disturbances of rhythm and modulation of speech, dysarthria, defective capacity to emit a meaningful sentence or proposition but with relatively preserved comprehension of speech. Four of these 6 patients had dense hemiplegias, and two had had hemiplegias during the acute phase of their illness.

Group B consisted of those patients whose aphasia was predominantly "receptive" in that their verbal outflow was of normal (or even increased) rate, propositions, sentences, and long expressions could be spontaneously emitted which had a normal rhythm and modulation. There was no dysarthria. They all had pronounced difficulty in understanding speech.

One patient (SU) was so severely aphasic in both respects that he could not easily be classified in this way. He had had three operations on his left temporal lobe for a recurrent pyogenic abscess in the last of which the anterior tip was resected. The dissection for drainage of the abscess was extended posteriorly to the occipital lobe. He was at the very limits of testability by this technique and did as poorly on visual as on the auditory task, requiring a 600 millisecond interval before he reached a 100 percent rate of correct responses in either modality. As classification was not easily decided, the data from this subject are excluded from further analysis.

In Table 19-3 are found the mean values and standard deviation at the 100 percent correct point for these two groups of aphasics compared with the control subjects. Fig. 19-3 and Fig. 19-4 show the performance of these groups compared with the control subjects for all other time intervals.

TABLE 19-3. 100 PERCENT CORRECT RESPONSE THRESHOLD (MSEC.)*

	Visual		Auditory	
	Msec.†	S.D.	Msec.†	S.D.
Control subjects (5)	115	±28.5	130	±47
Expressive aphasics (6)	175	±50.4	575	±192
Receptive aphasics (4)	306	±31.5	235	±57
Unclassified aphasic (1)	600		600	
Word-blindness + aphasia (1)	450		700	

* Directly determined experimental point.
† Each numerical value derived from an average of the 100% points for "high tone first" and "low tone first." A similar average was obtained of the 100% points for "green flash first" and "red flash first."

Table 19-4 lists the statistical analyses calculated at the 100 percent performance level with a two-tailed t-test. The probability values in Table 19-4 confirm the view that the performance of the expressive aphasics is worse on the auditory sequence discrimination and that the receptive aphasics do worse on the visual sequence discrimination.

INTERPRETATION OF RESULTS

There are several objections which might be raised concerning certain aspects of the performance of the control and aphasic subjects. In the first place, the control group contained a patient with a lesion in the *dominant* hemisphere —yet, this subject had normal temporal discrimination of order. It is important to note, however, that this was the only subject with a dominant hemisphere lesion who had no aphasia although he had a right hemiplegia. A clinical diagnosis of a capsular lesion had been made. There was no evidence of temporal lobe damage. This case thus serves to demonstrate that it is not a dominant hemisphere lesion itself which is related to disorders of discrimination of sequence, but a lesion in such a location which also produces aphasia.

It may be argued that these aphasic patients were merely demented and that their poor performance was a consequence of general intellectual impairment. A cursory examination of the data will dispel this objection as it can be seen that subjects BU, AN, and EL showed major defects for auditory temporal analysis but had an essentially normal response for visual analysis. Conversely, subject HA

TABLE 19-4. STATISTICAL COMPARISON*

	Visual			Auditory		
	t	d.f.	p	t	d.f.	p
Expressive aphasics *vs.* control	2.5672	10	<0.05	5.0165	10	<0.001
Receptive aphasics *vs.* control	9.5532	8	<0.001	3.0389	8	<0.02
Expressive *vs.* receptive	4.5845	9	<0.01	3.3820	9	<0.01

* Two-tailed test of significance.

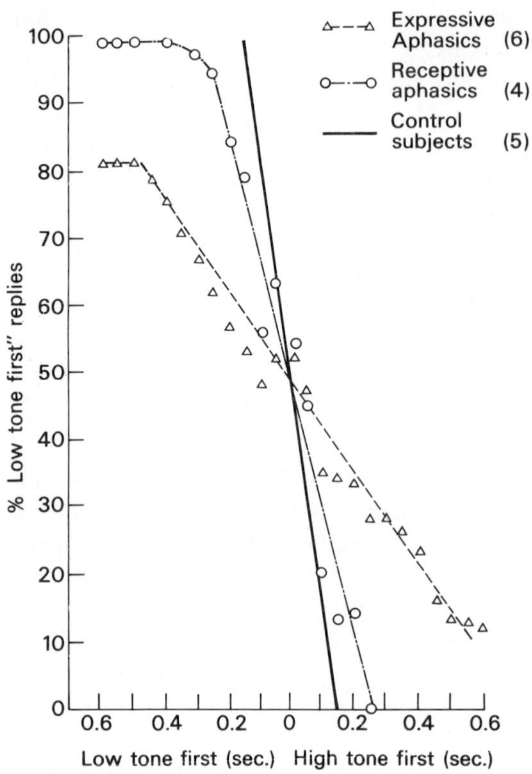

Fig. 19–3. Auditory sequence discrimination.

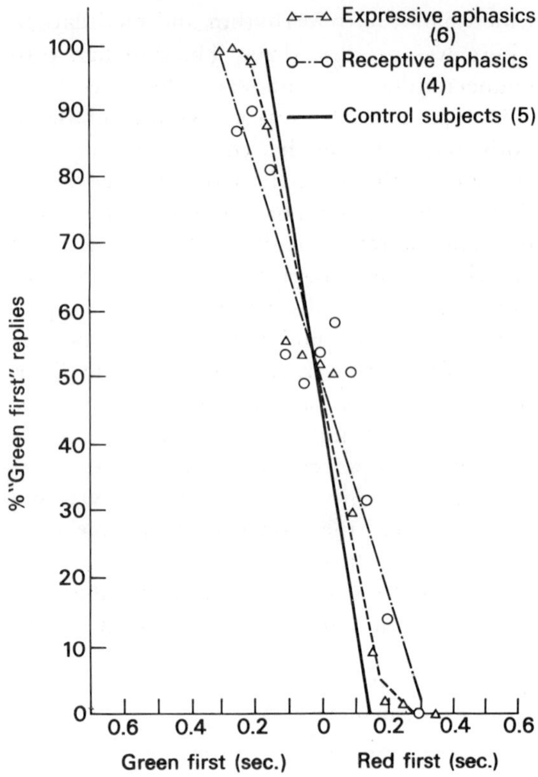

Fig. 19–4. Visual sequence discrimination.

had a normal response to auditory stimuli but had defective visual sequence discrimination. If the intellectual defect were of sufficient magnitude to produce a poor response in one modality it is then inconsistent with the normal performance in the other modality.

It might be argued that the poor performance of the aphasic group in both tasks was fundamentally due to a failure to understand the instructions or the nature of the discrimination. The design of the protocol, however, excludes this possibility for every subject reached a 100 percent rate of correct identification of sequence at *some* finite interval. This result proves that the subjects understood the task and could appropriately signal their reply. Furthermore, their performance levels at the shorter intervals showed a "normal" (Gaussian) distribution of correct replies (*see* figures 19-1, 19-2, 19-3, 19-4) indicating that the achievement of a 100 percent rate of correct replies was not just a matter of chance. This possible objection can also be rejected following analysis of the distribution of "simultaneous" or "don't know" replies. In figs. 19-5 and 19-6 are illustrated the frequency of such replies as a function of the interval between stimuli. For both modalities of sensation, the aphasic distribution contains a higher percentage of such replies. The distribution of simultaneous replies is "normal" (i.e. Gaussian) in the aphasics as well as in the control subjects, and this is further indication that they understood the instructions. The curves also show that even at intervals of 400–600 msec. the aphasic subjects were still somewhat uncertain as to the correct sequence and on occasion called the stimuli "simultaneous."

A similar argument applies to the objection that the aphasics were tone deaf—for if they were, a Gaussian distribution would be most improbable, and a 100 percent correct reply rate would never be achieved. Similarly, color blindness or difficulty in color identifica-

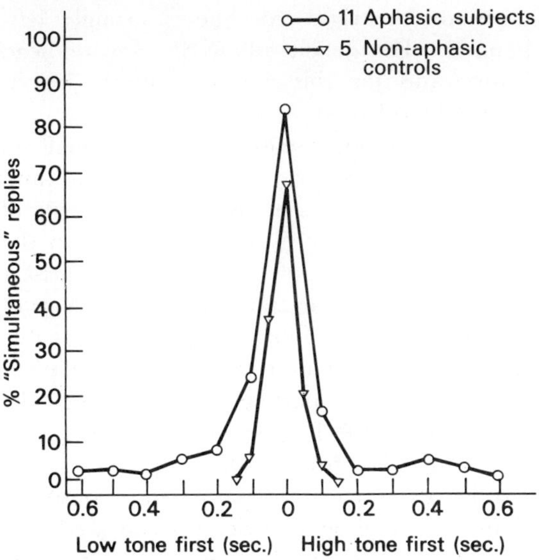

Fig. 19–5.

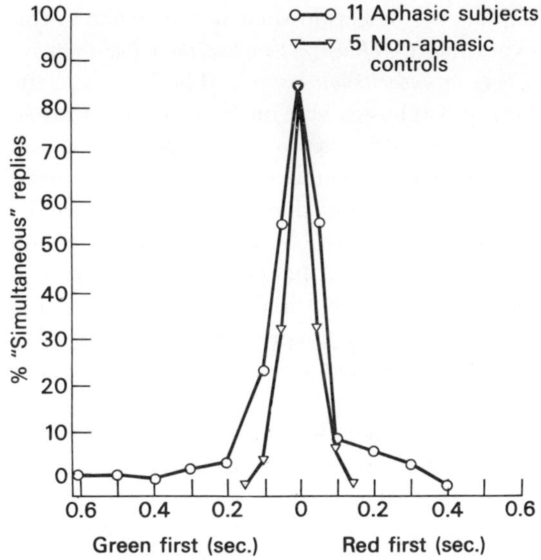

Fig. 19–6.

tion or in color naming would not account for these results. A hearing defect too can be excluded for the same reasons.

The slowness of aphasic replies, again cannot be an explanation as the subjects could receive as many pairs of flashes as they wished before signalling their reply. Their response time was not at issue.

It might be objected that the reason the aphasics made so many errors is that they received a random distribution of intervals. Perseveration of replies might well produce errors even at intervals at which they really could give correct discriminations. This too can be discounted as the subjects BU, AN, EL, and HA performed essentially normally on one of the two tests. Perseveration should play an equally great role in the two procedures.

Finally, any imbalance of intensities of sounds and lights was identical for control as well as experimental subjects.

It is clear, therefore, that none of these objections, either singly or in conjunction are sufficient to "explain" the outcome of these experiments. The results of this experiment are consistent with the hypothesis that the function of temporal analysis is performed in the hemisphere which is dominant for speech. The disturbances of temporal analysis of sequence which occur as a consequence of a lesion in the dominant hemisphere were theoretically anticipated. It was not possible, on the basis of the previously reported experiments, to make any predictions as to either the location of the essential areas within the dominant hemisphere or the manner in which these areas function. Further analysis of the details of the performance of these subjects may provide some information on these questions.

Table 19-4 shows that the "expressive" aphasics had more difficulty with the auditory sequence analysis than with the visual and that the "receptive" aphasics showed the reverse. The group of expressive aphasics had several subjects (BU, MAS) whose defects were almost exclusively in producing speech—comprehension being almost normal. The locus of lesions in this group is likely to be in the region of distribution of the middle cerebral artery in the Sylvian fissure. Thrombosis (the ætiology in all 6 cases) here usually produces damage to Broca's area as well as to the first temporal convolution and very likely parts of Heschl's gyrus. The lesions are, therefore, closely related physically to the primary auditory cortex. These patients had the more severe auditory sequencing defects in their performance in this experiment—*although they had the mildest clinical defects in understanding speech.* The lesions of the Group B aphasics were more posteriorly located (by clinical criteria) in the temporal lobe and these subjects had more severe visual sequencing difficulties. Two of these subjects (HA, GAL) had marked constructional apraxias. Although some auditory sequencing disturbance was clearly present in these subjects, it was less severe than in the "expressive" aphasics *yet these subjects had the most severe defects in understanding speech.*

From the view-point of these experiments, it might appear reasonable to think that the area for temporal analysis shows internal differentiation—the most anterior region being more concerned with auditory sequence (and possibly more concerned with motor sequencing too), and the most posterior being concerned with visual sequence analysis. If this view is correct, it is very difficult to understand why the expressive aphasics have such mild difficulties in comprehension of speech. Similarly, it is difficult to understand why the "receptive" aphasics have a greater and not a lesser disturbance.

It should be stressed at this point that the localizations of lesions in this group of aphasic subjects is on clinical grounds only and that anatomical precision cannot be expected. Yet, it seems most unlikely indeed that the clinical localization is inaccurate to such an extent that the dilemma can be so simply resolved.

In an attempt to clarify this problem, a patient (BRE) was studied whose primary defect is word-blindness. This patient is unable to read words or large numbers but is able to identify any letter or numeral rapidly. His comprehension of speech is essentially normal except that he will occasionally have difficulty if he is spoken to very quickly. He speaks fluently and has the barest trace of an occasional paraphasic difficulty. He has a constructional apraxia and is dysgraphic for words but can write letters and numbers. The performance of this subject (Table 19-1) shows a major defect for *both* auditory and visual sequencing tasks. His lesion is probably located in the angular gyrus on the right side (he is strongly left-handed). His deficit followed a severe head injury and for this reason multiple lesions cannot be ruled out.

It is thus not possible at the moment to correlate the relative defects in visual and auditory sequence analysis with the severity of any particular clinical manifestation with the possible exception of constructional apraxia which does occur in association with defects of visual sequencing ability. It is also not possible to find a correlation between the clinical severity of any particular defect and the magnitude of the 100 percent correct response threshold. To resolve these questions will require extensive neuropathological observations and much greater detailed knowledge of the anatomy of the dominant temporal lobe than is now available.

The performance of the expressive aphasic subjects on the auditory sequence task is so "poor" that one wonders how they can understand speech at all. These subjects did not get a 100 percent score until the two tones were separated by approximately 575 milliseconds. As phonemes occur approximately every 80 milliseconds, it could be cogently argued that comprehension of normal speech should be impossible. This paradox can be partially avoided if we appreciate that the comprehension of speech is a matter of probability. It may well be that perfect sequencing is not necessary for comprehension of speech but that a 75 percent correct rate will produce no detectable clinical disturbance of comprehension. Furthermore, the redundancy of the language serves as an additional safety margin. It is also known that more information is transmitted by the consonants than the vowels (written Hebrew, for example, usually omits vowels entirely—they are implied by the context) and this gives an added protection.

Finally, further information is received by word length, intensity, intonation, rhythm, etc. As the quantitative role of these factors is unknown, it is impossible to apply any correction to the 575 millisecond figure. These factors, however, may be sufficient to explain why comprehension of *speech* is still relatively preserved in the expressive aphasics, despite their poor performance with tones which carry much less helpful "information."[1]

The performance of the "receptive" aphasics who had major difficulties in comprehending speech showed a *less* severe disturbance of auditory sequence analysis than the expressive aphasics. It may well be the case that the functional defect in the receptive aphasics occurs *after* the phonemes or words are already sequenced. Indeed, several of these patients could repeat words and short phrases although they clearly did not understand them. That some defect in auditory sequence analysis is present does not necessarily mean that this mild defect is the cause of their comprehension failure. It must be recognized that after the phonemes of a word are properly sequenced, logically the next step is to compare this input sequence with the memory of that particular sequence and with the meaning of it. (Thus, the reader's auditory sequencing mechanisms may be intact but he will still not "comprehend" the words of an unfamiliar language.) A discussion of the physiological nature of this comparison with a stored "schema" (Brain, 1950, 1961) is beyond the scope of the paper.

The disturbances in speech which could occur at this later stage of input analysis may have nothing at all to do with temporal analysis. The "receptive" component of an expressive asphasic's difficulty may thus be *qualitatively* different (i.e. at an earlier stage of input data analysis) than the "receptive" component in Wernicke's aphasia.

DISCUSSION

A. Aphasia

It has been seen that the damage to certain areas of the brain disturbs the function of temporal sequence descrimination. Damage to the same areas is associated with aphasia—indeed, the defect in sequence discrimination was found *only when there was some degree of aphasia present.* Is this merely coincidence or does it reflect an *essential* relationship between the two observations? Further study of this phenomenon will be required before a definitive answer can be provided. There are, however, other observations which, when coupled with the experiments described here, suggest that this relationship may be of significance physiologically.

It is an everyday clinical observation that communication with aphasics is improved if they are spoken to slowly. Even with a reduced rate of verbal inflow, significant difficulty is present but much greater opportunity is allowed for inferring, from the words which have been correctly sequenced, the next word. When the speech rate exceeds the capacity of the patient to properly sequence, complete failure of communication might result on the receptive side. If this view is correct we should not look upon the aphasias as unique disorders of *language* but rather as an inevitable consequence of a primary defect in temporal analysis—in placing a "time-label" upon incoming data. Additional symptoms in the "receptive" aphasics may be due to defects at a later stage of analysis of the input pattern. Aphasia, thus considered, would be an epiphenomenon.

Similarly, one might reasonably expect a need for remarkably accurate programming

[1] An additional complication which must be considered is the work of Liberman, Delattre and Cooper (1952) which shows that certain consonants are correctly identified only when they are followed by particular vowels. These data can be taken to imply either that the vowel sound has a retroactive effect on the capacity to identify a preceding event (consonant), or that the consonant-vowel complex is normally identified as a unit. In support of the first explanation is the work of Treisman and Howarth (1959) on perception of visual and auditory stimuli and of Halliday and Mingay (1961) on cutaneous stimuli. Both groups of workers have shown that a warning stimulus can alter the threshold for perception of a stimulus which actually came *before* the warning. There is evidence in support of the second view (*see* Brain, 1950, 1961) that a whole word may be identified as a sound unit. In this case, using an estimate of 150 words per minute as an average figure for English speech, each word occupies approximately 400 milliseconds. Some defect in comprehension might then be detected if a subject could correctly sequence words only at a rate of every 575 milliseconds. The experiments reported in this paper do not permit a decision on the question as to whether it is word sounds or phoneme sounds which are sequenced—they only show that a defect in sequencing of *simple* visual and auditory elements exists in aphasics.

of verbal output. In this case there is not only a precise sequence of innervation to a large number of respiratory, lingual, facial, and laryngeal muscles, but a preceding selection of the proper sequence of words. A disturbance of central nervous system motor timing mechanisms would be expected to have perhaps more devastating effects on speech than on any other motor function. Thus, the aphasic dysarthria, facial apraxia, and other symptoms might be at least partially explained.

The area of the brain concerned with input sequence analysis of visual stimuli may be located somewhat more posteriorly than that for auditory analysis. If this is damaged and visual discrimination of order is disturbed, one might reasonably expect to see constructional apraxias and other "high level" visual disturbances. Indeed, 2 of the 5 patients with posterior lesions and receptive aphasias (HA, GAL) have clearly defined constructional apraxias and these subjects had poor performance on the visual task. The subject with word-blindness (BRE) who also had a severe visual sequencing difficulty also has constructional apraxia. The subject SU similarly has constructional defects, but he is so severely disabled that an accurate appraisal of any particular symptom is essentially impossible.

It may be objected that the list of special, "higher," or "cognitive" functions attributed to the dominant hemisphere is already so large that to locate yet another function (temporal analysis of sequence) in this overburdened hemisphere is intolerable. The hypothesis that the basic functions of temporal sequencing lie in the dominant temporal lobe may possibly serve to resolve this difficulty. It may be precisely because temporal sequencing is performed in this area that the "higher" functions *appear* to reside there.

In a series of papers, Walshe (1943, 1947) has logically demonstrated the impropriety of statements to the effect that "speech is *located* in such an area" or that "there is an area which performs constructional *eu*praxia." The hypothesis that temporal sequencing mechanisms are *located* or heavily centered in an area does not, I think, merely substitute a new set of words for the same concepts to which Walshe objects. We are, in fact, *not* saying that the symptoms (aphasia, dysarthria, and apraxia) "reside" or are "located" in the major hemisphere. Similarly, we are *not* saying that the normal execution of certain activities (euphasia, euarthria, and eupraxia) is located anywhere at all. We do suggest that there is a fundamental mechanism or process related to the requirements of "time-labelling" of input and output signals which *is* located in the dominant temporal lobe and that damage to this area and its radiations may result in symptoms of disturbance to these "higher functions." The "higher" functions are not in themselves "located" in the temporal-parietal lobe. Symptoms of inadequate function are not the same thing as functions. A symptom itself is not localizable—a function can be (*see* Walshe, 1947). A symptom, nevertheless, may be useful for localizing a *lesion*.

The fact that all the subjects who had defects in sequencing had not only some degree of aphasia, but had lesions in the temporal area[2] suggests that this area (and its connexions) is essentially concerned with time analysis.

B. Temporal Lobe Disease

This view is further supported by the notorious frequency of disturbances of subjective time sense which occur during temporal lobe seizures. The earliest papers on uncinate fits by Jackson (1888, 1890) describes a disorder in perception of time ("dreamy state"). The symptoms of disturbed appreciation of time interval as a consequence of a temporal lobe seizure can be exceedingly complex—subjective time being either accelerated or retarded or otherwise disturbed even during the course of one seizure (Efron, 1956, 1957). Seizures in these areas also produce speech arrest and word-blindness, and word-deafness is often seen in the post-ictal state.

Patients with damage to the temporal lobe also have memory disturbances which are

[2] Used in this sense, the word temporal is to be taken to include the first frontal convolution (Broca's area).

associated with disturbances of personal time sense. Symonds (1960) has analyzed a group of such patients and concluded that "The concept of a physical basis for memory must allow for the assumption, to begin with, that every moment of personal time has its physiological identity, and the further assumption that there are arrangements in the brain for recording these units of time. These constitute the personal clock, which provides for continuity of experience, without which memory in the ordinary sense could not exist." He then suggested that a "cinema film instead of being projected in the ordinary way were cut into short strips, and these strips were joined together in a random order instead of the proper chronological sequence, the result would have no meaning." Symonds' prediction can be confirmed by a viewing of the recent film "Last Year at Marienbad" directed by Alain Resnais. In this film the plot chronology was intentionally randomized for presumed "artistic" purposes and, as expected, the result had no meaning but conveyed a dream-like mood.

C. Déjà Vu

There is yet another symptom of temporal lobe dysfunction which may be attributed to a disturbance of the "time-labelling" mechanism —that is déjà vu. We have seen (Efron, 1963*a*, *b*) that information pertinent to the time of occurrence of an event which is received by the nondominant hemisphere may be transferred to the dominant hemisphere. Under normal conditions of life with the eyes freely moving, the head turning, and sounds being received bilaterally and from all directions, the two hemispheres receive essentially the same information about the events of the external world. The few milliseconds delay in the time of arrival of the data from the right hemisphere is not, apparently, subjectively detected. Suppose, however, that the delay in transmission from right to left hemisphere were, for a period of a minute, delayed by several hundred milliseconds. Under such conditions, the left hemisphere would receive information (and essentially the same information) twice—once directly, and the second time relayed after this delay from the right hemisphere. Normally an interpretation would be made that two different events have occurred. *Yet, as has been pointed out, the data are essentially identical.* It does not appear to be unreasonable to assume that under these conditions a person might have the following rapid, but unconscious interpretation: "Everything which I am perceiving *now* has already occurred once before (because it has already been 'logged-in' by the left hemisphere via the direct pathway). Yet, I cannot find any memory trace of that previous experience." A delay in the incorporation of data into a durable memory system is well established. In this case, the few hundred milliseconds might not be sufficient time for the memory (of the undelayed message) to be filed and retrieved. This subjective interpretation is clearly preferable to the alternative that "Everything is happening twice." The second interpretation requires an additional universe of similar events running on a parallel time scale. This latter conclusion is unacceptable as it requires that the subject discard his metaphysical principles of identity and causality. Thus, déjà vu may be explained.

After this state of delayed transmission has persisted for a few seconds, the subject has more information. He can then say "I am aware that a series of events are apparently occurring twice. As this is not acceptable (for the above reasons), the more likely alternative is that I am merely anticipating what will occur"—thus, clairvoyance may be explained.

The close relationship between déjà vu and clairvoyance, symptoms which, in some patients (Efron, 1956) occur simultaneously, may be explicable in this fashion. At any instant the two interpretations may even be equally valid. Dickens has most elegantly described the co-existence of déjà vu and clairvoyance in *David Copperfield*, "We have all some experience of a feeling which comes over us occasionally, of what we are saying and doing having been said or done before, in a remote time—of our having been surrounded, dim ages ago, by the same faces, objects, and circumstances—of our knowing perfectly what will be said next, as if we suddenly remembered it." Mullan and Penfield (1959) have called attention to the fact that déjà vu occurs primarily as a consequence of lesions in the nondominant hemisphere. It does not appear unreasonable to assume that a fit in this region may delay transmission of data to the dominant hemisphere—merely virtue of the fact that the interhemispheric pathways are overloaded with seizure discharges.

The preceding interpretations are based upon an implicit assumption—namely, that it is only after sensory data have reached the left hemisphere that one is "conscious" of the occurrence of an event. An "event" which is not occurring at any particular time (in relation to the "personal clock") can hardly provide the landmarks necessary for the continuity of experience and cannot be *subsequently* used to reconstruct reality. Even if these untimed events were stored in the memory, they would be of little practical value except possibly for their transient, short-lived consequence. One might not be any more *conscious* of them than of fleeting changes in excitatory states of spinal cord interneurones. To be conscious of something is to be conscious of something *now*. It is the thesis of this paper that the "now" is the moment of arrival of sensory data in the dominant temporal lobe. It may be argued that this view leads one to the untenable position that destruction of the left hemisphere should result in unconsciousness. This would be true *only* if no other region could perform the same function after the dominant hemisphere is destroyed or seriously damaged.[3]

The suggestion that déjà vu represents a disturbance of transmission of data from the non-dominant to dominant hemisphere is, at the moment, purely speculative. It is put forward, nevertheless, as it is consistent not only with the clinical and experimental observations but also with the hypothesis that has been elaborated in this paper. The speculation has additional merit in that it might be tested during neurosurgical operation by local anæsthesia of the corpus callosum.

In a previous paper (Efron, 1962*c*) on the Pulfrich effect, it was pointed out that at the point where the stereoscopic illusion fails (as a consequence of the excessive time taken by the sensory data from one eye to reach the level of consciousness), the subject "sees" two spots. In this case, we are dealing with an artificially introduced delay in one message going to both hemispheres. At any instant ("now"), the brain is presented with two "images" which are dissimilar. It reasonably concludes that there are two different *events* (spots) at *one* time.

It may be argued (*see* first paragraph) that temporal discrimination of order or "time-labelling" is necessarily present to some extent in all animals. Why should the function be so localized in man? Where is it located in lower animals? This question is only a concrete formulation of the more general question of cerebral dominance (encephalization). That the time analysis functions of the nervous system of man are localizable in the hemispheres is no more (or less) mysterious than that any other functions are performed in the cerebral hemispheres. Similarly, the idea that temporal analysis is performed in the dominant temporal lobe in the intact human is no more distasteful than the idea that the two hemispheres are different in their functions. Furthermore, it is not in conflict with the fact that unconscious temporal analysis takes place at every synapse. Implicit in Sherrington's concepts of the central excitatory and inhibitory state is the importance of the timing of impulses over the afferent arcs. The subsequent electrical analysis of synaptic action by Eccles (1957) and others has shown that the time-constant (RC) of the neural membrane determines the time course of the potential changes induced by each subthreshold stimulus. Thus, the membrane characteristics may be considered to serve as the elementary building

[3] It should be pointed out that the cardiac rhythm, normally determined by the rhythmic discharges of the sino-auricular node, is only momentarily stopped by destruction of that region. The migration of the pacemaker to the auriculo-ventricular region re-establishes the rhythm though at a slower rate. In this respect, it must be recalled that the aphasic patients could still sequence stimuli (after damage to their dominant hemisphere) but again at a slower rate.

blocks for more elaborate temporal analysis mechanism. The integration of spinal reflexes such as the crossed extension reflex requires a sequencing of activity which is ultimately dependent upon the time-constants of the individual neuronal membranes which in turn depends on their physico-chemical structure.

The apparent differences in the functions performed by the two hemispheres may be explicable on the basis of the genetic localization of the more complex temporal analysis mechanisms in the dominant hemisphere. Wyke and Ettlinger (1961) have shown that the efficiency of recognition is significantly greater when drawings are tachistoscopically exposed to the right visual field as compared to the left. Semmes, Weinstein, Ghent, and Teuber (1960) have shown that lesions in the dominant hemisphere frequently affect sensation bilaterally, whereas lesions in the nondominant hemisphere produce only contralateral sensory disturbances. They have called attention to the earlier observations of Foix (1922), Guillain, Alajouanine, and Garcin (1925) which demonstrated this phenomenon. Similarly, apraxias are frequently bilateral following dominant hemisphere lesions. Recent work by Goodglass and Kaplan (1962) on the gestural deficiencies in aphasics suggests that this deficiency is a consequence of an apraxia and not a defect of "communication." They also showed that the severity of the gestural deficiency is not correlated with the severity of the "aphasia."

Clinical as well as experimental observations thus strongly support the hypothesis which has been presented in this series of papers that temporal analysis of sequence, interval and simultaneity is performed in the left hemisphere in the right-handed subjects, as well as in the majority of left-handed ones. The localization of this particular function in the left hemisphere may make it more efficient for other tasks (requiring accurate temporal analysis of incoming or outgoing data) to be similarly "localized" in the same or nearby regions. Disorders of the central mechanism(s) for sequence analysis and control might thus account for certain essential aspects of the symptoms of aphasias, apraxias, and possibly other disturbances of "higher" functions particularly memory and consciousness. It is obvious but not trivial to point out that to "think" is to order our ideas sequentially and towards a purpose. Randomly occurring mental states or mental states triggered by chance external events, while they may well occur all too frequently, are neither purposeful nor can they be called "thinking."

Note added on proof: Prof. O. L. Zangwill has kindly called to my attention a monograph (*The Duality of the Mind* by A. L. Wigan, 1844, published by Longman, Brown and Green, London) in which the author suggests an explanation of déjà vu superficially resembling the one proposed in this paper. Wigan's thesis is that each hemisphere has a "consciousness" of its own but that one is normally dominated or suppressed by the other. Déjà vu, according to this view, results from the momentary loss of this suppression which in turn gives rise to a doubling or a duality of consciousness. This concept differs markedly from the speculation put forward in this paper. The only element in common between the two positions is the view that in man the right and left hemispheres have different functions—a fact which would not be denied by any neurologist.

REFERENCES

Brain, W. R. (1950) In: "Perspectives in Neuropsychiatry," edited by D. Richter. London, p. 127.

—— (1961) "Speech Disorders." London.

Eccles, J. C. (1957) "The Physiology of Nerve Cells." Baltimore.

Efron, R. (1956) *Brain*, **79,** 267.

—— (1957) *Brain*, **80,** 251.

—— (1963*a*) *Brain*, **86,** 261.

—— (1963*b*) *Brain*, **86,** 285.

—— (1963*c*) *Brain*, **86,** 295.

Foix, C. (1922) *Rev. neurol.*, **29,** 322.

Goodglass, H., and Kaplan, E. (1962) "Disturbance of Gesture and Pantomime in Aphasia." To be published in Brain.

Guillain, G., Alajouanine, T., and Garcin, R. (1925) *Rev. Neurol.*, **2,** 116.

Halliday, A. M., and Mingay, R. (1961) *Quart. J. exp. psychol.*, **13,** 1.

Heller, J. (1961) "Catch-22." New York.

Hirsh, I. J., and Sherrick, C. E. (1961) *J. exp. Psychol.*, **62,** 423.

Jackson, H. (1888) *Brain*, **11,** 179.

Jackson, J. H., and Beevor, C. E. (1889) *Brain*, **12,** 346.

Lashley, K. (1951) In: "Cerebral Mechanisms in Behavior," edited by L. A. Jeffress. Chapman, N.Y., p. 112.

Liberman, A. M., Delattre, P., and Cooper, F. S. (1952) *Amer. J. Psychol.*, **65,** 497.

Mullan, S., and Penfield, W. (1959) *Arch. Neurol.*, **81,** 269.

Semmes, J., Weinstein, S., Ghent, L., and Teuber, H. L. (1960) "Somatosensory Changes After Penetrating Brain Wounds in Man." Cambridge, Mass.

Symonds, C. P. (1960) Unpublished Hughlings Jackson Lecture, Montreal (quoted with permission).

Treisman, M., and Howarth, C. I. (1959) *Quart. J. exp. Psychol.*, **11,** 129.

Walshe, F. M. R. (1943) *Brain*, **66,** 104.

—— (1947) *Brain*, **70,** 329.

Wyke, M., and Ettlinger, G. (1961) *Arch. Neurol.*, **5,** 659.

20

A Pilot Study of Aphasia Among Bilinguals

WALLACE E. LAMBERT
SAMUEL FILLENBAUM

WALLACE E. LAMBERT, Ph.D., is with the department of psychology of McGill University, Montreal.
SAMUEL FILLENBAUM, Ph.D., is with the department of psychology of the University of North Carolina.
This research was supported by the Defence Research Board of Canada Grant D77-94-01-10.

The study of aphasia among people who speak more than one language has been undertaken in the main by specialists in aphasia, and several case reviews have been compiled. The course of aphasia among polyglots has been interpreted in terms of several different principles. First, cases have been reported which support the "rule of Ribot" (*see* 6, p. 76), which states that linguistic habits acquired early, as in childhood, are more resistant to aphasic damage than those acquired subsequently. The "mother tongue" is not only learned first but presumably is built up with more emotional meaning, thereby increasing its relative strength. An important paper by Pitres (5) offered a different generalization in order to account for his own observations of the effect of aphasia on polyglots. In essence, Pitres' is a habit strength principle which states that the language or languages most used before the aphasic insult will be the first to recover. The less well practised languages will be recovered less quickly and, if a language has been used very little before aphasia, that language might not be remembered or used at all afterward. Minkowski (4) presented several cases of bilingual aphasics which he proposed as exceptions to Pitres' principle and which also appear to be exceptions to the Ribot rule. Minkowski showed that an emotional or affective factor related to the use of one language might account for the survival of that language after the polyglot had suffered an aphasic insult. In short, cases have been presented which agree, and others which conflict with each principle. The conservative conclusion must be that aphasia can have various effects on the bilingual's languages, the particular post-aphasic pattern probably depending in some complex fashion on: the order in which the languages were learned, the comparative levels of skill attained in each, and the affective value each language has for the individual.

The study of the effects of an aphasic insult on the languages of a polyglot is also of interest and value to those who are primarily concerned with bilingualism itself. Thus, for example, the recent work of Weinreich (6), which indicates the relevance of data from polyglot aphasics to various theories about the verbal behavior of the "bilingual individual," makes it clear that our understanding of bilingualism would be greatly improved if data were systematically collected about the course of aphasia in bilingual patients.

Certain findings from our own and other research on bilingualism led us to a con-

From *Canadian Journal of Psychology* 13:28–34, 1959.

sideration of the data on aphasics. The point of departure was an hypothesis, developed by Weinreich (6) and Ervin and Osgood (1), which maintains that some bilinguals develop the same meaning for translated equivalents in their two languages, while others develop a different meaning for the concept in each language. The former would be characteristic of the "compound" bilingual and the latter of the "co-ordinate" bilingual for whom, theoretically, the two languages, or certain elements of the languages would function independently. This hypothesis is of value in understanding differences among bilinguals in their ease of switching from one language to the other, their control of interferences from the other language in any verbal situation, and their abilities to think and behave appropriately in the different linguistic contexts. This hypothesis was extended in a study by Lambert, Havelka, and Crosby (2) where it was concluded that the *learning contexts* in which the bilingual's two languages are acquired may well determine the functional independence of the languages. The more the learning contexts are "separated," either in time, cultural distinctiveness, or in distinctiveness of the setting of habitual usage, the more likely it is that bilingual "co-ordinateness" will develop.

There is the possibility that the functional relations of the bilingual's two languages have some systematic neural representation in those areas of the brain necessary to the functioning of language. The nature of this neural representation is necessarily largely a matter for speculation in view of how little is now known about language centres in the human brain. Our notion was that co-ordinate bilinguals should have more functionally separated neural structures underlying their languages than should compound bilinguals. Thus, the concepts "house" and "*maison*" which are more functionally independent for co-ordinate than for compound bilinguals would be "stored" in neural elements which have some sort of greater functional discreteness for the co-ordinate bilinguals.

It follows from this line of reasoning that any specific brain damage resulting in aphasia would be likely to affect all languages of the compound bilingual, but should lead to more selective disturbances for co-ordinate bilinguals. Thus, one would predict that if factors such as size and locus of brain damage could be held constant, co-ordinate bilinguals would be more likely to show aphasic damage in one language system, while compound bilinguals would be more likely to show aphasic damage in all languages known. It should be recognized that factors of size and locus of damage can never be "held constant," and that even with a large sample of patients only general trends can be expected to emerge from a study of bilingual aphasics.

The present work sought to examine some data on aphasia in polyglots, to determine (*a*) if any relation exists between language learning contexts and the nature of the aphasic disorder, and (*b*) to what extent these data fit the general principles previously suggested, particularly the principles of primacy and "habit strength." Most reported cases on polyglot aphasics are anecdotal and incomplete: factual information on the language proficiencies of a patient before brain damage is rarely available. Such information as there is, in nearly every case, is based on the recollections of the patient or his family. Furthermore, the hospital environment in most communities is unilingual and the bilingual aphasic's first speech efforts may be forced into the language spoken in the hospital, with relearning taking place in that language only.

As source material we used the cases of European polyglot aphasics presented in a recent review by Leischner (3), and cases of polyglot aphasics obtained from several hospitals and rehabilitation centres in Montreal. In the collection of our own fourteen cases we were no more successful in obtaining complete information than other researchers. Interviews were held with the patient and with members of his family in an attempt to elicit data on his premorbid and present language skills. Information was obtained as to the language history of the patient, the times, conditions, and circumstances of acquisition, and use of the different languages, and the relative fluencies of the patient in each language. Each patient was interviewed to determine the present state of his language skills. Conversation was carried out in both (or all) languages known, and attention was paid to his expressive and receptive difficulties in each, his ability to switch languages spontaneously or on demand, to answer questions, to use words, and to read in each language.

The extent to which the data fit such rules as a habit strength or primacy principle is summarized in Table 20-1, where European and Montreal cases are kept separate. It can be seen that the Montreal cases and European cases fall into substantially different patterns. The European cases in most instances fail to support either a primacy or a habit strength principle, while in contrast most of the Montreal cases are consistent with both principles (χ^2 values, corrected for continuity, for the difference between European cases and Montreal cases are 7.13, $p<.01$ (primacy) and 5.70, $p<.02$ (habit strength) respectively). In the European data there is evidence in seven cases for some affective factor which might account for the better survival of the language not first or better learned; in the Montreal data the one instance clearly involving some affective factor supports the importance of the first learned language. These apparent differences might be due to differences in the selection of cases: we investigated all bilingual aphasics available, cases reported in the literature may be the more dramatic ones taken as exceptions to expectation. We have no way of testing such a possibility.

The differences may also be interpreted, however, as evidence in favour of our original hypothesis. The typical pattern in the European patients is that the first learned language had been used for the greater (or greatest) period of time prior to aphasia, but a second language had also been acquired and used in the period prior to the aphasia. The language surviving aphasia best is characteristically a secondarily acquired language, a fact which conflicts with Ribot's generalization (primacy principle) and, to the extent that the second language is less known and used with less facility, with Pitres' (habit strength) principle as well. For the European patients the second language is typically learned in a context distinctly separated from the first, that is, the two languages are characteristically learned in a co-ordinate fashion. In Europe the polyglot may be forced to master the language of the new country of residence (its *only* language) and accordingly its acquisition (and retention after aphasia) will be of great personal importance. The seven cases in which an affective factor is evident suggest that a language which is emotionally important to the individual, although not used as often as another, may be the only language retained, or the one least damaged after aphasia. The typical Montreal case indicates that the first-learned language is also the one most used until the time of aphasia while the other language, learned early in life and used concurrently with the first, typically is not used as frequently as the first language. After aphasia, both languages are damaged but retain the order of dominance which was developed prior to aphasia. The affective factor is less apparent, perhaps because in Montreal a greater freedom of use of all languages known is possible. It is likely that the Montreal scene encourages the development of bilingual compoundedness since essentially the same con-

TABLE 20-1. SUMMARY OF INSTANCES OF SUPPORT FOR VARIOUS PRINCIPLES

	Primacy (Ribot)		Habit strength (Pitres)		Affective (Minkowski)
	Pro	Con	Pro	Con	Pro
European cases	5	17	6	14	7
Montreal cases	8	2	9	2	1

text for language learning is probably more likely to be used for all languages acquired. If we assume that the European and Montreal scenes encourage co-ordinate and compound bilingualism respectively, then the data offer some support for our hypothesis since the Montreal cases typically show a generalized disorder affecting both languages, while the European cases typically show a more specific-language disorder following aphasia.

A set of cases collected before the turn of the century by Pitres (5) was not mentioned or included in Leischner's 1948 review. Pitres' cases are of particular interest for our purposes because they were gathered in the southwest section of France, and because they include in all instances people who used French along with one or more languages, such as patois, Basque, Spanish, and Italian. In six cases, French was used most frequently and, with the exception of brief periods in two cases, was used continually throughout the patients' lives in France. It will be noted in Table 20-2 that these cases are strikingly similar to the Montreal cases in that both the Ribot and the Pitres principles are consistently supported, that is, the first learned language is the most used and also the one which returns first after aphasia. The generalization therefore seems appropriate that the language (or languages) which bilinguals use continuously from early life will probably be least vulnerable to aphasia. The Montreal cases are also consistent with this generalization in that two languages are more likely to be learned early in life and used concurrently in Quebec.

TABLE 20-2. PITRES' CASES OF POLYGLOT APHASICS

Primacy (Ribot)		Habit strength (Pitres)	
Pro	Con	Pro	Con
5	1	6	0

The Pitres cases also allow one further observation. The French people in the southwest section of France may learn a local patois and French in essentially the same context, much as Canadians may learn two languages in Montreal. That is, the patois and French may become "compounded" for these bilinguals. We would predict, then, that these two languages should be similarly affected by aphasia. Three of Pitres' patients are polyglots with French and patois as two of their languages. Two of the patients suffered complete aphasic loss for a long period during which *both* languages did not return, and after three years, in each case, French was only poorly used while the patois was not used at all. It appears that language training after aphasia was carried out in French, and the difference between the ability to use the two languages after this long period may have been due to the training only. It is possible that these languages were learned as a compound system and that both were similarly affected (in this case equally damaged) by the aphasia, as our theory would predict. The third case is also consistent with expectations. This person learned French and patois from early years and later acquired several other languages in work situations. Six months following aphasia this patient was able to use *both* French and the patois fairly well, but still could neither understand nor use the other languages.

In conclusion, although the results are consistent with the theoretical analysis of compound and co-ordinate bilingualism, much more detailed information about the language history of each patient is needed before alternative interpretations of the results can be excluded. For example, we argued that Montreal and that region of France where a local patois is used are likely to be situations which encourage the development of compound bilingualism. These social environments also allow the continual and concurrent use of two or more languages, and the difference in freedom of *usage* of languages known may also account for the differences in the effects of aphasia noted when Leischner's "European" cases are compared with our own cases and with those of Pitres.

SUMMARY

Several studies of the effects of aphasia among people who use more than one language were reviewed and three generalizations about the effects of aphasia in these cases were discussed. Classical cases of polyglot aphasics and new cases compiled in Montreal were analysed in order to test the hypothesis that the functional dependence or independence of polyglots' languages, determined by the manner in which the languages were originally learned, will determine, in part, how the languages are affected by an aphasic insult. Although the findings, derived from the analysis of cases, are consistent with the theoretical analysis, alternative interpretations cannot be excluded with the data available at present.

REFERENCES

1. Ervin, S. M., and Osgood, C. E. Second language learning and bilingualism. In C. E. Osgood and F. Sebeok (Eds.), Psycholinguistics. *J. abnorm. soc. Psychol.*, Suppl., 1954, 139–146.
2. Lambert, W. E., Havelka, J., and Crosby, C. The influence of language-acquisition contexts on bilingualism. *J. abnorm. soc. Psychol.*, 1958, **56,** 239–244.
3. Leischner, A. Ueber die Aphasie der Mehrsprachigen. *Archiv für Psychiatrie und Nervenkrankheiten,* 1948, **180,** 731–775.
4. Minkowski, M. Sur un cas d'aphasie chez un polygotte. *Revue neurologique*, 1928, **35,** 361–366.
5. Pitres, A. Etude sur l'aphasie chez les polyglottes. *Revue de médicine*, 1895, **15,** 873–899.
6. Wienreich, U. *Languages in contact.* New York: Linguistic Circle of New York, 1953.

21

Aphasia in a Congenitally Deaf Man

JOHN E. SARNO
LINDA P. SWISHER
MARTHA T. SARNO

JOHN E. SARNO, M.D., is director of the outpatient department of the Institute of Rehabilitation Medicine, and is with the department of rehabilitation medicine of the New York University School of Medicine.

LINDA P. SWISHER, Ph.D., is a research associate at the Central Institute for the Deaf, St. Louis.

MARTHA T. SARNO, M.A., is director of the speech pathology service of the Institute of Rehabilitation Medicine and is with the department of rehabilitation medicine of the New York University School of Medicine.

It has become the custom when introducing a paper on aphasia in the deaf-mute to quote J. Hughlings-Jackson who wrote, "No doubt by disease of some part of his brain the deaf-mute might lose his natural system of signs . . ." some ninety years ago (Hughlings-Jackson 1878). Since that time the subject has been treated by Grasset (1896), Critchley (1938), Leischner (1943), Tureen, Smolik and Tritt (1951) and Douglass and Richardson (1959). Each of these studies presented a single case of aphasia and speculated on the nature of this disorder in the "deaf-mute." Since the cases described including our own are so dissimilar, a useful comparison is not possible.

We would like to suggest at the outset that the term "deaf-mute" is not accurate since many who are born without hearing learn some speech. They are better referred to as the congenitally deaf and that term will be used in this paper.

Our observations suggest that aphasia in the congenitally deaf is analogous to that in the normal hearing. By extension this would imply that aphasia in the congenitally deaf results from pathology in the dominant hemisphere. Further, we suggest that the processes in the dominant hemisphere which subserve the faculties of speaking, comprehending spoken language, reading and writing in the normal serve analogous functions in the congenitally deaf and that only the methods and systems of communication are different.

In support of this thesis we are reporting a case of aphasia in a patient who seemed more ideally suited for study than those previously reported since he was in the older age group, congenitally deaf, right-handed, and a native speaker of English who sustained what appeared to be a stroke involving the left cerebral circulation. In all these respects he was typical of the majority of hearing aphasic patients seen in our clinic. Further, he used and understood both basic sign language and dactylogical (finger) spelling prior to his stroke as well as writing, ordinary reading and lip reading. Of importance, too, is the fact that he was available for thorough language testing.

Neither this nor any other presentation on this subject to date can be definitive since there is as yet no universally acceptable model of how and where language is encoded and decoded.

From *Cortex* 5:398–414, 1969.

Further, we do not know precisely what areas of the brain were damaged in the case here presented.

CASE REPORT

Medical History and Course

Mr. G. L. is a 69-year-old, right-handed man who was born with a profound hearing loss. On January 19, while at work, he suddenly slumped to the floor, did not lose consciousness but was unable to move his right arm or leg. He was removed to Bellevue Hospital where examination disclosed normal vital signs, an alert, cooperative man with right central facial weakness, moderate paresis of the right arm, milder weakness of the right leg (though he was unable to walk), symmetrical tendon reflexes which were 2+ at the biceps, 1+ at the knees and absent at both ankles. Fundoscopic examination revealed mild arteriolar narrowing and no hemorrhages. The right carotid pulse was stronger than the left. It was reported that he mimicked simple commands and tried to communicate by signs. It was apparent that there had been some restoration of motor function between the time of onset and his examination at the hospital.

The patient had been under treatment for hypertension for two years prior to onset and had also been treated for gout. Three years previously he had suffered a bout of renal colic and passed a calculus spontaneously. In 1952 he had a "nervous breakdown" which prevented his working for a period of two years, apparently because of depression and lethargy.

Diagnostic studies in the hospital revealed evidence of mild arteriosclerotic heart disease and hyperuricemia (two uric acid determinations, 8.5 and 6.8 mgm %). Lumbar punctures on January 19 and 20, 1968 were normal except for proteins of 63 and 81 mgm % respectively. Skull films, brain scan and echogram were negative.

It was concluded that the patient had sustained a left cerebral infarct, exact site undetermined, most probably on the basis of arteriosclerosis, hypertension and thrombosis.

In the subsequent 11 weeks after onset (January 19 to April 2, 1968) Mr. L. gradually regained sufficient motor power in the right leg to permit walking, although poorly, and isolated movement of all segments of the right arm but without significant function in that limb. Spasticity was moderate. The left-sided limbs remained normal, all sensory modalities were intact and there was no evidence of limb apraxia or tactile agnosia on either side. Right facial weakness was now minimal, eye movements were normal, there was no nystagmus or hemianopia. The tongue and uvula moved normally.

On April 2, 1968 he was discharged from the hospital to continue physical therapy as an outpatient. He improved over the next 12 weeks, learned to walk more proficiently but did not develop good hand function.

Audiometry

Testing was done in an IAC soundproofed room. A Beltone Model 12-D audiometer was used for conventional audiometric testing. Pure tones were presented to the right ear and to the left ear by air (125; 250; 500; 750; 1000; 2000;4000 and 8000 Hz) and by bone conduction (500–4000 Hz).

No responses were obtained by bone conduction testing. No responses were obtained at the right ear by air conduction and two (500 Hz at 110;750 Hz at 105 dB) were obtained at the left ear. However, Mr. L. indicated that these tones were felt rather than heard.

The results of this testing indicated that Mr. L. has no hearing for pure tones presented up to the limits of the audiometer.

Language, Cognitive, Psychosocial History

The patient and two right-handed sisters were deaf at birth. His parents were right-handed and had normal hearing. Mr. L. married a woman whose hearing had become severely impaired at ten years of age and they produced two sons of average intelligence and normal hearing. The patient's schooling was limited to a period of five years at the Lexington School for the Deaf in New York City which he attended between the ages of five and ten. Once, during his school years, he tried and rejected a hearing aid. His wife reports that his school attendance was irregular because he was not a well child and was kept at home for extended periods. His school records were destroyed by a fire but information from his family and friends suggests that Mr. L. was of average or better intelligence and a good student.

Mr. L. is reported to have used basic signs in communicating with his parents and his deaf siblings although he also *spoke* to his parents. The patient's wife states that he would speak in short phrases, frequently without phonation but with much lip articulation and that his vocabulary was "large." At work he would mouth what he had to say and only occasionally wrote word cues. He would frequently intersperse spoken words with basic signs and finger spelling when addressing his wife. We shall refer to this method of communication as the combined method. According to friends and relatives he had little difficulty communicating with them prior to his illness although some of his gestures were understood only by members of his immediate family. Apparently basic signs and finger spelling (French one-handed method) were learned at the age of seven, at the Lexington School, and he used his right hand. We were unable to determine which was learned first or how he communicated before going to school. His right hand was also used for writing which he avoided whenever possible despite his proficiency in this skill.

With regard to his receptive abilities, he is reputed to have been a good lip reader. He could understand both basic signs and finger spelling and he read the newspaper daily.

The patient worked for over 40 years as a craftsman in a company which manufactured fine leather handbags. He was the only deaf person employed by the company. When the specifications for a new design were complete, Mr. L. hand-produced the prototype model from which the company mass-produced the finished product. He continued to work after retirement age and was at work on the day he suffered his stroke.

Mr. L. was said to be a driving, perfectionistic, compulsive person. His family describes him as someone who was fastidious about the details of everyday life. In 1952 he suffered a "nervous breakdown." Although he was not bedridden he did not work for two years. According to his wife, he spent this time at home in a state of lethargy. A teacher of the deaf who knew both the patient and his wife described them as a neurotic, tense couple. She referred to the patient as stubborn and withdrawn. Mr. L. spent most of his leisure time improving and repairing his home. He was highly skilled in carpentry, plumbing and electrical work. He and his wife, had many deaf friends but he was less apt to encourage social contact than his wife.

His son reports that for a few years prior to the stroke Mr. L. began to show signs of forgetfulness and became less fastidious and compulsive than he had been.

Language Testing

Mr. L. was tested by members of the speech pathology service at eight weeks (March 14, 1968), 11 weeks (April 2, 1968) and 23 weeks (June 25, 1968) after his stroke. Most of the testing was recorded on video tape.

Certain general observations were made. As is characteristic of the language impaired patient, Mr. L. did not appear to be as severely impaired when engaged in ordinary conversation as he did under structured tasks. Throughout, he attended very well, had good social affect and tried hard to respond. Often, however, he showed marked frustration and impatience, would point to his right hand and shake his head when he could not express himself. (This may be analogous to the normal hearing severe aphasic who sometimes points to his mouth as if to explain his inability to speak.) At one point he complained of dizziness and confusion. He perseverated a great deal and seemed to have little awareness of his errors.

During the first meeting which consisted of

informal testing, it was obvious that Mr. L. had suffered severe damage to both expressive and receptive functions. This was borne out by later testing.

At 11 weeks (4/2/68) extensive language testing was done at the Institute of Rehabilitation Medicine. On the basis of history it was known that the patient had previously expressed himself by the use of writing, basic signs, finger spelling and the spoken word and often by a combination of the latter three. Our task was to determine the extent of impairment in these five expressive modes and in comprehension through finger spelling, basic signs, lip reading, the combined method, and reading. In addition we tested arithmetic calculation.

The patient's wife and his former teacher from the New York Society for the Deaf (T.N.) assisted in the administration and interpretation of tests.

EXPRESSION

Prior to language evaluation a test for repetitive movements was administered which requires the patient to imitate and repeat as rapidly as possible a number of oral movements, syllable groups, nonsense words and sentences carrying a preponderance of consonant clusters. Responses are timed, recorded on video tape and analyzed.

Mr. L. performed the non-speech oral movements, such as opening and closing the mouth, normally. Repetition of similar syllables (e.g. pa-pa-pa) was within normal limits but "pa-ta-ka" caused him great difficulty. He was able to sustain the vowel "ah" for a normal 22 seconds. He was totally unable to repeat the nonsense words (e.g. splasha) and difficult sentences, most likely as a result of his inability to hear them when presented. His ability to perform non-speech movements without difficulty indicated that he did not have oral apraxia. Also, a hearing aphasic with oral and/or verbal apraxia and scant verbal output would not do as well as our patient did.

Speech. Although the patient was reported to have used a large vocabulary and occasionally attempted during testing to say words along with basic signs or finger spelling he was unable to produce a single word. He often pointed to his mouth in frustration.

Finger Spelling. Mr. L. used his unaffected left hand to finger spell. His former teacher demonstrated that this was more difficult but entirely feasible. He was unable to spell his wife's name, the words "coffee," "wife," or "Woodside" (the section in which he lived) in response to questions and requests to spell specific words. He did finger spell the numbers of his home address correctly. He was not able to spell his name. After demonstration of this he tried again and got the first three letters of his six letter first name correct and eight letters of the twelve letter last name in approximately the right order.

When asked to imitate the examiner's finger spelling of his name he responded after each letter but his performance deteriorated progressively.

Throughout, he made errors of omission, substitution and reversals; some of the letters were unidentifiable.

Basic Signs. Performance in this mode was clearly better than finger spelling. In response to a question on what his breakfast had consisted of, he signed "coffee." When he tried unsuccessfully to finger spell it, he signed, "I'm confused, the heck with it." Although this was his best expressive mode, his wife indicated that he was much less proficient than he had been prior to his stroke.

Combined Method. His attempts to use this method were restricted by the marked impairments in speaking and finger spelling so that responses were essentially through basic signs. In response to the question, "Do you watch television?", he indicated that he no longer did because it made him dizzy and signed, "I get mad because I can't understand because it is fuzzy."

Writing. The patient was asked to write his name, address and age. The first two he did successfully but wrote *86 year* for his age (he is 69). He was able to copy a square and the words *hat* and *spend* but could not spontaneously write what he had eaten for breakfast, an invitation to a friend or a statement on some current event. He wrote with his left hand, poorly but legibly.

To summarize, the expressive hierarchy was as follows: Our patient was most severely damaged in speaking, somewhat less in writing and finger spelling; he was most intact in using the combined method since this employed basic signs, finger spelling and whatever small assists he could muster through verbalization. It is of interest that the same expressive hierarchy existed in his premorbid communication.

Since Mr. L. had always depended upon limb movements for communication, both through finger spelling and basic signs, it was thought important to rule out limb apraxia. In their study, Goodglass and Kaplan (1963) indicated that imitation as well as spontaneous gesture and pantomime should be disturbed in apraxia. We, therefore, required that the patient imitate the following movements, which he did successfully: Closing both eyes; using a toothbrush; using a pencil; sweeping, as with a broom; swimming; a variety of body movements such as, touch the right ear with the left hand. He was also able to correctly manipulate objects such as a comb and razor. On the basis of these tests we concluded that Mr. L. did not have limb apraxia and that his manual expressive impairments were aphasic in nature.

COMPREHENSION

Comprehension was tested by an informal conversation and the administration of the Token Test (De Renzi and Vignolo 1962).

Basic Signs. The following questions were asked by basic signs: Spell your wife's name; What did you have for breakfast?; Where does your wife live?; Where do you live?; How old are you?; Do you watch television? His responses indicated that he understood all of these questions.

Finger Spelling. He was much less responsive when finger spelling was used alone indicating that in comprehension, as in expression, he was more severely impaired in finger spelling than in basic language.

Combined Method, Lip Reading, Reading. The Token Test which is usually administered orally was given to Mr. L. three ways: by oral command to test his lip reading ability, by the combined method to test his comprehension of basic signs, lip reading and finger spelling together and by presenting the commands printed on cards to test reading. The test was considered appropriate since our patient would have had difficulty only with the lip reading mode premorbidly. To make our results more meaningful the lip reading version was given for comparison to a staff member who was congenitally deaf.

In the Token Test plastic tokens in two shapes (circles and rectangles), two sizes (small and large) and five colors are placed on a table in front of the patient who then manipulates them according to commands given by the examiner; these instructions become progressively more complete.

Before the actual test was begun visual agnosia was ruled out by having the patient match tokens according to shape and color.

The test is divided into five parts:

Part I (10 commands): e.g. touch the red circle.
Part II (10 commands): e.g. touch the small yellow circle.
Part III (10 commands): e.g. touch the yellow circle and the red rectangle.
Part IV (10 commands): e.g. touch the small yellow circle and the large green rectangle.
Part V (22 commands): e.g. put the red circle on the green rectangle.

The results of the Token Test are summarized in Table 21-1. His best mode of comprehension was reading. He did less well with the combined method and very poorly in lip reading.

Reading the commands from printed cards, Mr. L. completed all five parts although he had a high percentage of errors in Parts IV and V. With the combined method, he was 50–80% correct through Part III but then could go no further (on 4/2/68). As can be seen, his lip reading impairment was so severe he could not complete a single command while his control counterpart did quite well in Parts I, II and IV, had 30% correct in Part III and only one correct in Part V.

TABLE 21–1. CORRECT RESPONSES ON TOKEN TEST. COMPARISON SCORES OF LIP READING CONTROL/(R.W.) ARE NOTED

Token Test	Reading Mr. L.	Combined method Mr. L.		Lip reading Mr. L.		Lip reading R. W.
	4/2/68	4/2/68	6/25/68	4/2/68	6/25/68	4/2/68
Part I (10 commands)	9	8	8	0	No response	9
Part II (10 commands)	8	5	8	No response	Not given	7
Part III (10 commands)	10	6	3	Not given	Not given	3
Part IV (10 commands)	3	No response	2	Not given	Not given	5
Part V (22 commands)	6	Not given	Not given	Not given	Not given	1

Since we anticipated the relative difficulty of these modes of comprehension for the patient the tests were administered in the order that would minimize the effect of practice, i.e. lip reading first, the combined method next and finally by reading.

Reading was also tested by a standard method used at our institution. The patient is presented a series of statements printed in large boldface type. He then answers written, multiple choice questions about these items. He scored 40 out of a possible 100 points on this test, a result indicative of a moderate reading impairment. This was consistent with his performance on the Token Test although reading was his best comprehension mode on that test. Note that he was only able to respond correctly to the shorter, simpler instructions (Parts I, II and III) on the Token Test.

Summarizing the results of comprehension testing, it appeared that our patient was most intact in reading. He comprehended basic signs fairly well but below his premorbid ability. He was severely impaired in the comprehension of finger spelling and lip reading.

Although it was difficult to quantify, it was the impression of all observers that Mr. L. was generally more severely damaged in expressive than receptive modalities. He did best with basic signs and understood more than he could express.

Finally, calculation ability was tested and found to be severely impaired. On a test requiring the patient to count, add, subtract, multiply and divide he scored 23 out of a possible 100. He could not solve any of the written problems nor do multiple digit addition or subtraction.

On 6/25/68 the patient was again tested but refused to take the complete battery which had been administered on 4/2/68. A Ph.D. member of the staff who was congenitally deaf acted as communicant this time.

Some improvement was noted in his oral output. He now phonated more frequently and attempted spontaneous speech more often. He used the words "coffee" and "show" spontaneously and counted to ten.

Only mild improvement was noted in his ability to finger spell. He still misspelled his wife's name and the word "Woodside." In spelling his own name there were several letter repetitions, reversals and substitutions. On this occasion he successfully finger counted up to number ten.

Communication by basic signs showed greater improvement than finger spelling. For example, he was able through signs to explain that he watched television but did little reading. The quality and speed of performance were improved.

His ability to understand signs and finger spelling was definitely improved. His percentage of correct responses to signed and spelled words had increased. Of all input and output modalities, including speech but exclusive of reading and writing, this showed the greatest improvement.

Using the combined method, the repeat Token Test on 6/25/68 showed little improvement (see Table 21-1). He attempted Part IV though most of the responses were incorrect. Comprehension through lip reading showed no improvement.

DISCUSSION

Our patient suffered a motor stroke with aphasia involving all communication modalities. Presumably he sustained an infarction involving the left fronto-parietal region; one can say no more than this regarding localization and pathology.

In many respects he resembled hearing aphasics with strokes involving the dominant hemisphere. He had a history of hypertension, suffered the sudden onset of right hemiplegia without loss of consciousness, recovered some function of the limbs in a few hours but remained with hemiparesis and a profound aphasia. He had no sensory, visual or cognitive deficits so far as could be determined and no limb apraxia.

His behavior was typical of the hearing aphasic. He was depressed, frustrated, often angry. He would point to his right hand when unable to respond as though it was responsible for his aphasia very much as hearing aphasics point to their mouths.

There was also a striking similarity in the elements of his communication impairment with those of many hearing aphasics: he did better in a functional or conversational situation than in clinical testing (Taylor 1965); he was more impaired in expressive than in receptive modes. Using the combined method for comprehension he did moderately well on the Token Test and with reading did even better. To be sure, his lip reading ability was severely impaired but it had always been the least efficient of his comprehension modes. In contradistinction, testing revealed severe deficits in writing, finger spelling, the use of basic signs and speaking. He had letter finding difficulties in finger spelling which might be considered analogous to letter or phoneme losses in the hearing aphasic. He also used letters out of sequence, omitted or substituted them, all of which have their counterparts in the hearing group. The loss of spoken words was entirely equivalent. He had a tendency to perseverate on words or letters.

He seemed to have better recovery of comprehension than expressive skills. While there was significant improvement in his understanding of finger spelling and basic signs between 4/2/68 and 6/25/68, his output changed but little.

The degree of recovery noted on 6/25/68 was consonant with the severity of his impairment when he was first tested. That is to say, he improved but still had severe aphasia, as an experienced worker might have predicted. It should be noted here that all impressions of improved performance were documented by study of the video tapes done on 4/2/68 and 6/25/68.

The sum of neurological and language deficits in our patients have suggested to us that the areas and processes in the dominant hemisphere which subserve communication functions are the same for the congenitally deaf as for the hearing person. This assertion must eventually be substantiated by objective methods. However, it is reasonable to suppose that the congenitally deaf are born with the same anlage for developing communication skills as normal hearing people. The enunciation of words, the spelling of words with the fingers or the manipulation of the hands and arms to communicate whole concepts would all seem to be but motor variations of an underlying language process which is stable and immutable for all humans. Finger spelling is an alphabet which is signed rather than written. Is there a basic difference between the motor act of moving a pen to produce a series of letters and manipulating one's fingers to produce the same letters?

It is more difficult to equate finger spelling

with speaking. However, one can argue that the need to realize conceptualized thought is basic to the human species and that man has developed a variety of ways of expressing thought or emotion. The fact that the motor mechanism of speech is more complex than that of writing or finger spelling should not deter us from hypothesizing that they are motor variants of each other. The vocabulary and syntax for all are the same. Basic signs, on the other hand, have a "vocabulary and syntax" of their own but are still motor and the means of expressing thought or emotion.

This formulation would require that one consider the process of communication to be a function of at least three sub-processes. The following is an oversimplification of the problem but may clarify the concept: that (1) there is a level of language conceptualization which is closely related to or indivisible from the process of thought initiation; that (2) impulses from the brain areas where these are mediated stimulate a process of language organization from which stimuli are transmitted to the appropriate motor nuclei for (3) final expression. Decoding would represent the process in reverse: visual and auditory (and tactile in the case of braille reading) stimuli are organized into recognizable symbols and forms and interpreted at the highest level as meaningful language. Aphasia, then, reflects a disturbance in the organizational processes of communication.

As further support for this hypothesis of a basic, underlying communication process, one might evoke the theories of Chomsky (1967) and Lenneberg (1967) that man's language capacity is a function of biologically determined, species specific, innate brain processes, which require only experience in order to develop into functional communication. If such is the case, it is reasonable to suppose that although the congenitally deaf have a different developmental experience and may use different methods of communication, the basic process is the same as in the normal person.

Since the behavior of our patient violates neither our understanding of aphasia as seen in those with normal hearing nor any reasonable model of human communication, we are inclined to the view that aphasia in the congenitally deaf is entirely equivalent to that in normal hearing people.

SUMMARY

The case of a 69-year-old congenitally deaf man who had a stroke resulting in right hemiparesis and aphasia is presented. Investigation of his communication skills revealed deficits analogous to those seen in hearing aphasics. Results suggest that the congenitally deaf encode and decode language by the same fundamental processes as those with normal hearing.

Acknowledgments. The authors wish to thank Dr. D. Ballantyne and Miss Tanya Nash for their assistance in interpreting the patient's responses and Mr. Robert Wilson for his willingness to act as control for the Token Test.

REFERENCES

Alajouanine, T., and Lhermitte, F. (1964) *Non-verbal communication in aphasia,* in Disorders of Language, ed. by A. V. S. de Reuck and M. O'Connor, Little, Brown and Co., Boston.

Critchley, M. (1938) *Aphasia in a partial deaf-mute,* "Brain," **61,** 163–169.

Chomsky, N. (1967) *The general properties of language,* in Brain Mechanisms Underlying Speech and Language, ed. by C. H. Millikan and F. L. Darley, Grune and Stratton, N.Y.

De Renzi, E., and Vignolo, L. A. (1962) *The Token Test: a sensitive test to detect receptive disturbances in aphasics,* "Brain," **85,** 665–678.

Douglass, E., and Richardson, J. C. (1959) *Aphasia in a congenital deaf-mute,* "Brain," **83,** 68–80.

Goodglass, H., and Kaplan, E. (1963) *Disturbance of*

gesture and pantomime in Aphasia, "Brain," **86,** 703–720.

Grasset, J. (1896) *Aphasie de la main droite chez un sourd muet*, "Le Progres Medical," **4,** 281.

Hughlings-Jackson, J. (1878) *On affections of speech from disease of the brain*, "Brain," **1,** 304–330.

Leischner, A. (1943) *Die "Aphasie" der Taubstummen*, "Arch. fur Psych.," **115,** 469–548.

Lenneberg, E. H. (1967) *Biological Foundations of Language*, J. Wiley and Sons, N.Y.

Taylor, M. L. (1965) *A measurement of functional communication in aphasia*, "Arch. Phys. Med. Rehab.," **46,** 101–107.

Tureen, L. L., Smolik, E. A., and Tritt, J. H. (1951) *Aphasia in a deaf-mute*, "Neurology," **1,** 237–249.

22

Aphasia and Artistic Realization

THEOPHILE ALAJOUANINE

THEOPHILE ALAJOUANINE, M.D., is with the department of neurology and neuropsychology of the Hopital de la Salpêtrière, Paris.

The subject of this communication lies within the borderland of aphasia; and among the patients suffering from that severe neurological disorder I shall consider only that rare group whose activity before their illness was chiefly devoted to artistic realization. In what measure, and what way, that is altered by aphasia is exactly the question which I shall try to answer, by taking as examples the case-histories of three kinds of artist: writer, musician and painter. Thus my theme is to inquire what happens to productive literary, musical or pictorial activity after the onset of aphasia. Is the deterioration of artistic creation the same in importance in our understanding of the physiopathology of language, of the mental state of aphasia, or even of the psychophysiology of the artist? To that doubtless too ambitious programme, I hope to bring at least some precise material, in some way experimental, drawn from three histories concerning three great artists whom I have been privileged to follow myself over a long time, and whose work before their illness allows a precise comparison between their artistic production before and after their aphasia.

Let us consider first the case of the artist who uses the common tool of language, words and sentences, i.e. the writer. For his artistic creation (prose or poetry) he uses everyone's language. While M. Jourdain, the character of Molière's "Would-be gentleman" was amazed and delighted to know that his language was prose, and that he was thus using prose without being aware of it; conversely the writer makes more or less consciously or cleverly literary works by using everyday language in his own way. The way in which he uses language to dress his thoughts and to express their shades forms the peculiar artistic quality of literary work, and gives it both its individuality and its aesthetic value. That will be destroyed by aphasia.

There is in French literature a sadly famous example of a great poet crippled during his literary production by aphasia: Charles Baudelaire, who is perhaps, at least in my opinion, the greatest French poet of the nineteenth century. Suddenly, while his artistic creation was at its height, he suffered from a right-sided hemiplegia with aphasia. We do not know his exact medical history, but we gather from his friends that he was able to say just one word, a curse: "cré nom." He relied upon it to express quite different states of mind. One finds easily there the essential features so well expressed by Hughlings-Jackson: the preservation of a "leitmotiv word" (a curse as so frequently is the case), its use with various meanings, sometimes a purposeful one, sometimes an emotional one. But for our purpose one fact is sure: any artistic realization had been since forbidden to Baudelaire, though we do not know whether he ever

From *Brain* 71:229–41, 1948. Reprinted by permission of the Editor of *Brain*.

made any attempt to write with his unaffected hand.

I can afford more precise observations on a contemporary writer, whom I have followed for over ten years, and whose literary position I can only sketch, since he is still alive. When quite young, after he had attained a foremost rank in French contemporary literature by his poems, novels, essays on foreign literature (especially on English literature which he knows perfectly well and which he has interpreted to us in its newest expressions) he was suddenly affected by a right-sided hemiplegia with aphasia. The hemiplegia has remained severe, with a considerable spasticity, interfering with the gait and preventing any movement in the upper limb. Language, at first rather uniformly impaired in its verbal and graphic expressions, comprehension remaining quite good, improved gradually. Today, conversation is possible, but there is a synthetic reformation of the agrammatic type. He went through various phases during the rehabilitation process: at first wide, if not generalized, paraphasia, with a curious recurring utterance —"Bonsoir les choses d'ici bas"—he used to answer in an involuntary and automatic way every time he wanted to say anything. Even the customary "Bonsoir" was replaced by that melancholy expression. Then the "leit-motiv" sentence disappeared during the improvement of his voluntary speech, which was at first poor, slow, difficult and then more definite, despite his painful and at times impatient or disheartened attempts. At the present time, the trouble of synthetic construction remains the major element; the phonetic trouble has almost disappeared and the voluntary evocation of vocabulary is greatly improved. Written language has followed a parallel restoration. It is of course performed with the left hand and there is in it the same aggrammatism. On the contrary reading became rapidly possible, although slow. But if he can now, as before, read his favourite books in several languages (and before all English, Italian and Spanish, without any noticeable difference) he can write only sentences where the persistent trouble of synthetic construction forbids any literary production (at least the one he was used to for he did not employ that conventional agrammatism of some of the young literary schools).

Is the abolition of artistic activity in our patient due to a special deterioration of mental abilities caused by the disease? We have made a special study of that problem many times and we think it is not possible to correlate the inability of this writer to continue his work, with a deficiency of memory, reasoning, judgment or affectivity. His memory is remarkably preserved, of which I can give an example: once, while speaking with him about English contemporary literature, at a time when he was still very aphasic, he had just shown me an autographed book by James Joyce, and he wanted to refer to another author, upon whom he had also written an essay, but whose name he could not find despite his efforts. As I could not make out whom he meant, he stood up and walked uneasily to his library which contained several thousands of English books, and without any hesitation picked out the volume he wanted. It was by Coventry Patmore. His judgment can be evaluated by the way he saw through the press his works which were still unpublished at the time of his aphasia, and more particularly by the following fact: in the course of collecting some essays to be published, one of his friends, who was in charge of the publication, was of opinion that one of the chapters was of a lesser quality. He did not know how to make this understood by the patient without hurting his feelings. He was amazed to see the patient himself, despite his aphasia, realize that inferiority. The pages of the manuscript were turned before him, and at the place of dubious value, his friend asked him whether it should be omitted. As if he had understood, he pointed out the part in question, and said with effort—"not good"—finding at last the way to express his thought. I can add that the aesthetic taste of my patient does not seem to have been impaired by aphasia. Many examples show me that the characteristic trends of his literary personality have not been modified by the illness.

This, then, is an instance of a Broca aphasia in a writer which in spite of its marked improvement, and although it did not noticeably impair the aesthetic sense, judgment and memory, has abolished the possibility of literary artistic realization. The reason lies mainly in that disturbance of literary technique due to disease which converted that delicate artist and subtle grammarian into an agrammatist.

The next case-history concerns a musician. The artist who expresses himself by music uses a language which is not the common language made up of words and sentences. His is the musical language where instead of words the symbols comprise various sounds, united into melodic phrases, which are endlessly varied by the laws of harmony, instrumental technique and rich orchestral possibilities, just as the word assemblages—sentences of the poetic or prosaic speech—are endlessly diversified by the thoughts of the writer who uses them. To a spontaneous language, which, we are told, can be traced up to Amphion, the sons of man have given by the protean wealth of their sound-combinations unequalled powers of evocation, where each in turn sings joy or pain, pleasure or melancholy. Cleverly elaborated technique allows its extreme differentiation which seems endless. Just as it breaks the poet's calamus, so aphasia ruins Orpheus' lyre.

My second example is that of a famous musician whom I followed for over two years. He belonged to the pleasing class of musicians who have introduced a novel style, an original manner, and have expressed in a particular language a personality which will endure in the history of his art. At the peak of his artistic achievement, rich through an abundant and varied work, already classic, which expresses a delicate climate, Maurice Ravel is struck down by an aphasia. His aphasia is more complex than the writer's: it is a Wernicke aphasia of moderate intensity, without any trace of paralysis, without hemianopia, but with an ideomotor apractic component. The cause, though indefinite, belongs to the group of cerebral atrophies, there being a bilateral ventricular enlargement; but it is quite different from Pick's disease. Oral and written language are diffusely impaired, but moderately so, without any noticeable intellectual weakening. Memory, judgment, affectivity, aesthetic taste do not show any impairment to repeated tests. Understanding of language remains much better than oral or written abilities. Writing, especially, is very faulty, mainly due to apraxia. Musical language is still more impaired, but not in a uniform manner. There is chiefly a quite remarkable discrepancy between a loss of musical expression (written or instrumental), and musical thinking, which is comparatively well preserved. With the help of two musicians, a favourite pupil of the master and a neurologist with great musical ability we could study as precisely as possible musical tune recognition, note recognition (musical dictation), note reading and solfeggio piano playing, and dictated musical writing (copied or spontaneous). I apologize for giving such an analysis, but it seems to me essential in respect of the value of such a case-history.

Recognition of tunes played before our musician is generally good and prompt. He recognizes immediately most of the works he knew, and anyway he recognizes perfectly his own works. That recognition is not a vague one, for he is able to evaluate exactly rhythm and style as shown by the following facts. He immediately notices the lightest mistake in the playing; several parts of the "Tombeau de Couperin" were first correctly played, and then with minor errors (either as to notes or rhythm). He immediately protested and demanded a perfect accuracy. When playing the beginning of "La pavane de ma Mère l'Oye" which contains two exactly similar bars, one was omitted. The patient immediately stopped the pianist. He succeeded in explaining, in his halting speech, that the first bar was to link with the preceding part. The same is true for rhythm: if played too fast, he protests and has the music played again with its exact rhythm. Another remark: during these studies on musical interference of aphasia, my piano—because of the dampness of the winter—had become somewhat out of tune. The patient noticed it and demonstrated the dissonance by playing two notes one octave apart, thus showing again the preservation of sound recognition and valuation.

On the contrary analytic recognition of notes, and musical dictation, are quite faulty, or seemingly so, since he could name only some notes hesitatingly and with difficulty. His numerous mistakes are due, very likely, to aphasia itself, and to the difficulty of finding the name of a note, a trouble exactly similar to name designation for common objects. The fact that reproduction of notes played on the piano, without giving their name, is quite good, seems to confirm this opinion.

Note reading is extremely difficult. From time to time a note is read exactly. Most often reading is impossible. The same is true for solfeggio. The trouble of name-finding may partly explain the failure. But there is something more, since piano playing is almost impossible after reading. A component due to apraxia supervenes therein. Anyway a quite definite discrepancy is noted between deciphering musical signs, and their visual recognition. If an analytic deciphering is almost impossible, on the contrary the patient is able to recognize at first glance whatever piece he has to find, and that without any error.

Piano playing is very difficult, since in addition to difficulty in reading, our aphasic patient has to search for the location of notes on the keyboard. He sometimes misplaces notes without being aware of it. For instance he plays the *mi-mi* instead of the *do-do* arpeggio, and plays it again and again, until his fingers are placed on the proper keys. He plays scales quite well, both major and minor ones. Diesis and flats are well marked. There is just a praxic difficulty. He can play with only one hand (the right one) the beginning of "Ma Mère l'Oye." With both hands, he cannot decipher. He needs many exercises to play in that way. In spite of numerous exercises during a whole week he cannot succeed in playing the beginning of the "Pavan," even with separate hands. On the contrary he has a greater performance ability when he plays by heart pieces of his own composition. He suddenly gives a right idea of the beginning of "Le Tombeau de Couperin" which is, however, too difficult to finish. Seven or eight bars are played almost perfectly, and he plays them, transposing to the lower tierce, without any error. When attempting an unknown piece he finds a much greater difficulty: he cannot play more than two or three notes of a piece by Scarlatti, which he did not previously know.

Musical writing is very difficult, although better preserved than plain writing. He writes dictated notes slowly and with numerous errors, but copying is almost impossible and requires from the patient enormous effort. On the contrary, writing by heart a portion of his "Entretiens de la belle et la bête," though difficult and slow, is better performed than the other tests. Notes are better and more quickly placed, and he seems mainly disturbed by writing apraxia. Singing by heart is correctly performed for some of his works, but only if the first note or notes are given. He says that tunes come back quite easily, and that he can hear them singing "in his head." Musical thinking seems comparatively better preserved than musical language itself.

Though all artistic realization is forbidden to our musician, he can still listen to music, attend a concert, and express criticism on it or describe the musical pleasure he felt. His artistic sensibility does not seem to be in the least altered, nor his judgment, as his admiration for the romantic composer Weber shows, which he told me several times. He can also judge contemporary musical works.

Thus, in our musician, because of aphasia, and as already mentioned, because of a simultaneous apraxia, musical reading, piano playing, use of musical signs are much more impaired than expression and recognition of musical themes. Severe disturbance of realization, and difficulty of expressing a relatively preserved musical thinking, while affectivity and aesthetic sensibility are almost intact, are the main features of our composer's case-history. They explain why his work has been completely arrested by his cerebral affection.

And now here is the painter. The artist here does not use for his creation oral or written language. From his visual perceptions, and according to the way his hand can transcribe them, through drawing and colors, a particular aesthetic pleasure will emerge through the magic of a figurated art. From sensory images taken out of nature, and from the observation of the marvellous playing of light upon forms, a personal vision is suggested, in which are brought to life the expressions of a varied poetry, from the moving grace of a face, to familiar or grand life, from the charming melancholy of the luminous haze on a landscape to the merry glow of a bunch of flowers. What will aphasia do against the realization of that living and colored architecture? If it destroyed literary language in the writer, if it stopped sound expression in the musician, it leaves untouched plastic or figurated realization.

The painter who represents my third example is one of the most representative artists of the French contemporary school, because of the originality of matter, technical qualities of realization, and intense individualism of each of his works. He expressed the poetry of the Normandy coast, the glowing beauty of flowers or marine life, and the richness of feminine flesh. Poet and symphonist as much as a painter, he creates a climate where personal sounds vibrate, and gives to plastic art numerous resoundings, at first of a different nature: one often feels the bitter and sensual poetry of Baudelaire, and at times also the delicious polyphonic music of Debussy, mixing by a kind of sorcery their different languages to form his colored magic. His pictorial art is far from being only a purely sensorial expression; it contains numerous intellectual and affective components, which, however, are untouched by aphasia.

When he was 52, he was suddenly deprived of language after two short and transient aphasic spells. His aphasia is of the Wernicke type, without any phonetic trouble, without any right-sided hemiplegia, but with a slight hemianopic defect. Spoken language is much impaired, paraphasia is striking, voluntary vocabulary finding much disturbed, but understanding remains quite good because mainly of an intuitive grasp of the general meaning of conversation. Written language is impaired in a parallel way for reading as well as for writing. Writing is slow but has undergonc no deformation. Intellectual impairment is not to be found. Although oral or written conversation became very difficult especially when concerned with the aesthetic problems in which he used to be interested one can easily realize that memory judgment and taste are not at all impaired. But his always sharp affectivity is still sharper: he is irritable, sad, and disquieted by his illness, and he increases the isolation to which he was prone. His artistic activity remains undisturbed, even at a time when his aphasia had not yet diminished very much. He stopped drawing only for a short time when an apraxia—fortunately transient—supervened.

Artistic realization in our painter since his aphasia remains as perfect as before. According to connoisseurs, he has perhaps gained a more intense and acute expression. If one tries to analyze his production before and after his aphasia, one cannot find since his language deterioration any mistake in form, expression or color interpretation. There are no changes in the interpretation of sensorial data, no technical failure; neither is there any disturbance of thought. I am of the opinion that he lays emphasis on thematic characteristics with a poetical strength, in a completely unaltered manner, and that since his illness he has even accentuated the intensity and the sharpness of his artistic realization. Moreover, his activity and production have not slowed down, and he seems to work with the same speed. Perhaps, because of new affective conditions, his works are less regular. His preferred themes are the same without any duplication of the past ones. His inventive ability, his spontaneity seem untouched. Perhaps he is more prone, however, to use a previous model, or a discarded sketch. Anyway, his individuality has not been altered at all, as far as artistic realization is concerned, and every critic can discern in all of his works the hand of the artist he used to know.

It seems that our painter's artistic production goes on as if nothing had happened, and that in him the aphasic and the artist live together on two distinct planes. As he says himself when congratulated upon his artistic activity: "There are in me two men, the one who paints, who is normal while he is painting, and the other one who is lost in the mist, who docs not stick to life.

. . . I am saying very poorly what I mean. . . . There are inside me the one who grasps reality, life; there is the other one who is lost as regards abstract thinking. When I am painting I am outside my own life; my way of seeing things is even sharper than before: I find everything again; I am a whole man. Even my right hand that seems strange to me, I do not notice when I am painting. These are two men, the one who is grasped by reality to paint, the other one, the fool, who cannot manage words any more." Is it possible to describe better than our painter, with his faulty speech, the discrepancy he felt within himself between his speech abilities and expression through his representative art?

This last example shows—in contrast to what happens to the writer and the composer when deprived by aphasia of their artistic creative power—that a perfect preservation of pictorial artistic realization can occur despite a severe and persistent aphasia.

These are the facts I wanted first to analyze in some detail, to give all the data about the problems they suggest. We cannot think of drawing from these three histories all the conclusions they permit, so inexhaustible is psychological investigation in aphasia, furthermore, our goal is quite different.

It remains that three great artists are incapacitated by aphasia, as far as verbal and graphic expression is concerned. But concerning artistic realization they behave quite differently. Artistic production, completely preserved in the painter, is abolished in the writer and in the composer. These facts seem so definite that they do not need a long discussion, which could be endless, since neither Ruskin in England, nor Taine in France, have exhausted aesthetic problems. More modestly and more practically we simply want to stress what can be learned from these three cases as to the nature of intellectual impairment in aphasia, and its consequences in artistic realization, depending on the different nature and means of expression of the three arts.

Let us first remark, to avoid criticism about methodology in seeking to compare facts of too different a nature, that we are perfectly aware of the differences between the aphasias of our various artists. But has man ever seen two exactly identical aphasias? That does not depend only on the differences between the lesions (we do not consider anatomical or topographical conditions since our analysis is purely a functional one). We do not misjudge the various influences of somatic lesions on physiological and psychological processes which lie beneath language, but we believe that everyone's language is the expression of a complex whole, that goes beyond language itself, and expresses a totality and an individuality. Aphasia more or less respects that personality, as far as it remains unaltered by psychic troubles. These individual differences will help to differentiate each aphasic patient's language, even if gravely altered. Anyway the aphasia is different in each of our three cases. The writer has a Broca aphasia, the musician and the painter have a Wernicke's aphasia, complicated by a permanent apraxia in the composer and a transient one in the painter. But we know that if the phonetic troubles which characterize Broca's aphasia have a definite physiopathological and topographical value, as far as neurological interpretation is concerned, it is not enough to differentiate the aphasia with which it is associated. Language troubles are not of a different nature because a motor trouble which has to do with the organs of speech supervenes in these cases. That allows a comparison with the cases of the musician and of the painter whose language was impaired in a similar way, but without any phonetic syndrome. More important at first sight is the fact that our composer's aphasia was accompanied by apraxia, the role of which we have stressed in some of his troubles with musical expression, especially instrumental execution. On the contrary apraxia has nothing to do with his other defects in musical language. In reading, and in musical dictation, apraxia does not interfere, and cannot be blamed for the defect in artistic realization. Our musician might have remained a great composer, even if unable to play or to conduct his works. Is it not a similar example on a purely sensorial plane to the one given by Beethoven, deaf, going on with his work, without being able to hear it, or by Milton, finishing his admirable poetical work which he could not read?

The main fact is that our three aphasic artists have in common a language trouble that spares their personality, especially its aesthetic components that does not alter at all their sensibility, their memory, their judgment, or their taste, and where means of expression are much more altered than understanding. On the contrary they differ in that the writer and the composer are, consequently, annihilated as to their artistic production, while the painter is not affected. Although the same sensibility and aesthetic taste remain, although he is able to read his favored poet, even in a foreign language, our writer is no longer able to describe orally or by writing his emotion or his own artistic ideal. Although he possesses a relatively intact power of musical thinking, with excellent rhythm and recognition of style, and an unaltered aesthetic sensibility, our composer cannot give us any longer the expression (written or melodic) of his delightful musical language. As for our painter, although he explains only with imperfect and vague words the aims of his research for color values and the significance of his plastic figuration, he continues as well as before giving us speaking pictures as beautiful as ever.

This is the main fact that comes out of the comparison of our three artists. If, as Jackson said, one does not try to define whether intelligence is altered in aphasic patients, but only what form of intelligence is modified, one can say, doubtlessly, that the work of art, or at least its realization—that essentially intellectual manifestation—is not identically altered in aphasic artists. Since their similar language disturbance does not show any difference that may explain the fact, it is in the different nature of their art, and in the means they use to express themselves, that the reason of it is to be looked for. Being especially disabled in their expressive abilities by aphasia, as we have seen, our writer and composer are not able to express themselves by literature or music, for their technique is based on language and we have no reason to wonder at their failure in artistic realization. But since the painter does not suffer from his language deterioration, we have to consider the insignificant part played by language in plastic realization.

So we come to investigate technical means of the arts we consider in their relation with language. Art may be described as the expression of an individuality by way of appropriate technique. We have seen the almost complete preservation of each artist's individuality. Let us consider the differences between their technique.

Literary art is entirely dependent upon language in its outward expression. Nobody can deny it. Highest thinking, deepest sentiments are just immaterial facts of consciousness, if they are not clad in the flesh of language. When considering an aphasic patient's behaviour, while he uses his emotional or volitional speech, one cannot wonder at the aphasic writer meeting a considerable amount of difficulty in literary expression. Imprecision of aphasic speech, difficult adaptation of thinking to verbal or graphic expression, failure or slowing of realization are among the most important causes of failure. Difficulty in reaching abstraction for a writer who would not stick to material expression of a schematic tale is another main stumbling-block. Furthermore, if there is a synthetic disturbance, i.e. agrammatism, one may realize the presence of an invincible difficulty, because of the chief importance of grammatical construction and style in literary realization. The aphasic patient, with the involuntary use of ready-made sentences unadapted to what he wants to express, shows in some way a negative picture of literary art. One can say that his thinking itself is not noticeably impaired; realization of linguistic form, on the contrary, will remain quite unadapted. The aphasic patient, as Hughlings Jackson said, "is lame in thinking," one could add "he is lame in literary writing."

For the composer, who too has to master a language to express himself, the same is true. Musical language is made up of signs, where sounds represent a mere symbolism, but where the modes of musical phrases, with their intentional descriptive or affective meaning, represent a superior symbolism. Melodic forms are cleverly placed according to more or less conventional, arbitrary or individual patterns, in which may be recognized, superimposed on his thinking, the genius or technical ability of the author. Furthermore graphic transcription of a musical work needs a scriptorial expression similar to literary writing. That shows how many factors, of various levels, make artistic realization, as expressed in a musical work, and how such technique will be altered by aphasia as easily as the technique of literary expressions since we deal here also with an artistic expression through a language. That explains why, with a relatively preserved musical thinking that allows him to hear "inside himself" a musical phrase, or even to sing a tuneful theme, to hear and to appreciate a performance, our composer cannot however express his thoughts by writing or playing them. Musical expression is in him grossly impaired. Accordingly his artistic creation is completely destroyed, as it was in the writer, and, seemingly, in a somewhat similar way, with in addition an important apraxic component, as we have already stressed. So one may see the importance of unaltered means of expression in artistic realization. To conceive is nothing, to express is all. Pleasing musical themes, and likely poetical expressions remain, doubtlessly, deeply buried in many people, who have not found, for various reasons, chiefly technical ones, the necessary means with which to express them. The cause of the failure of both our artists appears to be a technical one. Mechanisms necessary to technical accomplishment of literary or musical works have been destroyed or altered by aphasia.

These two preceding examples are in agreement with all we know about interference of language impairment upon intellectual expression during aphasia. The particular point is that our third artist escapes such a disaster in the realization of his plastic work. Let us consider the reasons. Here, the painter will draw a figurated expression, aiming to suggest an interpretation of the world, from visual perceptions, forms and colors. That visual construction made up of drawing, composition, and color values, evokes in the observer various reactions, ranging from direct sensory impressions, more or less marked, to various emotions in which intelligence has a part (understanding, evaluation, comparison, discussion or realization and technique) but where visual sensations are prominent (harmony, expression, climate, visual satisfaction). We know that aesthetic pleasure, before a work of art, is not merely the result of sensorial function, but, unless we discuss some modern abstract painting, we cannot deny its main importance. Properly speaking, pictorial expression does not use a language, although sometimes the term of "pictorial language" is used. There is no plastic language, and the same is true for sculpture. There is a way of using drawing and color to express forms and light, and an art to emphasize them. This is not the use of a language made up of symbols, it is the use of a plastic reality, more or less transposed by particular technique into a climate which, in the painter, is the exact equivalent of the language. If the climate of a Rembrandt, of a Leonardo da Vinci, or of a Turner is immediately recognizable, it is so in quite a different way than is the language of Byron or Wagner. Because his climate is a direct one, without any symbolistic medium, we are conscious of it immediately, and we simultaneously take a part in the vision he gives us. On the other hand, the figurated expression of the musician, and to some extent that of the writer, is presented to us as a whole that flows through time, made of successive phases, which we have to remember to be able to gather. Aphasia, consequently, does not alter plastic expressive power, since it takes place outside language. Only visual agnosia, an "imperception" as Jackson used to say, by altering form and color perception would destroy their use in artistic realization. Of course, a concomitant apraxia would deprive the artist's hand of the power of laying on a canvas his personal vision. That happened in the case of our painter, fortunately only for a time. It is not without interest to notice that the most intellectual part of pictorial conception—the choice of a theme, the disposition of the subject, and the appreciation of values, i.e. everything that requires judgment—is not disturbed either. In addition to technique itself, the conceptual part of artistic realization remains unaltered by our painter's aphasia. But, as we have already mentioned, one may imagine that a painting, which is not made up of predominant sensorial components, but of abstract figuration, that is real ideograms, might be deeply altered by an aphasia. We would not, however, go so far as to hope that Picasso becomes aphasic, to show us that he can no longer paint in his present manner, but that he is still able to give us the fine paintings of his "blue period."

To summarize, we may state that the painter may continue with his artistic production despite aphasia, because it impairs a language but leaves him able to use his visual perceptions to create, through technical means, form and light values, a sensorial use of reality, but unable to use a language made up of symbols. In agreement with Jackson's idea that aphasia does not alter the whole of intelligence, but only part of it, artistic creation becomes impossible when aphasia disturbs techniques based on language, but preserves techniques based on visual perceptions. This fact also shows that a theory, such as the German authors' "Gestalt," cannot be applied to every case, or to every form of aphasia. On the contrary it seems to agree with Henry Head's view on the part played by alteration of symbolic thinking in aphasia.

If art, as one has said, is just "overcome difficulty," one must agree that aphasia creates for writers and musicians a major, insuperable difficulty: realization of an artistic language with deteriorated tools. The painter, with an impaired language tool, may use untouched visual perceptions and continue with his artistic creation.

This implies:

(1) The different nature of the psychophysiology in artistic realization in the writer and composer on the one hand and in the painter on the other.

(2) The main part played, in the disturbance caused by aphasia, by the alteration of technique which remains localized to language.

(3) The preponderance of altered means of expression in the failure of artistic realization, as compared with preservation of conceptual thinking.

(4) Intellectual interference in aphasia, as far as artistic creation is concerned, remains localized mainly to expressive means based on language.

Brain Disorders and Language Analysis

ALEXANDER R. LURIA

ALEXANDER R. LURIA, M.D., D.Sc., is head of the Neuropsychological Laboratory and is with the department of psychology at Moscow University.

Separate regions of the cortex form complicated systems for the analysis and synthesis of visual, auditory, kinesthetic and motor stimuli. Focal lesions of the brain produce a break-down in such analysis and synthesis and lead to a secondary disturbance of a whole complex of functions.

Lesions in the left temporal zone cause a break-down in the discrimination and generalization of sound patterns, and above all in phonemic auditory perception. This in turn affects pronunciation and writing, and also the structure of word-meanings. This failure at the lexical level affects the various parts of a word in different degrees: the roots of words, which carry the more concrete meaning, are lost, while suffixes, with their more abstract meaning, are retained.

Clinical observation of different cases throws light on the distinction between the "communication of events" and the "communication of relations." Lesions in the parietal and parieto-occipital areas produce a failure in dealing with "communications of relations," a failure to combine a number of elements into a single whole. When these lesions extend to the borders of the speech area, they entail a further break-down in operations that require the abstraction of a scheme of reference. "Communication of relations" necessitates precisely this operation and this explains why patients with parieto-occipital lesions are often unable to deal with such communications.

Lesions in the fronto-temporal areas affect the synthesis of successive elements and hence lead to a failure in "propositionizing."

In all cases of parieto-occipital lesion the "regulating" function of speech remains intact. Animal experiments have shown that ablation of the frontal sections of the cortex completely upsets the regulation of the animal's behavior. In man, frontal lesions interfere with the regulating function of speech without affecting other speech functions.

From *Language and Speech* 1:14–34, 1958.

Observation of aphasia—and more broadly of brain disorders of various kinds—has always provided invaluable material for analysis of the structure of human speech, and hence for a better understanding of some aspects of language structure. What is an indivisible whole in a normal person, and therefore difficult to analyze , in a pathological condition is split up and becomes accessible to analytical investigation, which is always concerned with the isolation of the basic components of a complex whole. The task of isolating such components in human speech and studying the complicated functional systems that directly depend on these components is the immediate purpose of utilizing pathological conditions of the brain for psychological and linguistic analysis.

Pathological conditions of the brain, and above all those which occur as a result of limited local affections, never produce a direct disintegration of the complex formation of language—morphology, syntax, lexicology or semantics. The time when research workers tried to find in the cerebral cortex special "centers" for understanding or pronunciation of words, for morphological, syntactic or semantic formations as well as for writing, reading and counting, has irrevocably gone. Attempts to correlate directly the various affections of the brain with various aspects of language was done by Head, and attempts to describe special forms of [illegible] nominal, syntactic and semantic aphasia [illegible] have no other value than as the initial summary of clinical observations; to [illegible] understanding [illegible] dynamic processes that have led to the emergence of the syndrome.

At present, thanks [illegible] achieved by normal morpho-physiology, [illegible] the clinical study of focal lesions and by the combined efforts of physiologists and psychologists in the study of syndromes which arise in localized affections of the brain, the position has radically changed; research workers can now formulate certain basic theses which make the data of brain pathology incomparably more fruitful for the analysis of normal functions.

It has been established by modern [illegible] physiology that separate regions of the cerebral cortex form the most complicated apparatus for specific forms of analysis and synthesis of "exteroceptive" or "proprioceptive" stimuli; Pavlov quite justifiably called these the "cortical analyzer terminals". Under normal circumstances the function of this apparatus proceeds with sufficient force, balance and mobility of the nervous processes and it guarantees the finest analysis and synthesis of visual, auditory, kinesthetic or motor stimuli. On the other hand, destruction of the brain tissue within the limits of one section or another, or such changes as can be observed in a limited break-down in the dynamics of the blood supply or of the cerebro-spinal fluid, alter the conditions of its functioning and reduce the strength of the nervous processes within the limits of the given functional system; the balance of stimulatory and inhibitory processes suffers and their normal mobility is replaced by pathological inertia.

Naturally, under any of these conditions normal function of the given "analyzer" is disturbed, the ability to differentiate stimuli in adjacent systems loses its precision, and the whole process of analysis and synthesis within the limits of the modality with which the particular cortical system is concerned, acquires an imperfect and sometimes even a pathological character. This disturbance of normal processes of analysis and synthesis within the limits of a given functional system (visual, auditory, kinesthetic or motor) is *a direct primary result of any focal lesion of the cortex.*

However, this immediate, primary effect of local lesions never remains an isolated one. The real units of brain function are those most complicated systems of temporal connections which lead to the well-known forms of adaptive activity and which in a human being assume the form of objective activity—active or passive speech, writing or reading, counting or the solution of cognitive problems. Every one of the very complicated functional systems that have been formed in the history of social development it includes in its composition many functional components and can normally be realized only in the presence of a number of physiological conditions. Naturally, in order to distinguish speech sounds a precise acoustico-articulatory analysis is necessary, just as the articulation of any word requires the conservation of those kinesthetic impulses that alone make possible the distinction between similar articulations. It is perfectly clear therefore that when the action of one analyzer which takes part in the realization of any of these activities is broken down, *then normal existence of the functional system as a whole becomes impossible, and there is a selective pathological effect on all that most closely depends on normal action of a given analyzer.* This break-down, which occurs as the result of a primary disturbance of the action of one of the analyzers, is *the secondary or systemic effect of the given lesion.* These secondary or systemic effects of the partial affection also constitute the basic content of the pathology of localized disturbances of cortical function. These effects include the symptoms of aphasia agnosia or apraxia, the study of which for analyzing the structure of the speech processes is the main subject of this article.

It would be wrong, however, to suppose that the complex speech system becomes equally disintegrated with the primary break-down of different components. The various components of speech activity do not occupy an equal place in the complicated functional system of speech; auditory analysis and synthesis, the kinesthetic differentiations required for precise articulation, analysis and synthesis of space and time relations—all this is necessary, but in different degrees, for the hearing and understanding of speech, for the active pronunciation of sound or words, for writing or reading. It is quite natural therefore that a defect in the action of one analyzer or another, arising as a result of a focal lesion of the brain, inevitably leads to a secondary disturbance of a whole *complex of functions*, normal realization of which depends on its conservation; therefore the disintegration of the speech system, which arises as a result of the primary disturbance of each of these physiological functions, will vary in character. Just as an experienced cardiologist can, according to the character of the disturbance in heart function, draw conclusions about the place in which the damage has occurred, so an experienced neurologist who is studying the character of speech disorders can with confidence deduce which of the primary defects lies at its base. And it is precisely because of this that the pathological method is so valuable for the discovery of those hidden peculiarities of the structure of speech and of the mechanisms on which language is based, and the analysis of which has inevitably escaped objective investigation.

TEMPORAL ZONE LESIONS AND DISINTEGRATION OF PHONEMIC ORGANIZATION OF SPEECH

Clinicians are well acquainted with cases where an affection of the postero-superior sections of the left temporal zone (in the right-handed patient), the so-called Wernicke area, leads to a break-down in the comprehension of speech; to the patient, words begin to sound like inarticulate noises and their meaning is no longer taken in. Such break-downs, as the outstanding linguist, Jakobson, has so aptly remarked, lead to disturbances of the elementary sound code of speech, and at the same time lead to a break-down in the normal designation of objects, in the process of writing and to peculiar disturbances in thinking. These disturbances of speech are widely known under the name of "sensory" aphasia, but the mechanisms which lead to this condition continue to provoke lively arguments. It has remained obscure precisely which of the primary break-downs lead to such disturbances of speech, whether it is a "defect of hearing" or a "defect of thinking", and it is difficult to explain the remarkable diversity of speech manifestations that are lost in such cases.

Analysis of a considerable number of cases of left temporal lesions, carried out by Soviet clinicians, physiologists and psychologists, during the last decades, offers a closer approach to the solution of some of these problems. Investigations have shown that a lesion of the area in which we are interested, which is a part of the cortical end of the acoustic analyzer system, does not produce (as was thought in classical neurology) any loss of hearing for any part of the frequency range, but inevitably leads to *damage in the process of differentiation and generalization of sounds, in other words, in the processes of sound analysis and synthesis.* This is evident from the fact that such patients easily form conditioned reflexes in response to sounds, but experience considerable difficulty when they are faced with the problem of differentiating complex groups of sounds, and these difficulties are very great both in the attempt to form differentiated reactions to chords which differ from each other by the presence of different components, and especially in attempts to work out a distinction between two series, in which sounds are arranged in different sequence (ABCD and ACDB) (Traugott, 1956, Babenkova, 1954, Kabelyanskaya, 1955, and others). It is characteristic that a corresponding differentiation of visual complexes remains in these cases relatively intact.

It seems, however, the most essential point is that this break-down of sound analysis and synthesis does not remain within the limits of elementary sound complexes, but is seen particulary clearly in the differentiation of similar phonemes; a break-down in phonemic auditory perception may be recognized with every justification as a basic symptom of a lesion in the region we are interested in.

As a result of work, the foundations of which were laid in the modern phonetic theory of Baudouin de Courtenay (1882), Shcherba (1912), Trubetzkoy (1939) and Jakobson (1956), it has become clear that the phonetic structure of language depends on a system of sound oppositions, which are variously arranged in different languages, but in which invariably one of the phonetic features (voice—voicelessness, accent—absence of accent, palatalization—absence of palatalization, etc.) plays a basic part, acting as a signal that differentiates meaning. The discrimination of these phonetic features, produced in the sound-complex by means of a variation in the articulatory processes, provides the mechanisms necessary for speech perception.

It is these systems of discrimination that are broken down in cases of lesions of the postero-superior sections of the temporal area of the dominant hemisphere, perhaps because this apparatus stands in the closest functional and morphological relation to the inferior sections of the kinesthetic and motor area of the cortex, which play a direct part in the act of articulation, and this part of the brain can be conceived of only as forming a single auditory-articulatory system.

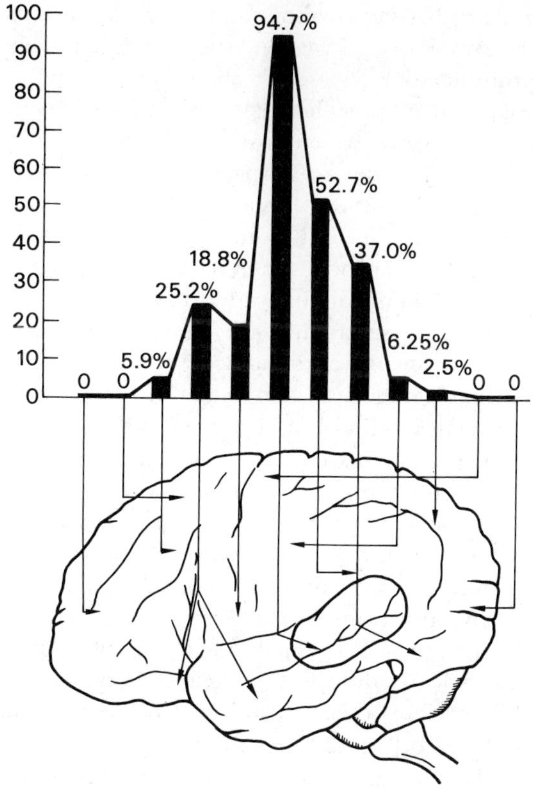

Fig. 23–1. Disintegration of phonemic acoustic perception in variously located brain damage (the columns show the percentage of break-downs in the total number of patients with corresponding location of the affection: each group comprises 60–90 cases).

The breakdown of phonemic auditory perception is a fundamental and persistent symptom accompanying lesions of the left temporal area, and may be easily revealed by simple experiments, such as asking the patient to repeat similar (but opposed) phonemes (e.g. /b-p, t-d, z-s/, etc.) or attempting to elicit from him definite differentiated reactions (e.g. raising the hand in response to the voiced /b/ and not raising it in response to the voiceless /p/). Fig. 23-1 gives a summary of results obtained during the war from the analysis of more than 800 cases of bullet-wounds of the brain, and it shows that the breakdown in phonemic auditory perception accompanies only lesions of the postero-superior sections of the left temporal area (or of parts adjoining them, in which case the break-down is a secondary effect), and is not typical of lesions of other sections of the brain. Further observations have made it possible to ascertain that this remains the most persistent symptom in residual phases of traumatic illness, is one of the early indications of the growth of a tumor in this area, and can be disclosed through stimulation by means of special sensitized probes even in the most serious cases of these lesions.

The break-down of phonemic auditory perception at once produces a series of *secondary disorders*: it inevitably leads to a break-down in the language system of all those formations in which it took part and which require precise phonemic auditory perception as an indispensable condition of their normal functioning.

The break-down of precise phonetic analysis

and synthesis leads above all to a break-down in the *pronunciation of words*, especially where this pronunciation does not have an automatic character. It is sufficient to ask the patient to repeat a word which is new and phonetically difficult in order to ascertain this. It leads to particularly severe break-downs in *writing*, even when the ability to copy a given text without difficulty is preserved; such a patient proves to be incapable of writing any word at dictation or spontaneously (again, provided it is not sufficiently automatized), has difficulty in distinguishing its component sounds, and substitutes similar but "opposed" phonemes.

Primary break-down of phonemic auditory perception leads, however, to more extensive consequences, exerting its own peculiar effect on the structure of the *meanings* of words, and essentially breaking down the language vocabulary formerly possessed by the patient. A patient with break-down of phonemic analysis loses the ability to take in words and to differentiate their meanings. If /telo/ and /delo/, /totʃka/ and /dotʃka/ come to sound similar, the meanings of these words cease to be clearly differentiated; if words with a complicated phonetic composition (e.g. with a consonant cluster) become for the patient insufficiently articulated groups, their meaning naturally ceases to be marked off from the meaning of other words, the superficial phonetic similarity, which is over-ruled by the precise phonemic structure of normal speech, is given free rein and the patient tends to class together words which have something in common in their sound, but which have never before been put into the same category of meaning. Thus /otʃen/ and /osen/, /kolos/, /golos/ and /xolost/, which were never formerly confused, easily begin to replace each other, and the basic meaning-structure of the patient's vocabulary disintegrates, giving way to phonetic connections no longer reduced to an orderly system. The disintegration of the phonemic structure of language inevitably leads to a break-down in its lexical structure; the break-down of the understanding of speech appears as a result not of intellectual disorder, but of the disintegration of the complex auditory function and it produces a failure of the power to use the systematized language code.

An essential fact is that the disintegration of the lexical structure of language caused by the break-down of phonemic auditory perception does not affect all morphological elements of a word to the same degree. Observations by Bein (1950) in recent years show that such patients lose the power to understand the roots of words, of which there are a great many in each language and for the precise understanding of which it is specially indispensable to differentiate them from many other complexes, phonetically similar but having a different meaning; on the other hand, suffixes of words, which are relatively few in a language and do not have such a multiplicity of possible phonetic connections, ordinarily remain considerably more comprehensible. Hence arises the paradoxical and apparently little-understood fact—so contrary to the widely held belief that in the pathology of these cases invariably those elements are earliest broken down which were last formed—that patients with the form of aphasia described lose the concrete meaning (attached to the root of the word) and retain abstract meanings, attached to such suffixes of abstract state, as *-ost (vidim-ost)* or *-ie (sostoyan-ie, obrazovan-ie)* in Russian, *-heit (Treu-heit)* or *-keit (Nachbar-keit)* in German, *-ance (vigilance)* in English or French, and so on.

The potential retention of abstract terms in patients with such disorders,[1] and the associated relative retention of abstract ideas, is one of the most interesting of those phenomena that allow a close approach to the analysis of formations which arose first on the basis of vocalic speech,

[1] The thesis just mentioned retains, of course, its significance only in the case of break-down of the phonemic structure of speech in adults who have already formed the semantic system of language. Early break-down (or underdevelopment) of phonemic hearing in a child, in whom the semantic system of language has not yet been formed, leads to considerably more general and serious disorders of mentation. This means only that in describing various forms of secondary disorder, which are the result of a partial affection, one must always keep in mind at what genetic stage this break-down took place and what system it found already in existence. This idea, already expressed by Vygotsky (1956), has a fundamental significance for evaluation of the systemic effect of disease, but a consideration of it is beyond the scope of this article.

but which, with the development of human mentation, have begun to take on a relative independence.

COMMUNICATION OF EVENTS AND COMMUNICATION OF RELATIONS

There is no doubt that the careful investigation of these phenomena which arise as a result of such disorders opens wide avenues for the analysis of important problems on the borders of phonetics and morphology on the one hand and the psychology of speech processes on the other. Information which a human being receives by means of language is not confined to the designation of single objects; the most significant information comes from *systems of words* or from whole communications. Since the time of Svedelius (1897) it has been customary to divide these communications into communication of events (of the type: "A dog bit the boy") and communication of relations (of the type "Socrates is a man" or "The circle is drawn under the square" or "This is the father's brother"). If the first type is expressed in European languages mostly by means of the inflexion system, the second type can be expressed both with the help of the most abstract forms of case relationship or with the help of special types of preposition or conjunction.

Linguistic analysis has always indicated a difference in the degree of abstraction in the two kinds of communication and the fact that in each of them the object, the visual perception and abstract thinking do not participate to the same degree. However, in spite of the facts which indicate that they originated at different epochs and that they have different logico-grammatical structures, the distinction between them has remained relatively formal.

In this problem of isolating the class of linguistic formations represented in the "communication of relations" and in analyzing peculiarities of their inner structure, pathology can offer considerable help. Already at the time of Head (1926), Gelb and Goldstein (1924), Van Woerkom (1925), Boumann and Grünbaum (1925) and of a number of other more specialized studies, it was noted that patients with disorders of the postero-parietal and parieto-occipital sections of the dominant left hemisphere show characteristic disabilities: although still able to understand everyday speech, they are incapable of understanding the meaning of complicated logico-grammatical combinations, which express certain abstract relationships. At the same time these patients show considerable difficulty in operating with spatial relations of objects; they lose their ability to operate with mathematical categories, easily confuse arithmetical symbols and find themselves in great difficulties when confronted with the necessity of analyzing numbers in structural arrangements. All these facts have been confirmed by research workers, who have given a closer description of the "parietal syndrome" (Konrad, 1932, Zucker, 1933, Klein, 1931, Gerstmann, 1932, Critchley, 1953, Hécaen, 1953, Zangwill, 1957, and others). The description of symptoms occurring with parietal affections leads us to believe that with the help of pathology we shall be able to isolate what is *specific* to the complex form—the "communication of relations". However, the theoretical interpretation and explanation of these facts has confronted research workers with considerable difficulties.

Some authors, adhering to the so-called "noëtic trend" (Goldstein, 1948, Van Woerkom, 1925, Grünbaum, 1925, and others) and in actual fact continuing the line of Pierre Marie, have been inclined to see behind these symptoms a break-down of the "general function of the intellect" or of "categorical thinking" (a view which explained very little and has rather obstructed the way to further research). Other authors, with a more analytical attitude (Konrad, Zucker, Critchley, and Zangwill), have not been satisfied with these somewhat too general principles and have begun to look for a more specific brain mechanism as the basis of these disabilities.

The solution of the problem has been materially advanced by observations that have stated the facts more precisely and have allowed us to make a step forward towards an adequate explanation of this most complicated syndrome.

A careful analysis of patients with limited lesions of the inferior parietal (or parieto-occipital) area has shown first of all that in these cases by no means all the forms of speech activity are broken down, and by no means all the forms of abstract thinking and behavior. These patients, while still able to understand everyday speech denoting events, also preserve abstract notions which express inner psychological states and moral values, as well as some abstract categories. They begin however to experience considerable difficulties every time they have to analyze a complicated figure and to coordinate its details into one whole, or to operate with numbers in structural arrangements; they confuse spatial direction when examining numbers of more than one digit and—a fact that is of particular interest for the problems with which we are directly concerned—they are nonplussed every time they are faced with a "communication of relations".

All this has compelled us to reject the global and clearly incorrect assertion of the "general lowering of the intellect" or "the loss of categorical thinking", supposedly resulting from these lesions, and, following our chosen direction, to seek the primary break-down of the higher nervous processes, which arises in the given local affection and which, as a secondary systemic effect, leads to the disorders just described.

Already experiments on animals have shown that lesions of the posterior sections of the cortex and especially of those areas which have acquired the name of "posterior intrinsic areas" (Rose, 1952, Pribram, 1957) break down the ability to react differentially to complex configurations of signs and considerably restrict the information that can be received by the animals; the work of Pavlov and his pupils with extirpations of the posterior sections of the cortex defined more accurately the physiological mechanisms which are at the base of these break-downs, and showed to what extent one set of functional systems may suffer a persistent heightening of sensitivity to stimulation whilst another distinct set of systems suffers a decrease in sensitivity.

Such break-downs in the processes forming the complicated systems of discrimination and occurring as a result of lesions of the parieto-occipital sections of the cortex have been described in great detail in man. Also, the basic disorder which occurs in these cases is illustrated by the phenomena of "simultaneous agnosia", widely known in clinical practice (and described by Wolpert, 1924, and Bálint, 1909) as well as by the phenomena of astereognosis which are similar in structure. The fact that patients lose their ability to "combine details into a coherent whole" (Head), that there is a loss of synoptic function, of the ability to "see elements in a single structure" (Goldstein) or to "transform the act of sequential observation into simultaneous observation" (Pötzl), all this only reflects those neurodynamic shifts which in these cases cause a break-down in the systematic activity of the cortex so that the patient, as Pavlov said, "finds himself in a condition to deal with only one point of stimulation at a time while the rest are inhibited".

We have had occasion to describe a patient whose bilateral lesion of the parieto-occipital area of the cortex led to his inability to combine two details simultaneously; in a tachistoscope he could not perceive two letters at once, nor could he make a point in the center of a cross or circle: one visual impression inductively inhibited the other and the simplest visual synthesis remained impossible for him.

Such a break-down of simultaneous synthesis can be quite justifiably regarded as the physiological basis of functional disorders, occurring in lesions of the parieto-occipital areas of the brain. However, if the lesion goes beyond the limits of the parieto-occipital areas of the cortex and reaches the border of the speech area, it may produce disorders which go far beyond the limits of the visual realm. They inevitably lead to a break-down of the more complicated mnemic operations, connected with abstraction of one signal and the synthesis of a series of elements in accordance with this abstracted signal. They also lead inevitably to a situation where *operations which use a definite complex code and which are linked by means of this code with the intellectual act become impossible.*

As has been shown by special research, affections of the parieto-occipital areas of the cortex lead precisely to the inability to isolate one signal and to produce a stable system of heightened sensitivity to stimulation whilst inhibiting irrelevant systems. They produce in the patients a significant break-down in generalization from visual figures which are similar in one parameter (e.g., color, shape, etc.) and different in others (Kok, 1957). Similar defects occur in these patients in their evaluation of space relations (Konrad, Zucker, Head, Critchley, Zangwill), in operations connected with counting off elements in space (compare finger agnosia and Gerstmann's syndrome) and finally in arithmetical operations (especially in those connected with the analysis of numbers in structural arrangement) and counting, especially of numbers exceeding 10. These operations always require the abstraction of a scheme of reference and comparison of a whole complex of connections with this scheme.

In all these cases, where the problem requires such complicated operations, affections of the parieto-occipital systems lead inevitably to their disintegration, at the same time conserving intact those operations which do not require such simultaneous observation of details and which can be realized by means of successive synthesis such as, for example, the beating out of rhythms, the reproduction of a

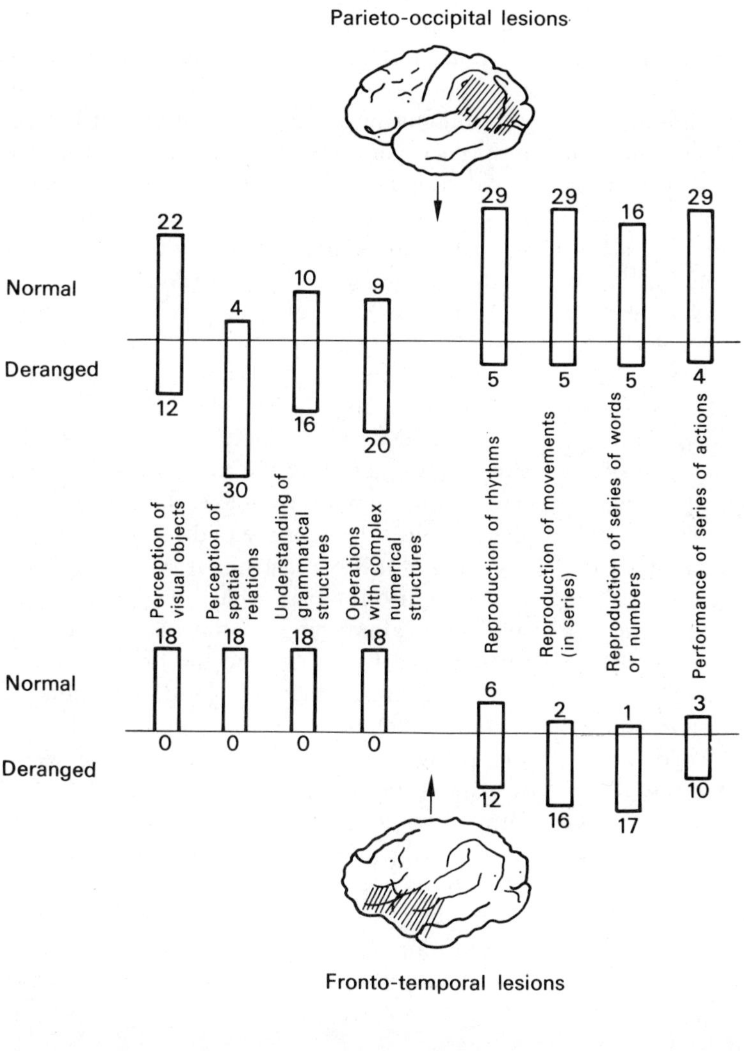

Fig. 23–2. Disintegration of the operations connected with simultaneous and successive synthesis in cases of affection of the posterior (parieto-occipital) and anterior (fronto-temporal) sections of the hemisphere. The columns show the number of cases in which a given operation could be carried out (upper columns) or could not be carried out (lower columns).

series of successive movements, of the words of a poem, etc. On the other hand, when the fronto-temporal systems are affected, with the analysis of which we have dealt elsewhere in detail (Luria, 1957a), operations associated with simultaneous synthesis remain completely intact, whilst operations which require a successive synthesis of elements (auditory or motor in the first place) into one complete structure, suffer considerably (see Fig. 23-2).

The above statement allows us to turn directly to the questions in which we are interested in this paper. We have already mentioned the two forms of language construction, which some linguists call "communication of events" and "communication of relations"; now we can return to their analysis from the new standpoint which has just been classified.

"Communication of events" in its simplest and purest form (of the type "A house is burning", "A dog bit a boy") depends on well-consolidated sequences of verbal relationships and does not require from the hearer a preliminary abstraction of one of the signals used in them, with the subsequent establishment of a complicated system of relations. Only in those cases where, as a result of inversion (e.g. "A boy was bitten by a dog"), the usual word order is affected and the order of communicated events ceases to coincide with the word order in a sentence,[2] does the preliminary analysis of construction become necessary; isolation and comparison of its separate elements and comprehension of this construction on the basis of "the combination of isolated details into a coherent whole" corresponds this time to the logico-grammatical code of the language.

The very opposite takes place in the understanding of a "communication of relations". Even the simplest "communication of relations" (if it is not of the most common type) is a complicated and peculiar problem, which necessitates a comparison of two elements together with the extraction of the basic signal and subsequent synthesis of the two elements into a specific structure.

A typical example of such a system is the construction "father's brother" and the opposite construction "brother's father". In both cases it concerns two objects, described as "brother" and "father". The construction as a whole does not refer to these objects, but to a third one, resulting from their logical combination: "uncle" in the first and "father" (defined from another, new relationship) in the second. In order to grasp this construction, which has developed relatively late, it is not sufficient simply to perceive two isolated designations; it is necessary to isolate the basic symbol ("father") and to grasp the meaning of the second symbol ("brother's"), having as a starting point its relation to the first. In some languages (e.g. Russian), which show these relations by means of the genitive attributive, it is necessary to carry out an operation of abstraction from the substantive meaning of the noun which is in the genitive and to convert it, according to its meaning, into a qualitive word (father's brother = paternal brother).

A completely analogous psychological construction is that of the communication of spatial relations expressed by means of a preposition, e.g. "a circle under a triangle" and its opposite "a triangle under a circle". In this case the simple designation of the two elements merely begins, but does not complete, the formation of the complex idea; for the understanding of the meaning of this construction it is also necessary to distinguish the basic object (e.g. "triangle") and to evaluate the spatial relation of the second object ("circle") to the first. A similar construction is that of communication of temporal relations (e.g. "summer following the spring" or "spring following the summer"), instrumental relations (e.g. "the earth is lighted by the sun" or "the sun is lighted by the earth"), the correct forms of which may be established only after an analogous operation of distinguishing the basic designation, and of establishing the meaning of the second object, and then in turn of establishing the meaning of

[2] In the case of separated and subordinate clauses; the following sentence may serve as an example of such a construction: To the school where Peter is studying, a woman came from the factory to talk about the preparations for the holiday.

the whole construction from the relation which has been analyzed.

After what has been said it becomes quite clear that these constructions which are very complex in form and came into being relatively late[3] are very vulnerable, and inevitably disintegrate when the basic condition, indispensable for their understanding, is unattainable as a result of the break-down of complex "simultaneous synthesis" and of the ability to combine isolated elements into a single analytic "unit".

This is why patients with parieto-occipital lesions, especially those located on the border of the "speech zones of the cortex", are often incapable of coping even with apparently simple "communications of relations)), are baffled by the task of "drawing a square under a circle" (ordinarily carrying out the task in an agrammatical way in the order in which the words are spoken and hence drawing a square, then under it a circle), and prove to be completely incapable of distinguishing between the two constructions "father's brother" and "brother's father", declaring that in both cases the brother and father are spoken of and consequently the constructions are identical; and readily accept the construction "the sun is lighted by the earth", in which the habitual order of words in an active construction is agrammatically adopted as being the correct one. This symptom, appearing distinctly in cases where the affection damages the most complex and most recently formed zones of the parieto-occipital region at its border with the temporal region, constitutes a basic symptom of so-called "semantic aphasia". For the analysis of this condition, problems in understanding the simplest logico-grammatical relations occupy the same place that problems in the differentiation of opposed phonemes occupy in the analysis of temporal "acoustic aphasia".

The close study of the changes that take place, in the cases we have considered, in the employment of the most complex codes of language (the phonetic code in one, the semantic code in the other case) consequently permits the use of focal lesions of the brain as a means for the analysis of complex linguistic phenomena and for the analysis of those functional formations which, without this method, would remain difficult of access to pathological analysis.

THE EFFECT OF FRONTAL LESIONS ON SPEECH

We have surveyed the analysis of those breakdowns in the complicated system of linguistic constructions caused by affections of the parieto-occipital systems of the brain which lead directly to the disintegration of simultaneous synthesis and to the break-down in the act of "combining isolated details into a single whole" which Head so rightly pointed out in his time.

The logic of our exposition requires us now to turn to disturbances of the speech structures which arise in cases of disintegration in another important function, which as all the data show (cf. Luria, 1957a), is provided for, in the first place, by the anterior fronto-temporal sections of the cortex, and which results in the *synthesis of successive elements into a single continuous series* or "dynamic system". Such disturbances of sequential synthesis and of acoustico-motor sequences directly linked with them, or, as they are often termed clinically, "kinetic patterns", do not remain without effect on the speech systems also. But in this case, as we have shown elsewhere (Luria, 1947, chap. 4) the disintegration of complex speech formations proceeds along a completely different course; the patient, revealing no noticeable defects in the distinguishing of the phonetic elements of verbal speech or in the grasping of logico-grammatical

[3] In some languages the emergence of such complex flexional or prepositional constructions goes back only as far as the XIVth-XVth centuries and in earlier records and documents such constructions are replaced by simpler ones, not requiring any complex analytic-synthetic effort. Typical examples of such simplification with the replacement of complex forms of government by simple paratactic constructions are the Greek: "They escaped the strength and arms of the Achaeans (instead of "the strength of the Achaeans' arms.") (Odyssey, VIII, 134); the German "mit Leidschaft und Liebe" (instead of "mit Leidschaft der Liebe") (Nibelungenlied, 1148,3); and the English "For yonder I hear Sir Guy's horn blow and (for 'which') has slain Robin Hood" (Ballad of Robin Hood).

relations in language, begins to display noticeable break-downs in smooth transition from subject to predicate, and consequently, in the realization of that "propositionizing" of which in his time Hughlings Jackson spoke so fully and in such detail. This break-down of sequential synthesis does not destroy single systems of stimulation but impedes the easy switching off of these stimulations and the transition from one system of innervation to another (in a pure form this break-down is seen in the so-called "pre-motor syndrome"). As a result of such disturbances there is a secondary affection of *internal speech,* which—as has been correctly affirmed by a number of psychologists—is predicative speech turned inwards (Vygotsky 1956) and the presence of which is absolutely indispensable for fluent predicative propositionizing. It is these affections which eventually lead to the appearance of that exceptionally interesting phenomenon which is widely known in clinical literature as "telegraphic style," and which Jakobson with full justification considers as a break-down of *contextual speech,* in many ways opposite to the break-down of the *"code of language"* (phonetic or logico-grammatical), with which we were concerned above. However, the limits of this paper do not allow us to concern ourselves in greater detail with this peculiar form of disorder, or, what is most important, to throw light on the primary neurodynamic conditions of its appearance in the same way as we have attempted to do with respect to the forms of speech disturbance dealt with earlier.

We shall therefore cut short our exposition and pass to the consideration of those forms of the pathology of speech which in many respects have special interest and which have not received the attention they merit. Up to now we have been concerned with the analysis of information provided by focal lesions of the brain for the analysis of the structure of the speech processes and in particular for the intensive study of the phonetic and morphological, semantic and syntactic side of speech. However, apart from these essential aspects of the speech process, which make possible the use of language as a means of communication and an instrument of thought, there is still another essential function of speech, which has received even scantier attention from linguists and psychologists. We have in mind the *regulating* function of speech, which, as we shall show below, remains relatively intact in the cases described above and which requires close consideration.

When an adult addresses some order to a child, he calls into action in the child a system of governing connections, which direct all its subsequent behavior and inhibit all irrelevant actions. The speech of the adult here regulates the behavior of the child. This regulating effect, which the speech of the adult exerts on the child's behavior, eventually becomes the source of complex new functional formations. In acquiring his own speech, at first external and later internal, the child begins to use it not only as an instrument of communication and thought, but as a *means of regulating his own behavior.* The child's own speech, which helps him in orientating himself in his environment, and creating a system of connections in which he reflects reality and formulates his desires, enables him to map out his own behavior and to regulate the course of his activity. Research carried out in recent years and treated by us in another place (Luria, 1957b) has made it possible to show what a complex path is traversed by the formation of this regulating function of speech before it becomes capable not only of setting in motion known and already consolidated actions, but of locking in the governing system of connections and checking all irrelevant actions, which do not relate to the fulfilment of the task formulated in speech. There is no doubt whatever that all the highest functional formations with which psychology is concerned—the accomplishing of conscious, purposive action, systematic active thought, voluntary memory—all these are in greater or less degree linked with the regulating function of speech. In all these cases external (or more often internal) speech locks in an existing system of connections, which in normal behavior become dominant, and which define the course of all the subsequent actions of the person, acquiring sometimes—as, for instance, was the case with Giordano Bruno—a strength which considerably exceeds the strength of vital instincts.

What does the study of pathological states of the brain contribute to the analysis of this very important but still little-studied regulating function of speech? Is that function broken down in equal degree in various brain lesions, or can we distinguish particular brain-systems, the preservation of which is absolutely indispensable for the regulating effect of speech on behavior?

The cases of focal brain lesions, which we have analyzed above, broke down the phonetic and lexical, semantic and syntactic side of speech, but did not yet lead to a distinct break-down of its regulating function. Patients suffering from the defects described above readily executed the doctor's instructions, formulated in speech, concentrated for a considerable time on carrying out the tasks he set and frequently revealed an exceptional persistence in the task of compensating for their defects, without which the restoration of the broken-down functions would be impossible. Special experiments (as yet unpublished), carried out recently, have shown that in all these cases the patient's speech, broken down in the phonetic or grammatical respect, continues to preserve its determining, directing role, ensuring at the same time intelligently directed behavior by the patient.

In order to study the pathology of the regulating function of speech, it is consequently indispensable to go beyond the limits of the forms of speech disorder studied by us, and as we shall see below, in general beyond the limits of what is clinically known as "aphasia".

For the successful solution of the question that interests us we should for a short time leave the description of speech disorders and consider the facts revealed by contemporary neurophysiology and psychology in studying the brain-mechanisms regulating the active behavior of animals.

All contemporary work which has studied the peculiarities of animal behavior after the removal of separate parts of the brain, beginning with the work of Franz (1907), Bianchi (1921) and Pavlov and ending with the latest researches of Fulton (1945), Pribram (1957) and Anokhin (1949)—despite the divergence in the positions from which they started—lead to one essential fact. Ablation of the *posterior sections of the major hemispheres* causes in the animal a break-down of accuracy in the operation of separate analysers, which leads to a defect in particular types of differentiation and the restriction of corresponding information coming from the environment, but never leads to a break-down of the general regulation of the animal's behavior, which remains just as expedient as before. On the other hand, ablation of the *frontal sections of the major hemispheres,* though not causing any noticeable break-down in the action of separate parts of the exteroceptive apparatus, sharply alters the whole behavior of the animal: it ceases to distinguish the essential in a situation, to assess its own experience, it reacts identically to those stimuli which are important for life and to those which are indifferent; it continues to make movements which have become senseless after it has found the bait it was looking for (as was the case in the experiments of Anokhin, Pribram and Shustin). Evidently it does not assess in its behavior the general situation and the effect of previous experience. All this justified Pribram in saying that the frontal sections of the brain have special functions, determing the expediency ("utility function"), the selective character of behavior ("preference behavior"), and allowed Anokhin to come to the conclusion that their function, closely connected with the regulation of motor behavior, consists in the creation of a complex "pre-initiatory afferentation", which includes signals concerning the successful completion of an act, and makes possible the realization of preference behavior.

The part played by the frontal sections of the brain in the regulation of complex forms of preference behavior is thus shown to be indisputable, and even if the physiological mechanisms which ensure this regulation remain up to the present obscure, the distinguishing of this function of the frontal portions should be considered among the important achievements of neurological science.[4]

If the purposive behavior of an animal is determined by that "pre-initiatory afferentation", which in fact regulates all its subsequent activity, then in a human being such "pre-initiatory afferentation" consists in a system of governing connections, formed by means of *speech*. Therefore it is natural that in cases of affections of the frontal systems in man, there should be a break-down not only of the system of synthetic "pre-initiatory afferentations" which determine his subsequent behavior, but in the first place a break-down of the system of "pre-initiatory afferentations" created on the basis of speech—in other words, a break-down of the regulating function of speech connections.

Protracted research into the disintegration of the structure of behavior in patients with lesions of the frontal portions of the brain, carried out by us together with a number of colleagues (Filippycheva, 1952, Meshcheryakov, 1953, Ivanova, 1953, etc.) have made it possible to describe the peculiar picture of disorders arising in these cases, which have never been classed as aphasia but which may be understood essentially as break-downs in the regulating function of speech.

As a rule, we do not observe, in patients with lesions of the frontal portions of the brain (however severe and massive these affections may be) any noticeable break-downs whatever in the structure of speech processes: the phonetic system and vocabulary, the semantic system and the grammar of speech of these patients proves as a rule to be completely intact both in its receptive and its expressive part. It is only in patients whose brain affection is situated in the postero-inferior sections of the left frontal area adjoining Broca's area that we observe a certain inactivity in speech, a break-down of monologue speech with preservation of responsive (dialogue) speech, which we have had occasion to describe elsewhere as a symptom of "frontal aphasia" (Luria, 1947).

And yet, despite its superficial intactness in these patients, the regulating function of speech proves to be severely disintegrated. This disintegration is revealed in patients with severe (and particularly bilateral) lesions of the frontal areas either by simple observation or in experiments involving their carrying out simple instructions. In many—the most severe—cases, such patients prove unable to carry out even the simplest instructions; though they may repeat in an echolalic way the experimenter's order "Raise your hand", they nevertheless make no attempt whatever to perform the required action. Sometimes the words of the experimenter may set in motion the action of the patient, but he proves to be powerless to stop it or to change the action once started to another. If such a patient is given the task of drawing a circle, he begins to carry this out, but then, submitting to the inertia of the stimulus in the motor regions of the cortex, he proves unable either to cease this movement or to change over to another action; when asked to draw a triangle, he correctly repeats this instruction, but continues through inertia to draw a circle. The inertia of an act once initiated and the weakness of the regulating effect of speech is displayed in experiments with the carrying out of a complex of instructions; in response to the request to draw a triangle, a circle and two squares, the patient begins to draw a number of triangles or a single triangle, accompanied by several circles, although in some cases the patient remains capable of repeating the instruction.

Particularly distinct data, indicating a significant break-down of the regulating function of speech, were gathered from these patients in special experiments, in which the speech of the experimenter did not set in motion the old, well-established connection, but locked in a

[4] It is interesting to note that Pavlov stresses the distinction of the functions of the occipital and frontal sections of the brain. "If you cut out the whole occipital part of the cerebral hemispheres of a dog," he writes, "you will get an animal which is in general quite normal. . . . It wags its tail when you stroke it. It will also show its pleasure, by sniffing in recognition at you. But such an animal will be unable to react to you if you stand at a distance. . . . Such a dog has very little use from its eyes and ears, but for the rest, is completely normal. But if you cut out the frontal part of the cerebral hemispheres . . . then you will have an obviously abnormal animal. It has no correct reaction to other dogs, nor to food, nor in general to surrounding objects. It is a completely ruined animal, evidently left with none of the signs of purposive behavior." I. P. Pavlov, Coll. Wks., III, 175-6.

new conditioned connection. If, as was shown by Meshcheryakov and Ivanova, such a patient was asked, in response to a flashing light, to press on a rubber bulb, or in response to a red light to press with the right hand, but in response to a blue light to press with the left hand, these instructions continued to regulate his action only for a very brief period, and the carrying out of the instruction would very soon cease, often being replaced by an inert repetition of stereotyped pressures, which would completely lose their relation to the preliminary signal and were carried out independently of it. Only by changing over to a prolonged insistence on the instruction by means of a frequent repetition of the command ("Press!" or "Don't press!") after each preliminary signal, was it possible to produce the formation of the required conditioned connection, but even this survived only a very short time, easily disintegrating in the course of the experiment and being replaced by persistent pressures which were not timed to the signal.

The break-down of the regulating role of instruction by speech appears most clearly in experiments with delayed reaction. When patients with a massive lesion of the frontal areas were asked to raise their hand in response to a knock produced 15–20 seconds after the instruction, they did so, but in cases of the most severe affection the regulating action of the instruction was broken down to such an extent that the movement set in motion by the instruction—the raising of the hand—was replaced by an imitative movement; the patient would reproduce the movement of the experimenter by knocking beside the place where the experimenter knocked. However, when such a patient was given the instruction, requiring the production of a reaction in accordance with speech connections already set up (e.g. "When the second hand of the watch reaches 25, raise your hand", or "When I count as far as 12, raise your hand"), the patient proved incapable of making the reaction; the best the patient could do was to declare "Now it's reached 25!" or "That's 12 now" but would make no movement. It is characteristic too that this fact is explained not by the break-down of memory (after the unsuccessful attempt the patient when questioned was easily able to reproduce the verbal instruction) but by heightened external inhibition, as a result of which the activity which had started (following the hand of the watch or listening to a series of numbers) inductively inhibited the influence of the instruction and produced a break-down of its regulating function.

A characteristic feature of these highly peculiar functional disorders is the fact that the phenomena here observed do not amount merely to the break-down of the regulating function of *another person's speech* (or more accurately, the systems of connections set up by it). Experiments were carried out in which we asked the patient to confirm by his own speech the effect of the instruction, making him declare the significance of the stimulus e.g. by saying every time the red lamp flashed: "I am to press!" and when the blue lamp flashed: "I am not to press!"—a method worked out with us by Khomskaya, the influence of which in ontogenesis has been described elsewhere (Luria, 1956, 1957b). These experiments showed that even the patient's own speech, easily passing over to an inert stereotype, and losing the required connection with the signal, in fact also ceases to display its regulating effect. In these cases the patient either begins inertly to alternate the responses "I am to press!", "I am not to press!", or (if his speech reactions were sufficiently strong) correctly reproduces the required responses, but ceases to make the movements corresponding to them, replacing them by inert stereotypes.

The break-down in the regulating function of speech proves characteristic of the whole behavior of such patients; it deprives their activity of the required purposiveness and leaves an imprint on the whole character of their broken-down intellectual processes.

The close study of this form of speech disorder, which is empirically well known to clinical workers, but which has not received the attention it merits, is still in its infancy. But there can be no doubt that systematic research into the method of formation of the regulating effect of speech in ontogenesis, how it is brought about in normal behavior and how it disintegrates in pathological conditions of the brain, will reveal a whole series of facts of considerable interest both for psychology and for that branch of science which deals with the pragmatic forms of speech activity.

We have thrown light here on only a few problems which are revealed to the psychologist when he uses the observation of pathological states of cerebral activity as a method permitting the discovery of some mechanisms of the speech processes which are internal and not easily approached by pathological investigation.

It would be a mistake—though unfortunately a common one—to think that pathological states of the brain return speech to stages it has once passed through and allow one to follow out the history of its formation in reverse. Pathological changes in cerebral activity break down one or another physiological condition, indispensable for the normal existence of speech processes; therefore in fact they never reproduce any of the earlier stages of speech development. But "breaking down and simplifying what is fused and indivisible in the physiological norm", they permit the use of this method as an important means of analysing the psychological construction of speech and the actual forms in which language is used.

REFERENCES

Anokhin, P. K. (1949). Problems of higher nervous activity (Moscow).

Babenkova, S. V. (1954). On the peculiarities of interaction of the signalling systems in the process of recovery of speech in various forms of sensory aphasia. *VII Conference of Inst. of Neurol., Acad. Med. Sci.* (Moscow).

Balint, R. (1909). Seelenlähmung des Schauens. *Monatsschr. f. Psychiatr. u. Neurol.*, **25.**

Badouin de Courtney (1882). Extracts from lectures on the phonetics and morphology of Russian (1st ed., St. Petersburg).

Bein, E. S. (1950). Psychological analysis of sensory aphasia. (Dissertation, Acad. Med. Sci., Moscow).

Bianchi, L. (1921). La mécanique du cerveau et la fonction des lobes frontaux (Paris).

Boumann, L. and Grunbaum, A. A. (1925). Experimentell-psychologische Untersuchungen zur Aphasie und Paraphasie. *Zeitschr. f. d. ges. Neurol. u. Psychiatr.*, **96.**

Critchley, M. (1953). The parietal lobes (London).

Ettlinger, G., Warrington, E., Zangwill, O. L. (1957). A further study of visual-spatial agnosia. *Brain*, **80.**

Filippycheva, N. A. (1952). Inertia of the higher cortical processes in local affections of the brain hemispheres. (Dissertation, Acad. Med. Sci., Moscow).

Franz, S. I. (1907). On the functions of the cerebrum —the frontal lobes. *Archives of Psychol.*, **2** (New York).

Fulton, J. F. (1945). Physiology of the Nervous System (Oxford).

Gelb, A. and Goldstein, K. (1924). Psychologische Analysen hirnpathologischer Fälle. *Psychol. Forschung*, **6.**

Gerstmann, J. (1932). Zur lokaldiagnostischen Verwertbarkeit des Syndroms: Fingeragnosie, Rechts-Links-Störung, Agraphie, Akalkulie. *Jahrb. f. Psychiatr. u. Neurol.*, **48.**

Goldstein, K. (1948). Language and Language Disturbances (New York).

Head, H. (1926). Aphasia and Kindred Disorders of Speech (London).

Hécaen, H., David, M., van Reeth, P., and Clement, J. (1953). Uber parietale Tumoren. *Wiener Zeitschr. f. Nervenheien*, **8.**

——, and Ajuriaguerra, J. (1956). Troubles mentaux au cours des tumeurs intracraniennes (Paris).

Ivanova, M. P. (1953). Disintegration of the interaction of the two signalling systems in the formation of complex motor reactions (Dissertation, Moscow State University).

Jackson, J. H. (1931). Selected Writings (London).

Jakobson, R., and Halle, M. (1956). Fundamentals of Language (The Hague).

Kabelyanskaya, L. G. (1955). State of the auditory analyzer in sensory aphasia (Dissertation, Acad. Med. Sci., Moscow).

Klein, R. (1929). Denkinhalt und Aphasie. *Zeitschr. f. d. ges. Neurol. u. Psychiatr.*, **129.**

——. (1931). Zur Symptomatologie des Parietallappens. *Zeitschr. f. d. ges. Neurol. u. Psychiatr.*, **135.**

Kok, E. P. (1957). Study of abstract and general concepts in patients with aphasia. (Dissertation,

Pavlov Inst. Physiol., Acad. Sci., Leningrad).

Konrad, K. (1932). Versuch einer psychologische Analyse des Parietalsyndroms. *Monatsschr. f. Psychiatr. u. Neurol.*, **84.**

Luria, A. R. (1947). Traumatic aphasia (Acad. Med. Sci., Moscow).

——. (1948). Restoration of the functions of the brain after war injury. (Acad. Med. Sci., Moscow).

——. (1950). Sketches of the psycho-physiology of writing (Acad. Pedagog. Sci., Moscow).

——. (1956). On the regulating function of speech in the formation of voluntary movements. *J. Higher Nervous Activity*, **6.**

——. (1957a) On the two aspects of analytico-synthetic activity of the brain cortex. *Proceedings of the Mechnikov University in Odessa*, **147.**

——. (1957b). On the genesis of voluntary movements. *Problems of Psychology*; **6.**

Meshcheryakov, A. I. (1953). Disintegration of interaction of the two signalling systems in the formation of simple motor reactions in local affections of the brain (Dissertation, Moscow State University).

Pavlov, I. P. (1951). Lectures on the action of the brain hemispheres. *Collected Works*, **III.**

——. (1951). Twenty years' experience in the study of higher nervous activity of animals. *Collected Works*, **IV.**

Potzl, O. (1928). Die Aphasielehre vom Standpunkt der klinischer Psychiatrie. Die optischagnostischen Störungen (Leipzig and Vienna).

Pribram, K. (1957). Neocortical function in behavior. *Symposium on Interdisciplinary Research in the Behaviorae, etc.* (Madison, Wis.).

—— (1957). On the neurology of thinking (Institute of Living, Hartford).

Rose, J. E. (1952). Cortical connections of the reticular complex of the thalamus. *Res. Publ. Ass. nerv. ment. Dis.*, **30,** 454–79.

Shcherba, L. Y. (1912). Russian vowels in qualitative and quantitative relation. (St. Petersburg).

Shustin, N. A. (1955). Break-down of nervous activity after removal of the frontal areas of the brain (Dissertation, Inst. Physiol. Acad. Sci., Leningrad).

Svedelius, G. (1897). L'analyse du langage (Uppsala).

Traugott, N. N. (1946). On sensory alalia and aphasia in childhood (Dissertation, Leningrad).

—— (1956). On the question of the peculiarities of auditory function in cases of breakdown of the cortical auditory analyzer. (Thesis, Conference on Questions of Comprehension of Speech, Leningrad.)

Troubetzkoi, N. (1939). Grundzüge der Phonologie Prague).

Vygotsky, L. S. (1956). Selected psychological studies (Acad. Pedagog. Sci., Moscow).

Van Woerkom, W. (1925). Uber Störungen im Denken bei aphasisches Patienten. *Monatsschr. f. Psychiatr. u. Neurol.*, **59.**

Wolpert, L. (1924). Die Simultanagnosie. *Zeitschr. f. d. ges. Neurol. u. Psychiatr.*, **93.**

Zucker, K. (1933). Uber die pathologischen Funktionen bei amnestischer Aphasie. *Monatsschr. f. Psychiatr. u. Neurol.*, **87.**

ADDITIONAL SUGGESTED READINGS ON: SYMPTOMATOLOGY

1. Fillenbaum, S., Jones, L. V., et al. Some Linguistic Features of Speech from Aphasic Patients. *Lang. Speech*, **4**:91–108, 1961.
2. Fry, D. B. Phonemic Substitutions in an Aphasic Patient. *Lang. Speech*, **2**:52–61, 1959.
3. Jones, L. V., Goodman, M. F., et al. The Classification of Parts of Speech for the Characteristics of Aphasia. *Lang. Speech*, **6**:94–107, 1963.
4. Street, B. S. Hearing Loss in Aphasia. *J. Speech Hearing Dis.*, **22**:60–67, 1957.

part II

TESTING

Introduction

As might be expected, testing in aphasia reflects our present-day knowledge and the diverse theories that exist on the physiology of language and the pathophysiologic entity we call aphasia. Few diagnosticians or therapists disagree that the ideal test for aphasia has yet to be designed. Taken as a whole, the articles in Part I could hardly point to any other conclusion. Each article in Part II, however, should contribute to the reader's fuller understanding of the contours of this problem. Some additional articles that may also prove useful are listed in the Appendix.

When one considers that almost all clinicians who evaluate patients administer diagnostic tests, the literature on the subject is quite limited. One of the first aphasia tests was published in 1898 (1). Early workers tended to use language achievement and intelligence tests, as exemplified by the battery designed by Weisenburg and McBride (11) in their study in 1935. Interestingly enough, in some intelligence tests, particularly when the test requirements are non-verbal, aphasics do as well or better than non-aphasic brain damaged patients.

The papers selected for this chapter seem to fall broadly into two categories—those describing the older, widely used tests and those presenting some of the tests more recently introduced. Today the tests most commonly used by speech pathologists are those designed by Eisenson (4), Schuell (8), and Wepman and Jones (12). Eisenson describes his approach to testing in Chapter 12 of the Travis *Handbook of Speech Pathology* (3). A factor analysis of the Schuell examination is included as one of the readings in this section (Reading 26). The Minnesota Test for the Differential Diagnosis of Aphasia (MTDDA) has the unique feature that test results classify patients in prognostic categories. The *Language Modalities Test for Aphasia* is described in a booklet by Wepman and his collaborators (12).

Another Schuell paper (Reading 25) re-evaluates the short version of the MTDDA and reflects the author's concern with the reliability and validity of the shortened version. In the article she proposes a method for using and interpreting the results of the short examination through the use of scaled tests.

Three articles (Readings 26, 27, and 28) comprise part of a controversy which began in 1959 (9) between the teams of Schuell and Jenkins and Jones and Wepman. In essence, the disagreement arose from differing conceptual models of aphasia, which were derived by each group from their respective test results. The technical and statistical details of the controversy are important, interesting methodological issues are raised, and the conceptual ideas presented should be stimulating and educative for the student.

Needless to say, the selection of papers for this part reflects the editor's view of the present state of the testing art in aphasia. Recent additions to the test armamentarium include the Porch Index of Communicative Ability (PICA), the Functional Communication Profile (FCP), The Token Test, and the Neurosensory Center Comprehensive Examination for Aphasia (NCCEA). The NCCEA, incidentally, contains a modified version of the Token Test.

The Token Test, the FCP, and the NCCEA represent in the editor's view the most useful combination of tests available at the moment. Using the principle employed in Pierre Marie's Paper Test, the Token Test defines the degree of receptive language disturbance by requiring the patient to manipulate objects according to oral commands of increasing complexity. De Renzi and Vignolo (Reading 29) believe that this test can detect latent aphasia. This entire problem was later studied by Boller and Vignolo (2). Subsequent studies demonstrate that the Token Test discriminates among aphasics, non-aphasic brain-damaged, and non brain-damaged hospitalized individuals (9).

The FCP focuses on the way a patient uses his residual communication skills. It gives a quantitative result but is a rating scale and not a test of performance. Its focus is the functional use of everyday communication behaviors.

The NCCEA is a test of performance; it was designed by its authors to produce a quantitative profile of specific deficits associated with brain damage in and around the so-called language centers of the dominant hemisphere. Benton's paper on test construction, included in this collection (Reading 24), is particularly valuable because it describes the NCCEA and, what is perhaps of equal importance to the student of aphasia, because it is a scholarly dissertation on the history of intelligence and aphasia testing as well as on the problems inherent in aphasia test construction. Chief among such problems is the question of what conceptual model one is to use in designing a test for aphasia. We are thus led back inevitably to the descriptive concerns of the readings in Part I. In order to broaden this circle, however, we recommend that the student examine the outline and psycholinguistic analysis of many well known aphasia tests in Appendix B of Osgood and Miron's *Approaches to the Study of Aphasia* (5).

REFERENCES

1. Bastian, H. C. *A Treatise on Aphasia and Other Speech Defects*. London, H. K. Lewis, 1898.
2. Boller, F., Vignolo, L. A. Latent Sensory Aphasia in Hemisphere—Damaged Patients: An Experimental Study With the Token Test. *Brain*, **89**:830, 1966.
3. Eisenson, J. Aphasia in Adults. In Travis, L. D. (ed.), *Handbook of Speech Pathology*. New York, Appleton, 1957, pp. 436–502.
4. Eisenson, J. *Examining for Aphasia*. New York, Psychological Corporation, 1954.
5. Osgood, C. E., Miron, M. S. (eds.) *Approaches to the Study of Aphasia*. Urbana, University of Illinois, 1963.
6. Porch, B. *Porch Index of Communicative Ability*. Palo Alto, California, Consulting Psychologists Press, 1967.
7. Sarno, M. T. *The Functional Communication Profile Manual of Directions*. Rehabilitation Monograph No. 42. New York, Institute of Rehabilitation Medicine, New York University Medical Center, 1969.
8. Schuell, H. M. *Minnesota Test for Differential Diagnosis of Aphasia*. Minneapolis, University of Minnesota, 1955.
9. Schuell, H. M., Jenkins, J. J. The Nature of Language Deficit in Aphasia. *Psychological Review*, **66**:45–67, 1959.

10. Swisher, L. P., Sarno, M. T. Token Test Scores of Three Matched Patient Groups: Left Brain-Damaged With Aphasia; Right Brain-Damaged Without Aphasia; Non-Brain Damaged. *Cortex*, **5**:264–273, 1969.
11. Weisenburg, T. H., McBride, K. E. *Aphasia: A Clinical and Psychological Study*. New York, Hafner, 1935.
12. Wepman, J. M., Jones, L. V. *Studies in Aphasia: An Approach to Testing*. Chicago, Education Industry Service, 1961.

Problems of Test Construction in the Field of Aphasia

ARTHUR L. BENTON

ARTHUR L. BENTON, Ph.D., is with the department of neurology of the University Hospital, University of Iowa.

The development of the test battery described herein was supported by Program-Project Grant NB-03354 and Research Grant NB-00616 from the National Institute of Neurological Diseases and Blindness, Neurosensory Center Publication No. 125.

I. GENERAL CONSIDERATIONS

I should like to open this discussion of problems of test construction in the field of aphasia by considering first an analogous problem, namely, intelligence test construction. There are many similarities between intelligence and language. Both are extremely complex concepts which are difficult to define in such a way as to secure the agreement of any large number of experts. Both are variables of great clinical and educational importance; therefore, whether he possesses a satisfactory definition or not, the clinician is forced to deal with these concepts as best he can. The potential development of both intelligence and language, as well as their actual level of function at any given time, are strictly determined by central nervous system factors. Yet, at the same time, both are cultural products, the social environment being an indispensable precondition for the development of each. Finally, both intelligence and language are frequently impaired, either in combination or separately, in adults with acquired cerebral disease and in children with congenital cerebral abnormalities. Given these basic similarities, it may be instructive to review briefly the development of test construction in the area of intelligence since, on the whole, it seems that we have been somewhat more successful here than in the area of aphasia.

The clinical application of tests of mental abilities has a history going back about 90 years. The impetus for their development appears to have come from a desire to probe for the presence of mental impairment in patients who were not obviously demented and also in aphasic patients. Of course, the concept of dementia goes back many centuries. But it was only during the latter half of the 19th century that physicians felt the need for defined procedures that would elicit, and also perhaps provide a quantitative measure of, behavioral expressions of dementia. Undoubtedly the controversial question of whether aphasia necessarily involved a deficit in intelligence stimulated the development of special test methods. The definitive description of sensory aphasia by Wernicke in 1874 must also have made it seem imperative to distinguish between specific loss of language comprehension and more general impairment in understanding.

However, the procedures and test methods that were developed were rarely standardized in the modern sense. Starting with a subjective criterion of what constituted normal perform-

From *Cortex* 3:32–53, 1967.

ance, the clinician defined pathological inferiority as any performance below that level without giving systematic consideration to the limits of normal variability or to the effects of such factors as age, sex and cultural level (although, of course, common sense and clinical experience must certainly have played a corrective role in many instances). Various clinics developed their own favored batteries of tests for memory, reasoning, practical judgment, calculation, reading and other abilities and utilized these tests for making judgments about their patients' mental status. No doubt this was useful within the context of any single clinic but the results usually meant little to other workers who used other tests. Criteria of normality varied from one place to another. In one clinic, failure to repeat 7 digits might be considered to indicate defective immediate memory while in another clinic the criterion was failure to repeat 5 digits. Perhaps each was a valid criterion in the respective clinic, the difference in norms being due to a difference in test administration or scoring performance or perhaps in the type of patient seen in the two clinics. But obviously the test results were not comparable. The unsatisfactory nature of this situation was realized and it was not long before standard mental status examinations or test batteries, designed to be used by all clinics, were proposed.

One such battery was proposed by the Würzburg psychiatrist, Rieger, who outlined an extensive battery of tests (which took about 100 hours to give) and who recommended its general use. Neither Rieger's battery (which was, of course, quite impracticable) nor other proposed test batteries were generally adopted. There were a number of reasons for this. Chief among them was that the assembling of a battery of tests such as this was essentially an armchair exercise. No explicit empirical standardization and no clear demonstration of clinical utility supported the tests. Consequently, there was no convincing evidence that a proposed battery was significantly superior to one's own battery. Thus, while it was readily conceded that the adoption of the same battery by a large number of clinics would be desirable, there seemed to be no compelling reason for adopting any particular battery of tests.

This was the state of affairs in intelligence testing and intelligence test construction when Alfred Binet entered the scene at the beginning of the 20th century. As we know, Binet was presented with a practical problem by the educational authorities of Paris, namely, how can one identify those children who were destined to fail in school because of lack of intelligence and who required special instruction.

Binet undertook to answer the question by developing a battery of mental tests to measure the hypothetical quality of intelligence in children. His tests were *objective*, that is to say, not only was the task explicitly outlined but the procedure for presenting it was exactly described and precise criteria for evaluating whether or not a subject's performance was satisfactory were listed. Moreover, his tests were *standardized*, that is to say, they were given to samples of boys and girls of different ages; those tests which did not show a progressive rise in performance level with increasing age and those which showed a significant sex difference were eliminated. The result was, as we know, a series of tests appropriate to children of different ages, ranging from age 3 years to the adult level.

We also know, of course, that the Binet scale enjoyed a phenomenal success. Bobertag in Germany, Burt in England and Terman in the United States standardized the tests for use in these countries and developed equivalent versions. In some countries the scale was merely translated and the French or American standardization was adopted without revision. This was certainly a mistake and must have led to many errors of interpretation. The scale enjoyed this unparalleled success because it was objective, because it was standardized and because its clinical utility was demonstrated. For whatever its limitations were (and it had many), clinical workers in different places at least could now obtain directly comparable results. In short, it established the possibility of meaningful communication among them.

One serious limitation of the Binet scale was that it had been standardized on children and therefore its application to adults sometimes produced results of questionable validity. Another limitation was that most of the tests of the scale were of a verbal nature and therefore were likely to underestimate the true intelligence of individuals who, for one reason or another, suffered a specific weakness of verbal skills.

Both of these limitations were overcome to some degree by the Wechsler scales, which were standardized on adults with due allowance for the effects of age on performance and which provided separate scales for "verbal" and "non-verbal" abilities. The Wechsler scales have many serious defects; it is not necessary to go into these here. The point to be made is that, despite these defects, the scales have enjoyed immense popularity. The reasons for their popularity are the same as those underlying the popularity of the Binet. The scales were objective, they were standardized and they had demonstrable clinical utility.

With this perspective in mind, let us turn to the problem of test construction and application in the field of aphasia. I think it is not inaccurate to say that we are today where intelligence testing was in 1900, i.e., in the pre-Binet stage. Many test batteries, some of them of excellent quality, have been devised and are used in the clinics in which they were developed. A few, such as the battery of Schuell (1965), have been adopted by other clinics but none has been so widely adopted as to make it generally recognized as a standard battery. In recent years important developmental work has been going on in a number of neurological centers, e.g., Berlin, Bucharest, Düsseldorf, Milano, Iowa City (cf. De Renzi, 1960; Kreindler and Fradis, 1961; Bay, 1964; Weigl, 1966; Spreen, Benton and Van Allen, 1966). It is not surprising that each of these centers is represented at this conference, for these are the centers which have been most keenly aware of the critical nature of the problem facing us and each has made intensive efforts to remedy the situation. Each has reported brief descriptions of a comprehensive series of tests which is used in that particular center and which *could* be used more widely. But none has been generally adopted. The history of clinical intelligence testing perhaps tells us why. Excellent as these batteries are, none of them have been published in *usable form*. None of them present standardization information, explicitly describe testing procedures, present exact criteria for scoring or offer detailed guides for the interpretation of performance. Moreover, none of them present convincing evidence that the battery possesses a degree of clinical utility which is significantly greater than any other series of aphasia tests which might be assembled.

I hope I am not misunderstood. I do not mean to say that the batteries of tests developed in many clinics are not well standardized and objective or do not possess great clinical utility. The point which must be made (and it is a simple one) is that there is little evidence in *published form* that they are well standardized, objective and useful. In brief, the batteries which each of us has developed falls short of accomplishing what the Binet scale or the Wechsler scales have accomplished.

The Binet scale and the Wechsler scales certainly are not the last word in intellectual testing. All of us are aware of their many deficiencies. But, at the same time, it seems to me undeniable that, if the field of aphasia testing could attain at least the Binet-Wechsler stage, a significant advance would be gained. However limited such a "universal" aphasia battery might be, at least it would establish the possibility of effective communication among us.

Let us consider some of the formidable prob-problems involved in developing such an examination.

The first problem which we encounter is of a conceptual nature, for our conception of language will determine what tests we employ to assess language disturbance. How should we conceptualize language? Should we analyze it in terms of different types of stimulus-response sequences, establish a classification on this basis and devise tests to assess each type of performance? Should we follow Jacksonian principles and conceive of language in terms of levels of performance which are defined not by specific modalities or specific modes of response but in terms of the complexity of the proposition? If we do, we should adopt a very different set of tests. Do we believe, following the tradition of Marie and Head, that there is only one basic language function and that the different clinical pictures we see represent essentially adventitious admixtures of a disturbance in the single basic function and various non-linguistic sensory or motor disabilities? Or do we believe, following the tradition of Wernicke, that there are different primary types of aphasic disorder—receptive and expressive, auditory and visual, central and conductive? Or, following the lead of some linguists, should we conceive of language in terms of basic grammatical categories? In each case, our fundamental preconception will determine the nature of our examination and of the specific tasks included in it.

Now, of course, quite the same conceptual problem arises in the field of intelligence test construction. What is the nature of intelligence? What is its structure? Is the nucleus of intelligence a single general ability which enters into all intellectual performances, as Spearman believed? Or is intelligence "multidimensional" in nature, consisting of a relatively small number of primary mental abilities, as Thurstone stated? Or is it simply the sum total of a large number of specific intellectual skills that the individual has developed during the course of his life as a function of his hereditary predisposition, his formal education and accidental circumstances? Obviously our fundamental conception of the structure of intelligence will determine our choice of test methods. If we believe that intelligence consists essentially of a single general ability, then theoretically the best measure is a single test (e.g., the Progressive Matrices of Raven) which assesses this ability most directly. If we adopt Thurstone's concept of multiple primary abilities, we would develop tests for each of 5, 6 or 8 abilities which have been derived from factorial analysis. If we accept the doctrine of specificity, our test battery will consist of many tests covering as broad a range of diverse abilities as possible.

How did Binet solve this conceptual problem? Very simply . . . he avoided it. At first, he offered some simple armchair definitions, such as anyone might come up with ("intelligence is the capacity to adapt to novel situations," etc.). However, when pressed to defend his scale as a measure of these hypothetical abilities, he retreated to a pragmatic (and circular) definition: "intelligence" is what the tests measure. In short, Binet was prepared to concede that the scale was of no theoretical significance and to defend it on the sole basis of clinical utility. The Wechsler scales are a similar mélange of tasks employed previously in clinical work and with no underlying conceptual basis. This is a grave deficiency of these scales which imposes severe limitations on their usefulness in clinical investigation. As we have seen, their popularity has been due to other factors.

Now we must face the difficult problem of whether it is possible to go beyond the pragmatic level in constructing a standard test battery for aphasia. Given the diversity of conceptual approaches to the problem of aphasia, it may not be possible to do so at the present time. This is a question which we must discuss today. If our answer is negative (i.e., if we see no possibility of achieving a single conceptual framework which is satisfactory to all schools of thought), then perhaps a standardized basic examination can be assembled on pragmatic grounds. For example, it is likely that all students of aphasia would agree that a test of visual object-naming is a necessary part of any aphasia examination, even though there are different conceptions about what information the test provides. On the other hand, probably only some students would consider that a test of tactile object-naming is a necessary part of an aphasia examination. No doubt all would agree that a test of oral language comprehension belongs in the examination. However, there would be considerable disagreement about the selection of items in such a test, depending upon how one defines "difficulty" or "complexity" (e.g., grammatical form, length of question, number of "bits of information" in the question, etc.). The status of tests of repetition of digits, words or sentences might well be controversial, valued by some but considered by others to be essentially irrelevant to the problem of aphasia.

I do not know the answer to this question.

But obviously, it is one which cannot be "wished away." Some kind of solution (or, at least, understanding) of the question must be achieved before a broadly acceptable standard examination for aphasia can be constructed.

The other problems involved in the construction of an aphasia examination are of a technical nature. They are not nearly as difficult as the conceptual problem in the sense that their solution is actually well within our capabilities while the conceptual problem may not be at the present time. However, these technical problems are quite formidable in the sense that their solution demands a great deal of labor. The construction of a technically adequate test battery to evaluate the status of language functions involves a number of tedious, time-consuming tasks: careful selection of items for each test in the battery; pilot testing to determine reliability, validity and level of difficulty; collection of normative data for performance on each test of appropriate groups of subjects, including assessment of the influence of such factors as age, sex and cultural status on performance level; determining the effects of practice or prior experience with the tests; considering whether two or more equivalent forms of the battery should be constructed in order to permit unbiased repeated examination of the same patient; correcting scores for the influence of age and educational level, when this is necessary; finally, transforming raw scores into standard scores or ranks so that one obtains a valid picture of an individual patient's strengths and weaknesses.

All these steps are necessary components in the development of an aphasia test battery designed for use within a single language community. The development of a standard examination designed for use in two or more language communities raises additional problems. The test battery must be standardized separately for each language community for it will be found that the same item does not necessarily have the same meaning or the same difficulty level in every community. Therefore the task is not one of simple translation of a test from one language to another but the more complicated one of constructing an essentially equivalent test in the second language.

Let me illustrate this problem by some specific examples. In standardizing a test of visual object-naming in our laboratory, we decided to select items on the basis of the age at which young children could name the object under the artificial condition of the psychometric testing situation. This we called the "acquisition age" of the name of the object. Thus we found that (at least in the case of children living in the midwestern section of the U.S.) the acquisition age for the word "key" was 4.1 years; for the word "jar," it was 4.6 years; for the word "shoe-lace," it was 5.2 years, etc. At the same time, Prof. De Renzi and Dr. Vignolo have been developing an Italian version of this visual naming test and, in the course of this, they have been standardizing the same items on Milanese children. Many of the items prove to have approximately the same acquisition age in the American and the Italian standardizations. However, other items prove to have lower or higher ages in one or the other language community. It is, of course, easy to understand why this should be so. For example, the age at which children in a given language community will learn the name of a safety razor will depend upon the relative prevalence of use by their fathers of safety razors as compared to straight razors or electric shavers. One of the items in our visual naming test is a toy rotary eggbeater representing the instrument which American housewives typically use to whip up various mixtures of eggs, cream, butter, etc. But this is generally a much less familiar object to Italian children since *their* mothers typically use the Continental egg-whisk (*fouet; frullino; Schneebesen*). Conversely, the Continental egg-whisk is not known by name to most American children.

These considerations may seem at first glance to be an academic exercise without clinical significance. I can assure you that they are not. Rochford and Williams (1962) have demonstrated that the naming of different objects and their parts shows a highly consistent order of difficulty in patients with nominal aphasia and in normal children. Recently we completed a similar study of the relationship between the errors made by aphasic patients in naming various objects and the "acquisition ages" of the names of these objects as determined in young children. The results disclosed extremely high correlation coefficients between the number of errors made by the patients and the age at which children learned the names of the objects. This held for both visual and tactile naming. It was as clear a demonstration of the "law of regression" as one could hope to make and fully confirmed the findings of Rochford and Williams.

What is true of visual object naming will hold, of course, for all the tasks in an aphasia examination. The difficulty of a specific test of language understanding will be determined by factors peculiar to each language such as the relative frequency in each language of the words in the proposition presented to the patient, the relative ease or difficulty of pronouncing the words in each language, and the grammatical form in which the proposition is stated.

It is evident, then, that a valid international aphasia examination will *not* consist of identical tests but rather of *essentially equivalent* tests, each of which has been standardized on the language population to which it is to be applied. It is equally evident that the development of such an examination is a task of considerable magnitude. However, the task can be done. I personally believe that the fruits would be worth the great effort which is required. If we should be successful, we would possess for the first time the means for a direct comparison of our individual findings. This, I think we would all agree, is a prerequisite for truly scientific intercourse among us and this has been lamentably lacking in the field of aphasia. Moreover, in the course of developing such an examination, we may well learn important new facts about aphasia. Finally, it may be anticipated that the very existence of an examination based on rigorous scientific criteria would have the effect of raising the quality of aphasia research throughout the world. This too, we would all agree, is a prerequisite for advancing our knowledge of this group of disorders of ever-increasing medical importance.

II. DESCRIPTION OF AN APHASIA EXAMINATION IN COURSE OF DEVELOPMENT

The construction of this battery of tests to evaluate language disorders was initiated at the Neurosensory Center of the College of Medicine, University of Iowa, in 1962 by Dr. Otfried Spreen and myself. In 1965, Prof. Ennio De Renzi and Dr. L. A. Vignolo of the University Clinic for Nervous and Mental Diseases in Milano began the development of an Italian language version of the battery.

The impetus for undertaking this major project was derived from several considerations: 1) to provide a fairly comprehensive examination that would include assessment of most of the areas of language function which are of clinical interest; 2) to provide sufficiently detailed tests for each area of language function so that a relatively exact measure of performance level can be obtained; 3) to include specific tests in the battery which could be employed to investigate current questions in the field of aphasia (e.g., the reality of the clinical pictures of conduction aphasia, central aphasia and transcortical aphasia; the nature of the pattern of recovery from aphasia; the nature of the pattern of loss in developing aphasia; the question of modality-specific aphasia); 4) to standardize and score test performances in such a way as to introduce necessary corrections for the effects of age, education and sex on performance and to make possible a direct and valid comparison of performances within the individual patient as well as among patients; 5) to include a series of non-linguistic control tests in the battery in order to insure valid interpretation of performance on the language tests; 6) to include a series of non-linguistic supplementary tests assessing various abilities in order to permit investigation of some of the non-linguistic intellectual deficits associated with aphasic disorders.

Selection of Tests

The selection of tests was based on theoretical and practical considerations. From the theoretical standpoint, it was believed that the traditional associationist approach still possessed sufficient validity to warrant formulation of certain test procedures along these lines. Thus, tests of tactile object-naming with the right and with the left hand were included as well as the more conventional test of visual object-naming. Analogous tests of reading and writing were included both in order to effect systematic variation in type of stimulus and mode of response and because of their importance for clinical purposes. Tests of language understanding were included for obvious reasons. Tests of repetition of sentences and digits were included with particular reference to the question of the concepts of conduction aphasia and transcortical aphasia. Verbal associative fluency and sentence construction were included with the hope that they might provide assessments of the status of "inner language" in aphasic patients.

The 20 tests of language function that comprise the nucleus of the battery are listed in Table 24-1. A brief description of each test follows:

1. *Visual Naming (VN)*. The patient is instructed to name 10–40 objects (not pictures); the actual number of objects presented depends upon the purpose of the test (clinical evaluation or specific research problem) and the level of the patient's performance.

2. *Description of Use (DU)*. The patient is instructed to tell the use of 10–20 objects from the basic set of 40 objects.

3. *Tactile Naming—Right Hand (TNR)*. The patient is instructed to feel the object with his right hand (without the aid of vision) and name it; 10–20 objects from the basic set of 40 are used; in case of failure, stereognostic capacity is evaluated by Control Test 1 (TMR).

4. *Tactile Naming—Left Hand (TNL)*. Same procedure as TNR.

5. *Repetition of Sentences (SRP)*. The patient is instructed to repeat tape-recorded sentences ranging from 1 to 26 syllables in length.

6. *Repetition of Digits (DRF)*. The patient is instructed to repeat tape-recorded series of digits ranging from 3 to 9 digits in length.

7. *Reversal of Digits (DRR)*. The patient is instructed to repeat in reverse order tape-recorded series of digits ranging from 2 to 7 digits in length.

8. *Word Fluency (WF)*. The patient is instructed to say all the words which he can think of that begin with a specific letter of the alphabet (e.g., "F," "A," "S"); 3 one-minute trials with 3 different letters are given.

9. *Sentence Construction (SC)*. Sets of 2 or 3 words are presented to the patient who is

TABLE 24-1. TESTS OF LANGUAGE FUNCTION IN THE APHASIA BATTERY

1.	VN	—	Visual Naming
2.	DU	—	Description of Use
3.	TNR	—	Tactile Naming, Right Hand
4.	TNL	—	Tactile Naming, Left Hand
5.	SRP*	—	Sentence Repetition
6.	DRF*	—	Repetition of Digits
7.	DRR*	—	Reversal of Digits
8.	WF	—	Word Fluency
9.	SC	—	Sentence Construction (Masselon Test)
10.	IN	—	Identification by Name
11.	IS	—	Identification by Sentence (De Renzi-Vignolo Token Test)
12.	RNO	—	Reading Names Orally
13.	RSO	—	Reading Sentences Orally
14.	RNP	—	Reading Names for Meaning
15.	RSP	—	Reading Sentences for Meaning (De Renzi-Vignolo Token Test)
16.	VGN	—	Visual-Graphic Naming
17.	WN	—	Writing Names
18.	WD	—	Writing to Dictation
19.	WC	—	Writing from Copy
20.	ART*	—	Articulation (Oral Repetition)

* Presented on tape.

instructed to make up a sentence with these words; 5 sets of words are given.

10. *Object Identification by Name (IN)*. The patient is instructed to point to objects (from the basic set of 40 objects) named by the examiner; the actual number of objects named depends upon the specific purpose of the test and the level of the patient's performance.

11. *Identification by Sentence (IS)*. This test, which is a slight modification of the Token Test of De Renzi and Vignolo, consists of 39 commands of progressively increasing complexity which assess the patient's capacity to understand oral language.

12. *Reading Names Orally (RNO)*. The patient is instructed to read aloud names of objects from the basic set of 40 objects.

13. *Reading Sentences Orally (RSO)*. The patient is instructed to read aloud 12 commands from the De Renzi-Vignolo Token Test.

14. *Reading Names for Meaning (RNP)*. The patient is presented with the written name of an object and instructed to point to it in a display of 10 objects.

15. *Reading Sentences for Meaning (RSP)*. The patient is presented with 12 written commands from the De Renzi-Vignolo Token Test and instructed to carry them out.

16. *Visual-Graphic Naming (VGN)*. The patient is instructed to write the names of 10 visually presented objects from the basic set of 40 objects; performance is scored in terms of accuracy of naming and not for graphic characteristics.

17. *Writing Names (WN)*. The patient's performance on Test 16 is scored for spelling but not for accuracy of naming; if the patient was not able to write the name of the visually presented object, the name is presented to him orally (i.e., writing to dictation).

18. *Writing to Dictation (WD)*. The patient is instructed to write 2 short sentences to dictation; performance is scored for spelling, punctuation, omissions and reduplications.

19. *Writing from Copy (WC)*. The patient is instructed to write 2 short sentences from copy; performance is scored as in Test 18.

20. *Articulation (ART)*. The patient is instructed to repeat clearly 30 meaningful and 8 nonsense words presented by tape; performance is scored in terms of the number of correctly articulated consonant or consonant blends.

Control Tests

These control tests are given to certain patients in order to determine whether their failure on certain language tests may be due to sensory or perceptual defect rather than to impairment in language. A brief description of these 4 tests follows:

C 1. *Tactile-Visual Matching, Right Hand (TMR)*. This test is given if the patient has made any errors in the test of tactile naming with the right hand (TNR), its purpose being to determine whether failure in the naming task may have been due to stereognostic defect. A series of objects is presented to the patient for tactile recognition with the right hand without the aid of vision; he is instructed to identify the object in a visual display set before him. The arrangement is illustrated in Figure 24-1.

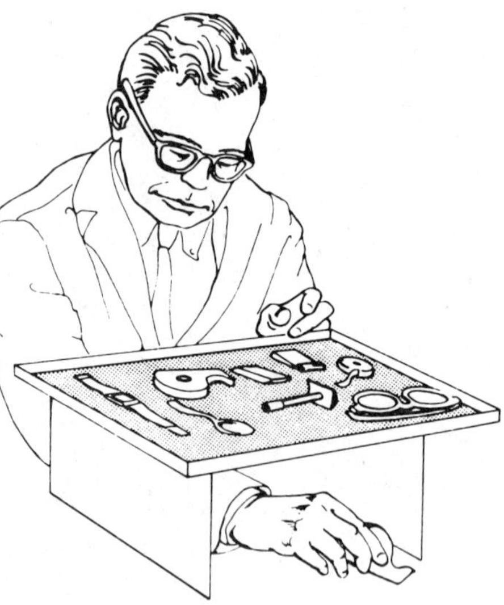

Fig. 24–1. Arrangement for test of tactile-visual matching, right hand.

C 2. *Tactile-Visual Matching, Left Hand (TML)*. This test, which is the same as Test C 1, assesses tactile recognition in the left hand and is given to any patient who has made one or more errors in the test of tactile naming with the left hand (TNL).

C 3. *Visual-Visual Matching (VVM)*. This test is given if the patient has made any errors in the tests of visual naming (VN) or identification by name (IN); two trays, each containing the same 10 objects, are set before the patient; one tray is in the standard position while the other is in the reversed position so that the locations of the objects are different on the two trays; pointing to an object on one tray, the examiner instructs the patient to point to the same object on the other tray. The purpose of the test is to determine whether the patient's failure on the language tests may have been due to impairment in visual recognition.

C 4. *Visual Form Perception (FP)*. This test is given if the patient has made any errors on any reading test (RNO, RSO, RNP, RSP); a visual display of 21 letters is set before the patient (Figure 24-2); 8 letters are then presented one at a time and the patient is instructed to identify the presented letter on the display; if he makes any errors, a second test is given to obtain a more precise estimate of his visuoperceptive impairment.

Supplementary Tests

As their name implies, these tests do not form an essential part of the language battery in the strict sense. They evaluate various aspects of praxis, perception, memory and reasoning and their purpose is to provide a fuller picture of the setting within which a patient's language disturbances appear. As such, they are considered to be useful both for the clinical evaluation and for investigative purposes. The 10 tests are as follows:

S 1. *Utilization Praxis, Right Hand (APR)*. The patient is instructed to demonstrate with his right hand the use of each of 10 objects from the basic set of 40 objects. If he does not understand the verbal instructions, the use of other objects in the basic set is demonstrated in an effort to communicate the nature of the task to him. His performance on each task is analyzed in terms of the component actions, e.g., his demonstration of the use of a knife is analyzed in terms of whether he grasps the handle, orientates the knife so that the blade is away from him and makes a cutting or spreading movement.

S 2. *Utilization Praxis, Left Hand (APL)*. This test, which is the same as Test S 1, employs other objects to assess demonstration of use with the *left* hand.

S 3. *Handedness Inventory (H)*. This test consists of a series of questions about hand preference in various activities and is presented orally to the patient or, when this is not possible, to a reliable informant; if doubt exists about the patient's understanding of the concepts of "right" and "left," he is asked to show how he would perform the activity mentioned, e.g., throw a ball or use a screw-driver. The supplementary questions about hand preference among members of the family are presented to the patient or a relative whenever it seems likely that reliable information on this point can be secured. The Inventory is shown in Table 24-2.

S 4. *Sound Recognition (SRC)*. This test consists of 13 tape-recorded familiar sounds which are presented to the patient with the instruction that he name the source of the sound. If performance on this sound-naming task is below the normal level, the test is repeated in the form of a non-verbal multiple choice task in which the patient must identify the source of the heard sound among 4 alternatives presented in visual form to him. Examples of this multiple choice task are presented in Figure 24-3.

S 5. *Three-Dimensional Block Construction (BC)*. This test of 3-dimensional block construction

Q W E R T Y U I O P

A W S D F G H J K L Z

Fig. 24–2. Visual display for test of visual form perception; individual letters are presented singly to the patient who is instructed to identify it on the display; actual height of letters is 5 mm.

TABLE 24–2. HANDEDNESS QUESTIONNAIRE

A.	Are you right-handed or left-handed?	Right - Left - Mixed
B.	Do you consider yourself *strongly* or *moderately* right-handed (or left-handed)?	Strongly - Moderately
C. 1	With which hand do you write?	Right - Left - Both
2	With which hand do you use a scissors?	Right - Left - Both
3	With which hand do you use a screwdriver?	Right - Left - Both
4	With which hand do you throw a ball?	Right - Left - Both
5	In baseball, do you bat right-handed or left-handed?	Right - Left - Both
6	With which hand do you use a hammer?	Right - Left - Both
7	With which hand do you use a needle in sewing?	Right - Left - Both
8	With which hand do you usually carry books?	Right - Left - Both
9	With which hand do you usually carry a suitcase?	Right - Left - Both
10	With which hand do you hold the toothbrush when you brush your teeth?	Right - Left - Both

Hand Preferences of Members of Family

Father:

Mother:

Siblings:

Brother 1 —	Sister 1 —
Brother 2 —	Sister 2 —
Brother 3 —	Sister 3 —
Brother 4 —	Sister 4 —

Husband/Wife:

Children (6 years and over):

Son 1 —	Daughter 1 —
Son 2 —	Daughter 2 —
Son 3 —	Daughter 3 —
Son 4 —	Daughter 4 —

involves the successive presentation of each of 3 block models to the patient with the instruction that he construct a replica which is exactly like the model (cf. Critchley, 1953; Benton and Fogel, 1962).

S 6. *Stereognosis, Right Hand (STR).* In this test the patient is required to identify abstract figures made of sandpaper haptically with the right *hand* and without the aid of vision, identification being accomplished by matching the haptically perceived form with the same form visually presented in a display (Figure 24-4).

S 7. *Stereognosis, Left Hand (STL).* Application of Test S 6 to the *left* hand.

S 8. *WAIS Block Designs (BD).* This subtest of the Wechsler battery is employed to assess higher-level two-dimensional constructional praxis.

S 9. *WAIS Picture Arrangement (PA).* This subtest of the Wechsler battery is employed to assess the patient's ability to organize pictorial information into a meaningful temporal sequence.

S 10. *Visual Retention Test, Multiple Choice Form (VRT).* This test of short-term visual memory involves the presentation of each of 15 abstract designs to the patient; after the design has been removed, the patient must identify it among 4 alternatives presented to him.

Standardization Procedures

The steps taken in standardizing test of visual object-naming (VN) may be described to illustrate the standardization procedures utilized in developing the tests in the battery. A total of 60 objects were presented for visual and tactile naming to a group of aphasic patients, a group of control patients and to children of various ages. On the basis of the findings, 40 objects were selected to form the test on the basis of the following criteria: 1) number of failures in visual naming of the item so that there would be a fairly wide range of difficulty; the actual percentage of failure ranged from 3.6 percent to 35.5 percent; 2) items that were appropriate for both visual and tactile naming;

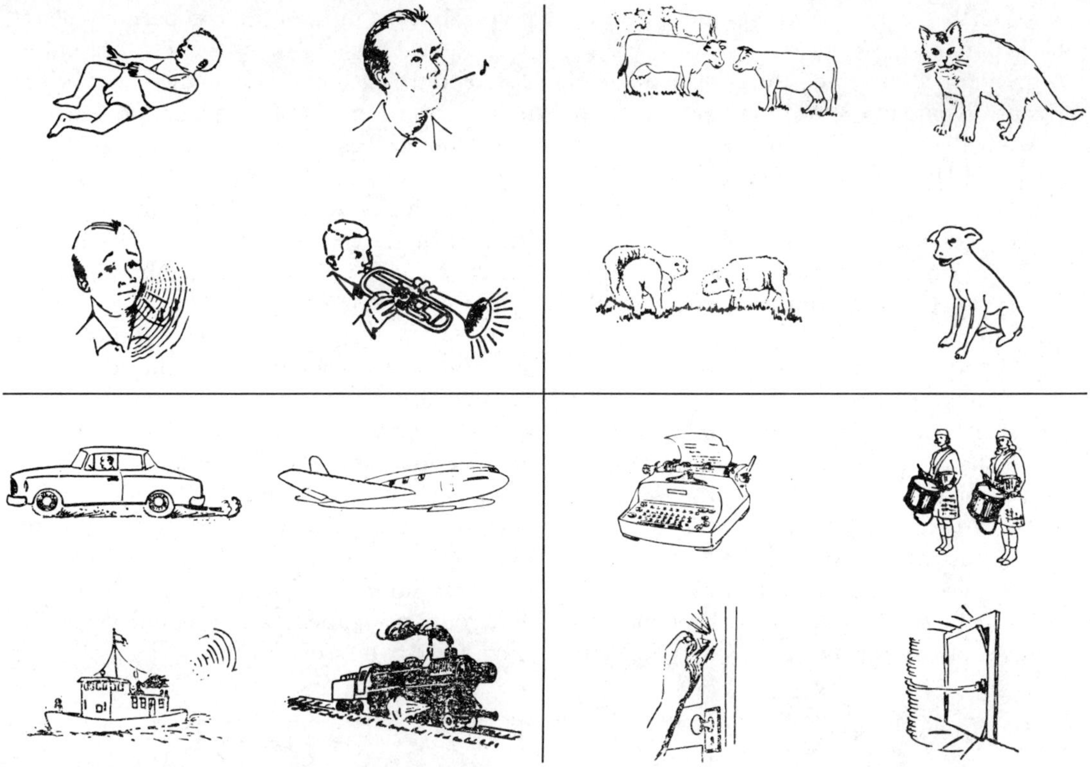

Fig. 24–3. Examples of multiple choice items on sound recognition test; patient hears tape-recorded sound (e.g., baby crying, boat whistle, drums) and is instructed to point to the source of the sound on the 4-choice card.

3) ease of scoring responses as correct or incorrect. This 40-item test was then divided into 4 subsets of 10 objects, each subset being of approximately equal difficulty level.

Administration of the test to control patients within the age range of 16–64 years indicated that there was no significant association between performance level and age or educational level and hence that no correction for these factors was necessary in establishing normative standards. However, on other tests (e.g., digit repetition, word fluency) corrections in score to control for the influence of age and education on performance were found to be necessary.

The test is administered in two forms:

1) For most clinical and research purpose, one or two trays (10–20 objects) are presented for visual naming. If the patient names all 10 objects on the first tray correctly, the test is terminated and he is assigned a score of 40. If he makes 1–9 errors in naming the objects of the first tray, the second set of 10 objects is presented and the assigned total score is twice the number of objects correctly named. Conversely, if the patient fails to name any object on the first tray correctly, the test is terminated and he is assigned a score of 0.

2) For certain specific research purposes, all 4 trays (40 objects) are presented (e.g., in studies of visual and tactile naming or of the relationship between frequency of errors in aphasic patients and the age of acquisition of the name of the object in children).

Development of Profile Sheets

A distribution of the raw scores of the control patients on each test was tabulated and appropriate corrections made for the influence of age and educational level on performance. Each distribution of corrected scores was then converted into a percentile rank distribution. Bay employed an essentially similar procedure of converting raw scores into ranks in his study of the performance patterns of 80 aphasic patients.

A profile sheet based on the performances of the control patients indicating the percentile rank equivalent of different raw scores was then constructed. It was found, however, that this profile sheet was unsuitable for evaluating the performances of aphasic patients because most of the scores of the "typical" aphasic patient fell below the entire distribution of scores of the control group. For example, the typical aphasic patient in our reference group correctly named 32 out of 40 objects on visual naming while the lowest score on this test for any control patient was 37. The typical aphasic patient was able to repeat 14 sentences correctly in the Sentence Repetition Test (SR); the lowest score made by a control patient was 16.

Thus it was evident that this profile sheet, which was developed on the basis of the performances of control patients, was not appropriate for the purpose of comparing aphasic patients with each other or for evaluating differential level of performance within the individual patient. However, it has proved to be useful for investigating the language performances of clinically non-aphasic patients, e.g., in comparing patients with lesions of the left and right hemispheres and in studying the decline of language functions in normal old age and in senile dementia.

In order to study language function in aphasia more precisely, we developed another profile sheet based upon the performances of what we designated as our "reference group" of aphasic patients. Within certain restrictions, this group consisted of all patients with a clinical diagnosis of aphasia who were referred to the Laboratory of Neuropsychology for evaluation. The restrictions consisted in excluding from the group any patient who was uncooperative or confused, whose disability was clearly limited

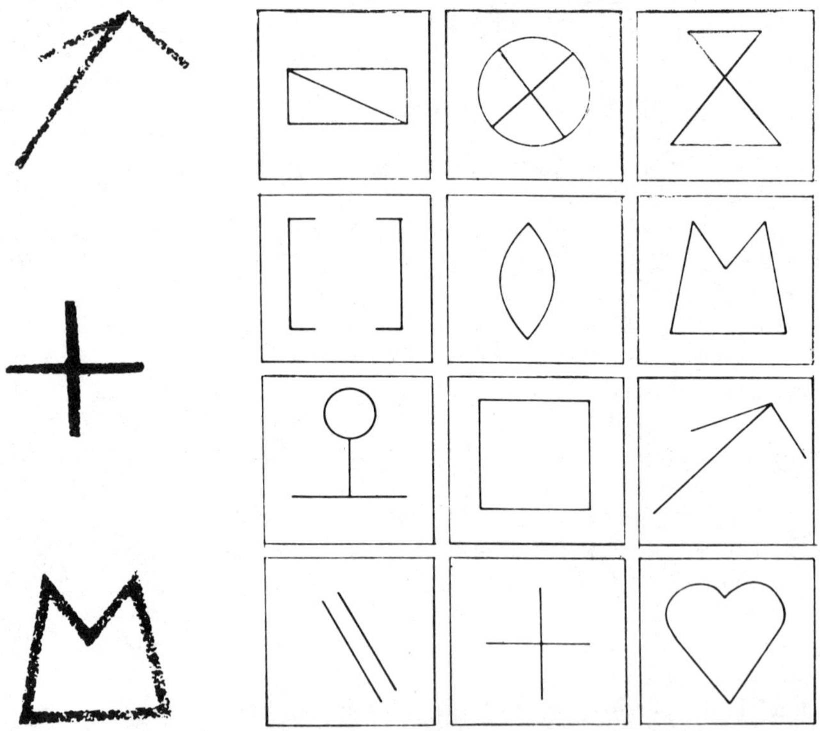

Fig. 24–4. a) *Examples of sandpaper figures used in supplementary tests of stereognosis (STR, STL); actual height of figures is 5 cm.*
b) *Visual display presented to the patient for identification of haptically perceived sandpaper figures; actual size of figures is the same as the sandpaper figures.*

to disturbances in articulation or whose concomitant dysarthria was so severe that his speech was not understandable.

The distribution of the raw scores of the patients on each test was plotted, the appropriate corrections for the influence of age and educational level were made and the corrected scores were converted into percentile rank scores, as in the first profile sheet. This new profile sheet was used as a basis for plotting the scores of individual aphasic patients (Figure 24-5). The individual profile gives an immediate indication of the overall severity of the aphasic disorder (as compared to our reference group of aphasic patients) and also of the pattern of performance of the patient on this battery of language tests.

Illustrative Profiles

Figure 24-6 shows the profiles of a young woman who presented with a relatively mild aphasic disturbance following a cerebrovascular accident and who recovered virtually completely from a clinical standpoint. "Anomia" was noted on the referral sheet as being the most prominent disability; actually, as the lower profile shows, her poorest performances were on the repetition and reversal of digits. On retest, she showed no aphasic deficits except inferior performances on the repetition tasks.

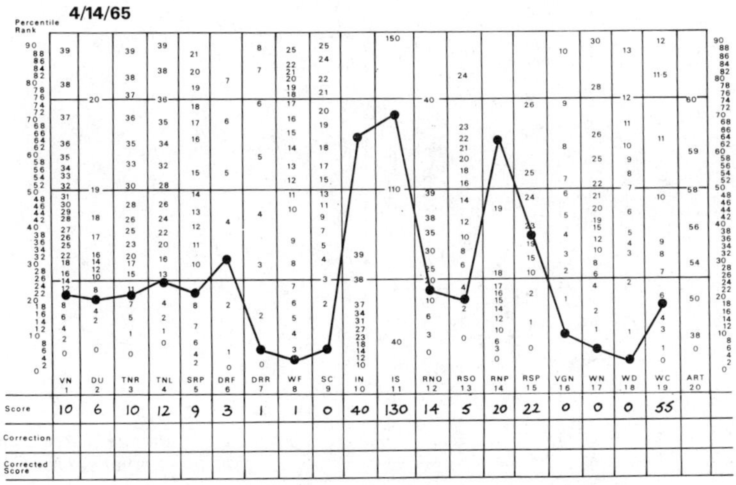

Fig. 24-5. (Case No. 63-5328). Profile of patient with clinical diagnosis of "expressive aphasia."

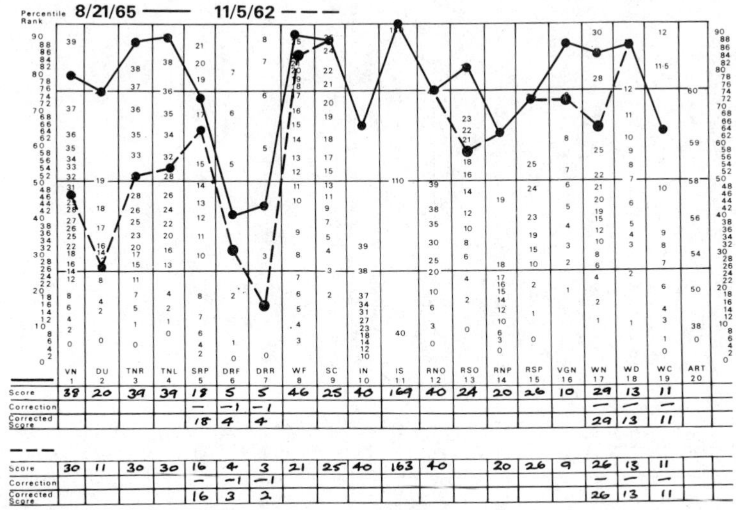

Fig. 24-6. (Case No. 62-26028). Profiles of aphasic patient initially referred with notation of "anomia" who showed virtually complete recovery from clinical standpoint.

8/13/65

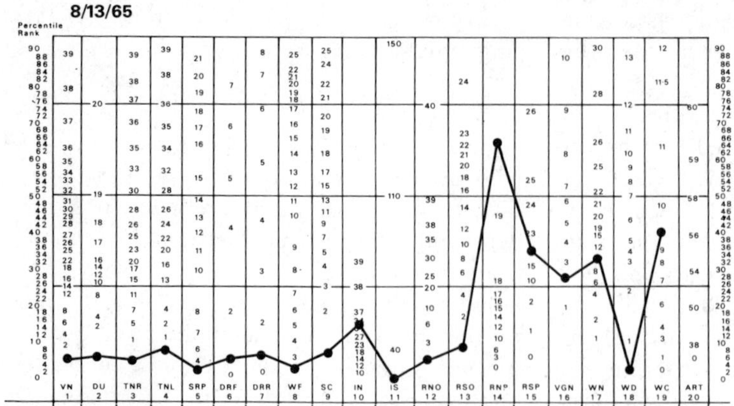

	VN 1	DU 2	TNR 3	TNL 4	SRP 5	DRF 6	DRR 7	WF 8	SC 9	IN 10	IS 11	RNO 12	RSO 13	RNP 14	RSP 15	VGN 16	WN 17	WD 18	WC 19	ART 20
Score	0	0	0	0	0	0	0	0	0	32	20	0	0	20	19	2	10	0	9.5	
Correction					2	1	1													
Corrected Score					2	1	1													

Fig. 24–7. (Case No. 62-22196). Profile of patient with referral diagnosis of "jargon aphasia."

12/10/65

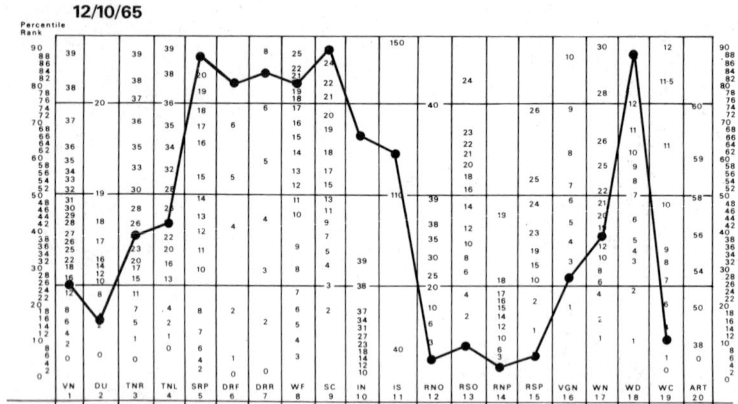

	VN 1	DU 2	TNR 3	TNL 4	SRP 5	DRF 6	DRR 7	WF 8	SC 9	IN 10	IS 11	RNO 12	RSO 13	RNP 14	RSP 15	VGN 16	WN 17	WD 18	WC 19	ART 20
Score	14	3	25	24	17	5	5	16	25	40	120	0	0	0	0	2	18	11	0	
Correction					4	2	2	4										2	2	
Corrected Score	14	3	25	24	21	7	7	20	25	40	120	0	0	0	0	2	18	13	2	

Fig. 24–8. (Case No. 65-16610). Profile of patient with referral diagnosis of "anomia"; note that all language performances involving vision are impaired.

2/14/66

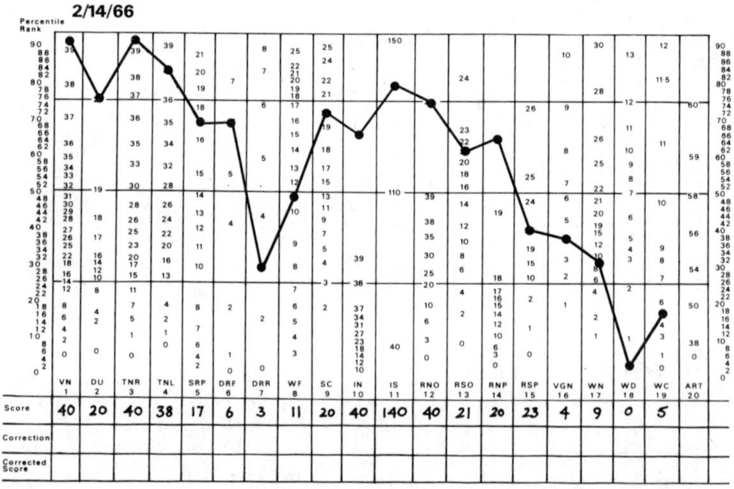

	VN 1	DU 2	TNR 3	TNL 4	SRP 5	DRF 6	DRR 7	WF 8	SC 9	IN 10	IS 11	RNO 12	RSO 13	RNP 14	RSP 15	VGN 16	WN 17	WD 18	WC 19	ART 20
Score	40	20	40	38	17	6	3	11	20	40	140	40	21	20	23	4	9	0	5	
Correction																				
Corrected Score																				

Fig. 24–9. (Case No. 66-1087). Profile of patient with referral diagnosis of "Gerstmann Syndrome."

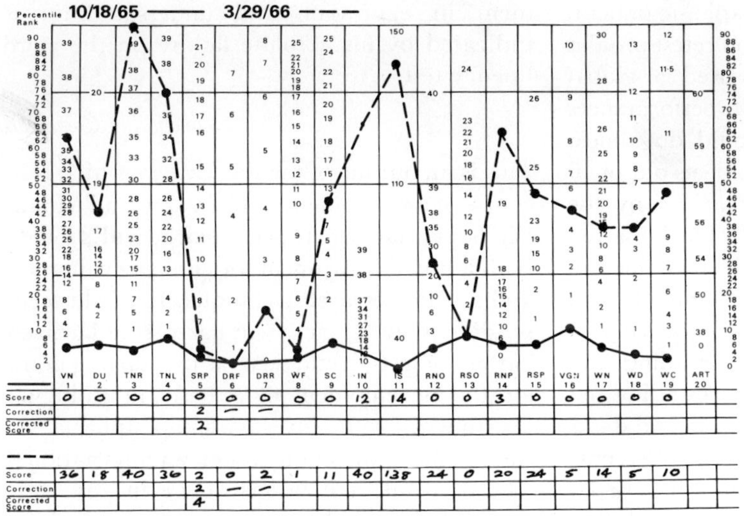

Fig. 24–10. (Case No. 65-14624). Profiles of patient with initial global aphasia who showed significant improvement over a period of 5 months.

Figure 24-5 shows the profile of a patient clinically diagnosed as a case of "expressive aphasia." It will be noted that all oral expressive performances, including the "inner language" performances involved in Word Fluency (WF) and Sentence Construction (SC), are severely impaired. Writing is also severely impaired. On the other hand, both oral and visual verbal understandings are less severely compromised but are nevertheless clearly defective. The profile fits the classic description of "motor aphasia."

Figure 24-7 shows the profile of a patient with the diagnosis of "jargon aphasia." It will be seen that, with the curious exception of Reading Names for Meaning (RNP), all performances are grossly defective. The profile fits the classic description of "Wernicke's aphasia."

Figure 24-8 shows the profile of a patient clinically classified as "anomia." However, the pattern of performance indicates that this is scarcely the picture of "pure anomia" or "amnesic aphasia." One notes that Description of Use (DU) is as severely impaired as Visual Naming (VN). In addition, all performances involving reading (i.e., visual discrimination) are severely impaired. It is also to be noted that Writing for Dictation (WD), i.e., via the auditory channel, is not impaired while Writing from Copy (WC), i.e., via the visual channel, is grossly defective. However, control test performances provided no evidence of gross visuosensory or visuoperceptive deficit. Visual-Visual Matching (VVM), Tactile-Visual Matching (TMR, TML) and Visual Form Perception were all performed perfectly. Nevertheless, the possibility of an interaction between a more subtle visual deficit and language performance, as postulated by Kok (1964) and by Bisiach (1966), should not be excluded.

Figure 24-9 presents the profile of a patient who was referred as having a relatively "pure", Gerstmann syndrome. She did in fact show severe finger agnosia, right-left disorientation, acalculia and agraphia. In addition, she manifested severe constructional apraxia and marked topographic disorientation. As would be anticipated, the profile shows that her writing is impaired, particularly writing to dictation and writing from copy. She also shows poor repetition of digits, which is not unexpected. She was considered on an impressionistic-clinical basis to be free from aphasia. The profile suggests why this impression was gained. Her naming performances, description of use of objects and identification of objects when the name is supplied by the examiner are fairly adequate. However, we also note that Reading for Meaning (RSP) is significantly impaired and that the "inner language" tests (Word Fluency and Sentence Construction) are performed quite poorly. Thus there would seem to be a significant impairment of language functions in this ostensibly non-aphasic patient.

Figure 24-10 shows the test and retest profiles of a patient who initially showed a global aphasia. On the first test, all performances were severely impaired; he could do almost nothing. He could identify 12 objects out of 40 when the name was supplied to him by the examiner, but that was about all. The impaired naming and reading could not be explained in terms of sensory deficit. He was examined again 5 months later and showed great improvement in naming, oral understanding, reading and writing. But some performances did not improve, e.g., repetition of sentences and digits and reading sentences aloud (RSO). We note also that tactile naming is somewhat better than visual naming. Furthermore, we see that "Description of Use" of visually presented objects is relatively poor. This raises the question, as in a case previously presented, of whether a subtle disturbance in visual recognition may not be a residual deficit. The extreme impoverishment of his "inner language" processes (despite his remarkable improvement in expression and understanding) is indicated by his absolute failure on the word fluency test.

Concluding Comments

This is an outline of the test battery which is in course of development in Iowa City and Milan. We hope that, when perfected, it will provide both a useful instrument for clinical evaluation and a valid research technique. It would seem possible that it, or a similarly standardized battery of tests, could serve as the starting point for the development of a basic multilingual instrument for the investigation of aphasia. Of course, the application of such an international battery would not be restrictive in any way. Certainly it would not preclude the utilization of special tests and approaches by any investigator or in any clinic. On the other hand, the uniform application of a standard examination such as this would go far towards establishing that level of *operational* understanding among workers which is a prerequisite for scientific communication in the field of aphasia.

REFERENCES

Bay, E. (1964) *Principles of classification and their influence on our concepts of language*, in Disorders of Language, ed. by A. V. S. de Reuck and M. O'Connor. Little Brown and Co., Boston.

Benton, A. L., and Fogel, M. L. (1962) *Three-dimensional constructional praxis*, "Arch. Neurol.," **7,** 347–354.

——, Meyers, R., and Polder, G. J. (1962) *Some aspects of handedness*, "Psychiat. Neurol.," **144,** 321–337.

Bisiach, E. (1966) *Perceptual factors in the pathogenesis of anomia*, "Cortex," **2,** 90–95.

Blackburn, H. L., and Benton, A. L. (1957) *Revised administration and scoring of the digit span test*, "J. Consult. Psychol.," **21,** 139–143.

Critchley, M. (1953) *The Parietal Lobes*. Edward Arnold and Co., London.

De Renzi, E. (1960) *Un test semeiotico per l'afasia e per le funzioni connesse*, "Arch. Psicol. Neurol. Psichiat.," **21,** 17–64.

——, and Vignolo, L. A. (1962) *The token test: a sensitive test to detect receptive disturbances in aphasics*, "Brain," **85,** 665–678.

Kok, E. P. (1964) *Modifications of speed of perception of pictures of objects in optic aphasia*, "Cortex," **1,** 328–343.

Kreindler, A., and Fradis, A. (1961) *The Bucharest symposium on aphasia*, "World Neurol.," **2,** 986–996.

Rochford, G., and Williams, M. (1962) *Studies in the development and breakdown in the use of names, I: the relationship between nominal dysphasia and the acquisition of vocabulary in childhood*, "J. Neurol. Neurosurg. Psychiat.," **25,** 222–233.

Schuell, H. (1965) *Minnesota Test for Differential Diagnosis of Aphasia*. Univ. Minnesota Press, Minneapolis.

Spreen, O., Benton, A. L., and Fincham, R. W. (1965) *Auditory agnosia without aphasia*, "Arch. Neurol.," **13,** 84–92.

——, ——, and Van Allen, M. W. (1966) *Dissociation of visual and tactile naming in amnesic aphasia*, "Neurology," **16,** 807–814.

Weigl, E. (1966) *On the construction of standard psychological tests in cases of brain damage*, "J. Neurol. Sci.," **3,** 123–127.

25

A Re-Evaluation of the Short Examination for Aphasia

HILDRED M. SCHUELL

HILDRED M. SCHUELL, Ph.D., (deceased) was director of the aphasia section of the neurology service of the Minneapolis Veterans Administration Hospital, and was with the department of neurology of the Graduate School of Medicine, University of Minnesota.
Research reported in the paper was supported by U.S. Public Health Service Research Grant No. NB-03364-05, from the Institute of Neurological Diseases and Blindness.

Several years ago, a short examination for aphasia by Schuell (1957) was published in *Neurology*. Since requests for reprints or permission to reproduce or translate have been continuous, a critical re-evaluation appears in order.

As the title was intended to suggest, the short examination was a clinical tool and not a standardized test. It was primarily designed to assist the neurologist in assessing aphasic disabilities as part of the neurological evaluation of the patient. Test items were selected from the *Minnesota Test for Differential Diagnosis of Aphasia,* which was then in experimental form. It was expected that when standardization procedures were completed, a short as well as a long form of the test could be developed.

The Short Examination was used successfully by some examiners and not by others. In general, the most sophisticated examiners reported the most consistent results, but this is true for any test instrument. The purpose of this paper is to consider possible sources of unreliability in the Short Examination and suggest an alternative procedure.

There are good reasons why a short test for aphasia cannot be completely satisfactory. In the first place, an adequate test must evaluate behavior in all language modalities lest important aspects of aphasic disability be overlooked. If any dimension of aphasic impairment is neglected misdiagnosis and corresponding errors of prediction may result.

The ability of many aphasic patients to respond appropriately to people, to situations, to visual cues, and to occasional words or phrases often obscures relatively severe impairment of auditory comprehension. If a patient has difficulty producing speech sounds, it is important to know if he can perceive differences between various sound patterns, and this is not usually obvious. Reading and writing may reveal impairment not observable in speech.

In the second place, an adequate examination must do more than specify major areas of disability. It must explore aphasic behavior within each language modality to determine why performance breaks down when it does. Reading is often disrupted simply because the patient does not have enough language. One cannot read Sartre, for example, with tourist French. Or reading may break down because verbal retention span is reduced, and the patient cannot hold on to a long enough string of words to perceive the meaning of a sentence or a paragraph. These are both language disabilities reflected in reading and have nothing to do with the visual system, which is an important diagnostic consideration.

To some aphasic patients, however, the

From *Journal of Speech and Hearing Disorders* 31:137–47, 1966.

printed page may appear as an array of random ink marks, one indistinguishable from another. Other patients may perceive letters and words, but often fail to discriminate between *b* and *d*, *m* and *w*, or *E* and *F*, for example. Still others have little or no difficulty discriminating letters in isolation, but tend to confuse words in context with words of similar appearance. *Store* may be read as *stone*, *mouth* as *month*, or *house* as *horse*, for example, even when the substitution results in a meaningless sentence. The nature of the impairment underlying a functional deficit, whether in listening, speaking, reading, or writing, is important diagnostic information.

Finally, aphasic impairment covers a wide range of severity in all language modalities. This range necessitates easy tests that make it possible to observe specific behaviors in patients who cannot perform on harder tests, and hard tests for patients who make no errors on easy tests. Between these extremes are patients who pass the easy tests and cannot perform on the hard tests, but require tests at some intermediate level.

Aphasia deals with one of the most complex and perhaps the only unique function of the human brain. It involves multiple variables in what appear to be underlying continuous distributions. Selection and ordering of information is possible, but the danger of oversimplification is always present.

A short examination may cover all language modalities and ask discriminating questions about the nature of observed deficits, and still fail to elicit an adequate sample of aphasic behavior from many patients for whom most of the tests on an abbreviated scale may be too easy or too difficult. To the extent that this occurs test results will be unreliable.

In summary, an adequate diagnostic test must sample relevant kinds of behavior in all language modalities over the entire range of aphasic deficit. Test reliability is always to some extent a function of test length. Length becomes particularly important when fine differential diagnosis is desired.

These considerations led to the decision not to include a short form on the current revision of the Minnesota Test, but to adopt a different strategy to reduce testing time. As an alternative the use of scaled tests, which permits the examiner to select appropriate items for each patient, is proposed.

SELECTING THE BEST TESTS FOR EACH SUBJECT

In the 1965 edition of the *Minnesota Test for Differential Diagnosis of Aphasia* (Schuell, 1965), tests in each language modality have been arranged in order of difficulty determined by the percentage of aphasic subjects failing each test. In other words, tests in each section were scaled for difficulty. The use of scaled tests enables the examiner to shorten testing time by obtaining a base line and a ceiling for each subject on each test section. This principle has been used in Binet testing for some sixty years, and today many standardized tests employ a similar method.

The procedure for the Minnesota Test is as follows. Before administering any test section the examiner estimates performance level in the language modality to be explored. He then selects the highest test he thinks the patient can pass and begins with this test. If the patient makes more than one error, the examiner goes back to an easier test until the criterion of not more than one error is met. This is the base line for the given test section. The examiner then proceeds to administer more difficult tests until the patient has failed 90 percent of the items on a given test. This is considered the ceiling in the modality tested.

A reasonable estimate of performance level in auditory comprehension and in spoken language can usually be derived from a preliminary interview with the patient. The best guess for performance in reading and writing is that it will approximate the level of speech. When this prediction does not prove true, the discrepancy serves to alert the examiner to begin searching for sources of interference that may affect language modalities differentially.

The method of obtaining a base line and a ceiling for each patient in each language modality selects the best tests for each patient. Each patient is given only the tests on which he can perform and upon which aphasic disabilities can be observed. A short test is obtained without the constraints imposed by arbitrary selection of a limited number of tests, of which only a fraction may be appropriate for any individual patient.

INTERPRETING TEST RESULTS

The Binet Method assumes that the subject has passed all the tests below the obtained base line and failed all tests above the obtained test ceiling. These are reasonably safe assumptions, and this method of reporting data may be used with the Minnesota Test. However, the total number of errors on a test section is not the most meaningful information for differential diagnosis. Investigators from Goldstein on have pointed out that the kinds of responses the patient makes provide more relevant information than the number of errors. With this rationale, a diagnostic scale was developed to summarize the critical information obtained from each test section, and present an over-all view of the pattern of impairment observed in each patient.

The Diagnostic Scale also provides a method of comparing diagnostic findings over a series of patients examined with different subsets of tests determined by obtained base lines and ceilings, and has been used to compare diagnostic findings across two languages.

Diagnostic ratings are completed after testing. It is essential that positive findings be documented by test evidence, since agreement between examiners is contingent upon clear operational definition of what is rated. The scale includes observations of auditory functions, visual and visuospatial functions, motor and sensorimotor functions, and use of language. The last deals with ability to use the words and rules of an acquired language for communication, and is not specific to any modality. In other words, you must know a word to understand it in a lecture or on the printed page, or to use it in speech or in writing. Probably all of us have had the experience of having to look up a rarely-encountered word more than once. In general the aphasic patient retains best and recovers first the words that are most common in the language. In addition to vocabulary, we learn the rules of a language. We must know the rules of German, for example, before we know whether to use *das, der,* or *die* before a given German noun. Most English speakers know, consciously or unconsciously, that we can say *a man,* but not *a men,* and that we say *you are,* but not *you is.* The ability of the aphasic patient to use the rules of his language usually correlates with the amount of language that is available to him. In other words the ability to combine words appropriately is related, to some extent at least, to size of vocabulary and length of verbal retention span.

Most investigators agree that the term aphasia should not be used unless some reduction of language can be demonstrated. If we accept this definition, it becomes meaningful to talk about simple aphasia, when no complicating conditions are present, and aphasia complicated by involvement of visual processes, sensorimotor processes, or by dysarthria, and so on. The advantages of this method of diagnosis are, first, that it makes it possible to describe any form of aphasia in a simple empirical manner; and second, that it is possible to demonstrate the interferences that are present with considerable precision, which facilitates agreement between examiners. This is the rationale of the Diagnostic Scale, which is presented below.

Diagnostic Scale

Rate as follows:

0 No information: appropriate tests could not be administered.
1 No impairment: performance within normal limits for age and educational level.
2 Mild impairment: occasional difficulties that do not disrupt performance.
3 Moderate impairment: consistent difficulties; performance possible, but limited or defective.
4 Severe impairment: almost complete disruption of performance.

	Rating
1. Auditory discrimination	( )
2. Auditory recognition	( )
3. Auditory retention span	( )
4. Visual discrimination	( )
5. Visual recognition	( )
6. Visual recall	( )
7. Spatial orientation	( )
8. Involvement of speech musculature	( )
9. Sensorimotor involvement	( )
10. Word finding	( )
11. Functional speech	( )
12. Functional writing	( )

The first three items on the scale refer to observable impairment of the auditory system. Relevant observations are as follows:

1. *Auditory discrimination* refers to ability to discriminate sounds and sound patterns used in speech. Does the patient frequently confuse the names of letters, or words, that sound alike, on appropriate tests?
2. *Auditory recognition* refers to ability to understand spoken words. Does the patient make errors pointing to objects or pictures named by the examiner? Can he demonstrate understanding of less common words appropriate to his educational level, on suitable tests? For example, some patients may be able to identify *window* but not *illumination, car* but not *transportation, recreation,* but not *isolation,* which is a somewhat less common although not a rare word.
3. *Auditory retention span* refers to ability to retain a series of words that are heard. Repetition of random series of digits is the most precise test for this. The examiner begins with two digits, pronounced at a rate of one per second, and proceeds to series of three, four, and so on, until the patient fails two series of any given length. Seven digits is usually considered normal for adults, although six is probably average for subjects over 50. Patients unable to repeat can be tested by being asked to point to common objects in a picture in series of gradually increasing length. Aphasic subjects who cannot repeat often have difficulty pointing to two or three objects named in a series.

The next four items refer to observations of visual or visuospatial disturbances. Relevant observations are as follows:

4. *Visual discrimination* refers to ability to discriminate learned visual patterns and is tested by matching. Does the patient make errors matching geometric forms, or matching letters of the alphabet? Does he tend to confuse letters that look alike, in isolation, or in words?
5. *Visual recognition* refers to reading vocabulary. Can the patient match words to pictures? Does he frequently confuse words that look alike? Is reading vocabulary significantly below the vocabulary level observed in speech, or on tests for auditory comprehension, for no apparent reason (such as educational deficit, foreign background, or reduction of visual acuity)? Visual recognition is not labeled defective on the diagnostic scale when reading impairment results from vocabulary deficit common to all modalities, in the absence of specific visual signs, such as confusion of letters and words with similar visual configurations.
6. *Visual recall* refers to retention of learned visual patterns. Does the patient have difficulty recalling letter forms? Does he produce reversals and distortions of letters? Does he often substitute one letter for another that looks somewhat similar? Does he tend to spell phonetically? Is spelling significantly below general vocabulary level for no apparent reason (educational deficit, etc.)? *Visual recall* is not labeled defective when writing reflects a language deficit common to all modalities, in the absence of specific visual signs, such as reversals, distortions, and substitutions of letters with similar visual configurations.
7. *Spatial disorientation* refers to impaired perception of relationships in space. On testing, impairment is shown by gross distortions on drawing and copying, by confusion of directionality on writing, and by difficulty on object assembly tests.

The next two items on the scale are related to production of speech sounds. It is important to remember that mispronunciations and even initial jargon may appear as a result of defective recall of auditory patterns. In the latter case errors are inconsistent, can usually be readily corrected by ear, and some connected speech is usually present that sounds normal.

8. *Speech musculature* includes relevant observations of gross movements of the speech musculature, usually in imitation of the examiner. Is phonation present? Is there evidence of difficulty swallowing? Is the palate elevated on phonation? Are palatal movements equal bilaterally? Can the patient protrude and retract the tongue? Can he elevate the tongue tip? Are lateral tongue movements equal?
9. *Sensorimotor involvement* refers to disruption of learned phonemic patterns in the absence of weakness of the musculature. The patient sometimes behaves as though he did not know where the tongue was in the mouth, or what to do to move it in a given direction or to a given position. Both auditory and proprioceptive feedback and control appear defective. Appropriate tests include repetition of phonetically edited monosyllabic words and repetition of phrases. Diadochokinetic movements are usually impaired initially but often improve as voluntary control is regained. Sensorimotor impairment is correlated with reduction of language throughout the course of recovery. Impairment that can be accounted for by weakness of the musculature is not designated as sensorimotor.

The last three items on the diagnostic scale refer to ability to use language for communication. They are concerned with the patient's ability to use the words and conventional rules that are learned as language is acquired. Occasionally a patient is found who has so much paralysis of the musculature that speech is almost unintelligible, but writing shows language to be intact. Such a patient is dysarthric rather than aphasic.

10. *Word finding* refers to ability to retrieve words from the memory store. Is the patient able to name common objects? Does he confuse words that are related in meaning? Does he frequently grope for words? Is language limited, or generally vague and imprecise, because vocabulary is limited? With mild word finding difficulty the patient may be able to name common objects, since common words are most resistant to aphasic breakdown, but may not have enough language to explain the use of an object or the meaning of a familiar term.
11. *Functional speech* refers to the ability to communicate in phrases and sentences according to the established conventions of the language. Normal speech contains many abbreviated utterances. The question is, can the patient use connected units of language in spontaneous speech, or does communication repeatedly break down because utterances are fragmentary and incomplete? Are sentences coherent, or does the patient get lost before he has succeeded in communicating the information he intended? One useful test is to ask the patient to produce sentences using given words, since this is something nonaphasic adults are able to do easily (Schuell, 1965).
12. *Functional writing* refers to spontaneous writing and is evaluated in terms of meaningfulness of content and use of acceptable linguistic patterns. The patient may be asked to write sentences using given words, and then to write a short paragraph describing a picture. Can the patient produce sentences in writing? Are sentences usually fragmentary and incomplete? Are sentences coherent? Does the paragraph consist almost exclusively of enumeration of objects? Is writing consistent with the educational or vocational level of the patient?

In using the diagnostic scale, the examiner must make allowances for nonaphasic conditions that may affect performance and, in some cases, make reliable diagnosis impossible. The patient may be too ill to respond. Scores may be depressed by hearing loss, reduction of visual acuity, absence of glasses, or educational deficit. It is better to use the zero rating, *no information,* than to make a judgment based on inadequate observations. It should be emphasized that the diagnostic scale designates the nature of the impairment that is observed. A diagnostic rating does not necessarily reflect the level of function in a given language modality. It is possible, for example, for the diagnostic scale to show no involvement of visual processes, at the same time that reading and writing are almost nonfunctional because of severe reduction of language. The diagnostic scale is an attempt to specify the underlying physiological processes that are impaired, and to document this impairment by appropriate observations.

Severity scale

A meaningful way to summarize test-retest findings is through the use of a scale indicating severity of aphasic deficit in each language modality. The Severity Scale presented in this section was initially developed to interpret test findings to individuals to whom scores obtained on various tests were not meaningful. It has since been used to evaluate changes that occurred with recovery or regression in patients examined with different subsets of tests determined by obtained base lines and ceilings, and with patients examined in different languages.

The Severity Scale and the Diagnostic Scale complement one another. The Severity Scale estimates the residual function in each language modality, and the level at which performance breaks down. It indicates what can be expected of the patient at a given time, as well as the functional limitations imposed by aphasia. It is sensitive to differences that occur over time. Comparison of test-retest ratings for 75 aphasic subjects using the Sign Test (Siegel, 1956), showed that the probability that differences between initial and final ratings in auditory comprehension, speech, reading, and writing were due to chance was $< .00003$ for each modality.

It may be argued that the Severity Scale is a clinical rating scale, and that clinical rating scales are notoriously unreliable. This is true when ratings are based on clinical impressions or intuitions, because these are not reproducible by other examiners who may have different frames of reference. If, however, a scale is used to summarize specifiable test results, and is documented by test findings, a high degree of reliability may result.

Correlations between severity ratings and number of errors made by 157 aphasic patients on corresponding sections of the Minnesota Test were all significantly high (.86 for auditory ratings, .80 for reading, .84 for spoken language, and .79 for writing). The probability that the clinical ratings were independent of test performance was essentially zero, with P still zero at the seventh decimal point, for each of the four measures. The scale for dysarthria was not included in the computations, since it was developed later. These findings indicate that the Severity Scale is a reliable tool for comparing aphasic involvement between subjects and for indicating test-retest differences, when it is used in conjunction with a test that permits adequate documentation of the behavior rated.

It should be emphasized that the Severity Scale designates level of impairment of basic language functions, but does not specify the nature of the observed impairment. It is in no sense diagnostic.

In contrast to the Severity Scale, the Diagnostic Scale indicates the nature and the overall pattern of deficit that underlies the aphasic impairment observed in an aphasic patient. The Diagnostic Scale remains stable, even with statistically significant changes in severity of aphasia, as indicated by the percentage of possible errors obtained on each test section on test and retest (Schuell, Jenkins, and Jiménez-Pabón, 1964).

The Severity Scale is as follows:

Auditory comprehension

0 No information.
1 No observable impairment.
2 Follows radio program or general discussion with only minimal difficulty.
3 Follows ordinary conversation with little difficulty.
4 Follows most conversation but sometimes fails to grasp essentials.
5 Follows simple conversations but requires repetition.

6 Follows brief statements with considerable repetition.
7 Usually responds inappropriately because he did not understand.

Reading

0 No information.
1 No observable impairment.
2 Reads average adult materials with only minimal difficulty.
3 Reads paper and short magazine articles.
4 Reads simple sentences and simple paragraph materials.
5 Reading vocabulary of 100 or more words: reads some phrases and sentences.
6 Matches words to pictures and some spoken to printed words.
7 No functional reading.

Spoken language

0 No information.
1 No observable impairment.
2 Converses easily with only occasional difficulty.
3 Conversational speech, with mild impairment of formulation or fluency.
4 Some conversational speech but marked difficulty expressing long or complex ideas.
5 Ready communication with single words and short phrases.
6 Expresses needs and wishes in limited or defective manner.
7 No functional speech.

Written language

0 No information.
1 No observable impairment.
2 Can write acceptable letter with only minimal errors.
3 Spontaneous writing present with mild impairment of spelling and formulation.
4 Can write short easy sentences spontaneously and to dictation.
5 Spelling vocabulary of 100 or more words; can write some phrases and sentences.
6 Can write name and a few words to dictation.
7 No functional writing.

Dysarthria

0 No information.
1 Normal articulation and fluency.
2 Minimal impairment; occasional or very mild slurring.
3 Mild impairment: mild slurring that does not interfere significantly with intelligibility.
4 Moderate impairment: speech is usually intelligible but listener has to follow closely to understand.
5 Severe impairment: speech is usually unintelligible.

CLASSIFICATION OF PATIENTS

It is possible to describe the performance of any aphasic patient, as has been pointed out, by listing the areas of deficit shown on the Diagnostic Scale. This procedure analyzes the overall pattern of aphasic deficit in a meaningful manner.

Some patterns of aphasic deficit are more common than others. Study of the course of aphasia in some 1,200 aphasic patients, many of whom were tested at the beginning and the end of a course of intensive therapy, and some of whom have been followed for periods of years, has made it possible to identify the patterns that have recurred most frequently in the population studied, and to predict the course of recovery associated with specific patterns.

The classification system presented with the short examination has been revised as a result of further experimental work (Schuell, Jenkins, and Jiménez-Pabón, 1964). The order of the groups was changed to permit a more logical arrangement, and two minor categories observed less frequently were added.

The revised classification system is as follows:

Major Categories

Group 1: Simple aphasia. Available language is reduced in all modalities, with no specific perceptual or sensorimotor involvement, and no dysarthria. Prognosis for recovery from aphasia is excellent. Most Group 1 subjects resume former occupations.

Group 2: Aphasia with visual involvement. Reduction of language is complicated by impaired discrimination, recognition, and recall of visual patterns used in reading and writing. The prognosis for recovery of language is excellent, as in Group 1. Reading and writing recover more slowly. Patients approximate former performance level, but rate tends to remain retarded, and occasional inconsistent errors tend to persist.

Group 3: Aphasia with sensorimotor involvement. Group 3 patients show severe reduction of vocabulary and verbal retention span in all language modalities, complicated by impaired perception and production of phonemic patterns. The prognosis is for limited but functional recovery of language. Patients learn to communicate through intelligible speech, usually common words and phrases, and later short sentences, but language continues to break down when longer or more complex responses are required. Normal articulation is usually achieved for common words and short language units, but continues to break down when longer sequences are attempted.

Group 4: Aphasia with scattered findings compatible with generalized or scattered brain damage. Some functional language is retained in speech or writing or both. Some visual findings and some dysarthria are usually present, although one system is often more severely involved than the other. Spatial perception may or may not be disturbed. Emotional lability is often present. Group 4 patients tend to have many physiological complaints, and personality changes sometimes occur. Patients sometimes work well when the clinician is present, and achieve more language or improved intelligibility, but tend to be incapable of consistent effort. Prognosis for recovery tends to be limited more by physiological and psychological status than by severity of aphasia.

Group 5: An irreversible aphasic syndrome. Group 5 subjects show almost complete loss of functional language skills in all modalities. They have difficulty pointing to common words named by the examiner and following simple directions. They cannot name common objects or give simple biographical information. They can sometimes match common words to pictures, but reading is nonfunctional. They sometimes learn to copy, and to write their names, but are unable to write simple words to dictation. They sometimes learn to repeat and to count. Some reactive speech usually emerges, but it does not become voluntary or functional.

Minor Syndromes

Minor syndrome A: Aphasia with partial auditory imperception. This syndrome is characterized by severe involvement of auditory processes, usually with some functional, normal speech present or recovered early. Patients frequently behave as though they were deaf. Early attempts at repetition may result in jargon. Although appropriate utterances may occur, patients have difficulty naming objects and expressing specific ideas. Reading and writing mirror language impairment. Patients often improve remarkably, but do not achieve normal language functions.

Minor syndrome B: Mild aphasia with persisting dysarthria. These patients resemble patients in Group 1, except for the presence of dysarthria. The prognosis for recovery from aphasia is excellent. Excellent articulation may be achieved, but conscious control must be exercised. Articulation continues to disintegrate whenever control is relaxed. The extent to which control is exercised after it is achieved varies from patient to patient, and appears to be related to personality traits.

It should be emphasized that neither classification of subjects nor prediction of outcome is reliable unless patients are neurologically stable when examined. Because achieving neurological stability usually requires about three months, it is frequently desirable to do a preliminary examination and initiate therapy before this time. It is the opinion of the author that active therapy should be deferred until the patient is taking notice of what is going on about him, and can sit up for two hours without fatigue. The essentials for the early period are sympathetic and supportive nursing and medical care, with counseling by the speech pathologist when indicated.

SUMMARY

A short examination for aphasia cannot provide an adequate sample of language behavior for reliable diagnosis over the whole range of aphasic disabilities. As an alternative the use of scaled tests is proposed, which permits the examiner to select an appropriate range of tests for each subject. In addition, a Diagnostic Scale and a Severity Scale have been presented. If the two scales are documented by test results, they permit comparison of diagnostic patterns and severity of functional deficits across aphasic subjects and over intervals of time, and constitute a concise and meaningful summary of the aphasic impairment observed in a given patient.

REFERENCES

Schuell, Hildred, A short examination for aphasia. *Neurology*, **7,** 625–634 (1957).

——, Jenkins, J. J., and Jiménez-Pabón, E., *Aphasia in Adults: Diagnosis, Prognosis, and Treatment.* New York: Hoeber (1964).

——, *The Minnesota Test for Differential Diagnosis of Aphasia.* Minn.: Univ. Minn. (1965).

Siegel, S., *Nonparametric Statistics.* New York: McGraw-Hill (1956).

A Factor Analysis of the Minnesota Test for Differential Diagnosis of Aphasia

HILDRED M. SCHUELL
JAMES J. JENKINS
JOHN B. CARROLL

HILDRED M. SCHUELL, Ph.D., (deceased) was director of the aphasia section of the neurology service of the Minneapolis Veterans Administration Hospital, and was with the department of neurology of the Graduate School of Medicine, University of Minnesota.
JAMES J. JENKINS, Ph.D., is with the department of psychology of the University of Minnesota.
JOHN B. CARROLL, Ph.D., is with the Division of Psychological Studies, Educational Testing Service, Princeton.
This investigation was supported by Research Grant B1984 from the Institute of Neurological Diseases and Blindness, Public Health Service.

This paper reports the results of a factor analysis of scores of 157 aphasic subjects on 69 tests. It represents a further attempt to explore relationships between sets of behaviors observed in a nonselected sample of aphasic subjects, and to achieve a more unified and meaningful description of aphasic impairment than an earlier scale analysis by Schuell and Jenkins (*35*) permitted. In this study the authors used the Guttman technique to analyze responses of 100 aphasic subjects to 18 tests. They reported an underlying dimension of aphasic language deficit which crossed language modalities and occurred in both the presence and the absence of other concomitants of brain damage.

Jones and Wepman (*21*) published results of the first factor analysis of aphasic responses in 1961, using scores of 168 subjects on 35 test variables, plus age and education. Five factors were extracted, and interpreted as follows:

Factor A, visual-to-oral transmission (principal task, reading).

Factor B, aural-to-oral transmission (principal task, repeating spoken words).

Factor C, visual-to-graphic transmission (principal task, copying printed words).

Factor D, aural-to-graphic transmission (principal task, writing spoken words).

Factor E, language-symbol comprehension (principal task, matching pictures to spoken and written words).

Jones and Wepman reported that all factors were intercorrelated, but concluded their data demonstrated the existence of several factors underlying the performance of aphasic subjects. They considered this conclusion incompatible with the hypothesis that language impairment in aphasia may be viewed as a unitary general disorder. Schuell and Jenkins (*34*) have elsewhere reviewed differences in selection of subjects, composition of test batteries, and intention of the two studies, and argued that there is no essential incompatibility between the findings.

Factor A (visual-to-oral transmission) on the Jones-Wepman analysis had varimax loadings above .20 on 22 out of 35 test variables; 10 of the 22 tests used auditory and not visual stimuli;

From *Journal of Speech and Hearing Research* 5:349–69, 1962.

four used graphic, not oral, responses; one used matching. Jones and Wepman commented that Factor A represented "some tendency toward a general factor."

Schuell and Jenkins (*35*) suggested that "the Guttman technique may isolate the items in a scale which are identical with those items appearing on the major factor in a factor analysis," and stressed the importance of "motor or perceptual deficits which may or may not coexist with the basic language deficit found in all the clinical groups described." In addition they pointed out that the diagnostic groups previously reported by Schuell (*31, 32*), and treated both independently and as a total population on the scale analysis, were based on observed patterns of coexisting deficits. Thus, in spite of procedural differences, the findings presented in both studies gave some evidence of a major dimension of language deficit not modality specific and some evidence for additional factors underlying the language performance of aphasic subjects.

PROCEDURE

Test Battery

The tests used in the present investigation were Form 6, 1955 Research Edition, of the Minnesota Test for Differential Diagnosis of Aphasia (*33*) and the Ammons Full-Range Picture Vocabulary Test (*1*), for a total of 69 tests comprised of 679 items.

On the Minnesota test, after four tests were excluded because not enough patients made errors on them for meaningful analysis of data, 68 tests, totaling 595 items, remained. Scores consisted of number of errors, except on four tests where responses were rated according to pre-established criteria. For tests with more than nine items, errors were grouped for coding in the middle and upper levels where differences were considered of least clinical importance.

All 84 items of the Ammons test were used. The test was administered in the standard way except that demonstration with nontest items was added before administration.

Subjects

Subjects were 155 aphasic patients admitted to the Neurology Service of the Minneapolis Veterans Administration Hospital between June 1955 and June 1958. These were consecutive admissions except for the following exclusions: patients who were neurologically unstable; patients with a psychiatrically confirmed diagnosis of psychosis or regression; patients who responded to no test items; and patients who were evaluated for diagnostic purposes but were not considered aphasic. In order to increase the number in one diagnostic group, records of two aphasic subjects tested by the senior author at Syracuse University, and made available through the kindness of Dr. Louis di Carlo, were included.

The test battery has also been administered to 50 hospitalized subjects without neurological findings. In general, nonaphasic subjects made occasional scattered errors which showed no consistent pattern.

Method

Distributions of scores on each of the 69 tests were studied so that the most appropriate statistic for expressing relationships between pairs of variables might be selected. As in earlier studies of data obtained from the Minnesota test, distributions were predominantly U-shaped and J-shaped. It was decided to use tetrachoric correlation coefficients for this and other reasons, as explained by Carroll (*8*). Each distribution was dichotomized as close to the median as possible, and tetrachoric correlations were computed by a procedure developed by Tucker[1] and programmed for the IBM 704 computer.

The resulting 69 × 69 matrix of tetrachoric correlations was subjected to a principal axis analysis. Communality was estimated for each variable by taking the highest of its intercor-

[1] L. R. Tucker, Notes on approximation of tetrachoric correlation, personal communication to John B. Carroll, April 4, 1960.

relations with all the other variables in the matrix. Eight principal axes exhausted 99% of the common factor variance as thus estimated. Projections of the test vectors on these eight axes were used as the basis for subsequent rotations. All eight axes were used in obtaining an orthogonal solution according to the normalized varimax criterion of Kaiser (*22*), and the first seven were used for an oblique solution according to the normalized oblimin criterion of Carroll (7), with equal weight given to the quartimin and covarimin components, that is, the parameter γ was set as equal to .5 (*14*, p. 325). In addition, a normalized oblimin solution based on all eight axes was obtained and subjected to minor graphical adjustments, but the resulting solution was so similar to the seven-factor solution, for all the major factors, that it is not worth while to present it here.

FINDINGS

All analyses resulted in virtually identical factor structures, although the loadings and relative order of a few tests changed somewhat. Each analysis showed five major factors identified by numerous tests, and two minor factors identified by only one or two tests. The five major factors are as follows: Factor 1,

TABLE 26–1. VARIMAX MATRIX SHOWING PRINCIPAL AXES FACTOR LOADINGS* OF THE 69 TESTS. THE FIVE FACTORS ARE AS FOLLOWS: FACTOR 1, LANGUAGE BEHAVIOR; FACTOR 2, VISUAL DISCRIMINATION (ON MATCHING, RECOGNITION, AND RECALL); FACTOR 3, VISUOSPATIAL BEHAVIOR; FACTOR 4, GROSS MOVEMENTS OF SPEECH MUSCULATURE; AND FACTOR 5, RECOGNITION OF STIMULUS EQUIVALENCE

Test		*Factor*				
Number	*Task*	*1*	*2*	*3*	*4*	*5*
Auditory						
1	point to items named	49	38	40	3	61
2	point to letters named	66	58	19	16	22
3	point to items named serially	67	56	24	− 4	27
4	repeat sentences	94	30	− 1	8	− 5
5	repeat series of digits	89	31	16	20	2
6	follow spoken directions	71	59	16	− 1	26
7	listen to sentences, indicate right or wrong	59	33	34	21	20
8	listen to short paragraph, answer questions yes or no	43	62	24	20	22
9	listen to long paragraph, answer questions yes or no	61	36	19	17	13
10	point to picture indicated by spoken word (Ammons)	36	44	19	18	51
Visual, Reading						
11	report or display visual difficulty	−43	−13	26	1	− 9
12	match geometric forms	13	22	84	16	43
13	match printed letters	8	11	61	25	54
14	identify irrelevant object in category	30	45	46	27	25
15	match words with pictures	45	35	54	7	43
16	match spoken, printed words	63	52	33	3	31
17	read sentences, check right or wrong	52	48	38	9	33
18	no task: reading rate timed on Test 17	49	59	38	0	12
19	read short paragraph, check questions yes or no	38	68	39	8	32
20	read long paragraph, check questions yes or no	48	71	28	1	25
21	read sentences aloud	74	50	26	1	17
Speech, Language						
22	imitate examiner: initiate, prolong phonation; alter pitch	6	11	22	68	3
23	imitate examiner: tongue movements	35	40	26	72	10

(continued on next page)

TABLE 26-1 (CONTINUED). VARIMAX MATRIX SHOWING PRINCIPAL AXES FACTOR LOADINGS* OF THE 69 TESTS.

Test		*Factor*				
Number	*Task*	*1*	*2*	*3*	*4*	*5*
Speech, Language (continued)						
24	imitate examiner: jaw movements	8	18	42	71	11
25	imitate syllables: palatal movements	28	−12	23	68	6
26	report difficulty swallowing (confirmed)	5	12	10	71	−2
27	repeat syllables rapidly	59	7	18	62	2
28	repeat monosyllabic words	82	20	22	34	5
29	complete sentences	93	22	17	7	13
30	count aloud to 20	77	34	15	44	−9
31	name days of week	86	31	18	32	−3
32	name months of year	91	28	19	12	−5
33	answer questions (one word)	96	16	6	7	14
34	name objects, pictures	91	26	20	0	19
35	give rhyming words	84	17	20	22	−7
36	define common words	89	29	7	18	16
37	supply biographical information	91	29	10	6	18
38	relate events	90	21	19	16	0
39	describe pictured situation	93	17	14	11	16
40	state similarity between pairs	91	27	7	8	16
41	explain proverbs	79	21	−2	−9	45
Visuomotor, Writing						
42	copy geometric forms	24	24	68	18	0
43	copy Greek letters	15	16	89	18	4
44	draw house	9	42	68	15	16
45	draw wheel exposed 10 sec	15	28	70	7	−4
46	write numbers 1 to 20	33	53	46	23	−2
47	copy letters exposed 2 sec	31	32	71	18	9
48	write names of pictured objects	60	64	29	6	12
49	write dictated words (equated with Test 48)	61	67	31	5	5
50	write letters dictated in random order	49	73	31	18	10
51	write dictated words (progressive difficulty)	54	75	25	15	10
52	spell words on Test 51 aloud	84	40	8	28	−10
53	write dictated sentences	64	68	29	7	−8
54	write sentences using given words	66	64	32	14	−13
55	write paragraph about picture	69	58	24	16	−19
Numerical, Arithmetic						
56	indicate coins for correct change	56	39	45	21	24
57	set clock	52	57	37	10	1
58	indicate correct answer to arithmetic combinations	36	62	40	19	8
59	solve simple arithmetic problems	58	61	21	28	19
60	solve problem in addition	27	63	44	21	1
61	solve problem in subtraction	33	66	28	17	8
62	solve problem in multiplication	39	38	34	21	15
63	solve problem in long division	43	44	45	36	10
Body Image						
64	name indicated body parts	90	22	17	10	21
65	point to body parts named	60	47	40	−1	43
66	follow directions involving body parts	75	47	31	−2	21
67	draw man	18	22	69	17	3
68	assemble manikin	−14	38	66	36	9
69	assemble manikin head	4	19	66	23	0
Percent of estimated common-factor variance		41.0	21.0	16.1	7.9	5.0

*Decimal points are omitted for all entries in the body of the table. Entries are given only for the five factors in the complete 69 × 8 matrix which was obtained. These factors account for 91% of the estimated common factor variance.

language behavior; Factor 2, visual discrimination (on matching, recognition, and recall); Factor 3, visuospatial behavior; Factor 4, gross movements of speech musculature; and Factor 5, recognition of stimulus equivalence. It is possible that the two minor factors were both severity factors, one representing severity of visuospatial and the other of motor involvement. Loadings of the tests on five major factors of the varimax solution are given in Table 26-1.

Factor 1: Language Behavior

Table 26-2 lists tests with critical loadings on Factor 1 (language behavior) on both the varimax and oblimin rotations. (Tests with low or negative loadings on Factor 1 may be seen in Table 26-1; none of these involved language; all had obvious visual, spatial, or motor components).

Since tests with highest loadings all required verbal responses, Factor 1 might appear to be a verbal output or "encoding" factor. The authors rejected this interpretation because of (a) the number of tests included on Factor 1, (b) the nature of the tests with high loadings, (c) the presence of tests not requiring verbal output, and (d) the interrelations between the tests with critical loadings on Factor 1 and Factor 4 (gross movements of speech musculature).

Number of Tests Included. On the varimax solution, Factor 1 had loadings above .40 on 45 out of 69 tests, loadings above .30 on 54 out of 69 tests, and accounted for 41% of estimated common factor variance in that solution. On the oblimin solution, where all loadings were smaller, Factor 1 had loadings above .30 on 34 tests, and loadings above .20 on 42 tests. It is concluded that a factor which permeates a battery of apparently diverse activities to this extent must involve a broad ability central to the entire battery. In the Minnesota test this ability is the use of language in the usual modalities: listening, reading, talking, writing, and dealing with numerical symbols. It seems reasonable, therefore, to conclude that Factor 1 represents the dimension previously identified through the Guttman scale analysis (*35*). (The 18 tests on the Guttman analysis had varimax loadings between .45 and .96 on Factor 1, with a median of .83, and oblimin loadings between .19 and .82, with a median of .64.)

Tests with High Loadings. The nature of the tests with critical loadings was the second reason for rejection of the "verbal output" interpretation for Factor 1. Even if one looks at only the verbal tests, it is clear that these involved kinds of integrations that cannot be attributed to organization of motor responses or to events in the outgoing pathways. The classical localization theory attributed "motor" or "atactic" aphasia to lesions in Broca's area, where motor patterns were assumed to be organized and stored, or in the corpus striatum, which was naively assumed to be the head of the motor tract (*2, 3, 6, 25*, pp. 581–875, *39*, pp. 265–324). Even this theory, however, recognized that all language events could not be accounted for in these terms; Broca, himself (*6*), was explicit on this point.

Responses to these verbal tests on Factor 1 involved vocabulary, auditory retention span (repeating sentences, repeating digits), and complex language formulation (describing a picture, giving information, defining words, and explaining similarities and proverbs). Tests chiefly dependent on coordination of movements were conspicuously absent. As evidence for this statement, and to permit comparisons to be made, obtained loadings on Factor 4, the only factor related to movements that emerged from the analysis, are included in Table 26-2.

The authors are in essential agreement with Jackson's (*19*) belief that internal and external language processes differ principally in that the latter demand innervation of outgoing processes, and the former do not. Lashley (*27*, p. 121) concluded that "the same central circuits whose activity constitutes internal speech are able to excite the overt movements."

Since the language tests in the present study were scored correct if responses were intelligible and appropriate regardless of presence or absence of articulation errors, the high loadings of these tests on Factor 1, together with their

TABLE 26–2. CRITICAL LOADINGS* ON FACTOR 1, LANGUAGE BEHAVIOR, ON BOTH THE VARIMAX (Var) AND OBLIMIN (Obl) ROTATIONS, WITH LOADINGS ON FACTOR 4, GROSS MOVEMENTS OF THE SPEECH MUSCULATURE, PRESENTED FOR COMPARISON. TEST CLASSIFICATIONS ARE SPEECH AND LANGUAGE (SpL); AUDITORY (Aud); BODY IMAGE (BI); VISUOMOTOR WRITING (VmW); VISUAL, READING (VR); AND NUMERICAL, ARITHMETIC (NA)

Test			*Factor 1*		*Factor 4*	
Task	*Number*	*Class*	*Var*	*Obl*	*Var*	*Obl*
answer questions (one word)	33	SpL	96	82	7	−7
repeat sentences	4	Aud	94	81	8	−9
describe pictured situation	39	SpL	93	76	11	1
complete sentences	29	SpL	93	75	7	−10
name months of year	32	SpL	91	75	12	−4
state similarity between pairs	40	SpL	91	72	8	1
name objects, pictures	34	SpL	91	73	0	−9
supply biographical information	37	SpL	91	72	6	−4
name indicated body parts	64	BI	90	72	10	−4
relate events	38	SpL	90	75	16	1
repeat series of digits	5	Aud	89	72	20	2
define common words	36	SpL	89	69	18	11
name days of week	31	SpL	86	69	32	11
spell words on Test 51 aloud	52	VmW	84	66	28	14
give rhyming words	35	SpL	84	67	22	8
repeat monosyllabic words	28	SpL	82	66	34	17
explain proverbs	41	SpL	79	58	−9	−1
count aloud to 20	30	SpL	77	62	44	16
follow directions involving body parts	66	BI	75	52	−2	−17
read sentences aloud	21	VR	74	49	1	−12
follow spoken directions	6	Aud	71	43	−1	−9
write paragraph about picture	55	VmW	69	44	16	3
point to items named serially	3	Aud	67	42	−4	−14
point to letters named	2	Aud	66	38	16	2
write sentences using given words	54	VmW	66	38	14	−3
write dictated sentences	53	VmW	64	39	7	−9
match spoken, printed words	16	VR	63	35	3	−10
write dictated words (equated with Test 48)	49	VmW	61	34	5	−12
listen to long paragraph, answer questions yes or no	9	Aud	61	43	17	0
write names of pictured objects	48	VmW	60	33	6	−3
point to body parts named	65	BI	60	33	−1	−15
listen to sentences, indicate right or wrong	7	Aud	59	39	21	3
repeat syllables rapidly	27	SpL	59	51	62	31
solve simple arithmetic problems	59	NA	58	29	28	18
indicate coins for correct change	56	NA	56	33	21	8
write dictated words (progressive difficulty)	51	VmW	54	26	15	−2
no task: reading rate timed on Test 17	18	VR	52	25	9	3
set clock	57	NA	52	28	10	−7
point to items named	1	Aud	49	22	3	−2
read sentences, check right or wrong	17	VR	49	23	0	−12
write letters dictated in random order	50	VmW	49	20	18	−2
read long paragraph, check questions yes or no	20	VR	48	16	1	−5

* Decimal points are omitted for all entries in the body of the table.

low loadings on Factor 4, are compatible with the interpretation that even tests which require verbal output are chiefly dependent on integrity of language; errors cannot be accounted for on the basis of defective organization of motor responses or involvement of outgoing pathways.

Tests not requiring verbal output. The third consideration arguing against the "verbal output" interpretation of Factor 1 involves the high loadings, on both solutions, of tests which required no verbal output. These tests, numbered and labeled as in Table 26-1, are cited below by categories in the order of the varimax loadings; in parentheses after each are first the varimax and then the oblimin loadings.

Tests for auditory comprehension:
66, follow directions involving body parts (75, 52);
6, follow spoken directions (71, 43);
3, point to items named serially (67, 42);
2, point to letters named (66, 38);
9, listen to long paragraph, answer questions yes or no (61, 43);
65, point to body parts named (60, 33);
7, listen to sentences, indicate right or wrong (59, 39);
1, point to items named (49, 22).

Visual and reading tests:
16, match spoken, printed words (63, 35);
18, no task: reading rate timed on Test 17 (52, 25);
17, read sentences, check right or wrong (49, 23);
20, read long paragraph, check questions yes or no (48, 16).

Visuomotor and writing tests:
55, write paragraph about picture (69, 44);
54, write sentences using given words (66, 38);
53, write dictated sentences (64, 39);
49, write dictated words (equated with Test 48) (61, 34);
48, write names of pictured objects (60, 33);
51, write dictated words (progressive difficulty) (54, 26).

Numerical and arithmetic tests:
59, solve simple arithmetic problems (58, 29);
56, indicate coins for correct change (56, 33);
57, set clock (52, 28).

These 21 tests did not require verbal responses and thus are evidence that the major factor is not a verbal output factor. They indicate, further, that the factor is not modality specific, since they include behavior involved in listening, reading, and writing, as well as speaking.

It seems probable that Factor 1 loadings were somewhat lower on these 21 tests than on the verbal tests because the former were necessarily less pure and response modes more heterogeneous. Tests for auditory comprehension required use of objects or pictures, or true-false choices, which are subject to guessing. (Multiple choice responses are even more ambiguous with aphasic subjects, who usually cannot retain instructions and alternatives simultaneously.) Since any unselected sample of aphasic subjects contains individuals with specific impairment of visual processes, the high language loadings on reading and writing tests are particularly significant. Matching and copying tests, on the other hand, were not found among tests with high loadings on Factor 1.

Tests common to Factor 1 and Factor 4. High language loadings on three tests with relatively high loadings on Factor 4 (gross movements of speech musculature) may appear contradictory to the interpretation presented here. These tests are shown in Table 26-3.

TABLE 26-3. TESTS WITH CRITICAL LOADINGS* ON BOTH FACTOR 1, LANGUAGE BEHAVIOR, AND FACTOR 4, GROSS MOVEMENTS OF SPEECH MUSCULATURE, FOR BOTH THE VARIMAX (Var) AND OBLIMIN (Obl) ROTATIONS

Test		*Factor 1*		*Factor 4*	
Task	*Number*	*Var*	*Obl*	*Var*	*Obl*
repeat monosyllabic words	28	82	66	34	17
repeat syllables rapidly	27	59	51	62	31
imitate examiner: tongue movements	23	35	14	72	59

* Decimal points are omitted for all entries in the body of the table.

Repetition of phonetically edited monosyllabic words had the highest language loading and the lowest motor loading of the three tests. Articulation, like perception, is facilitated by familiarity with the stimulus (*17*, *23*, *28*). Clinical experience has shown that many aphasic subjects in older age groups and subjects with educational deficits refuse to attempt repetition of nonsense syllables. Nonperformance may result from fear of an unfamiliar task, impaired perceptual discrimination, or impaired motor coordination. Although repetition of monosyllabic words is undoubtedly, facilitated by recognition of the word, more reliable and meaningful information is obtained than when nonsense syllables are used, because words elicit maximal and unequivocal responses.

The present findings suggest, therefore, that the speech mechanism is a functionally educated structure whose output is related to integration of language as well as to organization of movement patterns. The three tests with critical loadings on both Factor 1 and Factor 4 show an interesting progression of this interaction, and in that sense support rather than deny the rejection of the "verbal output" interpretation of Factor 1.

TABLE 26-4. CRITICAL LOADINGS* ON FACTOR 2, VISUAL DISCRIMINATION (ON MATCHING, RECOGNITION, AND RECALL) ON BOTH THE VARIMAX (Var) AND OBLIMIN (Obl) ROTATIONS, WITH LOADINGS FOR FACTOR 1, LANGUAGE BEHAVIOR, PRESENTED FOR COMPARISON. TEST CLASSIFICATIONS ARE VISUOMOTOR, WRITING (VmW); VISUAL, READING (VR); NUMERICAL, ARITHMETIC (NA); AND AUDITORY (Aud)

Test			*Factor 2*		*Factor 1*	
Task	*Number*	*Class*	*Var*	*Obl*	*Var*	*Obl*
write dictated words (progressive difficulty)	51	VmW	75	44	54	26
write letters dictated in random order	50	VmW	73	48	49	20
read long paragraph, check questions yes or no	20	VR	71	52	48	16
write dictated sentences	53	VmW	68	41	64	39
read short paragraph, check questions yes or no	19	VR	68	49	38	5
write dictated words (equated with Test 48)	49	VmW	67	39	61	34
solve problem in subtraction	61	NA	66	54	33	3
write names of pictured objects	48	VmW	64	39	60	33
write sentences using given words	54	VmW	64	39	66	38
solve problem in addition	60	NA	63	49	27	− 2
listen to short paragraph, answer questions yes or no	8	Aud	62	42	43	15
indicate correct answer to arithmetic combinations	58	NA	62	48	36	7
solve simple arithmetic problems	59	NA	61	40	58	29
follow spoken directions	6	Aud	59	36	71	43
read sentences, check right or wrong	17	VR	59	39	49	23
point to letters named	2	Aud	58	33	66	38
write paragraph about picture	55	VmW	58	35	69	44
set clock	57	NA	57	30	52	28
point to items named serially	3	Aud	56	29	67	42
write numbers 1 to 20	46	VmW	53	28	33	12
match spoken, printed words	16	VR	52	28	63	35
read sentences aloud	21	VR	50	26	74	49

* Decimal points are omitted for all entries in the body of the table.

Factor 2: Visual Discrimination (on Matching, Recognition and Recall)

In the oblimin solution Factors 1 and 2 were the most highly intercorrelated (Table 26-4). The writers interpreted Factor 2, visual discrimination (on matching, recognition, and recall), as one that represented the addition of visual events to language behavior. This is compatible with the viewpoint of descriptive linguistics (*26*), which holds that the spoken language is primary and that the written is derived from the spoken. Factor 2 is conceived as involving learned visual discriminations and the ensuing recognition and recall of learned patterns.

Some tests with relatively high loadings on Factor 2 involved recognition of objects and pictures. This seems to indicate that required processes were not essentially different from those involved in what are commonly regarded as reading readiness skills, that is, visual discriminations learned before reading and writing were acquired.

Tests with high loadings on Factor 2. Both reading and writing tests had high loadings on Factor 2. This finding offered no support for concepts of "pure alexia" or "pure agraphia" existing independent of each other (or independent of language, as the high loadings of reading and writing tests on Factor 1 demonstrate).

Translation from one modality to another did not seem to be the essential feature on Factor 2. Some tests required it, others did not.

Tests with low loadings on Factor 2. Tests which were negatively or minimally correlated with Factor 2 may be found in Table 26-1. Most of these tests involved movements of the speech musculature, or verbal responses on tests that did not employ visual stimuli.

There were three exceptions to this. The first two, matching letters and copying Greek symbols, used well-spaced letters .75″ high, in heavy black ink on a single line; stimuli were continuously available. Essentially these were simple tests that would be expected to reflect only severe visual impairment, usually combined with spatial disorientation. The other test, picture description, presumably had a low loading on Factor 2 because of its extremely high dependence on language (.93, .76).

Factor 3: Visuospatial Behavior

Factor 3 is a clear-cut visuospatial factor. Tests with high factor 3 loadings are shown in Table 26-5. They include matching, copying, drawing, and object-assembly tests.

Hebb (*16*, p. 17) wrote in 1949 that "simple perceptions are in fact complex, additive, the result of long learning processes, and partly dependent on motor activity." Bay (*4*) considered perception a highly complex achievement that depended on manifold dynamic processes in the nervous system, each of which could be disturbed and cause impaired perception. The basic argument is that visual perceptions are learned, that learning involves movements, which provide the proprioceptive information utilized in spatial perception, and that a continuous and dynamic feedback process operates.

Gooddy and Reinhold (*10*), like Bay, emphasized the dynamic aspect of spatial perception, and concluded, "Of the sensations which contribute towards orientation, vision and "feeling" (a term used to describe the perception of touch, posture, and joint and muscle change) are most important. "Feeling" is possibly more valuable than vision, for it is certainly a greater handicap to lose unilateral posterior column sensation than a homonymous field of vision." Critchley (*9*) pointed out the frequency of disturbances of spatial orientation in parietal lobe syndromes, although he added the caution that poor performance on drawing tests was not necessarily related to parietal lobe deficiency.

The authors consider that Factor 3 emerged as separate from Factor 2 because tests loading on it are dependent on proprioceptive as well as visual information. Brain-injured patients sometimes show severe spatial disorientation even when visual acuity, at least in some parts of the visual field, is well preserved.

TABLE 26-5. CRITICAL LOADINGS* ON FACTOR 3, VISUOSPATIAL BEHAVIOR, ON BOTH VARIMAX (Var) AND OBLIMIN (Obl) ROTATIONS. TEST CLASSIFICATIONS ARE VISUOMOTOR, WRITING (VmW); VISUAL, READING (VR); AND BODY IMAGE (BI)

Test			*Loading*	
Task	*Number*	*Class*	*Var*	*Obl*
copy Greek letters	43	VmW	89	61
match geometric forms	12	VR	84	38
copy letters exposed 2 sec	47	VmW	71	45
draw wheel exposed 10 sec	45	VmW	70	45
draw man	67	BI	69	53
draw house	44	VmW	68	46
copy geometric forms	42	VmW	68	51
assemble manikin	68	BI	66	31
assemble manikin head	69	BI	66	53
match printed letters	13	VR	61	16
match words with pictures	15	VR	54	16
write numbers 1 to 20	46	VmW	46	22

* Decimal points are omitted for all entries in the body of the table.

Errors on tests with high loadings on Factor 3 included horizontal and vertical reversals of letters, on both matching and writing tests. On reproducing letters and writing numerals to 20, subjects who scored low on the group of tests loading on Factor 3 frequently appeared not to know where to begin the letter or in which direction to proceed. Some patients corrected errors by comparing the result with the given stimulus and sketching in corrections, thus showing ability to make visual discriminations.

Tests with high loadings on Factor 3. Tests with high loadings on Factor 3 included three copying tasks, writing numerals to 20, three matching tests, three drawing tests, and two object-assembly tests. This exhausted the copying, matching, and object-assembly tests in the matrix.

Tests with low loadings on Factor 3. Tests with negative or low loadings on Factor 3 (as shown in Table 26-1) were all speech and language tests.

Factor 4: Gross Movements of Speech Musculature.

Factor 4, gross movements of the speech musculature, was a small factor with critical loadings on only six tests. The authors considered this factor reflected the kind of gross motor impairment which sometimes occurs with brain damage. If there is paralysis or paresis of the speech musculature, all structures tend to be affected to some extent, and there is usually attendant difficulty swallowing, as Jackson (*19*) pointed out in 1864. Patients who scored low on this entire group of tests had dysarthria, in addition to various amounts of language deficit.

Tests with high loadings on Factor 4. Tests with high loadings on Factor 4 (Table 26-6) included phonation, imitating movements of the tongue and jaw, palatal movements, confirmed reports of difficulty in swallowing, and rapid alternating movements. Only two of these, tongue movements and alternating movements, were correlated with Factor 1, as previously reported.

Tests with low loadings on Factor 4. Tests with negative or low loadings on Factor 4 were all tests with high loadings on Factor 1. This substantiates the view that impairment of the speech musculature is not an essential component of reduction of language in aphasia.

The critical point is that this syndrome generally represents paralysis or paresis of the musculature, as has been pointed out, and this is not necessarily related to language deficit.

TABLE 26-6. CRITICAL LOADINGS* ON FACTOR 4, GROSS MOVEMENTS OF THE SPEECH MUSCULATURE, ON BOTH THE VARIMAX (Var) AND OBLIMIN (Obl) ROTATIONS. ALL TESTS BELOW ARE IN THE CLASSIFICATION OF SPEECH, LANGUAGE

Test		*Loading*	
Task	*Number*	*Var*	*Obl*
imitate examiner: tongue movements	23	72	59
imitate examiner: jaw movements	24	71	64
report difficulty swallowing (confirmed)	26	71	61
imitate examiner: initiate, prolong phonation; alter pitch	22	68	51
imitate syllables: palatal movements	25	68	48
repeat syllables rapidly	27	62	31

* Decimal points are omitted for all entries in the body of the table.

Such paralysis usually results from bilateral cerebral damage. This damage may be scattered, and leave language functions virtually intact. It may be generalized, and result in less efficient operation of all language processes.

Factor 4 does not represent what was meant by "motor aphasia" in the early or later literature. Broca's (*6*) definition contained the words, "without paralysis of the musculature," and so did the definitions of the other localizationists (*2, 3, 29, 39*). In the present analysis, an articulatory disturbance without paralysis or paresis did not emerge as a separate factor. It is presumably represented by the three tests previously cited (tongue movements, alternating movements), and repetition of monosyllabic words) which had inversely related loadings on Factor 1 and Factor 4, suggesting that motor components on required tasks decreased in importance as language components increased.

Bastian (*3*) considered Broca's area a kinesthetic rather than a motor center. Without subscribing to this theory of localization, the senior author (*31*) has long considered that impaired organization of movement patterns in the absence of paralysis is a sensorimotor disturbance resulting from impaired auditory as well as impaired proprioceptive feedback mechanisms. This position is supported by the fact that patients with such impairment respond better, clinically, to intensive auditory stimulation than to more direct techniques for motor control. It is also consistent with the clinical observation that as recovery occurs, language units which are strongly reinforced contain no articulatory errors, although errors recur when new units, or longer ones, are attempted.

These observations appear to support the hypothesis that the impairment Broca described does exist, but is not, as he thought, independent of other aspects of language deficit. None of the data support the idea of a sensory and motor dichotomy, or a division of aphasia into motor or sensory categories. Paralysis or paresis of the speech musculature may or may not exist with aphasia; this is true also of paralysis or paresis of the arm and leg. Impaired organization of speech patterns is correlated with the amount of over-all language deficit present in all modalities, and is inseparable from it.

Factor 5: Recognition of Stimulus Equivalence

The authors were inclined at first to consider Factor 5 (recognition of stimulus equivalence) a matching factor, similar to Factor E on the Jones-Wepman (*21*) analysis, which included nine matching tests and writing words to dictation. Jones and Wepman regarded comprehension of symbols as the common variable on these tests. Neither of these concepts seemed adequate to explain the tests on Factor 5 in the present study, and a further explanation was sought.

Tests included on Factor 5. Table 26-7 reports the tests with important loadings on Factor 5. High loadings were observed on two tests (matching forms and matching letters) that involved identical visual stimuli; on four tests (matching words to pictures, pointing to objects and to body parts named by the examiner, and the Ammons Full-Range Picture Vocabulary Test, a similar task) that involved word comprehension; and on explaining proverbs. The latter test involved comprehension, but not to any greater extent than many other tests that did not appear on Factor 5.

It was the proverbs test that suggested the notion of stimulus equivalence. On the matching tests, the task is obviously to determine that the form on one card is equivalent to the form on another card. Pointing to an object when its name is spoken or presented on a card involves recognition of symbolic equivalence. Explaining a proverb essentially requires recognition of the equivalence between common situations and experiences.

Taking account of stimulus equivalence is obviously one kind of integrative behavior the brain performs, although the mechanism is not known. Klüver (*24*, p. 169) reported: "Facts of equivalence come to light not only when the organism is studied along pathological, physiological, biochemical, and anatomical lines, but also when behavioral and psychological mechanisms are analyzed. Not only do heterogeneous stimuli often produce the same behavioral effect, but the same stimuli may be dealt with by diverse actions and reactions. We find such facts of equivalence on all levels of behavior, ranging from reflexes to the most complex reactions of normal and abnormal personality."

McCullogh (*20*, pp. 100, 101) interpreted stimulus equivalence as an ability to pull out universals. Such ability obviously enters into symbolic, as well as nonsymbolic, behavior.

TABLE 26-7. CRITICAL LOADINGS* ON FACTOR 5, RECOGNITION OF STIMULUS EQUIVALENCE, ON BOTH THE VARIMAX (Var) AND OBLIMIN (Obl) ROTATIONS. TEST CLASSIFICATIONS ARE AUDITORY (Aud); VISUAL, READING (VR); SPEECH, LANGUAGE (SpL); AND BODY IMAGE (BI)

Test			*Loading*	
Task	*Number*	*Class*	*Var*	*Obl*
point to items named	1	Aud	61	46
match printed letters	13	VR	54	71
point to picture indicated by spoken word (Ammons)	10	Aud	51	32
explain proverbs	41	SpL	45	20
point to body parts named	65	BI	43	28
match words with pictures	15	VR	43	38
match geometric forms	12	VR	43	61

* Decimal points are omitted for all entries in the body of the table.

TABLE 26-8. INTERCORRELATION* OF FACTORS: FACTOR 1, LANGUAGE BEHAVIOR; FACTOR 2, VISUAL DISCRIMINATION (ON MATCHING, RECOGNITION, AND RECALL); FACTOR 3, VISUOSPATIAL BEHAVIOR; FACTOR 4, GROSS MOVEMENTS OF THE SPEECH MUSCULATURE; AND FACTOR 5, RECOGNITION OF STIMULUS EQUIVALENCE

Factor	*1*	*2*	*3*	*4*	*5*
1	100	61	37	30	32
2	61	100	55	27	45
3	37	55	100	58	36
4	30	27	58	100	14
5	32	45	36	14	100

* Decimal points are omitted for all entries in the body of the table.

Tests with negative loadings on Factor 5. Tests with negative loadings on Factor 5 included almost all kinds of behavior sampled by the battery except reading comprehension. Factor 5 loadings on the latter ranged from .12 to .32 on the orthogonal solution, and from .08 to .14 on the oblique. The highest loadings on reading tests, on both solutions, was obtained on comprehension of a short paragraph.

Intercorrelation of Factors

Intercorrelations of the five factors in the oblimin solution (Table 26-8) are interesting, although cautious interpretation is necessary. In any analysis of performances of brain-injured patients generally positive correlations would be expected over almost any set of behaviors examined: gross damage tends to deteriorate all performances; limited damage may leave all performances relatively intact. In addition, all subjects in the present study were aphasic, which probably further increased the probability of obtaining generally positive correlations.

Beyond this gross positive relationship, however, one would predict higher correlations between some variables than others; this would indicate genuine behavioral relations that result from common experiences and training, on the one hand, and neurological contiguity or contingency, on the other.

Thus, on the present analysis, Factor 1, language behavior, was most highly correlated with Factor 2, visual discrimination (on matching, recognition, and recall). It was not identical with it, however, since not all language behavior involves visual discrimination. Factor 2 was highly correlated also with Factor 3, visuospatial behavior, but not identical with it, since Factor 3 required proprioceptive as well as visual information. Factor 3 was most highly correlated with Factor 4, gross movements of the speech musculature, on which proprioceptive processes also were represented to some extent. Correlations between Factor 5 and other factors were fairly flat. Some relationship with visual processes was apparent, perhaps because of the nature of the tests on this battery that had high stimulus-equivalence loadings.

It may be noted that the intercorrelation matrix for the first four factors has some of the characteristics of what Guttman (*13*) calls a simplex structure. These factors were arranged in the order of decreasing sums of squares of factor loadings, but there is no special meaning to the order in which they appear; they can be arranged in any arbitrary order. As it happens, however, the factors arrange themselves in such a way that each factor tends to be most highly correlated with the adjacent factors in the matrix, and this is the characteristic of Guttman's simplex structure. If the pattern of intercorrelation of factors found in this study proves to be reliable, its importance lies in the implication that the sources of deficit, conceived as both functionally and spatially related systems, are ordered in the following manner: language behavior → visual discrimination → visuospatial behavior → gross movements of the speech musculature. Such a structure would imply not only a primary language deficit plus additional deficits, as has already been suggested, but also an ordering of the specific deficits in the systematic fashion given, and corresponding neurophysiological arrangements in the brain. Because the evidence is fragile, depending on one particular pattern that may have arisen by chance, and because the number of possible spatial arrangements consonant with such a pattern is so large, little more can be said at the present time.

DISCUSSION

Factor 1 has been interpreted as relating to language behavior in all modalities tested. In the literature (*2*, *15*, *30*, pp. 135, 150, 168, 258 ff., *39*) impairment of language, as opposed to impairment of articulatory processes, has traditionally been labeled anomia, paraphasia, or amnesic aphasia, when it refers to errors in words; and telegraphic speech, agrammatism, or syntactical aphasia, when it refers to errors in inflection or sentence structure. These errors have been dichotomized, probably on the basis of the obviousness of the presenting symptoms. In the experience of the senior author, these errors are inseparable: both are found in the same patients and both correlate with the over-all severity of language deficit.

The present battery contained no tests requiring specified syntactical usages or transformations. Goodglass,[2] who with Hunt (*12*), Berko (*11*), and others, has devised such tests and administered them to aphasic subjects, recently reported that subjects whose verbal responses did not exceed five words made more errors on the two transformations tested than did subjects who made longer verbal responses. This is what would be predicted if there were a correlation between syntactical errors and severity of language deficit. The present authors would expect such tests to load heavily on Factor 1. In other words, impaired structural usage, like vocabulary, is an aspect of language impairment that can be identified and studied in aphasia.

Other aspects of language behavior which appeared on Factor 1 were vocabulary, auditory retention span, and ability to deal with language formulations at various levels of complexity, in all modalities.

The first of these dimensions, vocabulary, has been analyzed more comprehensively in previous studies (*18*, *37*, *38*). In general, these studies show a relationship between vocabulary reduction in aphasia and word frequency. Schuell and Jenkins (*36*) further demonstrated that confusions of words associated in meaning appear in all modalities, while other kinds of errors (such as articulatory errors, and confusions and distortions of letter forms) are appropriate to some modalities, but not to others. In the present analysis, there were substantial loadings on Factor 1 for vocabulary tests in all modalities: pointing to objects named by the examiner; matching words to pictures, and matching printed to spoken words; naming; writing words in response to visual and auditory stimuli; and spelling, both oral and written.

Tests for auditory retention span also ranged over all modalities: repeating sentences; repeating digits; pointing to items named serially; following directions; and writing sentences to dictation (all of these tests contained items which were equated for vocabulary difficulty but progressive in length). Tests involving more complex language formulations included auditory and reading comprehension of paragraph materials; defining words, and explaining similarities and proverbs; describing a picture in speech and in writing; and writing sentences and a paragraph spontaneously. All of these tests had high loadings on Factor 1.

In terms of the present findings, it is possible to define Factor 1 as a factor which is identifiable in listening, speaking, reading, and writing, and which includes vocabulary, retention span, and ability to deal with language formulations of various degrees of complexity.

The findings do not support the concept of a sensory-motor, receptive-expressive, or input-output dichotomy in aphasia. Factor 1 included tests in all modalities; Factor 2 included reading and writing tests, and correlated highly with Factor 1; Factor 3 included matching, as well as copying and drawing; Factor 5 involved matching, and verbal output.

Factor 4 was the only pure output factor. Tests on this factor included only imitation of gross movements of the speech musculature; as soon as language was involved, even on such a simple task as repetition of monosyllabic words, Factor 1 loadings exceeded Factor 4 loadings. The reasonable explanation that Factor 4 represented the presence of paralysis or paresis of the speech musculature, and almost nothing more, is substantiated by the exceedingly high Factor 4 loading on difficulty in swallowing, a common part of this syndrome.

The occurrence of dysarthria with brain damage is not really a controversial point. Motor processes involve complex integrations at many anatomical levels between the cortex and the brain stem. Accordingly, many forms of dysarthria occur, in both the presence and the absence of aphasia. Patients with spastic

[2] H. Goodglass, Applications of psycholinguistic research to clinical diagnosis in aphasia; paper read at twelfth annual Veterans Administration Medical Research Conference, Cincinnati, 1961.

paralysis, Parkinson's disease, multiple sclerosis, bulbar polio, or cerebellar disease, may have dysarthric speech from lesions at various sites; these lesions may result in impaired coordination and control of movements, but frequently leave language behavior otherwise intact. There is general agreement in the literature concerning distinctions between aphasia and dysarthria. At the same time, scattered or generalized brain damage may produce both aphasia and dysarthria, which are not related, as the present findings show. The essential criteria of the presence of both are, first, that a language deficit, as defined by Factor 1, should exist; and secondly, that some paralysis or paresis of the musculature can be demonstrated.

It is further necessary to distinguish between aphasic impairment and dysarthrias that result from loss of control of higher over lower motor centers, as, for example, in some kinds of extrapyramidal or cerebellar involvement. The quality of the observed disturbance, and its independence of language impairment, are probably the best differentiating criteria.

Lastly, dysarthria must be differentiated from articulatory impairment that results from disturbances of feed-back mechanisms essential to language, when no paralysis is present. This kind of deficit is correlated with existing language deficit. On the present analysis, it is considered to be represented by the subgroup of tests with loadings on Factor 1 and Factor 4, previously discussed.

It is theoretically possible that lesions in the occipital lobe could result in perceptual disturbances affecting reading, and that, with the rest of the brain intact, the patient could speak normally, and even write fairly well, by spelling words as he wrote them and utilizing learned movement patterns and intact proprioceptive feedback mechanisms. This is certainly not a usual finding, but rare cases have occasionally been reported; when well documented they provide important information concerning little-understood cerebral mechanisms.

It is doubtful that lesions disrupting auditory processes can result in impairment confined to one language modality, because language itself is so highly dependent on auditory integrations. Bocca (*5*), for example, found that length of message and meaningfulness were not only important dimensions in auditory perception, but the ones most frequently affected by temporal lobe tumors in the dominant, as contrasted with the nondominant, hemisphere. This interdependence presumably accounts for the high loadings of all the tests for auditory comprehension on Factor 1. Patients with severe auditory imperception sometimes have (or recover) some residual speech, but severe language limitations can usually be demonstrated in all modalities. It is probable that auditory comprehension did not appear as a separate factor because it is such an integral part of all behavior identified by Factor 1.

It would seem meaningful to talk about aphasic behavior in terms of the factors identified here: to say that language breaks down, in all modalities, at some approximate level; to determine whether or not additional deficits of visual discrimination, involving matching, recognition, and recall, or visuospatial behavior were present, describe what was observed, and evaluate the severity of the deficit; to describe any demonstrable paralysis or paresis of the musculature, or articulatory impairment existing in the absence of observable paralysis or paresis; and to specify whether or not the subject recognized stimulus equivalence. It is possible that failure on the group of tasks included on Factor 5 may indicate impairment of mental functions extending beyond the language deficit.

SUMMARY AND CONCLUSIONS

This paper presented a factor analysis of test scores for a nonselected sample of aphasic subjects on 69 tests, comprised of 679 items and including tests for auditory comprehension, visual and reading performances, speech and language performances, visuomotor and writing performances, and performances involving numerical relations, arithmetic processes, and body image. Tetrachoric correlations were used as a basis for determining principal components. Varimax and oblimin rotations, as well as graphic solutions, resulted in identification of five factors:

Factor 1, language behavior. This factor included all language modalities tested and accounted for 41% of test variance.

Factor 2, visual discrimination (on matching, recognition, and recall). Both reading and writing tests had high loadings on this factor; Factor 2 correlated most highly with Factor 1 ($r = .61$).

Factor 3, visuospatial behavior. This factor involved both visual and sensory processes, and correlated most highly with Factor 4 ($r = .58$) and Factor 2 ($r = .55$).

Factor 4, gross movements of the speech musculature. This factor appeared to reflect paralysis or paresis of the speech musculature. A subgroup of tests showing interrelations between Factor 1 and Factor 4 was considered to reflect sensorimotor involvement related to impairment of auditory and proprioceptive feedback mechanisms.

Factor 5, recognition of stimulus equivalence. This factor was considered to reflect integrative processes involved in symbolic, and probably also in nonsymbolic, behavior.

The authors consider these findings support the following conclusions:

There is a dimension of general language deficit in aphasia that is not modality specific.

Reading and writing performances may be further impaired by disturbances of visual discriminations, involving matching, recognition, and recall.

Visual performances may be further impaired by the addition of sensory disturbances related to perception of spatial relationships.

There may be a syndrome of gross motor impairment characterized by paralysis or paresis of the speech musculature and difficulty in swallowing; this is not necessarily related to language deficit.

In the absence of paralysis or paresis of the speech musculature, there may be impairment of articulation that is correlated with language deficit, and considered to result from impairment of auditory and proprioceptive feedback mechanisms.

Recognition of stimulus equivalence plays a part in symbolic as well as other kinds of behavior.

There is no support for the hypothesis of a sensory-motor, a receptive-expressive, or an input-output dichotomy in aphasia.

These findings confirm the hypothesis that the general dimension of language impairment (*35*) isolated by the Guttman technique is essentially the same as the major factor which appeared on the varimax and oblimin solutions in the present factor analysis.

These findings confirm the hypothesis of Jones and Wepman (*21*), and previous findings reported by Schuell and Jenkins (*35*), that additional variables compatible with brain damage may play a role in aphasic behavior, and must be taken into account in the evaluation and treatment of aphasic conditions, as well as in the formulation of conceptual models of aphasia.

REFERENCES

1. Ammons, R. B., and Ammons, Helen S., *Full-Range Picture Vocabulary Test.* Missoula, Mont.: Psychol. Test Specialists, 1948.
2. Bastian, H. C., On different kinds of aphasia, with special reference to their classification and ultimate pathology. *Brit. med. J.*, **2,** 1887, 931–936, 985–990.
3. ——, *A Treatise on Aphasia and Other Speech Defects.* London: Lewis, 1898.
4. Bay, E., Disturbances of visual perception and their examination. *Brain*, **76,** 1953, 515–550.
5. Bocca, E., Clinical aspects of cortical deafness. *Laryngoscope*, **68,** 1958, 301–309.
6. Broca, P., Remarques sur le siege, le diagnostic et la nature de l'aphèmie. *Bull. Soc. anat. Paris*, 1863, 379–385, 393–399.
7. Carroll, J. B., Biquartimin criterion for rotation to oblique simple structure in factor analysis. *Science*, **126,** 1957, 1114–1115.
8. ——, The nature of the data, or how to choose a correlation coefficient. *Psychometrika*, **26,** 1961, 347–372.
9. Critchley, M., Discussion on parietal lobe syndromes. *Proc. roy. Soc. Med.*, **44,** 1951, 337–341.
10. Gooddy, W., and Reinhold, Margaret, Some

aspects of human orientation in space. *Brain*, **75,** 1952, 472–509.

11. Goodglass, H., and Berko, Jean, Agrammatism and inflectional morphology in English. *J. Speech Hearing Res.*, **3,** 1960, 257–267.
12. ——, and Hunt, J., Grammatical complexity and aphasic speech. *Word*, **14,** 1958, 197–207.
13. Guttman, L., A generalized simplex for factor analysis. *Psychometrika*, **20,** 1955, 173–192.
14. Harman, H. H., *Modern Factor Analysis*. Chicago: Univ. Chicago Press, 1960.
15. Head, H., *Aphasia and Kindred Disorders of Speech.* Cambridge: University Press, 1926.
16. Hebb, D. O., *The Organization of Behavior; a Neuropsychological Theory*. New York: Wiley, 1949.
17. Howes, D. H., The intelligibility of spoken messages. *Amer. J. Psychol.*, **65,** 1952, 460–465.
18. Howes, D., and Geschwind, N., Statistical properties of aphasic language. *Nat. Inst. Hlth prog. Rep.*, Grant M 1802, 1960.
19. Jackson, H., Loss of speech. . . . *Brain*, **38,** 1915, 28–42.
20. Jeffress, L. A. (Ed.), *Cerebral Mechanisms in Behavior* (Hixon Symposium). New York: Wiley, 1951.
21. Jones, L. V., and Wepman, J. M., Dimensions of language performance in aphasia. *J. Speech Hearing Res.*, **4,** 1961, 220–232.
22. Kaiser, H. F., The varimax criterion for analytic rotation in factor analysis. *Psychometrika*, **23,** 1958, 187–200.
23. King-Ellison, P., and Jenkins, J. J., Visual duration threshold as a function of word frequency. *Tech. Rep.* **6,** Off. Nav. Res., contr. N8-66216.
24. Klüver, H., Functional differences between the occipital and temporal lobes with special reference to the interrelations of behavior and extracerebral mechanisms. In L. A. Jeffress (Ed.), *Cerebral Mechanisms in Behavior* (Hixon Symposium). New York: Wiley, 1951.
25. Kussmaul, A., Disturbances of speech. Vol. **14** in H. von Ziemssen (Ed.), *Cyclopaedia of the Practice of Medicine*. New York: William Wood, 1887.
26. Lamberts, J. J., Basic concepts for teaching from structural linguistics. *Engl. J.*, **49,** 1960, 172–176.
27. Lashley, K. S., The problem of serial order in behavior. In L. A. Jeffress (Ed.), *Cerebral Mechanisms in Behavior* (Hixon Symposium). New York: Wiley, 1951.
28. Liberman, A. M., Some results of research on speech perception. *J. acoust. Soc. Amer.*, **29,** 1957, 117–123.
29. Lichtheim, L., On aphasia. *Brain*, **7,** 1884, 433–484.
30. Pick, A., *Die Agrammatischen Sprachstörungen.* Berlin: Springer, 1913.
31. Schuell, Hildred, Clinical findings in aphasia. *Lancet*, **80,** 1960, 482–490.
32. ——, Diagnosis and prognosis in aphasia. *Arch. Neurol. Psychiat.*, **74,** 1955, 308–315.
33. ——, *The Minnesota Test for Differential Diagnosis of Aphasia.* (res. ed.) Minneapolis: Univ. Minn. Print. Dept., 1955 (out of print).
34. ——, and Jenkins, J. J., Comment on "Dimensions of language performance in aphasia." *J. Speech Hearing Res.*, **4,** 1961, 295–299.
35. ——, ——, The nature of language deficit in aphasia. *Psychol. Rev.*, **66,** 1959, 45–67.
36. ——, ——, Reduction of vocabulary in aphasia. *Brain*, **84,** 1961, 243–261.
37. ——, ——, and Landis, Lydia, Relationship between auditory comprehension and word frequency in aphasia. *J. Speech Hearing Res.*, **4,** 1961, 30–36.
38. Wepman, J. M., Bock, R. D., Jones, L. V., and Van Pelt, Doris, Psycholinguistic study of aphasia: a revision of the concept of anomia. *J. Speech Hearing Dis.*, **21,** 1956, 468–477.
39. Wernicke, C., The symptom-complex of aphasia. In A. Church (Ed.), *Diseases of the Nervous System.* New York: Appleton, 1908.

27

Dimensions of Language Performance in Aphasia

LYLE V. JONES
JOSEPH M. WEPMAN

LYLE V. JONES, Ph.D., is director of the Psychometric Laboratory at the University of North Carolina, Chapel Hill.

JOSEPH M. WEPMAN, Ph.D., is with the department of psychology and is director of the Speech and Language Clinic of the University of Chicago.

Different phases of the research reported were supported by grants from the Department of Health, Education, and Welfare through (a) the National Institutes of Health, Neurological Diseases and Blindness Council (Grant B-710), (b) the National Institutes of Mental Health (Grants M-1849 and M-1876), and (c) the Office of Vocational Rehabilitation (Grant 168).

Attempts to classify language deficit consequent to cortical insult are prominent in the literature concerning aphasia (for example, *5*, *9*). Critical of such classificatory systems is the recent paper by Schuell and Jenkins (7) who present evidence which they interpret to be "more compatible with the theory of a single dimension of language deficit than with the multiple dimensions or topologies suggested in the past." Currently, then, it is not clear whether qualitative distinctions can usefully be made among aphasia disorders. If they can, there appears no general agreement concerning the appropriate form of such distinctions.

Before embarking upon an exploration of the nature of language performance in brain-damaged patients, it is imperative to define the language act, as well as to specify carefully a population of subjects to which conclusions pertain. The primary source of differences among conceptual systems for viewing performance in aphasia clearly appears to be one of diversity of definition, either of the domain of language performance or of the criteria of aphasia.

From *Journal of Speech and Hearing Research* 4:220–32, 1961.

Every complete language act consists of a stimulating situation, a system of central processes, and a response. The stimulating situation, or input, may be actor initiated or initiated by means external to the actor. The sensory mode of stimulation may be dominantly visual, aural, kinesthetic, somesthetic, etc. The mode of response may be graphic, oral, or gestural. The content of response is attributable both to characteristics of the stimulus and to the interpreting and mediating central processes.

Systematic investigation of the nature of residual language skills following cortical damage would appear to provide unique advantages for understanding normal as well as disturbed language processes. The extent to which clusters of language skills are concomitantly affected by brain damage should cast light on the organization of these skills in successful performance of language acts.

Factor analysis is a statistical tool appropriate for defining such clusters of skills. Just as factor analysis has served to discover separate verbal abilities for normal subjects (for example, *2*), so it may be possible to identify "islands" of language performance which sometimes remain intact in brain damaged aphasia patients. For this purpose, specially devised tests must be developed, assessing a variety of language acts. To be differentially sensitive to possible differences among aphasia patients the level of difficulty of tests must be established appropriately. Test materials should be of sufficient ease so that among brain intact adults performance would be near perfect. Among brain damaged adults, in order optimally to distinguish among different levels of performance, the proportion of subjects passing a typical item should be nearer .5 than either 0 or 1.

TEST MATERIALS

A battery of test materials was constructed to meet these objectives. A film strip is used for presenting all visual materials. Auditory stimulus items are presented orally by the examiner. Specification of types of items presented appears in Table 27-1. Kinds of responses utilized for the various stimuli are listed below:

Visual Stimuli

a. Reads or names
b. Writes word or name
c. Matches word to picture or picture to word
d. Matches word to word or picture to picture

Auditory Stimuli

a. Repeats after examiner
b. Writes word spoken by examiner
c. Matches spoken word to picture
d. Matches spoken word to printed word

A shortened version of the test battery, the Language Modalities Test for Aphasia (*8*), has been prepared for general use in the assessment of aphasic disorders.

SUBJECTS

Results reported here are based upon the test performance of 168 selected subjects from 19 different hospitals and clinics throughout the northeastern United States. Subjects were selected only if (a) the medical record displayed attested medical diagnosis of brain damage; (b) the hospital or clinic record noted language disability consequent to the brain damage; (c) subjects retained sufficient ability to follow test instructions; (d) subjects displayed no more than mild dysarthria. Evidence regarding (c) and (d) was obtained from an interview with the subject and administration of a screening test.

The patients studied included 147 male and 21 female; 124 were in-patients, while the remaining 44 were out-patients. The cause of brain damage had been diagnosed as cerebro-

TABLE 27-1. CATEGORIES TESTED AND EXAMPLES OF EACH CATEGORY IN BOTH VISUAL AND AUDITORY MODALITIES

Visual		*Auditory*	
Category	*Example*	*Category*	*Example*
Pictures	baby	Consonant Sounds	p
Letters	M	Letter Names	dee
Geometric Forms	O	Geometric Forms	circle
Number, Arabic	4	Numbers	four
Number, Printed	Four		
Arithmetic Signs	+		
Words	Bread	Words	man
Special Words	You	Special Words	at
Sentences		Sentences	
a. 3-word	Women prepare food.	a. 3-word	He has that.
b. 5-word	He has it for us.	b. 5-word	She takes her dog out.
Tell-a-Story Picture			

vascular accident for 130 cases, external trauma for 29 cases, and as tumor extirpation for six cases. No cause was listed for three patients. Right hemiparesis was reported for 130 subjects, left hemiparesis for five, bilateral paralysis for three, no paralysis for 25, while the medical records of the remaining five gave no information concerning paralysis. In terms of premorbid educational level, 15 were college graduates, 46 completed high school but not college, 51 completed grade school but not high school, and 23 failed to complete grade school. Educational history of 33 subjects is unknown. Subjects ranged in age from 14 to 76, with mean age of 51, standard deviation of 15.

SCALING OF RESPONSES

Responses from aphasia patients, when in error, nevertheless display a range of distinct qualitative characteristics. A response may be judged erroneous as a result of faulty articulation, of the appearance of an inappropriate word or phrase, or of simple refusal of the patient to offer a response. To accommodate for such qualitative differences, the following scoring categories were utilized for each oral or graphic response to test items.[1]

Code Number	*Values*
1	Correct response
2	Self-corrected response
3	Single articulatory or spelling error
4	Two or more articulatory or spelling errors (response recognizable as correct word or number)
5	In-class word substitution
6	Out-of-class word substitution
7	Jargon or unintelligible response
8	Automatic response
9	No response

For the purpose of precisely specifying the characteristics of language loss in aphasia patients, maintenance of such distinctions regarding form of errors is thought to be equally important with recognition of the mode of stimuli and form of response for which errors occur. However, to factor analyze a set of variates representing test performance, quantitative rather than qualitative scores are required.

To derive quantitative indices of performance, the categories of response were subjected to analysis by the method of optimal scaling (*1*, *3*). The method depends upon selecting scale values for the response categories which maximize the correlation ratio for the sum of squares between patients to the total sum of squares computed from these scale values. The resulting scale, then, has the effect of discriminating optimally between subjects, in the sense that between-subject variance is maximum relative to within-subject variance.

Scaling was accomplished separately for various subgroups of test items (see Table 27-2). For the purpose of deriving scale values for response categories, the within-subject variance was defined over all items within each item class. Since the test was administered in two forms, presented on successive days, the within-subject variance includes variance due to the sampling of items, variance due to instability of performance during a test session, and day-to-day variability of a subject. The within-subject variance thus is a good measure of the variance which detracts from test reliability. Indeed, the scaling method may be regarded as one which maximizes reliability of the subtests (item classes).

From results of the scaling analysis, Table 27-2, it is seen that the correlation ratios are sufficiently high to make possible clear quantitative distinctions among subjects' performances. In most cases, the order of size of the scale values corresponds closely to that conjectured when category designations (1, 2, . . . , 9) were assigned. The one consistent discrepancy is the inversion of scale values for categories 7 (jargon) and 8 (automatic phrases). For auditory stimuli especially, 7 is closer to 9 (no response) than is 8. This would indicate that the tendency toward jargon response appears frequently in conjunction with the

[1] In the revised Language Modalities Test for Aphasia, scoring categories have been redefined and collapsed, so that six rather than nine are used.

TABLE 27-2. SCALE VALUES OF THE NINE SCORING CATEGORIES (C_1, C_2, . . . C_9) DETERMINED FROM EACH OF 10 CLASSES OF TEST ITEMS INVOLVING PICTURES (P), FIGURES (F), NUMBERS (N), LETTERS (L), SIGNS (Sn), WORDS AND SENTENCES (W-S), AND SOUNDS (Sd); NUMBER OF ITEMS IN EACH OF THE 10 CLASSES; AND CORRELATION RATIO FOR EACH OF THE 10 CLASSES

C	*Visual Stimuli*						*Aural Stimuli*			
	Oral Response			*Graphic Response**			*Oral Response*		*Graphic Response*	
	P	*FNLSn*	*W-S*	*P*	*FNLSn*	*W-S*	*SdFNL*	*W-S*	*FNL*	*W-S*
Number of Items										
	8	36	96	8	20	16	24	72	82	36
Scale Values										
C_1	.567	.608	.586	.659	.430	.476	.496	.568	.593	.664
C_2	.132	.136	.122	.090	.023	.050	.027	.537	.106	.048
C_3	.040	.049	.134	.232	–.099	–.057	.066	.020	–.001	.145
C_4	.012	–.027	.025	.112	–.044	–.152	–.023	–.061	–.010	.060
C_5	.089	.038	.011	.081	–.047	.004	–.085	.007	–.018	.018
C_6	–.175	–.101	–.084	–.100	–.026	–.041	–.133	–.118	–.057	–.026
C_7	–.459	–.401	–.266	–.294	–.496	–.486	–.436	–.489	–.294	–.034
C_8	–.363	–.328	–.297				–.234	–.286	–.057	–.034
C_9	–.528	–.574	–.676	–.623	–.744	–.712	–.692	–.579	–.738	–.702
Correlation Ratio										
	.721	.637	.768	.661	.593	.721	.618	.611	.483	.659

* No graphic responses to visual stimuli were scored in category 8.

tendency toward failure to respond. Jargon and response failure are more often associated within the same subjects than automatic phrases and failure of response.

Other departures from the conjectured ordering are confined to categories 2, 3, 4, 5, and 6, and are not consistent from scale to scale. The scale values for these categories are close together numerically, when compared with the full range of the scale, and it is apparent that the large contribution to discrimination is being made by categories 1 and 9, "correct" and "no response." Taking into account the smaller contribution of the middle categories, it may be concluded that the scales are sufficiently similar to justify adopting a single coarse scale to quantify all responses for purposes of item analysis.

Category	1	2	3	4	5	6	7	8	9
Scale Value	6	1	1	0	0	–1	–4	–3	–7

It can be shown that the correlation ratios based upon this approximate scale are only slightly smaller than the maximal values displayed in Table 27-2. The economy of adopting a single one-digit scale for all item classes would appear to override the slight loss in discrimination among subjects.

ITEM DIFFICULTY

Several measures of difficulty of item classes have been determined, both in terms of proportion of correct responses and mean scale values of scoring categories. The measures agree in distinguishing several item classes as markedly more difficult than others. For the subjects studied, the task of providing written response to aurally presented sentences is most difficult, with mean proportion of words correctly written, $P = .25$. Other difficult tasks are graphic response to pictures (demanding the written name of whatever is pictured), written response to aural words, oral response to visually presented geometric forms and to arithmetic signs, with mean proportion correct, P, ranging from .26 to .29. It is to be noted that all of these item classes demand a translation from a given stimulus to a response mode of a distinct kind. The easiest items, on the other hand, involve copying of short visual stimuli (geometric forms, letters, arithmetic signs, numerals), $P = .73$, or repeating of short auditory stimuli (numbers, letters, prepositions, and pronouns), $P = .66$.

FACTOR ANALYSIS

Two sets of factor analyses have been performed, one on 35 test variables, the other on 37 test variables. The lists of test variables overlap considerably; the second list differs from the first most importantly in its inclusion of items involving matching responses (typically matching a visual or aural language stimulus to one of four alternative pictures). Because of this addition, the 37-variable problem will be discussed here. In no case is interpretation of results from the 35-variable study inconsistent with that from the 37-variable study.

Four distinct forms of analysis were completed, based upon performance of the 168 subjects on the 37 variables (defined in Table 27-4) included in the study. Two were graphical, one orthogonal and one oblique graphical solution having been obtained. Two were analytic, a varimax (orthogonal) solution (*6*) and an oblimin (oblique) solution.[2] Since the initial analyses were completed, still further solutions have been obtained, an oblimax solution and a hierarchical solution.

For each of the test variables, a score was defined for each subject by summing the scale values of his responses for all items within the class represented by that variable. The distribution of such scores then was normalized separately for each of the 37 variables. Product-moment correlation coefficients were computed among the 37 variables, with $N = 168$, utilizing the IBM 650. A principal axes factor solution then was obtained on the ORACLE, a digital computer located at Oak Ridge, Tennessee. The principal axes solution was based upon communality estimates

$$h^2_{ii} = 1 - 1/r^{ii},$$

where r^{ii} is the diagonal element for variable i in the inverse of the 37×37 complete matrix of correlations among the 37 variables (see *4*, p. 89).

[2] J. B. Carroll, Solution of the Oblimin Criterion for Oblique Rotation in Factor Analysis, unpublished manuscript, 1958.

TABLE 27-3. PRINCIPAL AXES FACTOR LOADINGS.* VARIABLE IDENTIFICATIONS (VI) ARE GIVEN BY NUMBER IN THE LEFT HAND COLUMN

VI	Factor *1*	*2*	*3*	*4*	*5*	*6*
1	272	−462	280	−219	−045	−064
2	018	−366	−097	−060	147	−492
3	913	213	−049	079	−195	−034
4	879	287	−181	101	−115	−100
5	904	256	−167	090	−136	004
6	885	297	−160	090	−102	−044
7	902	236	−161	077	−086	−058
8	882	278	−204	095	−071	−046
9	893	261	−111	071	−110	068
10	879	231	−141	093	−188	−031
11	898	182	−158	096	−056	−052
12	895	236	−151	048	014	−007
13	891	225	−169	094	−057	−042
14	617	−517	181	409	−025	−030
15	562	−604	179	397	004	008
16	548	−541	273	374	064	−016
17	520	−597	210	324	−018	−044
18	623	−490	−070	−187	−262	147
19	625	−453	−154	−163	−149	010
20	623	−396	−108	−195	070	−262
21	720	−349	−171	−220	−084	−037
22	660	−362	−194	−297	−061	−072
23	819	205	409	−097	086	−051
24	774	285	426	−064	061	−012
25	739	164	467	−139	029	023
26	714	291	445	−066	027	−037
27	749	323	429	−131	−062	−058
28	790	392	167	−040	107	027
29	799	389	168	−106	118	006
30	827	−212	−216	028	324	093
31	818	−156	−173	−044	316	177
32	835	−026	−158	011	428	084
33	815	−056	−210	018	378	074
34	623	−291	−091	−283	068	−008
35	648	−400	010	−062	−191	196
36	675	−390	164	−279	−012	070
37	508	−383	066	−078	−189	143
$\Sigma a^2/37$	.557	.119	.050	.032	.025	.014

*Decimal points are omitted for all entries in the body of the table.

TABLE 27-4. VARIMAX FACTOR MATRIX,* GIVING STIMULUS, RESPONSE, VARIABLE IDENTIFICATION BY NUMBER, ITEM, NUMBER OF ITEMS, FACTOR, AND h^2, IN THAT ORDER, LEFT TO RIGHT

S	*R*	*VI*	*Item*	*N*	Factor *A*	*B*	*C*	*D*	*E*	*F*	h^2
		1	Age		16	−25	−26	02	−49	−14	65
		2	Education		−10	−11	13	04	16	59	64
V	O	3	Nouns	8	83	35	18	04	28	−04	96
V	O	4	Verbs	8	89	26	10	11	19	04	96
V	O	5	Adjectives	8	88	27	12	13	25	−05	97
V	O	6	Abstr nouns	8	88	29	10	14	20	−01	96
V	O	7	Abstr verbs	8	86	28	13	16	24	02	95
V	O	8	Abstr adjectives	8	88	25	10	18	20	01	96
V	O	9	Pronouns, prepositions	8	83	32	12	16	25	−11	95
V	O	10	Color names	4	85	27	14	06	26	−03	94
V	O	11	Names of sounds	4	82	26	17	19	25	03	94
V	O	12	Sentences†	23	81	31	11	26	23	00	94
V	O	13	Sentences**	9	84	27	14	19	23	01	94
V	G	14	Nouns	4	24	12	81	10	33	07	92
V	G	15	Verbs	4	15	07	83	13	36	06	93
V	G	16	Adjectives	4	11	18	81	14	30	08	90
V	G	17	Pronouns, prepositions	4	10	10	77	08	38	11	88
V	M	18	Pictures	8	25	05	28	04	78	−06	87
V	M	19	Numbers	12	30	01	25	11	70	10	82
V	M	20	Arithmetic signs	8	28	13	22	20	58	39	82
V	M	21	Nouns, verbs, adj	12	40	10	18	18	69	15	85
V	M	22	Sentences	4	34	08	11	18	71	20	84
A	O	23	Nouns, verbs, adj	12	46	77	18	15	21	02	95
A	O	24	Abstr nouns, verbs, adj	12	47	77	15	12	13	−05	93
A	O	25	Pronouns, prepositions	8	36	76	17	09	24	−06	90
A	O	26	Color names	4	43	76	14	06	11	−04	89
A	O	27	Names of sounds	4	48	78	08	−01	16	−04	93
A	O	28	Sentences†	21	63	60	03	23	08	−06	91
A	O	29	Sentences**	11	61	63	−01	24	12	−03	92
A	G	30	Nouns, verbs, adj	12	50	13	30	59	42	09	94
A	G	31	Pronouns, prepositions	4	47	20	23	60	42	00	93
A	G	32	Sentences†	15	54	26	21	65	28	08	96
A	G	33	Sentences**	5	55	19	21	62	30	09	93
A	M	34	Geometric forms	4	26	18	10	27	60	14	75
A	M	35	Numbers	4	28	12	36	09	64	−13	81
A	M	36	Nouns, verbs, adj	8	16	36	25	18	68	04	85
A	M	37	Sentences	4	17	12	31	02	57	−09	69
$\Sigma a^2_i/37$					.315	.138	.101	.061	.162	.019	.797

* Decimal points are omitted for all entries in the body of the table.
† Only syntactic words from sentences.
** Only semantic words from sentences.

Several criteria agree in suggesting that six principal axes are sufficient to account for nonrandom common variance for this problem. It is reassuring that the varimax solution was relatively invariant for this study when the largest 6, 7, 8, 9, or 20 principal axes were included for rotation. (Twenty characteristic roots of the 37 × 37 reduced correlation matrix were positive.) Projections of the 37 variables upon the first six principal axes appear in Table 27-3.

Despite dissimilarities in sizes of loadings and in correlations among factors, all solutions are in essential agreement in displaying five clearly defined common factors and a sixth, doublet factor.

Simple structure is most striking for the oblique solutions. However, the sizable correlations among factors lead to difficulties of interpretation, and the orthogonal varimax solution is presented here.[3] The solution appears in Table 27-4.

(In the following informal tables and in Table 27-4 these abbreviations are used: variable identification by number, VI; stimulus, S; response, R; factor loading, Ldg; aural stimulus, A; visual stimulus, V; oral response, O; graphic response, G; matching response, M.)

Factor A

For all analyses, Factor A is defined best by all items demanding oral response to visual stimuli. (For the oblique solutions, no other classes of items are prominently represented on the factor.) Since such items formed the most numerous item class, this factor accounts for more common variance than does any other, 40 percent of common factor variance, 32 percent of total variance. The defining items, together with their loadings as obtained on the varimax solution, are listed in Table 27-5.

TABLE 27-5.

VI	S	R	Item	Ldg
4	V	O	Verbs	.89
5	V	O	Adjectives	.88
6	V	O	Abstr nouns	.88
8	V	O	Abstr adjectives	.88
7	V	O	Abstr verbs	.86
10	V	O	Color names	.85
13	V	O	Sentences*	.84
9	V	O	Pronouns, prepositions	.83
3	V	O	Nouns	.83
11	V	O	Names of sounds	.82
12	V	O	Sentences†	.81
28	A	O	Sentences†	.63
29	A	O	Sentences*	.61
33	A	G	Sentences*	.55
32	A	G	Sentences†	.54
30	A	G	Nouns, verbs, adjectives	.50
27	A	O	Names of sounds	.48
24	A	O	Abstr nouns, verbs, adj	.47
31	A	G	Pronouns, prepositions	.47
23	A	O	Nouns, verbs, adj	.46
26	A	O	Color names	.43
21	V	M	Nouns, verbs, adj	.40

* Only semantic words for sentences.
† Only syntactic words for sentences.

All items which involve oral response to visual stimuli display loadings on Factor A in excess of .80. It is tempting to interpret the factor as one representing *the transmission and translation from visual stimulus to oral response.*

Note that, following the visual-oral items in order of size of loadings on Factor A are the four items demanding oral or graphic response to aurally presented sentences, all of which exhibit loadings in the range .55 to .62. This finding is consistent with the interpretation of Factor A as a visual-oral transmission factor if such transmission can be considered to play a function in oral or graphic response to sentences. The finding suggests that the probability of correct oral repetition of an aurally presented sentence is enhanced for individuals able to maintain a visual image of the sentence after hearing it. Only then could the visual-oral transmission function be relevant to the task. In addition, that graphic response to spoken sentences is represented on the factor suggests the functions both of visual retention and of subvocal oral response as possible intervening steps between aural stimulation and written response. (Even on the oblique factor solutions, these variables, particularly 28 and 29 which entail oral response to aurally presented sentences, exhibit positive projections on the vector representing Factor A.)

Many of the remaining variables exhibit substantial Factor A loadings on the orthogonal varimax solution. This represents some tendency toward a general factor, in the sense that all tasks on the test tend to be positively correlated. Seven of the 37 variables, however, exhibit loadings less than .20.

Factor B

Factor B contributes 18 percent of common variance, 14 percent of total variance, and is

[3] Results of the other analyses are available from the authors upon request. The varimax solution given in Table 27-6 is that which resulted from an input of six principal axes.

TABLE 27-6.

VI	S	R	Item	Ldg
27	A	O	Names of sounds	.78
23	A	O	Nouns, verbs, adj	.77
24	A	O	Abstr nouns, verbs, adj	.77
25	A	O	Pronouns, prepositions	.76
26	A	O	Color names	.76
29	A	O	Sentences*	.63
28	A	O	Sentences†	.60

* Only semantic words from sentences.
† Only syntactic words from sentences.

represented primarily by the variables shown in Table 27-6.

Those variables with highest loadings on Factor B include those variables demanding oral response to aural stimuli. All such variables exhibit loadings of .60 or greater; no other variable exhibits a loading as great as .40.

Factor B would seem to represent *the transmission of aurally received stimuli into orally produced response.*

That this transmission ability can play a part in the success of patients on items other than those which require oral response to aural stimuli is suggested by loadings of items requiring oral response to visual stimuli (loadings of .25 to .36), of items requiring matching of visual alternatives to aurally presented words (.36), and of items requiring graphic response to aurally presented sentences (.19 and .26). In each case, it is tenable that by "reauditorization" patients would better be able to perform the assigned tasks, and that aural to oral transmission is necessary for this process. The test variables which exhibit near-zero projections upon Factor B include only those involving graphic response to visual stimuli or matching response to visual stimuli, tasks in which the aural-oral channel could not be anticipated to play a prominent role.

Factor C

Factor C accounts for 14 percent of the common-factor variance, 11 percent of total variance. Only four variables exhibit loadings in excess of .40, and these exhaust the items which demand copying of visual stimuli (Table 27-7).

TABLE 27-7.

VI	S	R	Item	Ldg
15	V	G	Verbs	.83
14	V	G	Nouns	.81
16	V	G	Adjectives	.81
17	V	G	Pronouns, prepositions	.77

Factor C apparently involves *transmission from visual stimuli to graphic response.*

Other variables, with loadings between .22 and .39 include the majority of the matching variables, both auditory and visual stimuli, as well as all variables demanding graphic response to auditory stimuli. Conjecturing the possibility of a visual image of a word instigated by aural stimulation, it is reasonable that these tasks might be aided by intact visual-graphic transmission.

Factor D

The four variables with projections on Factor D in excess of .40 are listed in Table 27-8. Factor D accounts for approximately 7 percent of common variance, 6 percent of total variance.

TABLE 27-8.

VI	S	R	Item	Ldg
32	A	G	Sentences*	.65
33	A	G	Sentences†	.62
31	A	G	Pronouns, prepositions	.60
30	A	G	Nouns, verbs, adj	.59

* Only syntactic words from sentences.
† Only semantic words from sentences.

This list includes all test items which involve written response to aural stimulation. It appears to reflect *aural to graphic transmission.* No other variables display loadings greater than .25.

Factor E

Factor E accounts for 18 percent of common factor variance, 15 percent of total variance, second in prominence only to Factor A. The variables which display loadings of .40 or greater are as shown in Table 27-9.

TABLE 27-9.

VI	S	R	Item	Ldg
18	V	M	Pictures	.78
22	V	M	Sentences	.71
19	V	M	Numbers	.70
21	V	M	Nouns, verbs, adj	.69
36	A	M	Nouns, verbs, adj	.68
35	A	M	Numbers	.64
34	A	M	Geometric forms	.60
20	V	M	Arithmetic signs	.58
37	A	M	Sentences	.57
1			Age	−.49
31	A	G	Pronouns, prepositions	.43
30	A	G	Nouns, verbs, adj	.42

All nine matching tests head the list of defining variables for Factor E; five tests require matching of visual stimuli to visually presented alternatives, while four require matching of auditory stimuli to visually presented alternatives. These variables have in common their dependence upon the need for comprehension of symbols. The task demands correct matching of a verbal symbol to a pictorial representation of that denoted by the symbol. Variables 30 and 31 are the only two which require written response to spoken words. With comprehension of word meaning, it is tenable that the likelihood of correct response is enhanced.

Factor E clearly represents *an ability to comprehend language symbols*, since aural as well as visual stimuli are prominently involved. Factor E, in a central way, represents aphasia as distinct from the agnosias and apraxias which depend upon input-output modalities.

Factor E is the only factor on which age is prominently represented. The loading of age, —.49, indicates a tendency for older patients to perform less well on the tasks which define the factor. The finding may reflect the general deterioration of comprehension abilities which accompanies increasing age of the nervous system, an effect probably accentuated by cortical damage.

It is instructive to note, from Table 27-4, the nature of other variables with nonzero projections on Factor E. Loadings between .20 and .40 are displayed by several variables involving graphic response to visually or aurally presented words and sentences, as well as variables which require oral response to visually presented words or sentences. In the case of each such variable, it is tenable that comprehension of the stimulus, understanding the words, would enhance the likelihood of correct response.

Factor F

Accounting for only about 2 percent of the variance, Factor F displays only two appreciable loadings (Table 27-10).

TABLE 27-10.

VI	S	R	Item	Ldg
2			Education	.59
20	V	M	Arithmetic signs	.39

Variable 20 requires selection of correct answers among alternative choices presented as possible solutions to arithmetic problems, also presented visually. Addition, subtraction, multiplication, and division are represented, each indicated by its conventional sign (+, −, ×, ÷). This arithmetic variable appears, with all other matching tests, on Factor E, but it alone is displayed on Factor F, together with number of years of premorbid education.

One might view Factor F as a rather trivial doublet, representing a relationship between education and arithmetic, expected to appear for intact individuals as well as aphasic patients. Such a view probably is in error. The arithmetic problems presented are so simple that individuals with even some grade school experience would be anticipated to perform correctly. There is little question, however, that among brain-intact subjects the tasks would be performed with greater alacrity by those with greater educational experience. It would appear from these results that such individuals are less likely to lose their arithmetic skills after brain damage than are individuals whose education was less and whose initial arithmetic experience may have been narrow.

Remaining Factors

No principal axes factor beyond the sixth accounts for more than 1 percent of common factor variance, and all may be considered residual factors.

DISCUSSION

Results of this study clearly demonstrate the existence of several dimensions which underlie test performance of aphasic patients, and thus argue against the hypothesis that language disturbance after brain damage may be viewed as a unitary, general disorder. It follows from the findings that a single test score is not a sufficient indicant of degree of aphasic disorder. Performance of aphasic patients may differ in kind as well as in extent. As a consequence, useful information is provided by separate scores representing the possible transmission channels which mediate language acts, and a separate "comprehension" score also will be of value. The correlations among these scores will be far less than unity in the population of aphasic patients from which the 168 cases of the present study were selected.

The results are in sharp contrast to those presented by Schuell and Jenkins (7), and critical assessment of the results of those investigators thus is appropriate. The Schuell and Jenkins conclusions appear to result from two major sources: (a) a highly restricted selection of tests upon which the primary analysis is based, and (b) an inappropriate method of analysis used to test for "the existence of a single hierarchy of language functions."

Schuell and Jenkins analyzed performance of 100 aphasic patients on 29 tests, seven of which involved visual presentation of stimuli, 22 of which depended upon aural stimulation. For the major analysis, 18 of these tests were selected; the criterion for selection was high correlation of a test with the remainder of the battery. Remaining among the 18 were only three tests which required visual presentation, 15 of which required aural stimuli. The criterion for selecting among the 29 tests (already designed to emphasize certain functions, for example, matching to aural stimulation) clearly served to further increase the homogeneity of the test materials. The functions required on the 18 tests do not adequately represent the various transmission functions (11 of the 18 tests require a matching response to aural stimulation, and no more than two tests require use of any of the transmission channels defined by Factors A through D of the present study). Thus the selection of tests predisposed towards finding a single, general aphasia factor.

Whether such a single factor would emerge from the 18 tests remains unclear. No analysis was performed which yields an appropriate test of this. As Carroll[4] has demonstrated, the Guttman scale analysis which was employed by Schuell and Jenkins is inappropriate for an investigation of the dimensionality of a psychological domain. A high "coefficient of reproducibility" may be obtained from factorially complex tests, even when multiple factors are represented.

While test selection and methodological choice are sufficient reasons to question the generality of the Schuell and Jenkins findings, other difficulties remain to be briefly noted. (a) Of the 100 patients, 17 failed essentially all items presented them. The failure to reject these patients beforehand serves artificially to accentuate the relations among the tests. (b) Difficulty of tests was rarely moderate for those

[4]J. B. Carroll, A Note on Reproducibility and Dimensionality, unpublished manuscript, 1958.

selected for the major analysis. The distributions of scores suggest that some items were too easy, others were too difficult to enable sharp discrimination among patients or among distinct components of language tasks. (c) A score of *one* was assigned if a test was performed without error, otherwise (if one or more errors occurred) *zero* was assigned. The failure to discriminate degree of error may further serve to camouflage distinctions among language functions.

SUMMARY

Six factors were found sufficiently prominent to warrant interpretation when intercorrelations among 37 variables on an aphasic sample were subjected to varimax factor solution. Of these six factors, four appear to represent input-output transmission functions: Factor A, visual to oral transmission; Factor B, aural to oral transmission; Factor C, visual to graphic transmission; Factor D, aural to graphic transmission; Factor E, in contrast, transcends stimulus modality. It is defined by variables which require the matching, from one symbol system to another, of symbols with equivalent meaning. Factor E is interpreted as representing ability to comprehend language symbols. Factor F appears to represent ability to perform simple arithmetic operations, a function strongly affected by the educational attainment of the patient.

It should be emphasized that essentially the same factors appeared from several alternative factor solutions. The solution presented here is entirely analytic, and involved no subjective judgments of the investigators other than those required in interpreting and deriving conclusions from the final results.

The finding of relatively distinct interpretable factors of aphasic test performance strongly suggests that variables corresponding to the factors should be given explicit attention when testing for aphasia. Without adopting this strategy, two patients might receive the same score on a composite test for entirely different reasons. Only by distinguishing performance on each of the abilities reflected by the factors can one learn relative strengths and weaknesses in language performance of aphasic patients, information vital to useful diagnosis and treatment.

Acknowledgments. The authors are extremely grateful to Dr. Henry F. Kaiser, University of Illinois, for supervising computational aspects of varimax solutions on the IBM 701, University of California at Berkeley, and on the Illiac, University of Illinois, as well as to Dr. John B. Carroll, Harvard University, for supervising computational aspects of the oblimin solution on the IBM 704, Massachusetts Institute of Technology. The oblimax solution and a hierarchical solution on the 37 variables were performed by Mr. John Horn, University of Illinois. (Harman, *4*, provides excellent discussion of the alternative factor methods.)

The authors are indebted to the Oak Ridge Institute for Nuclear Studies, and to Mr. C. T. Fike, ORACLE Applications Program, University Relations Division, for supervision of coding and computations of the principal axes factor solution.

REFERENCES

1. Bock, R. D., Methods and applications of optimal scaling. Univ. North Carolina, *Psychometric Lab. Rep.*, No. 25, 1960.
2. Carroll, J. B., A factor analysis of verbal abilities. *Psychometrika*, **6,** 1941, 279–308.
3. Fisher, R. A., *Statistical Methods for Research Workers*, (10th ed.) Edinburgh: Oliver and Boyd, 1946.
4. Harman, H. H., *Modern Factor Analysis.* Chicago: Univ. Chicago Press, 1960.
5. Head, H., *Aphasia and Kindred Disorders of Speech.* New York: Macmillan, 1926.
6. Kaiser, H. F., The varimax criterion for analytic rotation in factor analysis. *Psychometrika*, **23,** 1958, 187–200.
7. Schuell, Hildred, and Jenkins, J. J., The nature of

language deficit in aphasia. *Psychol. Rev.*, **66,** 1959, 45–67.
8. Wepman, J. M., and Jones, L. V., *The Language Modalities Test for Aphasia.* Chicago: Univ. Chicago, Ind. Rel. Ctr, 1961.
9. Wiesenburg, T., and McBride, K., *Aphasia: A Clinical and Psychological Study.* New York: Commonwealth Fund, 1935.

28

Comment on "Dimensions of Language Performance in Aphasia"

HILDRED M. SCHUELL
JAMES J. JENKINS

HILDRED M. SCHUELL, Ph.D., (deceased) was director of the aphasia section of the neurology service of the Minneapolis Veterans Administration Hospital, and was with the department of neurology of the Graduate School of Medicine, University of Minnesota.
JAMES J. JENKINS, Ph.D., is with the department of psychology of the University of Minnesota.

We welcome the opportunity to comment on the study by Jones and Wepman concerning dimensions of language performance in aphasia. Jones and Wepman[1] conclude that their findings are "in sharp contrast" to those previously reported by us (*3*). It appears to us that they have misinterpreted our findings. We, therefore, should like to clarify our hypothesis and to suggest that the two studies, theirs and ours, complement each other to provide a comprehensive description of aphasic performance.

We concluded our data did not support classical descriptions of aphasia which are based on a sensory and motor dichotomy, or isolation of "pure" defects, each as alexia, agraphia, and acalculia. Our study pointed out that such logical categories were not empirically determined, and demonstrated that analysis of data, obtained from performance of a large sample of aphasic subjects on a substantial battery of tests, was compatible with the hypothesis of a single dimension of deficit crossing all language modalities. We welcome the data-oriented approach of Jones and Wepman, and are gratified that their extensive research, utilizing a different test battery, an even larger aphasic population, and a different statistical tool, similarly rejects historical a priori classifications. We trust the ghosts of classical analyses will be laid for all time. The congruence of the two studies in this respect is extremely convincing.

The Jones-Wepman discussion, however, has introduced a new issue: a general factor of language deficit versus multiple factors. It is implied that we support a general factor of deficit and determination of a single quantitative subject-score, while Jones and Wepman recognize more dimensions and argue for multiple scores and more detailed analysis. This is reminiscent of the older controversy concerning the structure of intelligence, with advocates of a "general" factor on one side, and advocates of "group" factors on the other. With the fine acuity of hindsight, it is now possible to see that both sides were "right." Virtually all factor analysts now recognize group factors, and almost all analysts expect to find some level of a general, or second-order, factor in analysis of a broad range of intellectual activities. Both factorially-pure test batteries and factorially-complex general tests have been found useful, depending on the purpose of the psychometrics. General tests are normally used successfully for populations with a wide range of intellectual abilities. We predict that something of the same sort will be found

From *Journal of Speech and Hearing Research* 4:295–99, 1961.
[1] See Reading 27: "Dimensions of Language Performance in Aphasia," Lyle V. Jones and Joseph M. Wepman.

true in the current apparent disagreement, and, with this in mind, propose to examine some of the differences between the two studies, in an effort to examine the sources of disagreement and to clarify our position concerning language deficit in aphasia.

TEST BATTERIES

An important difference between the two studies is certainly, as Jones and Wepman suggest, differences between the test batteries from which the data were obtained. The Wepman battery was constructed to sample selected stimulus-response relationships at a uniform level of difficulty: it was considered that items should be passed by half and failed by half the subjects. Such a battery should be most sensitive to covariations of different kinds of tests, but, on the other hand, places limitations on the kinds of tests used, the population studied, or both, in order to maintain a specified difficulty level.

The Minnesota Test, on the other hand, was a research battery, constructed and revised over a period of years, to study the break-down of language processes in aphasia as comprehensively as possible, and to examine changes which occurred with recovery or regression. In general, items were retained which appeared to discriminate between aphasic and nonaphasic populations, between segments of aphasic populations, and between performances of subjects at various stages of recovery.

Significant differences between the batteries resulted from these points of view. In the Minnesota battery, when two tests appeared redundant (i.e., measured the same function, were of the same difficulty level, and, in the main, passed and failed the same patients), one of the two was dropped to make room for new material. An example of this was two language tests: one, free word association, and the other, simple sentence completion. It seems obvious now that the same processes were sampled in both tests, but once it was not so apparent. The free word association test was dropped and the sentence completion test retained because instructions were easier for aphasic subjects to follow, and administration time was shorter for the latter than for the former. Elimination of redundant tests tends to minimize group factors. On the other hand, in order to sample break-downs of performance at higher levels, the Minnesota battery includes serial responses (counting to 20, giving days of the week, months of the year) in the absence of specific cues, and includes tests requiring formulation of oral and written responses without specific cues (answering simple questions, giving autobiographical information, defining low-frequency words, expressing ideas, explaining similarities, writing sentences to use given words, and writing a paragraph to describe a picture). There are no such tests in the Wepman battery, and while these tests are generally difficult for aphasic subjects, they are considered important in wide-range appraisal of language deficit. The lack of such tests in the Wepman battery tends to minimize general factors.

PATIENT POPULATIONS

Subjects in the Jones-Wepman test were selected by means of an interview and by use of a screening test which required performance at a given level. The Minnesota population was selected only to the extent that subjects who responded to no test items, subjects who missed no test items (and so were not diagnosed as aphasic), patients not neurologically stable, and patients with a medically-confirmed diagnosis of psychosis, were excluded. The wide range of the Minnesota battery permitted inclusion of subjects at both ends of the continuum who would presumably have been excluded by Wepman criteria.

METHOD OF ANALYSIS

Jones and Wepman consider the Guttman scale analysis technique an inappropriate test for a general factor. This is not the place for defense of the Guttman technique, nor are we qualified for such a task. The following explanation of the background of the study and choice of method is pertinent, however.

In work with severely impaired aphasic patients, who are without functional speech, reading, or writing, certain regularities were observed during recovery. With a given set of materials, auditory recognition (pointing to object named by clinician) usually preceded repetition; next the word could be elicited by a well-established association or a question; this, in turn, tended to precede naming. Not until considerable basic vacabulary was available was it possible for patients to express longer or more complex ideas. It was further observed that gains tended to cross modalities at all levels. It was to test the validity of these clinical observations, that is, to ascertain if any such hierarchical order could be demonstrated, that scaling of tests was undertaken.

Previous analyses of obtained findings for successive samples of patients, tested on various forms of the Minnesota Test, had shown that characteristic distributions of errors were not normal curves but rather were U-shaped or J-shaped. Tests at one end of the continuum tended to be passed by most patients, tests at the opposite end failed, while intermediate tests tended to separate patients into two readily discriminable groups (passing or failing) of varying proportions. This seemed to indicate that most tests were sets of homogeneous items cutting through a continuum (or continua) of deficit at a particular level. Phi coefficients and Guttman scaling were preferred to usual product-moment correlation techniques because the latter are based on the assumption of a normal distribution, a criterion these data did not meet.

To criticize the Guttman technique on the grounds that a scalable hierarchy may not be a general factor is, of course, admissible. Concerning this point, we commented as follows (*3*):

The question of factorial purity of the dimension discussed here may well be raised. It is conceivable that the dimension may be factorially complex when viewed in the context of many other tests. At the present time the authors are of the opinion that this question can only be decided by further empirical studies. The work of Gage on opinion poll data (1947) indicates that at least under some circumstances the Guttman technique may isolate the items in a scale which are identical with those items appearing on the major factor in a factor analysis. Whether this is true of the present findings is a point to be resolved by future work.

Rejection of the Guttman technique on the basis of Carroll's hypothetical demonstration (Interim Conference, Symposium on Aphasia, Social Science Research Council, Boston, 1958) is to beg the question and ignore the nature of the hypothetical tests used in the Carroll demonstration. The difficulty levels Carroll assumed *forced* these tests to scale, as is shown by computation of the minimal reproducibility of the assumed test data. Minimal reproducibility indices presented in our data (*3*) show that the latter data were not similarly "forced."

Selection of tests included in the analysis was largely determined by the hypothesis to be examined. Tests were selected from Forms 4, 5, and 6 of the Minnesota battery. Tests were necessarily eliminated from consideration which were not common to all three forms of the test. In addition, tests which were not primarily language tests (matching pictures, colors, forms; phonation, imitations of movements of speech musculatures; copying and drawing) and tests directly designed to measure other skills (numerical relations, arithmetic processes, spatial orientation, and body image) were excluded from the analysis as having little bearing on the language hypothesis.

Of the remaining tests, some were obviously more reliable than others; tests requiring true-false discriminations, for example, are more susceptible to guessing than certain other tests, but were retained to sample responses of subjects who could not speak or write. It is not necessary or desirable in a comprehensive battery that all tests should scale, nor do high phi coefficients assure scalability or reproducibility. Briefly, the tests sampled the various domains of language function which classical categories would have segregated, and yet, surprisingly, the tests were scalable.

The final list of "difficulties" cited critically by Jones and Wepman is a little puzzling.

Certainly inclusion of the homogeneous and uniformly low-scoring Group 1 subjects would contribute to reproducibility. This was explicitly stated, and analysis was repeated with patients in other diagnostic categories, both separately and combined, with Group 1 subjects omitted. These data were included in our article, and showed reproducibility of scaling essentially unchanged.

Distribution of test difficulty has already been commented on in relation to construction of the tests. Jones and Wepman suggest that a wide range of difficulty indicates the tests must have been discriminating poorly. This is completely untrue. In the first place, a wide range of difficulty is essential in this kind of scale, and, in the second place, no distribution discriminates more sharply than a U-shaped distribution at its optimal level.

The next question was why detailed scores were not utilized, instead of pass-fail treatment of subtests. It was considered that use of a range of possible scores for each test, to establish scalability of language deficit, was open to criticism on the grounds that manipulation of cutting scores would increase the likelihood that some cutting point might be found which by chance would permit the test to scale. Such scaling would of course be spurious to some unknown degree. It was therefore decided to test scalability by setting an arbitrary cutting point. That the tests scaled, not only under this handicap but also over all diagnostic categories included, is remarkable evidence for the pervasive nature of the dimension identified. As was pointed out later in our study, adjusting cutting points for tests previously found scalable on a pass-fail basis further improved reproducibility of the scale. This finding indicates that we did not fully exploit the sensitivity of the scores in our first analysis; however, we preferred to establish the reproducibility of the scale before manipulating scoring procedures.

One further point needs to be restated, lest readers conclude, from the hypothesis of a unitary language deficit crossing modalities, that we advocate measuring that deficit alone. The senior author has pioneered in the development of a classification system (*1*, *2*) which repeatedly has proved valuable in diagnosis, prognosis, and treatment of aphasic patients. This system is based on observed patterns of impairment which are differentiated by the presence or absence of specific motor or perceptual defects which are found in some subjects and not in others. In "An Investigation of the Nature of the Language Deficit in Aphasia," this was restated (*3*):

> The reader should not assume that the tests in any of the scales given above are sufficient to form a test battery for diagnosis and prognosis in aphasia. It obviously is important to have tests with very high visual requirements, to test for motor malfunctions and hearing loss, and to investigate the patients' functioning on tests of mixed abilities which are important in everyday life (for example, spatial orientation and mathematical competence).
>
> It should be re-emphasized here that the classification system described earlier in the paper is actually based on the presence or absence of specific motor or perceptual deficits which may or may not co-exist with the basic language deficit found in all the clinical groups described, and that while prognosis appears to be related to the over-all pattern of injury incurred in the brain, the recovery of language, when it occurs, progresses systematically and relatively independently of the superimposed defects, as indicated by the congruence of clinically observed recovery patterns and ordering of tests obtained on the clinical scale.

DISCUSSION

Turning from discussion of the previous study, we should like to comment on the Jones-Wepman study itself. We find support for our hypothesis in their analysis. The "sizable correlations among factors," which lead to difficulties of interpretation in their study, are, we consider, a reflection of general language reduction across modalities. That reading (Factor A) is somewhat different from repetition (Factor B) supports the reasonable view that the tasks are differentially affected by visual deficits, and that duration or continued availability of the stimulus plays a role in determining the probability of the correct response for patients who can utilize such stimuli.

In a study currently in press (*4*), we have reported research on a test involving pointing to pictures of objects named. The test was first presented with auditory stimuli alone and repeated with combined auditory and visual stimuli. The presentations correlated highly (+.80), with the second task proving easier, as expected. Departures from perfect agreement in ordering of subjects were in the main attributable to the fact that subjects in Groups 3 and 5, who showed cerebral involvement of visual processes, did not benefit as much as other subjects from added visual cues.

We are pleased that "copying" (Factor C), and "arithmetic" (Factor F) fall out as relatively independent of the language function; this is in agreement with our rationale for excluding such tests from an inquiry into general language deficit. We regard "writing to dictation," the prominent tasks on Factor D, as a complex of visual and visuomotor skills and auditory recall; hence we should have expected these tests to load on language factors as they do.

We cannot yet say whether the Jones and Wepman "comprehension of language symbols" (Factor E) is most closely allied with the general language deficit which we see in aphasia. It seems probable that it is, judging from the nature of many of the tests found scalable in our study, but the heavy reliance of this factor on picture matching as a response modality raises some questions.

We do not expect residual differences of opinion to be resolved by this discussion. What is obviously required is further searching, critical work. There is now in process a factor analysis of data obtained from the 73 tests on Form 6 of the Minnesota battery administered to 157 aphasic subjects. We trust this will help us integrate our findings more closely with those of Jones and Wepman and enable us to move another step forward in the precise description of aphasia.

Finally, to avoid misunderstanding, we should like to recapitulate the conclusions stated in our earlier study. We believe that classical divisions of aphasia into sensory and motor dichotomies and isolated pure defects are in error; we consider current evidence compatible with the hypothesis of an underlying general language deficit crossing modalities. We do not believe either identification or assessment of this general language deficit constitutes adequate information about any aphasic patient. We strongly advocate a comprehensive battery of tests, over a wide range of difficulty levels, to evaluate perceptual and motor disabilities and the effects of these deficits on various language performances; we consider this information essential for diagnosis, prognosis, and treatment of aphasia.

We realistically expect that, over a large sample of aphasic patients, many dimensions of impairment resulting from brain damage are identifiable, and need to be studied, in addition to the common or general dimension of language deficit. We further expect that, at a given level of language deficit, language tests may be arranged in subgroups which show systematic regularities in aphasic performance in various modalities as well as systematic differences in the performance of various segments of aphasic populations. We do not believe this is in conflict with the notion of a general dimension of language deficit present in aphasia.

We trust finally that this will be a rich and exciting field of further inquiry.

REFERENCES

1. Schuell, Hildred, Diagnosis and prognosis in aphasia. *Arch. Neurol. Psychiat.*, **74,** 1955, 308–315.
2. ——, A short examination for aphasia. *Neurology*, **7,** 1957, 625–634.
3. ——, and Jenkins, J. J., The nature of language deficit in aphasia. *Psychol. Rev.*, **66,** 1959, 45–67.
4. ——, ——, Reduction of vocabulary in aphasia. *Brain*, **84,** 1961, 243–261.

29

The Token Test: A Sensitive Test to Detect Receptive Disturbances in Aphasia

ENNIO DE RENZI
LUIGI A. VIGNOLO

ENNIO DE RENZI, M.S., and LUIGI A. VIGNOLO, M.D., are with the Clinica delle Malattie Nervose e Mentali of the Università di Milano, Italy.

A routine clinical examination of a patient with aphasia sometimes fails to reveal the slightest receptive disorders: this happens most often either in very mild sensory aphasics or in aphasics whose disturbances seem limited to a frank expressive syndrome. In such case the examiner is compelled to challenge the language comprehension of the patient with subtler tests: in so doing, however, he almost always finds himself giving tasks which involve other intellectual functions than language alone. Consequently, if the subject fails, it is hard to decide how far his errors are due to a difficulty in "decoding" the semantic structure of the message and to what extent they are simply due to a lack of the capacity of grasping its intellectual implications. A typical illustration of this ambiguity in tests of verbal comprehension is given by Head's (1926) Hand-Eye-Ear Test, which was designed expressly to get aphasics into trouble and yet turned out to be quite difficult also for a certain number of normal individuals (Goldstein, 1950), and even for some subjects of the highest intellectual level (Weisenburg and McBride, 1935). Our own experience confirms the difficulty such tasks present for organic brain patients, even including those who are free from defects in the language area.

From *Brain* 85:665–78, 1962. Reprinted by permission of the Editor of *Brain*.

Another widely used test is Pierre Marie's Paper Test, which consists in a series of commands connected by no logical link, to be performed in their correct order by the patient: "Here are three papers, a big one, a middle-sized one, and a little one. Take the biggest and rumple it up and throw it on the ground. Give me the middle-sized one. Put the smallest one in your pocket." This test deserves the popularity which it enjoys, for two reasons—one practical and one theoretical—which will repay further attention and should be borne in mind in designing any set of tests of receptive processes in aphasics. The practical reason, at first sight trivial, in fact reflects a principle of considerable importance: it is that Marie's test does not require any special equipment and can be applied at any moment at the patient's bedside. The theoretical reason is that its difficulty lies entirely on a linguistic level and not on an intellectual level. The orders are, in fact, extremely elementary from a conceptual standpoint and they would prove very easy even to a child. However, their comprehension is made hard by the fact that they refer to objects—the three papers—of the same nature, which can be identified only through the quantitative relations that exist between them: "big," "middle-sized," "little." From the linguistic standpoint this means that the three objects are not denoted by three clear-cut and simple semantic entities, as they would be if a separate concrete noun applied to each, but, on the contrary, by words representing a much subtler distinction, namely different degrees of the attribute "size." From this point of view the alternative test proposed by Pierre Marie himself is not as good: "Stand up, knock three times on the window with your fingers, come back in front of the table, turn once around the chair and sit down." It is clear that here the operations which the subject is required to perform involve simpler discriminations among more tangible features of the environment and, consequently, simpler and more definite linguistic denotations. This task, moreover, shows very clearly the weak point shared by both of Marie's tests, that is, the need for the patient to remember accurately a complex sequence of commands, in order to perform the tasks correctly. As a result, carelessness and confusion in the performance may sometimes be due to a defect of fixation rather than to misunderstanding, especially if aged patients are being tested.

Another test to reveal slight receptive defects is the one proposed by Thomas and Charles Roux (quoted by Ballet and Laignel-Lavastine, 1911). It consists in pronouncing before the patient a certain number of syllables, one of which forms part of the name of an object which is meanwhile shown to him. The syllable may be the first, the last, or an intermediate syllable of the given name. The patient has to recognize which syllable is the one. Such a test is undoubtedly subtle, but it requires great attention and a skill in analyzing the syllabic structure of words, i.e. in spelling words, which is not necessarily within the reach of all subjects.

Passing over various other kinds of examination—for example, Kleist's test (Kleist, 1922–1934), not very different from that of Thomas and Roux—we cannot escape mentioning the important work of Weisenburg and McBride (1935), who have systematized a conspicuous number of tests for aphasics, some of which are suited to the examination of slight receptive disorders. The book of the American authors undoubtedly constitutes a mine of information for anyone who seeks suggestions and advice as to the examination of aphasics, although there is perhaps the risk of becoming confused among such a wealth of tests and of not knowing which are the most useful. Moreover, the most penetrating tests suggested by Weisenburg and McBride were derived from intelligence tests and their solution must therefore imply to some extent the overcoming of difficulties which are not merely verbal, but also conceptual. Language Intelligence tests such as the Opposite Test, the Part-Whole, the Analogies, the Absurdities, and so on, are quite typical in this sense. It seems clear, for example, that if we lack any other evidence (as may be the case in subclinical aphasia) we shall be in doubt how to interpret a failure to identify the absurdity included in a statement such as this: "When there is a collision, the last car of the train is usually damaged most, so the guard thinks it would be best if the last car were always taken off before the train starts." Now, this is exactly the sort of test we may be tempted to employ in cases of subclinical aphasia; yet the chances are that, in this event, we shall end up by adding more and more perplexities to our initial problems.

Finally, if it is to be clinically useful in revealing slight receptive disorders, a test must have certain qualities that can be briefly listed under the following headings:

(1) The test should require only a reasonably short time.

(2) It should require neither special apparatus nor specific printed material, for often neither will be available when needed.

(3) It should be made up of orders so short as to be easily memorized by any normal adult, regardless of his age.

(4) It should include the least possible difficulty on an intellectual level, so that any individual may be able to perform the tasks correctly, independently—within reasonable limits—of his I.Q.

(5) It should contain, on the contrary, considerable difficulties on a linguistic level.

At this point, we must define more accurately what we mean by the phrase "difficulties on a linguistic level." It must first of all be realized that we do not refer to the use of unusual words and syntactic forms, since the comprehension of these depends mainly upon previous experience and the ability of the subject to profit by it; hence an intellectual or "culture" factor is involved. The difficulty must lie, on the contrary, in the lack of redundancy of the message transmitted to the patient and in the necessity, which this entails, of grasping its significance from the semantic value of every single word he hears. Lack of redundancy to this extent rarely occurs in everyday conversation, where the comprehension of speech is aided by a whole series of factors—some linguistic and some extra-linguistic—which contribute towards orienting the expectancy set of the hearer in a given direction, so that he merely needs to understand some elements of the question in order to respond with an adequate answer. These contributory clues to the understanding of speech could be classified as follows:

(1) Clues coming from the *situation* in which the patient finds himself and from the relation that traditionally binds him to the person he communicates with. If such a person is a physician, the patient will expect to be asked certain particular questions—questions, that is, that are usually asked during a medical examination. As Ombrédane (1951) rightly points out, comprehension of a command such as "Put out your tongue" is made easier by the fact that this is a usual request when it comes from a doctor. No wonder, therefore, that it may be understood perfectly well by severe aphasics, who are unable to grasp the meaning of other equally simple but not so obvious orders.

(2) Clues given by the *nature of the objects* with which the patient is invited to perform. Such clues exist when the order represents the most usual way of dealing with the object. If I put a pencil before a patient, the operations I can require him to perform are quite narrowly limited: I can tell him to write, to draw, to take the pencil, to hand it to somebody; but he can virtually ignore the possibility that I shall tell him to eat it, to light it or to tie a knot in it, requests which would rightly be more expected if he had before him, respectively, an apple, a cigarette or a piece of string.

It should be noted also that the comprehension of orders concerning an object lying in front of the patient is made easier by the very fact that such an object *is there*. In this connexion we might recall a test suggested by Luria (1959), in which the examiner invites the patient to pick up various objects one by one from a selection of objects he has before him, and from time to time gives the trick-command to take up an object which is not there.

(3) Clues given by the *verbal context*. Words in proposition are not uttered at random, but each of them calls for other words, according to rules determined by linguistic laws and by the nature of things. When the hearer has grasped some elements of a proposition, he can often fill in the blanks with some confidence, by referring to the words that come before and after those he has failed to understand. As Miller (1956) points out, "if one perceives enough of speech, to discover the fundamental set-up of the phrase, the number of words that can be replaced (in the perceptive blank) is much reduced; therefore, the possibility arises of making an exact guess. For example, in the statement "he threw . . . out of the window," we can immediately reject all nouns which connote objects that one cannot throw. Then, we can give our preferences to objects which people use to throw, such as balls, stones, bombs and so on. So we come to a very limited number of possibilities."

Moreover, when we talk, we use many words, circumlocutions and turns of phrase which are not strictly necessary to the communication of our thought and which serve mainly to embellish its expression, to add emphasis or superfluous precision, to make it clearer or more interesting to the hearer, and which are therefore redundant as far as the essential of our communication is concerned. Consider, for instance, one of the items of a test for aphasia currently used in our clinic (De Renzi, 1960). The patient is asked the following question: "Could you tell me the name of the animal the farmer milks every day in the stable?" It is obvious that this sentence—uttered, as it is, with a questioning note—could be cut down to "the animal the farmer milks in the stable." Probably even the fragment "animal farmer milks" would suffice for the understanding of the entire question. In Marie's test, quoted above: "Stand up, knock three times on the window with your fingers, come back in front of the table, turn once around the chair and sit down," the fragments "stand up" and "come back in front of the table" are, strictly speaking, redundant, because both actions are already implied by the orders that come next.

The foregoing considerations suggest a way in which to enhance the sensitivity of a test for inapparent receptive disorders. At the level of the relation between examiner and patient no facilitation problem arises, provided that the typical requests of a medical examination are avoided. At the level of the characteristics of the material with which we will examine the patient, we can choose between two alternative courses. We can, for example, modify the operations for which the objects are habitually used, going as far as to switch the habitual use of an object with that of another. If a pencil and a toothbrush are on the table, we may ask the subject to draw a square with the toothbrush and to brush his teeth with the pencil. Alternatively, we can choose objects that are poorly differentiated, both in reality and in language, such as pieces of paper of various shapes, going on the principle that the concept, and therefore the verbal expression, "piece of paper" is far less specific than "toothbrush."

Finally, at the third level—that of verbal context—every effort must be made to give commands in a non-redundant form, that is to say, in such a way that the understanding of every single word of the sentence becomes indispensable to the right performance of the order. It must be made impossible for the hearer to deduce or to reconstruct any word he may miss by following the clues contained in the words which precede or follow it.

THE TOKEN TEST

We hope to make some contributions to the semeiology of receptive language functions by putting forward a test based on the above-mentioned principles. The material of the test consists of tokens like those used in card games. As far as shape is concerned, there are two types of token: circles and rectangles. As far as size is concerned, there are also two types: the large ones and the small ones. Finally, there are five types of token as far as color is concerned: red, blue, green, yellow and white. Summing up, we have four rows of five tokens each: large circles, small circles, large rectangles and small rectangles; and in each row we have a red, a blue, a green, a yellow and a white token (Figure 29-1). The peculiar characteristic of the test material is that, when all the 20 tokens are present, it is not enough to use a single word in order to identify a particular token, but, on the contrary, at least three specific words are required, namely a noun and two adjectives. Thus, we will have to say, for example: "the large red rectangle," "the small red circle," and so on. If, however, large tokens only are used, two specific words—a noun and a color adjective—will suffice to identify a particular token, for we can then say merely: "the white circle," "the green rectangle," and so on. None of the specific qualifying words is redundant, that is to say, each of them must be decoded correctly in order to choose the right token. Moreover, if

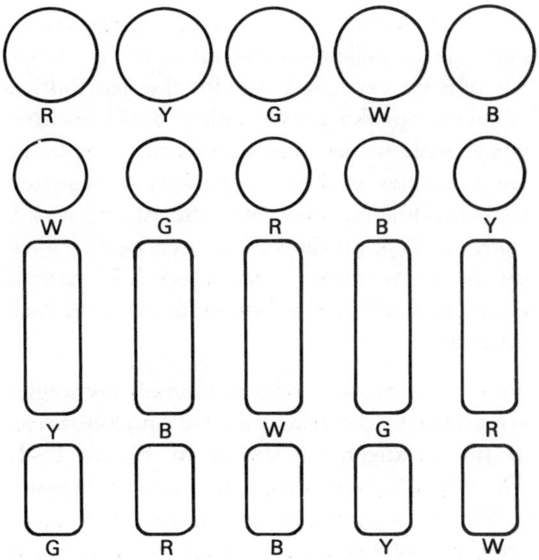

Fig. 29-1. R = red, B = blue, G = green, Y = yellow, W = white. Colours are distributed entirely at random.

only two out of the three elements of the connotation are understood, they do not give any clue concerning the third element: when I am told that I must take the large rectangle I still have no clue whatsoever as to which of the large rectangles—the red, the blue, the green, etc.—the order is about. Finally, the fact that the material is constituted by tokens and not, for example, by cigarettes or pencils is quite important. Tokens, like pieces of paper, are objects that can be denoted by an abstract noun, such as "circle" and "rectangle." We will come back to this point later, when we will come to discuss the results of the test.

The test is built up of five parts, progressively more and more difficult. In the first four parts, commands are expressed in an elementary grammatical and syntactic form: verb, object. In the fifth part we have tried to make the test more difficult by introducing grammatical particles or other more complex syntactic structures, the exact understanding of which is always necessary to a correct performance. Before starting one must make sure that the patient has no agnosic disturbances as far as form and color recognition is concerned and understands the meaning of the words "circle" and "rectangle" and of the five colors to be eventually called forth.

First part. Large rectangles and large circles only are arranged on the table in two rows. There is no particular rule for the distribution of colors. Speaking with a clear and measured voice, without any special prosodic emphasis, the examiner invites the patient to take ten different tokens, one after the other, saying simply: "Pick up the yellow rectangle," "Pick up the white circle," and so on. The patient must put back each token in its place on each occasion.

Second part. Small circles and small rectangles are added to the tokens already on the table, in the arrangement shown in Figure 29-1. Three specific words are now necessary in order to identify a particular token. Ten commands are given, of the type: "Pick up the small white rectangle," "Pick up the large blue circle," and so on.

Third part. Large tokens only are placed before the subject, as in the first part: here, however, the patient is invited to take two of them, for example: "Take the red circle and the green rectangle." Ten commands are given, connoting 20 different tokens.

Fourth part. All tokens are on the table again, as in the second part, and the patient is asked to take two of them every time: "Take the white large circle and the small green rectangle." Ten performances are required.

Fifth part. Large rectangles are put in the first row before the patient and large circles are put in the second row. There is no particular rule for the distribution of colors, except that the yellow rectangle must be near the green one, so as to allow item 7 to be applied. Orders are as follows:

(1) Put the red circle on the green rectangle.

(2) Put the white rectangle behind the yellow circle.

(3) Touch the blue circle with the red rectangle.

(4) Touch—with the blue circle—the red rectangle.

(5) Touch the blue circle and the red rectangle.

(6) Pick up the blue circle or the red rectangle.

(7) Put the green rectangle away from the yellow rectangle.

(8) Put the white circle before the blue rectangle.

(9) If there is a black circle, pick up the red rectangle.

N.B. There is no black circle.

(10) Pick up the rectangles, except the yellow one.

(11) When I touch the green circle, you take the white rectangle.

N.B. Wait a few seconds before touching the green circle.

(12) Put the green rectangle beside the red circle.

(13) Touch the rectangles, slowly, and the circles, quickly.

(14) Put the red circle between the yellow

rectangle and the green rectangle.

(15) Except for the green one, touch the circles.

(16) Pick up the red circle—no!—the white rectangle.

(17) Instead of the white rectangle, take the yellow circle.

(18) Together with the yellow circle, take the blue circle.

(19) After picking up the green rectangle, touch the white circle.

(20) Put the blue circle under the white rectangle.

(21) Before touching the yellow circle, pick up the red rectangle.

As one can see, this last part is quite different from the others. In the former four parts, in fact, orders comprised only a verb (always the same) and an object, so that the attention of the patient was allowed to concentrate entirely on the task of identifying the latter element of the order. On the contrary, most of the statements of the fifth part include a new grammatical element, i.e. a preposition, a conjunction or an adverb. These are small enough additions to the message, as far as its length is concerned, but they suffice to give the message a much greater linguistic subtlety and to change radically the meaning of the action that the patient is required to perform. Now it is not enough to understand the isolated meaning of the new particle, but it is also necessary to grasp its contextual meaning, i.e. to determine to which other element of the sentence it refers. In some cases it is essential to pay attention to the position that such a grammatical element occupies within the sentence, since a small displacement is sufficient to reverse the meaning of the command. This is illustrated by the two following items: "Touch the blue circle with the red rectangle" and "Touch—with the blue circle—the red rectangle."

A particular emphasis has been put on prepositions denoting spatial relations between objects, for these are quite difficult for aphasics to understand, as Ombrédane has shown by his Cat and Chair Test. The same prepositions are usually understood by patients with spatial agnosia, with except for the terms "right" and "left," which have not been included in our test for this reason. A special remark should be made about the prepositions "before" and "behind." A normal subject dealing with the tokens arranged in the forementioned order on the table may interpret "before" as connoting either a position "nearer to" himself or a position "farther from" himself. This possibility should be remembered during the examination, and it is advisable that the examiner wait until both items 2 and 8 are performed before scoring them.

A small group of 4 statements—items 9, 12, 20, 22—include a subordinate clause, that modifies, limits or suspends the command expressed in the main clause. Here the subject, in order to understand well, must keep in mind both principal and subordinate information until the message is over, so as to be able to put them in their adequate reciprocal relation and treat the command as a whole. Consider, for example, item 9: "If there is a black circle, pick up the red rectangle." The meaning of the main clause "Pick up the red rectangle" is completely altered by the condition introduced by the subordinate clause "If there is a black circle," for, as there is no black circle, the meaning of the order turns out to be: "Do *not* take the red rectangle."

Summing up, here we have a number of messages, sufficiently elementary from a conceptual standpoint, short and easy to memorize (the longest of them contains 19 syllables against the 48 syllables of Pierre Marie's test), which, however, make two kinds of demand upon the comprehension of the patient: one arises out of the difficulty of identifying a particular token specified by three independent features and the other from that of grasping the semantic complications introduced by the "small instruments of language."[1]

[1] It should be noted that the test has been originally designed for and applied to Italian patients. The orders presented here are the same, translated into English as accurately as possible: therefore, they should be considered merely as a demonstration of the degree of difficulty of the different items. It would be convenient, perhaps, to substitute or modify some of them, so as to make them convey, in English, differences of meaning comparable to those involved in the original Italian text.

RESULTS

All aphasics who, at a normal clinical examination of aphasia, already show clear disturbances in the understanding of speech have serious difficulty in the performance of the Token Test. The test, however, is not made for them, but rather for those aphasic patients in whom receptive disorders seem very slight or altogether lacking during normal conversation: they are mild sensory aphasics, or motor aphasics with a defect apparently confined to the expressive side.

Among this latter type of patients we have selected 13 "pure" motor aphasics—at least 5 of which could be classified as cases of "anarthrie" as defined by the French authors—and 6 sensory aphasics at a stage of very good regression of the symptoms: none of them showed any difficulty of understanding during a normal conversation. Each of these patients had been examined also with a complete test for aphasia used in our clinic (De Renzi, 1960), and most of them had no receptive difficulty throughout all the 54 items of that battery. Thus, their language comprehension appeared to be unimpaired despite an investigation far more thorough than a routine clinical examination of aphasia.

In each of these cases, the Token Test has revealed clear disturbances in the understanding of oral messages. As would be expected, the mildest aphasics perform the first part quite well, and often even the second and third part—although some errors may appear quite unexpectedly here and there—but in the fourth and fifth part mistakes become very frequent. We will deal later more broadly on the nature of such mistakes. Here it pays to insist on the extreme sensitivity of the test, an example of which is the following case of presenile cerebral atrophy, which, we think, deserves the qualification of latent aphasia, at least in the sense that, on the clinical level, none of the neurologists who had previously examined him had suspected the presence of language disturbances. The patient was a 60-year-old mechanical engineer, who had been suffering for six months from a conspicuous reduction of his working capacities and from memory defects. The neurological and general medical examination showed no evidence of disease. The psychological examination, on the contrary, revealed a certain mental deterioration, with lowered associative power, poor capacity for original judgment, amnesia for recent facts, disturbances in calculation and apathy with some tendency towards depression. At the Wechsler test he had an I.Q. = 92, with, however, an M.D. = 66 percent; at the vocabulary subtest he obtained a high score: 13. At the Weigl test he succeeded in classifying only according to color. The pneumoencephalography showed a conspicuous dilation of both lateral ventricles, especially of their temporal horns, without displacement. The cerebrospinal fluid was normal. The patient seemed to understand everything he was told and expressed himself correctly from a linguistic standpoint. Reading and writing were good. At the Token Test, he started making a great number of mistakes in the second and third part, and ended up with gross and frequent errors in the fourth and fifth part. Such mistakes were not due to a fixation memory defect, because the patient repeated the order to himself correctly aloud and yet performed it wrongly, thereby showing that he had grossly misunderstood its meaning. We tried to check the presence of aphasia with further examinations: among the Weisenburg and McBride battery of tests, the patient did well in the Sentence Completion, both Oral and Printed—except for one slight perseveration. Opposites were easily identified. Oral Analogies and Oral Absurdities gave him considerable trouble. He had a very hard time in building up sentences with three given words (from Terman's Test), and he often failed altogether. The best evidence of aphasia was provided, however, by his poor performance in Ombrédane's tests, that is the Cat and Chair Test and Caran D'Ache's cartoons.

In this, as in the other cases where the test has been applied, one could object that mistakes depend more on a general intellectual defect than on true aphasia. From a theoretical standpoint, such an hypothesis seems rather improbable, since, as we have already said, the orders employed are conceptually very simple and do not involve any unusual or odd linguistic form. On experimental grounds, moreover, we have observed that the test is performed quite well even by non-aphasic subjects with intellectual deterioration, provided that their mental condition leaves them a certain capacity for concentration. Finally, at least three of the patients with anarthrie who have shown poor comprehension in this test, performed well in non-linguistic tests.

It might be interesting to try to analyze qualitatively the types of mistake most frequently encountered. One could discover, for example, whether certain linguistic elements appear to be recognized worse than others by aphasics. This kind of analysis is quite simple so far as parts one to four are concerned. In order to make classification easier, it will be convenient to represent by capital letters the various parts of the message and to underline the letter corresponding to the part which has been misunderstood. For example, the statement "Take the small white circle" can be outlined thus: V (verb)—A' (size adjective)—A" (color adjective)—N (noun). If the patient takes the small white rectangle instead of the small white circle, we will write: V—A'—A"—N, underlining the N. The verb is always identical and therefore it may be overlooked.

It should be noted that if the subject were to choose entirely at random he would have a 50 percent chance of guessing the right noun and the right size adjective—because only circles and rectangles, and large and small tokens are there—but he would have only a 20 percent chance of guessing the right color adjective, since 5 colors occur in the test. Even leaving aside this aspect of the problem, we must consider that nouns are presented sixty times during the first four parts of the test, while adjectives are presented ninety times. This means that we should expect the greatest number of errors to fall within adjectives in general, and color adjectives in particular. On the contrary, the total count of errors reveals that—speaking in absolute figures—they affect nouns more often than adjectives. In fact, in parts one to four, the performances of all the patients submitted to the test show 152 errors due to misunderstanding of nouns vs. 104 errors due to misunderstanding of adjectives. One might jump to the conclusion that nouns represent a weaker category than adjectives, but we think that such an hypothesis, tempting as it may be, must be discarded, and that the unequal distribution of errors must be attributed to the peculiar type of noun employed in the test. In fact, by applying to the same patients another version of the test, where several objects, like pencils, thimbles, toothbrushes and so on, of five different colors, are used instead of tokens, we have noticed that the understanding of nouns was far less affected than that of adjectives.[2] The reason for this fact is that there is, we think, an important difference between a noun such as "pencil" and a noun such as "circle" or "rectangle," as employed in the test: the former is indissolubly bound to a very specific object, which it denotes in its whole, indivisible unity, while the latter identifies an attribute of the token—its form—like the adjective "red" identifies its color and "large" its size. In this sense, "circle" and "rectangle" are really adjectives pretending—so to speak—to be nouns. If such an equivalence between the nouns denoting form and the adjectives denoting color and size is true, then the purely formal distinction noun vs. adjective seems senseless here and should be substituted by the distinction between "verbal expressions denoting form," "verbal expressions denoting color" and "verbal expressions denoting size." The results of the test reveal that verbal expressions denoting form are understood worse than the others. A tentative explanation for this fact could be that shape is possibly a more abstract concept than color or size, geometrical conceptions—and their linguistic equivalents—being learned later than size and color-discrimination in childhood.

In the fifth part of the test, as we have said above, other grammatical elements—preposi-

[2] Incidentally, we must say that the test, thus modified, is definitely less sensitive.

tions, conjunctions, adverbs—have been introduced; and it would be interesting to know whether aphasics find it more difficult to grasp the meaning of such elements than that of the "nouns" and adjectives which appear in the same commands. It must be pointed out however, that the test, in its present form, has not been designed specifically to answer this question. Furthermore, it has not been applied to a sufficiently large number of cases to afford us any firm conclusion. What follows is, therefore, no more than a hint for future research.

In every item of part five, expressions denoting form, color and size ("nouns" and adjectives) on the one side, and grammatical particles on the other are unequally represented. In fact, there are two "nouns," two adjectives and one particle in almost every item. Consequently, if mistakes were determined by mere chance, they should fall on the group of the expressions denoting form, color and size more often than they would on the particles, according to a four-to-one ratio. On the contrary, we find 120 errors on particles vs. 101 errors on "nouns" and adjectives: this means that wrong performances are due a little more often to misunderstanding of the particle. Some of them appear particularly weak: they are spacial prepositions such as "on," "under," "before," "behind," the disjunctive particle "or," the contradictory "—no!—," the conditional "if." However, while it seems sensible to us to believe that grammatical particles are impaired in aphasia more easily than expressions denoting form, color and size—because they have a merely connecting function, because they have no semantic independence, and finally because they have been acquired late in the development of language—we do not feel able to determine which of them are more impaired and which are less impaired on the basis of the present results. It is hard to see how prepositions, conjunctions and adverbs could be evaluated in terms of their abstract difficulty. It seems, rather, that they must be considered within a given context, and it must be admitted that contexts are not the same throughout the Token Test: commands differ from each other in respects both structural and conceptual. For example, an order such as "Instead of the white rectangle, take the yellow circle" is probably easier than the conceptually similar "Take the red circle—no!—the white rectangle," because in the first case the adverb is put at the beginning of the order and therefore raises the expectation of a correcting message to come, whereas in the second case it shows up after the order has been given, cancels it quite unexpectedly and compels the hearer to switch his attention towards a completely different task. On the other hand, the order "If there is a black circle, take the red rectangle" contains a little conceptual trick: for the first time during the test, a command refers to an object which is not on the table, and coming, as it does, after so many positive orders, it ends up inviting the patient to do nothing at all. This overall experimental context, rather than the use of a conditional clause, may be responsible for the difficulty of the item.

At all events, it seems to us that the Token Test, if analyzed from this viewpoint, might provide some interesting data for that linguistic approach to aphasia which many contemporary authors consider to be promising and from which Wepman *et al.* (1956) and Goodglass and Hunt (1958) have already obtained fruitful results.

The Token Test, however, must be considered above all as a practical clinical tool, endowed of great sensitivity and contaminated as little as possible by intellectual difficulties.

Acknowledgment. The authors wish to thank Dr. Hugh Thomas for his helpful suggestions in reading the English text.

REFERENCES

Ballet, G., and Laignel Lavastine (1911) Aphasie. *In* "Bronardel and Gilbert." Nouveau traité de médecine Paris. Vol. **31,** (Semiologie Nerveuse). p. 55.

De Renzi, E. (1960) *Arch. Psicol. Neur. Psich.*, **21,** 17.

Goldstein, K. (1950) "Trastornos del Lenguaje" (Spanish Translation). Barcelona.

Goodglass, H., and Hunt, J. (1958) *Word*, **14,** 197.

Head, H. (1926) "Aphasia and Kindred Disorders of Speech." Cambridge.

Kleist, K. (1922–34) Kriegsverletzungen des Gehirns in ihrer Bedentung für die Hirnlokalisation und Hirnpathologie. *In*: "Handbuch der ärztlichen Erfahrungen im Weltkriege 1914/1918," edited by O. von Schjerning. Leipzig. Vol. **4,** p. 343.

Luria, A. R., and Yudovich, F. I. (1959) "Speech and the Development of Mental Processes in the Child." London.

Miller, G. A. (1956) "Langage et communication" (French Translation). Paris.

Ombrédane, A. (1951) "L'Aphasie et l'élaboration de la pensée explicite." Paris.

Weisenburg, T., and McBride, K. E. (1935) "Aphasia, a Clinical and Psychological Study." New York.

Wepman, J. M., Bock, R. D., Jones, L. V., and Van Pelt, D. (1956) *J. Speech Dis.*, **21,** 468.

30

A Measurement of Functional Communication in Aphasia

MARTHA L. TAYLOR

MARTHA L. TAYLOR (Sarno), M.A., is director of the speech pathology service of the Institute of Rehabilitation Medicine, New York University Medical Center, and is with the department of rehabilitation medicine of the New York University School of Medicine, aided by a grant from the Vocational Rehabilitation Administration, Department of Health, Education, and Welfare, Washington, D.C.

Since the central subject of this presentation is the measurement of verbal behavior in the patient with aphasia, perhaps it would be appropriate to begin by defining the term *aphasia*.

Some regard the disorder simply as an impairment of speech associated with brain damage whether congenital or acquired; others as a reflection of generalized diminution of intelligence, memory, and judgment with accompanying verbal dysfunction. Unfortunately, the term has been used to refer to infinite numbers and kinds of impairments without recognition that those actively engaged in studying aphasia use the term in a very restricted sense.

The term alone does not indicate the degree of impairment, the linguistic features which are impaired, a prognosis for recovery, or a method of treatment (*1*). *Aphasia* is as general a classification as demyelinating disease, central nervous system disease, or heart disease. In this presentation, *aphasia* shall refer only to an acquired impairment of verbal behavior caused by brain damage which impairs the linguistic features involved in encoding or decoding language. It is characterized by a reduction and/or dysfunction in vocabulary and/or syntax in oral-aural language use. The words *expressive* or *receptive* are used to qualify when the patient's aphasic difficulties tend to cluster in encoding (expressive) or decoding (receptive) language skills. The term excludes those communication disorders due to neuromuscular impairment of the speech musculature, dysfunction of the peripheral sense organs, mental deficiency, organic mental syndrome, or psychopathology. While deficiencies in writing, gesture, calculation and reading (paralanguage systems) often accompany aphasia, isolated losses in these skills without concurrent oral-aural dysfunction do not independently constitute an aphasic symptom (*2*). By restricting the definition in this way, one can immediately sort out the large number of brain-damaged patients, many of whom have left hemiplegia, who exhibit defects of mentation and perception so often confused with aphasic symptoms. This definition is in keeping with the linguist's view that language is primarily an oral-aural event (*3*).

The relevant information carried by the term *aphasia* is limited. The term tells us that the patient's verbal impairment (1) is one of input and output, (the transmission and reception of spoken language) rather than the mechanics of sound production; (2) it is

From *Archives of Physical Medicine and Rehabilitation* 46:101–07, 1965.

acquired; (3) its etiology is brain damage; (4) the individual's control over the vocabulary and/or syntax of the language is reduced; and (5) disorders of perception, mentation, or social behavior may or may not accompany the verbal impairment (*2*).

The research tools used to analyze and describe verbal behavior are derived from the sciences of linguistics and behavioral psychology. The linguist's science is based entirely on the analysis of language as it is said. He does not prescribe what should be said or attempt to establish a "correctness" of language usage. The linguistic scientist is dedicated to the rigorous description of language from observations made of speakers using the language in natural context. His raw data consist of samples of natural speech which require his analysis over long periods of time. Since speech is an event in time which is momentary, verbal samples are documented on tape recordings which are studied until precise observations can be described (*4*). The linguistic features of the sample are described and classified according to the phoneme, morpheme, and syntax systems of the language.

Knowledge of natural speech utterances has increased rapidly in recent years through psycholinguistic research. An impressive series of papers in the measurement of natural speech in normals has appeared in psycholinguistic literature (*5*). The linguist has long recognized that spoken language produced in natural situations is markedly different in its linguistic characteristics from that language which is elicited through questioning or testing. This disparity of language usage obtains as much to brain-damaged persons as to normal speakers. I will differentiate these two kinds of language, hereinafter, as:

Clinical performance: Verbal performance under test or other task oriented conditions. A measure is clinical when the conditions or stimuli used to obtain the sample are not representative of natural language usage.

Functional performance: Verbal performance under conditions which simulate the natural use of language. A measure is functional when the conditions or stimuli used are informal and they sample language usage without task presentation. The fact that functional and clinical language operate differently should not be misunderstood to mean that natural language is random. It obeys its own set of rules. In fact the pathology of language, far from being a random disturbance, obeys a set of rules. The disorders of language display their own peculiar order and require a systematic linguistic comparison with our normal verbal code (*6*).

When we direct the aphasic patient to write his name, he is performing a clinical act since a task has been presented to him. On the other hand, when he signs his name on a check at the bank, he is performing functionally. Here the language behavior is natural to the situation.

Generally when aphasic patients are evaluated, they are clinically tested by a so-called aphasia test. Many of these examinations have appeared on the scene since World War II. They are designed to discover and describe whatever language residuals a patient may have in each modality and are in many ways similar to standard verbal intelligence tests. The results of these tests, however, tell us nothing about what the patient does in his attempts to circumvent his verbal impairment (*7*). The test results can often be extremely misleading. A patient who may not respond to any of the formal test comprehension items may respond appropriately when casually asked a question (*7*). In addition, clinical language tests do not take into account that many aphasic patients (1) use gestured signals to communicate; (2) may respond accurately though inconsistently; (3) may have intact vocabulary and syntax in oral language except that they require greater time to respond orally; and (4) that the more specific a task, the more difficult it is for an aphasic to perform (*7*). These tests are usually insensitive to the minimal impairments of some patients whereas severely impaired patients cannot perform any item. Less than 20 percent of the patients in our program can pass the screening section of the most widely used aphasia test.

Standard practice, then, in the language evaluation of aphasia measures clinical performance rather than the unforced, voluntary,

FUNCTIONAL COMMUNICATION PROFILE

EVAL (Blue)	RE-EVAL (Red)	RE-EVAL (Red)	RE-EVAL (Red)
Date ________	Date ________	Date ________	Date ________
M ___ ___% (.)	M ___ ___% (.)	M ___ ___% (.)	M ___ ___% (.)
S ___ ___% (.)	S ___ ___% (.)	S ___ ___% (.)	S ___ ___% (.)
U ___ ___% (.)	U ___ ___% (.)	U ___ ___% (.)	U ___ ___% (.)
R ___ ___% (.)	R ___ ___% (.)	R ___ ___% (.)	R ___ ___% (.)
O ___ ___% (.)	O ___ ___% (.)	O ___ ___% (.)	O ___ ___% (.)
Overall ___ ___.___%	Overall ___ ___.___%	Overall ___ ___.___%	Overall ___ ___.___%

	NORMAL	GOOD	FAIR	POOR	O	
MOVEMENT						Ability to imitate oral movement
						Attempt to communicate
						Ability to indicate "yes" and "no"
						Indicating floor to elevator operator
						Use of gestures
SPEAKING						Saying greetings
						Saying own name
						Saying nouns
						Saying verbs
						Saying noun-verb combinations
						Saying phrases (non-automatic)
						Giving directions
						Speaking on the telephone
						Saying short complete sentences (non-automatic).
						Saying long sentences (non-automatic)
UNDERSTANDING						Awareness of gross environmental sounds
						Awareness of emotional voice tone
						Understanding of own name
						Awareness of speech
						Recognition of family names
						Recognition of names of familiar objects
						Understanding action verbs
						Understanding gestured directions
						Understanding verbal directions
						Understanding simple conversation with one person
						Understanding television
						Understanding conversation with more than two people
						Understanding movies
						Understanding complicated verbal directions
						Understanding rapid complex conversation
READING						Reading single words
						Reading rehabilitation program card
						Reading street signs
						Reading newspaper headlines
						Reading letters
						Reading newspaper articles
						Reading magazines
						Reading books
OTHER						Writing name
						Time orientation
						Copying ability
						Writing from dictation
						Handling money
						Using writing in lieu of speech
						Calculating ability

ESTIMATED TOTAL SPEAKING VOCABULARY: 0 1-50 50-100 100-500 500-1000 over 1000

DEPARTMENT OF PHYSICAL MEDICINE AND REHABILITATION, NEW YORK UNIVERSITY MEDICAL CENTER,
Speech Therapy Service, New York, New York

Fig. 30-1. Form sheet for functional communication profile

and habitual utterances which characterize spoken language (*6*). These clinical tests clash with the most elementary requirements of linguistic methodology (*6*). They are more often a measure of potential than actual language use.

The notion of measuring "function" in language is relatively new in the practice of speech pathology. It is not new to the physiatrist who appreciates that the results of range of motion and muscle testing and the patient's actual use of these residuals for the activities of daily living do not necessarily correlate. Many patients with adequate muscle function do not use these residuals for feeding, ambulation, and dressing activities. Others with great limitation of movement seem to defy clinical measures by achieving self-sufficiency in spite of their limitations. This is analogous to the disparity between clinical and functional performance in the aphasic patient.

Ideally, a functional measure of language usage in everyday life could be obtained if one could follow a patient in the course of his everyday life and make firsthand observations of his verbal behavior. Since this is not possible, the examiner must rely on estimates made on the basis of informal interaction with the patient, and information obtained from the patient's family.

In an effort to measure functional language performance in aphasic patients, a scale called the Functional Communication Profile (Figure 30–1) was designed about eight years ago. The Profile attempts to measure the second dimension of language performance not otherwise accounted for in clinical testing. It consists of a list of 50 integrated communication behaviors considered common language functions of everyday life. Such items as handling money, indicating floor to elevator operator, and saying greetings are included. It was designed to encompass as much functional information as possible in the simplest, most visible manner. The form makes no reference to symptomatology or diagnostic labels and, therefore, avoids the confusion and ambiguity which exists in the nomenclature. Ratings of each behavior are made on a continuum along an eight-point scale on the basis of informal interaction with the patient in a conversational situation. In this natural context the examiner rates what functional use the patient makes of his residual language.

On the scale, the rating of *normal* represents the patient's estimated premorbid level of language proficiency estimated according to known social, educational, and personality factors in his history. The *normal* estimated for the patient establishes a frame of reference against which to measure change. This baseline is vital to functional measurement. "Each person's manner of using language is something individual and personal, which he never altogether shares with the rest of the community; it is something which reflects his total personality, in the same way as his handwriting or bodily mannerisms." (*8*) An item is rated as *normal* when it is estimated that the patient performs the act precisely as he did premorbidly. This means that the ratings take into account (1) speed, (2) accuracy, (3) consistency, (4) voluntary control without benefit of external cues, and (5) compensatory function for the behavior (i.e., a patient who cannot say the numbers of the floor to the elevator operator but who can point to the appropriate floor number would be rated as functionally adequate although not normal).

Each rating is assigned a weighted score which is converted into percentages in each of the five modalities: movement, speaking, understanding, reading and a miscellaneous category which includes writing and calculation. There is also provision made for an overall score which is a reflection of the sum of all of the scores. It can be used as a single measure of an individual's communication effectiveness in everyday life. An overall score of 62 percent, for example, indicates that the patient's overall verbal effectiveness is rated at 62 percent of his premorbid level.

Ratings are indicated by filling in the blocks along the eight-point continuum for each item in blue at the time of evaluation. At monthly intervals, changes in language function are indicated in red. The color coded profile permits the clinician to follow the course of recovery across time in visible form. With this

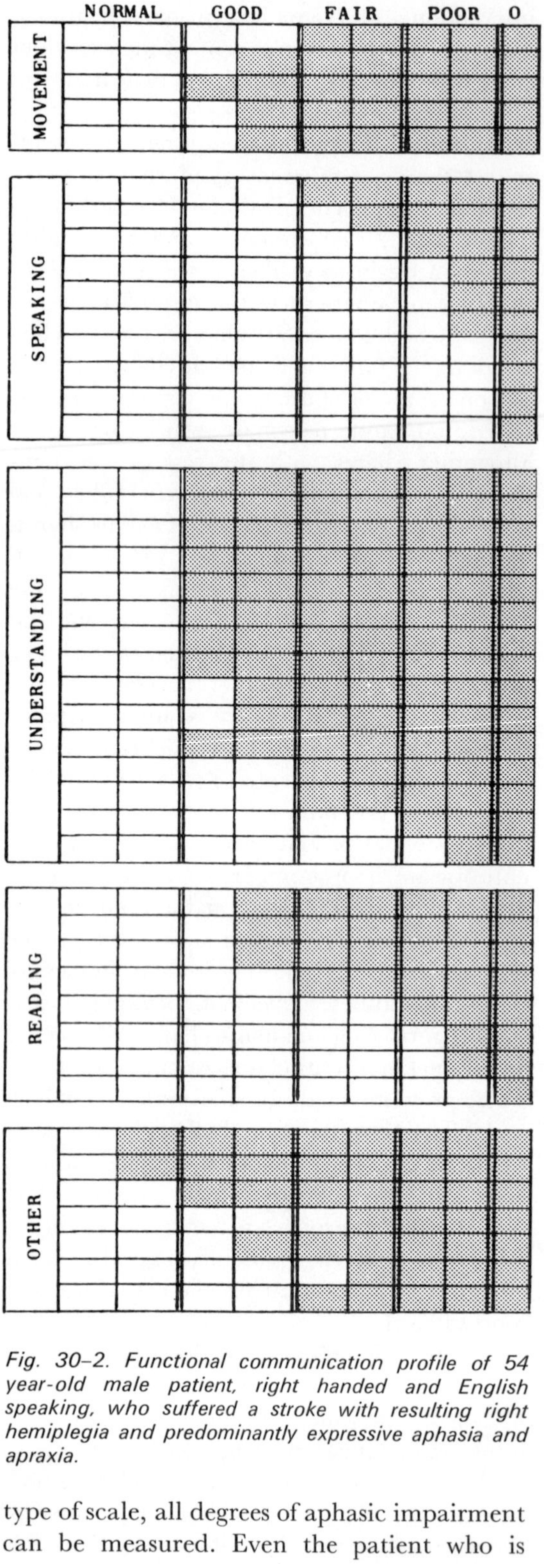

Fig. 30–2. Functional communication profile of 54 year-old male patient, right handed and English speaking, who suffered a stroke with resulting right hemiplegia and predominantly expressive aphasia and apraxia.

type of scale, all degrees of aphasic impairment can be measured. Even the patient who is nonverbal but who points for his needs will achieve a percentage score. Likewise, since the Profile is based on function, it differentiates patients with impaired affect from those who retain at least some awareness of a verbal world.

We have routinely used the Functional Profile on our aphasic population for eight years. Recently computer-based studies have been in progress to examine the tool's information-giving potential more systematically (*9*).[1] The pilot study findings and the work in progress offer promising indications of the reliability and predictive value of the Profile.

The original form grouped the items according to expressive or receptive function. The first step in the pilot study was to submit the items to factor analysis. The analysis established that the items clustered into five major groups rather than expressive and receptive groups. The factors were movement, speaking, understanding, reading, and other, a miscellaneous category including writing, calculation and telling time. The Profile was then redesigned in accord with the factor analysis and the items were redistributed into the five present groups. No changes were made in the items themselves. The overall score, instead of the separate expressive and receptive scores, was derived from the fact that in the mathematical analyses, a single factor accounted for 95 percent of the variability in the data. The revised form allows us to obtain single factor percentages as well as a single overall score.

The Profile visually differentiates among types of verbal impairment. Figure 30-2 shows the Profile of a patient who displays an understanding score of 75 percent of normal and approximately 50 percent of normal in every other factor except speaking, where function is greatly impaired. Results of our preliminary studies immediately suggest that this distribu-

[1] Mathematical analyses were conducted by Dr. Louis J. Gerstmann, Research Scientist, Data Processing and Computation Laboratory, New York University, College of Engineering. This work was supported in part by National Institutes of Health under Grant No. FR-00002, and in part by the Vocational Rehabilitation Administration under Grant RT-1.

tion of impairment signals the presence of verbal apraxia. Note the very high loading in understanding and the great imbalance in function between speaking and all of the other factors. In spite of the fact that this patient exhibits losses of vocabulary and syntax, his greatest deterrent to normal communication rests with his impairment in controlling the motor movements for speech.

Often patients with damage to the non-dominant hemisphere display verbal impairment which is not aphasic in nature. These disorders are generally related to impaired memory, disorientation, and judgment. Figure 30-3 illustrates the verbal behavior of a left hemiplegic patient without aphasia. The lowered scores in all factors except the other category might mislead the observer to believe that the reduced function reflects an aphasic impairment. However, the significantly greater reduction of function in the other category is not consistent with aphasic Profiles. Since time orientation, copying, and writing are disproportionately lower than other factors, the distribution of impairment suggests signs of organic mental syndrome rather than aphasia.

In a pilot group of 52 subjects who had had a cerebrovascular accident, who were right handed and right hemiplegic, and native speakers of English, overall scores were plotted from the time of evaluation to the time of discharge. The results of these preliminary analyses give indications of the direction that our future study might take. Regression analysis on this group demonstrated that the single best predictor of recovery was the amount of time in treatment. Since the average length of treatment in the group was only a little over three months, there is strong indication that language retraining, at least in our program, should continue for a longer period of time. Those patients who were admitted with higher understanding scores and lower speaking scores made greater functional recovery than the reverse. These preliminary studies give us reason to believe that the identification of patterns of function on the Profile may supply us with a set of prognostic tools. The studies in progress also show that there is no clear-cut dichotomy between expressive and receptive language functions but that a common factor underlies the verbal behavior of aphasic patients. We shall be anxious to see in our continued study whether

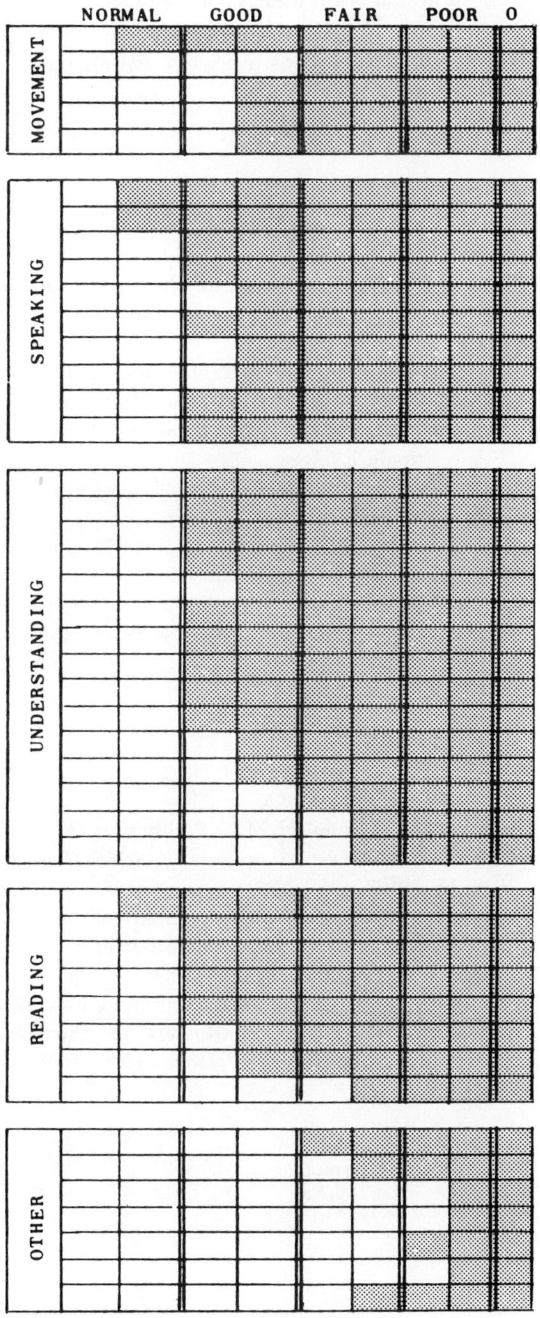

Fig. 30-3. Functional communication profile of patient who had a stroke with left hemiplegia but no aphasia.

the five subscores increase at different rates during treatment thereby refining an objective index for deciding who will benefit from language training.

We can begin to see that what might appear to be clinical judgments of aphasic verbal behavior are useful and quantifiable as research data. A subjective measure, when submitted to scientific method, appears to provide us with a reliable and objective research measure of language function. The revised Functional Communication Profile offers some strong support for certain linguistic principles and theoretic models of aphasic behavior presented in the research literature.

REFERENCES

1. Taylor, M. L., Linguistic Considerations of the Verbal Behavior of the Brain-Damaged Adult. *The Linguistic Reporter*, Vol. **6,** No. 3, (June) 1964.
2. ——, Evaluation and Rehabilitation of Brain-Damaged Patients With Verbal Impairment. Seminar, University of Tokyo, School of Medicine, Tokyo, Japan, 1964.
3. Hall, R. A., *Linguistics and Your Language.* New York, Doubleday, 1962, p. 36.
4. Sturtevant, E. H., An Introduction to Linguistic Science. New Haven, Conn., Yale University Press, 1947, p. 30.
5. Pollack, I., and Pickett, J. M., The Intelligibility of Excerpts from Conversation. *Language and Speech*, 1963, Vol. **6,** Part 3, pp. 165–171.
6. DeReuck, A. V. S., and O'Connor, M., Ciba Foundation Symposium, *Disorders of Language.* Boston, Little, Brown and Co., 1964.
7. Osgood, C. E., and Miron, M. S., Approaches to the Study of Aphasia. Urbana, Illinois, Univ. of Illinois Press, 1963.
8. Critchley, M., Articulatory Defects in Aphasia. *J. Laryng.* **66**:1–17 (Jan.) 1952.
9. Taylor, M. L., A Rating Scale for Aphasic Adults Based on a Functional Frame of Reference. ASHA, Vol. **5,** p. 777 (abstract).

ADDITIONAL SUGGESTED READINGS ON: TESTING

1. Brown, J. R., Schuell, H. M., A Preliminary Report of a Diagnostic Test for Aphasia. *J. Speech Hearing Dis.*, **15**:21–28, 1950.
2. Orgass, B., Poeck, K., Clinical Validation of a New Test for Aphasia: An Experimental Study on the Token Test. *Cortex*, **2**:222–243, 1966.
3. Piercy, M., The Effects of Cerebral Lesions on Intellectual Function: A Review of Current Research Trends. *Brit. J. Psychiat.*, **110**:310–352, 1964.
4. Sklar, M., Relation of Psychological and Language Test Scores and Autopsy Findings in Aphasia. *J. Speech Hearing Res.*, **6**:84–90, 1963.
5. Spiegel, D. K., Jones, L. V., et al., Test Responses as Predictors of Free-Speech Characteristics in Aphasic Patients. *J. Speech Hearing Res.*, **8**:349–362, 1965.

part III

RECOVERY AND REHABILITATION

Introduction

The subject of recovery and rehabilitation in aphasia is of great interest since many workers in the field are motivated by a desire to treat the aphasic patient and thousands have already received more or less effective speech therapy. Few valid conclusions on the efficacy of treatment are permissible today, however, because we know very little about the pathophysiology of aphasia and less about the recovery process. One must ask, therefore, how we know with reasonable certainty what we are treating, and, lacking an understanding of the natural elements of recovery, how can we assist the process?

Put another way, although the end product of damage to human communication faculties has been well described, one is unable to explain the observed losses in the absence of a thorough understanding of normal language processes. Contemplation of the process of recovery is equally difficult since one can argue persuasively that the involved brain cells are destroyed and the functions they served are now irretrievably lost. One can argue, on the other hand, for the pluripotentiality of brain tissue or for a concept of language organization not wholly dependent on anatomical factors.

One must seriously question whether or not the effort to *teach* the aphasic has any grounds for success. For, attempts to teach necessarily imply that there is a residual communication system in the aphasic's brain which can increase its capacity, as in the developing child. What is more likely is that the aphasic's communication centers have been damaged and can neither function spontaneously nor be trained to function again.

The reader will do well, therefore, to approach the subject of recovery and rehabilitation critically. It should be noted that views on the subject are multiple and many studies present only hypotheses.

Some problems that plague most studies to date are the lack of a careful description of the patient population according to type and severity, of objective measures of improvement, and of controls. These requirements may well be met in future studies.

Although there are a few early references to aphasia therapy before 1940, it was not until World War II that treatment attracted much attention. Some of the major studies supporting the effectiveness of speech therapy are included (Readings 33, 34, 35), but none meets the criteria suggested above. They were included because of their historical value and because each touches on one or more of the following questions: What is spontaneous recovery? What constitutes recovery from aphasia? What are the temporal factors in recovery? Does treatment influence recovery and, if so, what kind? Can aphasics learn? Vignolo's paper, for example, draws conclusions about the spontaneous evolution of recovery, about the importance of time elapsed from onset, and about the length of time treatment should be administered.

Since many readings deal with multiple aspects of the problem, it is difficult to categorize clearly and distinctly those selected. Articles primarily addressed to the process of recovery precede those concerned with rehabilitation.

The paper by Culton (Reading 31) deals exclusively with the problem of spontaneous recovery and is included for that reason.

In an approximate manner, a few of the papers are concerned with prognosis. Wepman (Reading 36) points up the importance to recovery of the patient's capacity to self-correct. Tikofsky and his group (Reading 37) relate electroencephalographic findings to improvement in patients receiving speech therapy, and Sands and others (Reading 38) suggest the prognostic importance of time and the age of the patient at onset in recovery from aphasia.

In two papers (Readings 39 and 40) their authors address themselves to exploration of the problem of the aphasic's ability to learn. These papers are included since they are among the few experimental studies extant on learning in aphasia.

A number of papers were chosen because they dealt with actual techniques of treating aphasics and the theoretical bases for treatment. Wepman is represented by two additional papers in this section. The first (Reading 32) is one of the earliest of its kind and describes his ideas concerning stimulation, facilitation, and motivation as a basis for treatment. The second (Reading 43) is, in a sense, a repudiation of most methods of treatment (including his own) and considers a psychotherapeutic approach as the most fruitful method of management. Reading 42, which sets forth a specific psychotherapeutic modus operandi, is included for this reason. Hildred Schuell's paper describing her method of treatment (Reading 41) is a contribution of one of the great clinicians in the field of aphasiology. The therapeutic system outlined in her paper has been the basis for much of the aphasia therapy used in this country.

A number of books and book chapters have discussed methods and rationales for treatment. Wepman (3) details the recovery and rehabilitation process in a series of 68 traumatic aphasics. Schuell (2) presents guidelines for management in her textbook and Eisenson (1) explains his views on aphasia rehabilitation in the Travis *Handbook of Speech Pathology*. So varied are the techniques and methods of treatment, an exhaustive review is impossible.

This collection ends with the first controlled study of the effects of speech therapy in a group of severe aphasics (Reading 44). The urgent need for studies of this type cannot be over-emphasized if we are to accumulate objective information on the nature of recovery in aphasia and the efficacy of treatment.

REFERENCES

1. Eisenson, J. Aphasia in Adults. In Travis, L. E. (ed.), *Handbook of Speech Pathology and Audiology*. New York, Appleton, 1971, pp. 1219–1252.
2. Schuell, H. M., Jenkins, J. J., et al. *Aphasia in Adults*. New York, Harper, 1964, pp. 315–386.
3. Wepman, J. M. *Recovery from Aphasia*. New York, Ronald, 1951.

31

Spontaneous Recovery from Aphasia

GERALD L. CULTON

GERALD L. CULTON, Ph.D., is with the department of speech pathology and audiology of the University of Akron, Ohio.

Most authors agree that the majority of dramatic changes in aphasia are confined to the immediate posttraumatic period (Granich, 1947; Nielson, 1957; Schuell, 1955, 1965). Therefore, the speech pathologist who initiates early remedial treatment may not know the degree to which the language retraining program affects the "recent" aphasic because the client may be experiencing spontaneous recovery of language function at the same time. Weisenburg and McBride (1935) recognized this dilemma some 30 years ago when they pointed out the need to compare spontaneously recovering aphasics with aphasics receiving language retraining.

Opinions differ regarding the importance of studies of spontaneous recovery from aphasia. Head (1926) believed that observation of patients with different types of aphasias would show that some types improve more rapidly than others. Eisenson (1949) and Wepman (1951) stressed the importance of the aphasic's age and psychological adjustment as factors influencing improvement in language function, as well as physiological improvement. The similarity between the temporary and permanent language symptoms of "recent" aphasics has caused others to avoid early evaluations and predictions. Schuell (1954) prefers not to attempt a prognosis until physiological factors have stabilized causing the language problem also to become more stable and predictable. Brain (1961) stated that because both permanent and transitory symptoms may be equally severe in the early stage of aphasia, it is impossible to distinguish between them.

There are also differences of opinion concerning the relationship between aphasia and intellectual function. The trend has been to accept the hypothesis that aphasics exhibit reduced intellectual function, but the reduction is generally considered no greater than the deficit exhibited by other brain-injured but not aphasic individuals (Anderson, 1951; Bauer and Becka, 1954; Boone, 1959; Weisenburg and McBride, 1935). Some investigators have found differences between the performances of aphasic and nonaphasic brain-injured subjects on intellectual tasks which do not involve language (Anderson, 1951; Bauer and Becka, 1954; Weisenburg and McBride, 1935); others have not found such differences (Boone, 1959; Shontz, 1957). Eisenson (1963) and Zangwill (1964) indicated that the intellectual losses in aphasics improve spontaneously. Although the relationship between language and intelligence is not clearly understood, there is some agreement that aphasics are hampered intellectually and that some spontaneous improvement of intellectual function occurs in aphasics.

This study attempted to isolate, measure, and analyze certain language abilities as they changed during the weeks immediately following the onset of aphasia, in the absence of

From *Journal of Speech and Hearing Research* 12:825–32, 1969.

specific language retraining. We also attempted to measure intellectual changes during the same time period.

METHOD

Subjects

Group I. These 11 subjects made up the group of primary interest since they had been aphasic less than 30 days. The subjects were obtained from hospitals in Denver, Colorado, where no clinical speech services were readily available. Since this investigation focused upon spontaneous recovery, we tried to locate persons who could not otherwise have received the attention of a speech clinician. It was felt that the testing program provided an evaluative service for these aphasics as well as a referral service for future speech retraining.

Nine of the 11 Group I subjects were aphasic as the result of CVAs. One case resulted from a left subdural hematoma and one from a gunshot wound of the left temporo-parietal region. The subjects were seven males and four females ranging in age from 18 to 78 years, with a mean age of 54.36 years. The length of time from the onset of aphasia to the initial test administration for these subjects varied from one to four weeks with a mean of two weeks. The subjects were, therefore, labeled as "recents."

Persons were not included as Group I subjects unless they met the following criteria:

1. On a short screening test, they must have been judged aphasic.
2. The aphasia must have resulted from CVA or head trauma, according to medical diagnosis.
3. The onset of aphasia must not have occurred more than 30 days prior to testing.
4. They must not have previously experienced aphasia.
5. They must have passed screening tests of hearing and vision.
6. They must not have had any formal language retraining prior to testing, nor were they allowed to receive such retraining during the testing period.

Group II. These 10 subjects had been aphasic for some time. All had become aphasic subsequent to CVAs and all had received language retraining. The subjects were nine males and one female ranging in age from 36 to 73 years, with a mean age of 57.5 years. The length of time since onset varied from 11 to 48 months with a mean of 27 months. Since the usual period of spontaneous recovery encompasses only the first three to six months after onset, all Group II subjects were considered as having stabilized physiologically and were, therefore, labeled as "stables."

Criteria for the inclusion of Group II subjects were essentially the same as for Group I except that differences in elapsed time since onset for Group II were longer (6 months vs. 30 days), and that it was necessary to withhold the "stables" from language retraining only during the testing period since their stability of function was the factor under observation.

Measures

Each subject was required to participate in four evaluation sessions at two-week intervals. The battery comprised eight different language tasks and an intelligence measure. The language tasks were constructed by the investigator, while J. C. Raven's *Standard Progressive Matrices Test* (1938) was selected as the performance intelligence measure.

Language tasks. Since the design of this investigation required several test administrations, it was necessary to test rapidly and efficiently, employing an alternate forms arrangement. This procedure was used to reduce subject boredom and lessen the effects of learning from repeated testing. Therefore, a short battery of tasks was developed (alternate forms) to which a pass-fail criterion of one point per correct response was applied. Each form (A and B) consisted of eight tasks, with each task having 10 potential correct responses. Thus, each administration of the language tasks resulted in eight separate task scores and a total score which compared the subject's performance with the perfect score of 80. This procedure allowed direct comparisons between each of the tasks over the four administrations on the basis of the number of correct responses. The eight language tasks created for this investigation were:

1. Auditory Decoding: Recognizing Pictured Objects by Name.
2. Auditory Decoding: Following Directions.
3. Visual Decoding: Matching Printed Word to Picture.
4. Visual Decoding: Reading Comprehension-Sentences.
5. Oral Encoding: Naming-Oral Response to Pictures.
6. Oral Encoding: Answering Simple Questions.
7. Graphic Encoding: Writing Letters and Numbers from Dictation.
8. Graphic Encoding: Writing Words from Dictation.

Intelligence measure. The most common objection to intelligence testing with aphasics is that the verbal emphasis of most tests hampers subjects with speech and language problems. Therefore, an intelligence test of the performance type which required little verbal communication between examiner and subject was needed. The *Mental Measurements Yearbook* favorably evaluated one such measure, the Raven Test, as useful for estimating the intelligence of those having communication disorders (Bortner, 1965). Zangwill (1964) reported successful use of the Raven Test with aphasic subjects indicating that it seemed little affected by the classical forms of aphasia.

Although the Raven Test was used in this study, the usual scoring procedure was altered somewhat. Instead of obtaining a percentile score according to the subject's age, we scored the total number of correctly completed designs. Differences between the total scores on the two test administrations constituted the point of comparison for the test-retest analysis.

Testing schedule

Language tasks. It was essential that the language testing of both groups (I and II) be identical since the test-retest reliability of the language tasks had not been previously determined and so that inter-group differences could be attributed to factors other than methodological variations in testing.

The eight language tasks were administered to each subject in both groups at two-week intervals until four administrations had been completed. All eight language tasks were given in the same order at each session. The alternate forms arrangement was used, with the first administration always employing Form A. Therefore, each subject in both groups received the same language task forms in the same order, with the same time interval between administrations.

Intelligence measure. As with the language tasks, the test administration schedules for the Raven Test were kept identical for Groups I and II so that intergroup differences in scores could be attributed to actual changes in the subjects' behavior. Each subject took the Raven Test twice, with a six-week interval, immediately following the first and last administrations of the language tasks.

RESULTS

The Spearman rank correlation method (Ferguson, 1966) was used to determine the reliability of the language tasks. Table 31-1 contains the results of that analysis. The Group II ("stables") test-retest reliability coefficient for Form A, which included administrations one and three, was 0.90, while Form B test-retest reliability, including administrations two and four, was 0.95, both significant (>0.01).

TABLE 31-1. RANK CORRELATION ANALYSIS OF TEST-RETEST RELIABILITY AND INTER-FORM RELIABILITY FOR GROUP II (N = 10)

Administration and Form	Group II
Test-Retest Reliability	
1A-3A	0.90
2B-4B	0.95
Inter-Form Reliability	
1A-4B	0.97
2B-3A	0.94
1A-2B	0.98

The analysis of interform (A and B) reliability with Group II subjects also provided significant results (>0.01) with correlation coefficients of 0.97 between administrations one and four (A^1—B^4), 0.94 between administrations two and three (B^2—A^3), and 0.98 between administrations one and two (A^1—B^2).

Recovery of language function

Figure 31-1 is a graphic representation of the mean scores for Groups I and II on all eight language tasks. The two graphs again clearly indicate that Group II subjects were highly stable throughout the testing period on all tasks. Group I subjects were quite changeable,

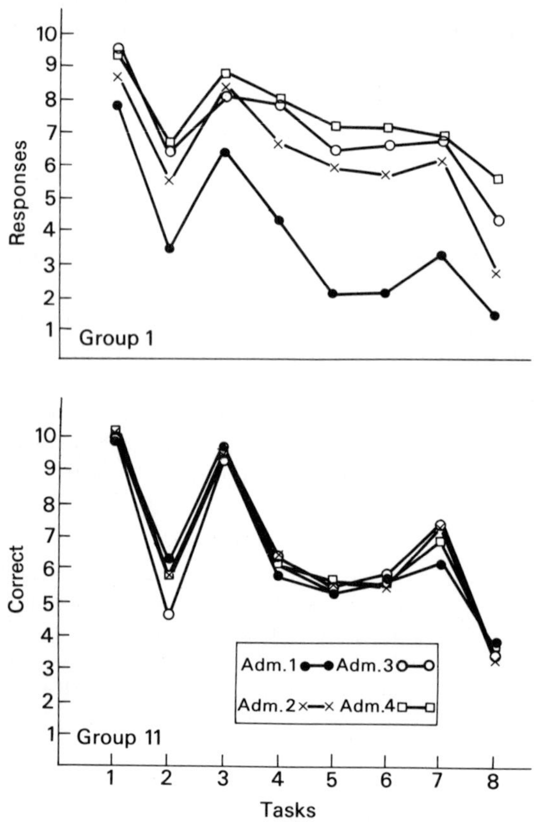

Fig. 31–1. Total mean scores on all eight language tasks and four administrations for groups I and II. Adm. 1 ●——● ; Adm. 2 ×——×; Adm. 3 ○——○ ; Adm. 4 □——□.

with an increase in mean scores on each task. Even though Group I subjects improved in mean scores, the configuration remained essentially the same over the four administrations, with Tasks 1 and 3 being easier than Task 2 (Figure 31-1). Tasks 4 through 7 remained in practically the same rank order while Tasks 5 and 8, on nearly all administrations, were the most difficult. Figure 31-1 also demonstrates a similar configuration of task performance for the stable, Group II subjects. A comparison of task difficulty indicates that both groups found Tasks 8 and 5 to be the most difficult (mean of means 8=3.52, 5=5.34) and Tasks 1 and 3 to be the easiest (mean of means 1=8.75, 3=7.86). Only minor variations existed in the order of difficulty for the four tasks of average difficulty (Tasks 2, 4, 6, and 7). The order from easy to difficult was Tasks 4, 7, 2, and 6 in Group I; and Tasks 7, 4, 6, and 2 in Group II.

The median chi-square test (Edwards, 1962) was employed to examine differences in the amount of recovery which occurred between the language task administrations (Table 31-2). The increase in correct responses between administrations one and four, which reflects the entire testing period, was significant ($\chi^2=6.545$). A significant increase was also noted between administrations one and two ($\chi^2=6.545$) reflecting rapid early improvement in language task performance. The overall chi-square ($\chi^2=6.18$) which encompassed all four administrations was not significant, as were those obtained between administrations two and three, and three and four (χ^2's$=$ 0.727).

Recovery of intellectual function

The results of initial and final intelligence test administrations are presented in Table 31-3. Again, Group I subjects showed a sizable mean improvement while Group II subjects showed little change. The mean change for Group I was statistically significant ($t=4.76$, $df=10$) while the change for Group II was not ($t=0.808$, $df=9$).

TABLE 31-2. MEDIAN CHI-SQUARE ANALYSIS OF THE FOUR ADMINISTRATIONS OF LANGUAGE TASKS WITH GROUP I SUBJECTS

Administrations	χ^2	*Median*	df	p
All Four 1, 2, 3, 4	6.180	50	3	NS
1 and 2	6.545	31	1	0.02
1 and 4		31		
2 and 3	0.727	55	1	NS
3 and 4		70		

TABLE 31-3. DIFFERENCES IN INTELLIGENCE TEST SCORES BETWEEN ADMINISTRATIONS 1 AND 2 FOR GROUPS I AND II

	Means		
Groups	*Initial Test*	*Final Test*	*Difference*
I	12.90	21.63	8.73
II	19.00	20.20	1.20

DISCUSSION

The results of this study confirm that there is a period of spontaneous recovery of language function in persons who have recently become aphasic. Persons who had been aphasic for some time did not experience improvement within the time dimensions of this study. The "recent" aphasics reflected spontaneous recovery by increases in the overall total scores of subjects, and by increases in mean scores on each of the eight different language tasks. These findings provide experimental support for the many clinical references in the literature to spontaneous recovery of language function in recent aphasics.

Rapid spontaneous recovery of language function was noted in the first month following the onset of aphasia. Although an increase in mean scores was noted, further significant improvement was not evident during the second month. This is somewhat incompatible with the predominant notion that significant spontaneous recovery of language function continues to occur three to six months after the onset of aphasia.

This study also supports the hypothesis that "recent" aphasics exhibit spontaneous recovery of intellectual function. The "stable" aphasics in this investigation did not change in intellectual function during the testing period. These findings are consistent with those of Berry and Eisenson (1956), showing that intelligence test scores of aphasics improve with time, and with Weisenburg and McBride (1935), that there are concomitant intellectual problems with aphasia which are reduced as the aphasia lessens in severity.

Acknowledgment. The original study was completed as a doctoral dissertation at the University of Denver under the direction of Daniel R. Boone. The author wishes to thank Darrel Teter, David Minear, and Roger Burgraph for their assistance in gathering subjects for the investigation.

REFERENCES

Anderson, A. L., The effect of laterality localization of focal brain lesions on the Wechsler-Bellevue subtests. *J. clin. Psychol.*, **7,** 149–153 (1951).

Bauer, R. W., and Becka, D. M., Intellect after cerebro-vascular accident. *J. nerv. ment. Dis.*, **120,** 379–384 (1954).

Berry, M. F., and Eisenson, J., *Speech Disorders.* New York: Appleton, Century, Crofts (1956).

Boone, D. R., Communication skills and intelligence in right and left hemiplegics. *J. Speech Hearing Dis.*, **24,** 241–248 (1959).

Bortner, M., Critique of Raven Test. In *Mental Measurements Yearbook*, 6th ed. Buros, O. K. (Ed.), N.J.: Gryphon, 764–765 (1965).

Brain, R., *Speech Disorders.* Washington: Butterworth (1961).

Edwards, A. L., *Statistical Methods for the Behavioral Sciences.* New York: Holt, Rinehart and Winston (1962).

Eisenson, J., Prognostic factors related to language rehabilitation in aphasic patients. *J. Speech Hearing Dis.*, **14,** 262–264 (1949).

——, Aphasia, Ch. 24 (I), *Voice and Speech Disorders: Medical Aspects.* Levin, N. M. (Ed.), Springfield, Ill.: Charles C. Thomas, 851–873 (1963).

Ferguson, G. A., *Statistical Analysis in Psychology and Education.* New York: McGraw-Hill (1966).

Granich, L., *Aphasia: A Guide to Retraining.* New York: Grune and Stratton (1947).

Head, H., *Aphasia and Kindred Disorders of Speech.* (I) New York: Macmillan (1926).

Nielsen, J. M., Motor aphasia with recovery: Report of a case with autopsy verification. *Bull. Los Angeles neurol. Soc.*, **22,** 148–149 (1957).

Raven, J. C., *Standard Progressive Matrices.* London: H. K. Lewis (1938).

Schuell, H., Clinical observations on aphasia. *Neurology*, **4,** 179–189 (1954).

——, Diagnosis and prognosis in aphasia. *A.M.A. Arch. Neurol. Psychiat.*, **74,** 308–315 (1955).

——, *Minnesota Test for Differential Diagnosis of Aphasia.* Minneapolis: Univ. Minnesota (1965).

Shontz, F. C., Evaluation of intelligence potential in hemiplegic individuals, *J. clin. Psychol.*, **13,** 267–269 (1957).

Weisenburg, T., and McBride, K., *Aphasia.* New York: The Commonwealth Fund (1935).

Wepman, J. M., *Recovery from Aphasia.* New York: Ronald (1951).

Zangwill, O. L., Intelligence of aphasia. In *Disorders of Language.* De Reuck, A.V.S., and O'Connor, M. (Eds.), Boston: Little, Brown (1964).

A Conceptual Model for the Processes Involved in Recovery from Aphasia

JOSEPH M. WEPMAN

JOSEPH M. WEPMAN, Ph.D., is with the department of psychology and is director of the Speech and Language Clinic of the University of Chicago.

The history of aphasia therapy for any large number of patients does not extend beyond the early nineteen-forties. With the influx of war-injured adults, many of them flown almost directly from the battlefields, it was necessary to develop treatment without reference to theory. Concomitantly, the increased tensions of life for civilian populations during the war years produced a growing number of cerebrovascular accidents due to hypertension. The therapy programs developed and utilized in army hospitals and in Veterans Administration installations became available for many patients in private environments. The consequences of this increasing amount of aphasia therapy has been twofold: (1) There has been a tremendous increase in the number of therapists and (2) therapy of all kinds has been applied with little or no knowledge of its effectiveness or its expectations. Aphasia therapy, therefore, has been opportunistic rather than planned and the results obtained have been neither uniformly good nor uniformly bad. Since expectancy or prognosis for recovery has not been evaluated, the known product of all of the activity in therapy has been in terms of the resolution of defects in individual patients.

The backlog of experience on individual patients now seems great enough that it should be possible to fix several useful points in the therapeutic process. With these in mind we should be able to view therapy more rigorously and begin to understand the answers to many of the questions that have been of concern for the past decade.

Three sources are available for the determination of an overall concept that might account for recovery from aphasia. First, the patient—his personality, his intellectual propensities, his behavior in therapy and in life—needs to be scrutinized. Second, the therapist—his role in the treatment process, as well as his training and background—needs to be studied. Third, the therapeutics that have been utilized by different therapists must be considered. By extracting what is known from each of these primary areas some fundamental considerations should be available to permit the construction of a working model that will permit a more scientific approach to the problem.

As yet we know very little that is factual concerning either the personality structure or the intellectual potential of the aphasic patient. Various researchers hold widely differing opinion in both areas. Some hold that brain damage produces a change in personality which tends to make all such patients very much alike (*3*). Others hold that only the overt manifestations of behavior change while the basic personality remains the same (*12*). Neither view has been substantiated, but both are now being studied. A similar condition

From *Journal of Speech and Hearing Disorders* 18:4-13, 1953.

exists in regard to the problem of intellectual ability following cortical insult. Research has been reported on brain-injured patients that indicates a particular kind of deterioration (*11*), or an inability to abstract (*3*). Such a list of separate intellectualizing factors can be extended almost indefinitely, yet no research has shown to this time any universal or holistic picture of the intellectual function after brain injury that is ultimately useful in planning therapy.

Still another area which should be ultimately productive of valuable data for the aphasia therapist is the manner in which the cortex functions. The recent Hixon Symposium (*8*) on cerebral mechanisms of the cortex reported on a vast amount of recent research in this area. Sperry, however, in his discussion of brain function (*10*) epitomized the level of direct value to be gained when he pointed out that "despite steady advancement in our knowledge of the brain, the intrinsic nature of mind and its relation to cerebral excitation remains as much an enigma today as it was a hundred years ago." Interest in neuropsychology at this level continues, however, and while direct factual material useful to the present planning of treatment is lacking, many theoretical concepts are forthcoming. As will be seen later these constructs may give extremely useful leads in the present context.

Probably the most important area of study for the present purpose is the clinical observations made during therapy itself. It is notable, for example, that patients showing all varieties of language disturbances seem to get some resolution of their problems, seemingly regardless of the particular approach used with them. Still other patients with a similar variety of symptoms do not seem to improve or do so only to a very limited degree. To illustrate this rather vital point it has been shown that the expressive language disorders are more amenable to therapy than are the receptive disorders (*12*, *1*). Yet, at the same time, some patients with comparatively mild expressive problems do not respond to therapy while other patients who have exhibited severe receptive disorders have responded extremely well. In fact it has been observed that there is little if any relation between the severity of brain damage and the degree of recovery.

The usual explanation for these noted discrepancies has been in terms of either the neurological deficit or the personality of the patient. Since both of these can only be represented as unknowns in our present state of knowledge they become convenient scapegoats for our failures. Neither seems adequate to the present writer. If the neurological deficit is the reason for the failure then there should logically be some definite relationship between either extent of damage and severity of the disorder or location and extent of damage in the cortex and the presenting symptom. Neither of these conditions have been seen to be valid in our observation of patients, excepting in a very gross way.

With regard to the unknown vector of the personality of the patient, it would seem that we would need to know much more about personality structure itself, before we could reasonably accept it as the major determinant of recovery. Too many psychologists hold such widely diverging opinions for any such generic term as "personality" to be meaningful in this regard. Patients have been seen whose general personality characteristics seem to be approximately the same and yet who differ almost completely in their recovery process. Not only do they differ markedly between themselves, but they differ noticeably from time to time in their individual patterns of recovery.

STIMULATION

It appears to this observer that the best defined parameter along which patients differ is in their ability to be stimulated. Whether this difference in "stimulatability" is a physiological factor, a psychological factor or a combination of both cannot be determined by observation. Perhaps this is the function that Head (*5*) called "vigilance" or that Halstead (*4*) has called the "p factor" or perhaps it is related to the psychological characteristic called "drive" or "need." Whatever it may be, it is observable in almost every patient. Some patients can be stimulated and others cannot. Some patients can be stimulated in certain areas of behavior, others in different areas, some in all areas, while still others in no area. Here, too, there seems to be little if any relation between the variables of severity of symptom, type of language disorder, length of time since trauma, beginning of therapy, age of the patient, etc. To this writer this appears to be the first needed signpost. To what degree can the patient be stimulated? In what area of language can he be stimulated? What kind of response is generated by different kinds of stimulation? These may be the most useful questions to be asked as a treatment program is planned.

Another observation bears upon the question of stimulation. It has been noted by the writer in visiting centers in different parts of the country that aphasia therapy is rarely the same thing in any two places. Some therapists follow a fairly rigid, educative approach. Drill, repetition of exercises, work books, daily lesson plans, etc., make up a bulk of the work being done. Others lean more heavily upon a more psychological approach, permitting the patient to select his area of language and guiding him through the difficult spots as they occur. There seem to be all varieties depending for the most part upon the training and background of the therapists rather than upon the needs of the patient. At different times the writer has used almost every kind of approach in his own clinical practice. What is important is that patients seem to get better or do not get better in approximately the same proportions, regardless of the approach used with them. This may mean that patients who fail to improve in one treatment center might be more likely to respond under some other therapeutic regime. Or, it may mean, and this is more likely true, that some of these patients could not be properly stimulated or were not so stimulated. For with the great variations of approach being used it seems most probably true that what is being done with the aphasic patient in each treatment center is a stimulation process rather than an educative one. Some therapists, in other words, are stimulating their patients by one technique, while others are using different techniques, but in the final analysis all therapists, regardless of their particular approach, are doing what might be called "stimulation therapy." If this is true the content of our therapy is of less importance than the manner in which it is conducted.

This factor has been of concern for some time; its implications are extremely important in the entire recovery process. The content of therapy has received possibly as much attention as any other single factor in the training of therapists. Many therapists are considered to be trained when they have in their possession a list of techniques and a knowledge of the material that has been found useful with patients. In fact, knowledge of this sort has at times become so primary that the needs of the patient, his personality and even his desires have been overlooked in order to instill in therapists particular approaches and specific content material. If it seems maximally useful to consider the patient and his ability to be stimulated, then therapists must be concerned with the patient and their ability to stimulate them rather than with techniques or content. A new orientation to therapy will be necessary and a different training for therapists will become vital.

One final factor bears on the point of stimulation as one of the important considerations necessary in planning aphasia therapy. A common observation during the recovery process is the tendency for patients to develop language forms quite unrelated to the therapy. Vocabularies are used which can only be considered as old recall patterns produced by cerebral function much in the manner in which they were produced prior to the trauma. The implication from this is quite clear. Therapy may have succeeded in stimulating the patient to efforts on particular language forms which when completed have permitted the patient to function in language generally rather than specifically. For example, one patient, a surgeon, exhibited a marked verbal apraxia and an extremely slow recovery of voluntary language. While still working on simple naming of common objects he one day demonstrated that words quite far removed from the vocabulary used in therapy, such as the names of technical surgical instruments, were used with facility.

Examples like this can be duplicated many times. The implication seems to be that the content of therapy served only to stimulate the patient to produce the integrations necessary for language, but did not convey specific new learning or new vocabulary to the patient.

FACILITATION

The second parameter of our conceptual chain relates to the state of the organism. Sometimes the patient seems ready to produce the integrations necessary for use in language, at other times he seems quite unready. He acts as though at times his cortex was able to symbolize, while at other times the integrations necessary could not be made. Whether, as Hebb (*6*) postulates it, we conceive of cortical function as a network of cells in which the individual is able to produce a connected pathway leading to a motor act, a final common pathway of response, or if we utilize Kohler's (*5*) concept of positive and negative electrical fields, or McCullough's (*5*) reverbating circuits, or Sperry's (*10*) concept of the "motor-end product," to note just a few of the existing theoretical frames of reference, there must at all times be a readiness of the individual organism. Aphasia therapy as we conceive it has as its role that of facilitating the organism as it prepares to function. It so stimulates the patient that when he is ready to produce language, he becomes able to do so. Facilitation, then, becomes a concept related to the physiological state, the ability to increase the flow of energy into the system which permits it to form new integrations for language, utilizing the nervous tissue present which seems incapable of spontaneous function.

Another way of stating this, physiologically, might be that aphasia therapy reduces the impedance against function by its stimulation effect. The impedance here might be thought of in terms of the destruction through trauma of the pathways which formed the previous integrations necessary for language response, which leave the patient with sufficient cortical tissue for response but insufficient intact pathways for the particular act he wishes to perform. Unless these new pathways be formed the impedance will be too great for successful integration.

In brain injured patients there are varying degrees of cortical insult. One patient may have sufficient cortex remaining for new pathways to be formed easily with almost any kind of stimulation. Other patients may have more serious disruptions and destructions of cortex which obviate all but a few pathways. Still others may have their most serious loss in particular areas which serve as the nucleus for auditory reception or for verbal expression and only in these areas will the patient have his greatest disability. Facilitation of cortical function through therapy then is seen as the change that must take place in the organism before the integrations for language can be formed. Perhaps what was said earlier about stimulatability can now be translated into "facilitatability" of the individual. The difference lies in the stage of the process. Stimulation is what is done externally to the patient which produces some heightening of his efforts. Stimulation, however, cannot effect a change in the patient unless he is in a state or set or condition which permits the integration to be made. When such a state does exist the stimulation has its effect and the patient's efforts are facilitated.

Some clinical evidence for such a process being operative does appear to be present. Patients regardless of their particular facade of aphasia symptoms respond accurately at some times and at others seem quite unable to respond. One of the truisms that has been developed in aphasia therapy is the timing of therapy to take advantage of this apparent shift of ability within the patient. Therapists are told that when a patient seems to be able to respond without frustration or without more than minimal frustration, therapy should be stressed. Conversely, at those times when patients seem to be easily frustrated and even may respond with apparent catastrophic reactions, therapy should be discontinued. Evidently what is happening to these patients is that at times their systems are in a state of readiness to respond; it is possible at these times to facilitate their behavior, to assist them. At other times when their frustration tolerance is low they are incapable of being stimulated; it is impossible to facilitate their behavior. In our present state of knowledge we are quite incapable of describing what the difference may be in cortical function between these two states. The observation seems none the less valid, however.

It remains, then for us to do more than apply a given set of instructions or to attempt to view aphasia therapy as the application of a given series of techniques which, if properly applied, will cause definitive changes in the patient. Contrariwise, its inference would be that being clinically aware of the state of the organism by the behavior of the patient at any given moment is of more concern than the content of therapy. Clinical adroitness or clinical maturity would be more important then than any amount of technique, even if we conceded that there was a given technique or approach that was more valuable than any other.

Facilitation is a bimodal concept. It is first the consequence of stimulation, that factor which assists the nonintegrated cortical structure to function in a more integrated manner. At the same time it is the physiological lowering of the impedance against organized cortical action. One is reminded of Bertrand Russell's statement on electricity (*9*):

> Some readers may expect me at this stage to tell them what electricity really is! The fact is that it is not a thing, like St. Paul's Cathedral; it is a way in which things behave. When we have told how things behave when they are electrified, and under what circumstances they are electrified, we have told all there is to tell.

This is about the only explanation that can be given for the concept of "facilitation" as we use it here. It is not a thing, but people do behave in certain ways when they are stimulated at some times and in other ways when they are stimulated at other times. Stimulation is felt to be valuable and useful and meaningful when the organism is in a state in which the stimulation can have a productive end. This is a state of facilitation. The individual is at that time facilitatable as the product of stimulation.

Some patients seem to be constantly in this state, that is, their integrative level is approximately ready to function, they need only the added cues and clues of the therapist to set their own cortical processes into constructive action. They are easily stimulated and there is an immediate facilitation of their own efforts. Other patients have varying degrees of cortical readiness, that is, the disruption of the cortical function was more or less severe or widespread or more specialized nervous tissue was effected by their particular insult. With these patients it requires a greater degree of stimulation, even when the readiness to function is apparent. It may take more astute clinical adroitness, more thoroughly conceived frustration material.

While it would seem that any material would be useful and consequently the material itself need be given little thought in our therapeutic plans, this does not seem to be true. What must be carefully considered is the factor of frustration. Not only the level of frustration tolerance in the patient, but the actual act of frustration itself. It has been found to be maximally useful in this regard to analyze very carefully the particular language deficit presented by the patient. Thus on a very gross level if we conceive of the patient as an organism with a trimodal input system consisting of auditory, visual and tactual pathways by which he can receive stimuli from his environment and likewise a trimodal output system by which he can express himself, consisting of oral, graphic and gestural pathways of expression we can rather readily measure his deficit. Since our usual goals are to rehabilitate him as a useful (to himself at least) individual in society we should work most directly toward establishing a means of communication for him by selecting the particular path which is best retained after the trauma, whether it be an aural input and a graphic output or a tactual in-put and a gestural expressive path, and developing that pathway until he is able to communicate his attitudes and thoughts with some ease and facility. To do this we must be able to construct a training program which frustrates him just beyond his presenting ability, that he may be led or guided toward his goal of communication. This does not mean that we should avoid the other pathways or deal exclusively with the best retained, but that we should give an added emphasis to that direction of his behavior. This should be the pathway by which it is simplest and easiest to facilitate his own efforts for it is along this path that the least disruption of cortical tissue must have taken place.

MOTIVATION

It should be recognized at this point that the dual concept of "stimulation-facilitation" does not completely explain the recovery process. That is, a mere stimulation of a neural system which is physiologically capable of functioning is not enough, for it is evident clinically that a psychological state of readiness must also exist before maximal learning of the formation of new, operative neural integrations are possible. The most commonly used term which expresses this concept is "motivation."

Motivation, as the third link in our conceptual chain, indicates the level of goal-directed behavior possessed by the patient. Motives are here defined as goads to action; goals to be achieved, consciously recognized or not as the case may be. As with the concept of facilitation, motives are not observable entities but are inferences drawn from the behavior of the individual by which we can account for behavior. Hull (*7*) hypothesized that:

> . . . there is a goal gradient which can be quantitatively defined . . . rewards and punishments, pleasures and pains, act in some way to reinforce some acts and to inhibit others; goals offer rewards and failures to reach them punishment.

The aphasic patient, like the rest of us, functions best when he reaches a psychological state of high motivation.

A middle-aged patient exhibiting a marked receptive-expressive aphasia, for example, showed a definite plateau in recovery. New gains in language had not been achieved for some time and it seemed that no particular intensity of stimulation, of the type previously used quite successfully, seemed to move him. By a review of the patient's pretraumatic behavior, his vocation and his avocation, it was seen that the usual background data had been used directly in the compilation of therapeutic work material. One area that had not been used, however, or had at best been given only a minor emphasis early in therapy, was the patient's love of outdoor sports as a participator. Attempts to use this area previously had met with considerable resistance. The patient's self-concept, it was felt, was not sufficiently stable that he could talk or work in the area of his previous love of active sports. At this later date, however, there had been a considerable reduction in his hemiplegia. He was now able to walk quite successfully without a cane and had become especially facile in the use of his left hand. Reintroducing the area of sports (fishing and hunting especially), first as a vocabulary area and later as direct activities to the limit of his ability, became so motivating that the plateau was left behind and language therapy could be continued upon measurable and meaningful levels.

This case history illustrates a number of important things about aphasia therapy, but most importantly it stresses the vital need for understanding the patient's background, his interests and his capability of accepting these previously highly motivated areas of behavior in his posttraumatic state. Language areas which might be very stimulating at one time may be almost detrimental at another. The therapist, then, must be constantly aware of the patient's readiness to act in a particular area. This readiness may be both a function of the physiological state as well as the psychological state of the patient.

It has been argued that all patients are motivated to speak, to read, to write again. This is undoubtedly true. Some degree of motivation to resolve all parts of the language problem, and to be able to use communication meaningfully, is present at all times. In some patients, however, it is to be noted that the desire for other behavior may be more highly motivated than that of language. It is, for example, a common experience that patients express a real need for increased function in their paralyzed arms and legs before they express a need for improved speech or language. Unless some effort is made toward reducing their realized anxiety in this direction, language therapy may fail because of a lack of sufficient motivation, or put another way, motivation for other functions may be greater than for language recovery. With these same patients, however, when physiotherapy is prescribed, when exercise, heat, massage, braces, etc. that make up the physical rehabilitation becomes a part of the program, the patients seem more immediately available, psychologically, for language therapy.

It is for such reasons as these that the present writer has become such an advocate of the team approach as the most useful method for total therapy. Patients that see themselves as permanently physically debilitated and visualize themselves as never again being able to function as whole people tend to develop withdrawal characteristics secondary to their brain damage. These patients seem almost unable to be motivated for language therapy, per se. Thus, the patient may be in a position where his cortex is again capable of integrated behavior and we may be ready and willing to provide the proper stimulation for language recovery and yet lack of the proper psychological set or motivation may block every effort.

The concept of motivation can be considered in still a different light. As aphasia therapists we may believe that the most desirable immediate goal in therapy falls along the pathway of auditory reception and verbal expression. This may be our best considered opinion from our knowledge of the patient and his ability to perform at the time. With this in mind we may set out a program designed to assist him to recover communication facility along this pathway. The patient, however, may have other ideas, which because of his aphasia he cannot verbalize, about his communication needs. He may have been a person who always utilized as his language modality of choice a visual reception and a graphic expression. He may, internally, be highly motivated to attain his previous proficiency in these areas and along this path. Regardless of our concept that the best retained pathway is the direction which should be given to the therapy, maximal motivation may exist in this less well retained pathway. If so, it is along that road that we must travel. At the very least, we must be prepared to accept as our goal what the patient feels to be his greatest need. For unless we can strike the highest level of motivation and satisfy the need of the patient our attempts to assist may be quite meaningless for this particular patient.

The patient's motivational level and the effect it has upon the recovery process is probably easiest seen in the in-patient hospital environment. In one such aphasia center patients were being seen with a reasonable amount of success being obtained in some patients, but what appeared to be an inordinate amount of withdrawal and negativism observed in a great number of other patients. At that time each patient was being seen individually for language therapy while he was being treated for his physical debilities by his ward neurologist and under the latter's guidance was receiving physiotherapy, occupational and corrective therapy as they seemed indicated. It was evident that something was lacking in the overall approach. Many patients did not seem to improve under the stipulated regime. Social group therapy was then added to the program. As the patients came to know one another in a free and relaxed environment, as their self-concepts changed through the interpersonal relationships developed, there seemed to be an almost dramatic change in their language progress. They became less withdrawn and negativistic toward participation in their individual therapy and the over-all tone of the program for the entire group seemed heightened and improved. This increased activity and progress seems understandable to the writer only on the basis of increased motivation. For some of the patients the motivational improvement seemed to come from the acceptance of the other patients, for others it seemed to originate in the opportunity for competition with other patients after acceptance was assured. But without question the entire group, almost to a man, showed increased motivation and a lessening of the psychological blocks toward recovery.

French (*2*) in his recent book on the integration of behavior points out that "it is impossible to understand most behavior unless we discover its motives." The motivation of the aphasic patient like the motives that move all others must be understood before we can hope to achieve reasonable success in therapy. The needs of the patient should be one of the first interests as we plan therapy for any patient. In part this can be understood only by studying his pretraumatic history. In part these may be hidden because of the patient's inability to communicate. But by careful observation of the patient's behavior as we work with him we can see the success we are obtaining at meeting his needs as we attempt to assist him in his resolution of his language deficit. Thus the concept of the patient's motivation must be always with us or we will blindly follow our own needs and overlook those of the patient.

CONCLUSION

Three concepts, stimulation, facilitation and motivation, form the constructs which are believed important in the recovery process. They are inextricably interrelated. One cannot produce therapeutic changes without the other. Aphasic patients left to their own devices tend to plateau in the resolution of their language deficits. With this plateauing comes the development of a whole series of so-called secondary reactions to their condition. Accepting their disability usually means a withdrawal from the social environment. Anxiety and depression become increasing problems. A sense of worthlessness, feelings of futility and an overall attitude of insecurity becomes pervasive. In sheltered environments they tend to become overly dependent, invalidized and infantilized. Therapy that is supportive as well as instructive is the only way in which these patients can again regain a wholesome self-concept which permits them to function in society as whole people. They must be stimulated to action. Their physiological readiness must be utilized. Their motivational levels must be understood and constructively used.

Stimulation, as used here, means any and every kind of outside, external persuasion, used by those in the patient's environment to provide the individual with stimuli to which he may react. Therapy is organized, goal-directed stimulation, based upon a recognition of the patient's needs, his drives, his motivation. As stimulation is provided at a time when the organism is capable of response it tends to facilitate neural integrations. If the direction of the stimulation at the proper time is in keeping with the patient's psychological state of readiness, if the stimulation is within the modality of language which meets the patient's needs, if the stimulation provides the end reward by realizable and recognizable goals of achievement, then success in therapy is more likely to follow.

Aphasia therapy reduced to its primary function becomes in this conceptual structure a process by which the therapist provides stimulative material in the area of a patient's greatest need at a time when his nervous system is capable of utilizing it for the facilitation of cortical integrations leading to language performance. Facilitation is seen as the physiological strength of the drive to motivate action. It is the increase in neural activity that comes about because the patient has been stimulated at the time when he can make use of the stimulation. Motivation in its simplest terms is seen as the amount of goal-directed behavior the patient possesses. When all three concepts are operating at their maximal level, aphasia therapy has its greatest and perhaps its only real chance for success.

REFERENCES

1. Butfield, E. and Zangwill, O. Re-education in aphasia. *J. Neurol. Neurosurg. Psychiat.*, **9,** 1946, 75–79.
2. French, T. *The Integration of Behavior.* Chicago: Univ. of Chicago Press, 1952.
3. Goldstein, K. and Scheerer, M. Abstract and concrete behavior. *Psychol. Monogr.*, **53(2),** 1941, 1–151.
4. Halstead, W. *Brain and Intelligence.* Chicago: Univ. of Chicago Press, 1947.
5. Head, H. *Aphasia and Kindred Disorders of Speech.* London: Cambridge Univ. Press, 1926.
6. Hebb, D. O. *The Organization of Behavior.* New York: John Wiley, 1949.
7. Hull, C. L. In Murphey, G., ed. *Historical Introduction to Modern Psychology.* New York: Harcourt, Brace, 1949.
8. Jeffress, L. A., ed. *Cerebral Mechanisms of the Cortex. The Hixon Symposium.* New York: John Wiley, 1951.
9. Russell, B. *Dictionary of Mind, Matter and Morals.* New York: Philosophical Library, 1952.
10. Sperry, R. W. Neurology and the mind brain problem. *Amer. Scient.*, **40,** 1952, 291–311.
11. Wechsler, D. *The Measurement of Adult Intelligence.* Baltimore: Williams and Wilkins, 1941.
12. Wepman, J. *Recovery from Aphasia.* New York: Ronald Press, 1951.

Reeducation in Aphasia: A Review of 70 Cases

EDNA BUTFIELD
OLIVER L. ZANGWILL

EDNA BUTFIELD, F.C.S.T., is principal of the West End Hospital Speech Therapy Training School, London.
OLIVER L. ZANGWILL, M.A. (Cambridge), is head of the department of experimental psychology at the University of Cambridge, England.

The problem of reeducation in aphasia and kindred disorders has attracted the interest and challenged the skill of both neurologists and psychologists for the past fifty years. Among the earlier discussions of the subject, those of Mills (1904) and Froeschels (1914) are worthy of special mention. But it was only with the war of 1914–18 that the problem took on real practical urgency and large-scale explorations of the possibilities for reeducation in aphasia were undertaken. This work was developed above all in Germany and is especially associated with the names of Poppelreuter, Isserlin, and Goldstein. Poppelreuter's work (1917) is, unfortunately, not available, but Isserlin (1941) has reported briefly on the work undertaken by Feuchtwanger at the Brain Injuries Institute in Munich. Of 178 cases of aphasia given reeducational treatment at this center, complete recovery was reported in 10.1 percent, marked improvement in 25.3 percent, some improvement (partial recovery) in 55.6 percent, and no significant change in 9 percent. The great majority of the cases were traumatic, and these gave consistently better results than the few cases in which the aphasia was due to cerebral disease. Thus, all the cases who recovered completely or showed marked improvement were traumatic, and the group of cases who recovered partially included only 8 cases whose aphasia was due to disease. On the other hand, 50 percent of the patients who showed no improvement were cases of aphasia due to cerebral disease. The outcome of the reeducational work undertaken by Goldstein and his colleagues has not been presented in quantitative form, but valuable records of the technique, course, and outcome of reeducation in individual cases are available (Goldstein, 1919). Goldstein (1942) has more recently summed up his experience of the problems and methods of reeducation in a useful review. Other contributions to the German literature of this period worthy of mention are those of Froeschels (1915), Gutzmann (1916), and Reichmann and Reichau (1919), Retraining work with cases of aphasia in civil life has been described by a number of authors, but all this work has been on a very limited scale (Franz, 1924; Singer and Low, 1933; Weisenburg and McBride, 1935). Weisenburg and McBride, who stress the need for more extensive studies, have presented a useful review and discussion of the whole field in their book on *Aphasia* (1935, pp. 92–100; 385–412).

An objective appraisal of the outcome and value of reeducation in aphasia is far from easy

From *Journal of Neurology, Neurosurgery and Psychiatry* 9:75–79, 1946. Reprinted by permission of the Editor and authors.

in view of the lack of controlled studies. We are seldom able to compare in a controlled manner the course and outcome of the disorder in two equated groups of patients of which only one group has been given formal re-education. In consequence, we possess no definite standards whereby to assess spontaneous recovery of cerebral function as opposed to the effects of re-education. This is a particular disadvantage in the study of traumatic cases in which, as is well known, spontaneous recovery is to be expected much more frequently than in cases of cerebral disease. Nevertheless, there is a certain amount of indirect evidence in favor of re-education of the traumatic case. Thus Frazier and Ingham (1920), in a review of the effects of gunshot wounds of the head, mention 16 cases of residual aphasia in which re-education treatment had been given. They conclude that "although we have seen no evidence of the development of new language centers on the normal side of the brain, improvement has been marked in every patient of this group, the aphasic symptoms of some of which had previously remained stationary for several months" (1920, pp. 31–2). We may also mention that one of Goldstein's war cases made little progress for 3½ months after his injury, but considerable progress in the first two weeks of training which was then begun. In addition, there is evidence that re-education may appreciably hasten the natural course of recovery. Thus Weisenburg and McBride, in reviewing the outcome of retraining in their own cases, conclude that "re-education increases the rate of improvement and aids in overcoming specific disabilities and also in helping the patient to find new ways of achieving the results he is unable to achieve in a normal manner" (1935, p. 412). Lastly, all workers with practical experience agree as to the value of re-educational work for the aphasic patient's adjustment and morale.

We shall present in this paper the principal results in 70 cases of dysphasia[1] and kindred disorders of language referred to us for investigation and re-education in this unit. This figure represents roughly 75 percent of the total cases of dysphasia referred for investigation. In the remaining cases, formal re-education was deemed inexpedient on account of unfavorable prognosis, gross defects of comprehension, or complicating psychiatric symptoms. The bulk of the concrete retraining work was undertaken in 28 cases by Mrs. H. Mitcheltree, sometime speech-therapist to this unit, and in 42 cases by one of the present writers (E. B.)

Cases.—The cases comprised 66 organic acquired dysphasic syndromes and 4 developmental dysphasic conditions. Service patients numbered 37, and civilians 33. Thirteen of the patients were women.

In order to provide some measure of control for the influence of spontaneous recovery, we have divided the 66 cases of acquired dysphasia into two groups. In Group 1, reeducation in all cases was begun less than six months after the onset of the disorder. In Group 2, on the other hand, reeducation was begun more than six months after the onset of the disorder. In 4 cases in this group the interval was over a year. In view of the fact that spontaneous improvement is in general liable to be both limited and slow after six months, it is permissible to ascribe the greater part at least of any improvement made by the patients in Group 2 to reeducation. It has unfortunately been possible to include only 14 cases in this group, and the available material is thus too limited to allow any determinations to be made of the statistical significance of the results. We nevertheless believe that a broad comparison of the outcome in the two groups will prove instructive.

The great majority of the patients in both groups were young adults between 20 and 45 years of age. Only 3 were under 14, and all but 11 under 45. The ætiology of the dysphasic condition was traumatic in 37 cases, vascular in 19, and neoplastic in 10. In Group 2, 5 of the 14 cases were traumatic and the remainder vascular. The average age of the vascular cases was slightly higher than that of the traumatic, 53 percent of the former falling within the 30–44 year age range as compared with 27 percent of the latter. In the cases of cerebral tumor, the time-interval elapsing before reeducation was begun has been computed as from the date of operation.

The distribution and severity of symptoms in speech, reading, writing, and calculation are shown in Table 33-1. The figures represent totals of cases in each group with impairment in the corresponding language field. In each case the degree of disability has been rated as severe, moderate, or mild.

A classification of the disorders of speech proper is

[1] We propose henceforward to use the term "dysphasia" to cover all varieties of central language disorder apart from dysarthria and total aphasia.

TABLE 33-1.

	Speech		Reading		Writing		Calculation	
	Group 1	Group 2	Group 1	Group 2	Group 1	Group 2	Group 1	Group 2
Severe	28	6	20	6	32	8	20	6
Moderate	13	1	15	3	11	1	13	4
Mild	9	6	10	4	5	4	9	2
Total	50	13	45	13	48	13	42	12

TABLE 33-2.

	Mixed	Expressive	Receptive	Amnesic
Group 1	6	22	14	8
Group 2	2	8	2	1
Total	8	30	16	9

given in Table 33-2. Three of the 66 cases have been excluded in view of the fact that these patients showed no disturbance of oral speech at the time re-education in other fields was begun. The remaining cases have been classified in terms of the four-fold scheme advocated by Weisenburg and McBride (1935). This distinguishes (1) mixed expressive-receptive conditions; (2) predominantly expressive conditions; (3) predominantly receptive conditions; and (4) amnesic conditions. The second group includes, in addition to cases of the classical motor-aphasic type, a number of milder defects defined by Head (1926) as verbal aphasias. The third group is largely made up of cases of the type defined by Head as syntactical aphasias, but includes a few with defects of the semantic type. The fourth group corresponds to Head's class of nominal aphasias.

Methods and Procedure

The program of re-education was formulated in every case on the basis of careful individual examination and testing. Examination methods cannot be described in detail here, but were based on the procedures developed by earlier investigators (cf. Zangwill, 1945). It is sufficient to state that special attention was given to the nature, severity, and distribution of defects in the various language fields, to the patient's learning capacities, and to his psychiatric condition generally. The methods of retraining were adapted in large part from those recommended by earlier workers, in particular Goldstein (1919, 1942). Direct methods of reeducation were found of principal value in the predominantly expressive speech disorders and it was often found necessary in these cases to begin with preliminary training in the use of the appropriate muscles (lip and tongue exercises). Thus the patient was shown first how to imitate, and then how to make, a number of positions and movements of the lips, tongue, palate, and larynx. After the necessary facility and control of these movements had been established, speech training proper was begun. This consisted in teaching the patient to imitate simple speech movements of the therapist, using visual and tactual aids where necessary. Thus the use of a mirror, whereby the patient could scrutinize his own mouth movements, was often helpful; and allowing the patient to touch first the therapist's mouth and then his own whilst pronouncing a particular sound was sometimes of value in correcting persistent errors of articulation. In cases where the patient could repeat, though not spontaneously produce, the necessary speech sounds, systematic repetition of these sounds was used as a method for reestablishing voluntary control. The proper association between every speech sound and the movements necessary to produce it was always stressed. This was made possible in certain cases by associating the required movements with some purposive act already within the patient's control. Thus the patient might be taught to pronounce the *p* sound by puffing out smoke.

As the patient's speech improved, every effort was made to develop it within a more natural setting, and exercises in reading, naming, describing pictures, and simple conversation formed part of the speech-therapist's routine. The less formal atmosphere of the occupational therapy department was also very favorable for flexible exercises of this type.

Retraining in the cases of predominantly receptive dysphasia was in most cases along a more round-about route. Although little could be done directly in cases with any degree of word-deafness, disorders of reading could be profitably approached along indirect lines (compensation and substitution). In several cases of dyslexia, for example, it was found that the patient could recognize letters if allowed to trace their outlines with his finger-tip. This served as a basis for systematic re-education. The patient was first requested to trace the outline of large block-letters and to spell out simple words in this manner. When this method of recognition had become relatively automatic, the patient was given normal reading material and instructed to carry out cursive writing movements in reaction to it. These writing movements eventually became extremely rapid and abbreviated and finally dropped out, but were prone to reappear with unfamiliar or difficult words. In favorable cases this technique led to the restitution of accurate, if slow, reading. Some patients, on the other hand, made little progress along these lines, and the use of non-symbolic visual cues, such as picture series suggested by Goldstein (1942), in which letter outlines are derived progressively from pictures of concrete objects, was found of greater help. In general, we have no hesitation in stating that our methods were often purely empirical and adapted by trial-and-error to the individual case. Patients with less severe dyslexic defects were retrained by a method of progressive practice. Reading material of graded difficulty was provided, and systematic exercises in reading both silently and aloud undertaken daily. Special instruction and help was given with words or phrases found to present special difficulty, and complementary exercises in writing were generally undertaken. Thus the patients were often asked to write down from memory the gist of the material which they had read. The patients were also encouraged to study illustrated magazines and the like in their own time.

In the case of writing, reeducational work was indicated, especially in patients who had not lost the capacity to form and copy letters, but who presented dysgraphic symptoms in the context of a more generalized dysphasic syndrome. These patients were given systematic exercises in copying, spelling, and dictation, and occasionally instruction in grammar. In patients who had lost the capacity to form letters as such (whether as a primary agraphia or as part of a constructional apraxia), no satisfactory method of reeducation was discovered. Retraining in cases of gross acalculia was achieved to a limited extent by the use of highly-concrete procedures comparable to those used in teaching young children. In milder cases, progressive practice in mechanical arithmetic (e.g. Kraepelin's adding tests) and simple exercises in arithmetic of the ordinary scholastic type were regularly given. The patients were also given practice in handling money in simple concrete situations. The duration of reeducation varied considerably from case to case. As a rule, every patient undertook two sessions daily with the speech-therapist, each lasting half an hour. But many of our patients engaged in supplementary work of a re-educative character in the occupational therapy department or in their own time. This work was carefully coordinated with the formal sessions. The total number of such sessions was 25 or under in 22 cases, 26 to 50 in 22 cases, 51 to 75 in 12 cases, and over 75 in the remainder. The smallest number of sessions in any one case was 5, and the largest 290.

Formal re-education was terminated when the patient had improved to a point at which little or no practical disability remained, or, in the less responsive cases, when the language condition appeared to have become more or less stationary despite prolonged re-education. At this point, careful psychological re-examination was undertaken. The various language functions in regard to which re-education had been attempted were rated on a three-point scale as much improved, improved, or unchanged. These ratings were based on the following criteria: (1) the opinion of the senior member of the clinical staff of the unit in charge of the case; (2) the results of repeated psychometric testing; and (3) the patient's work record in the speech-therapy department. It must be borne in mind in assessing the results that progress ratings are based on the original degree of impairment of the affected language functions. They do not therefore necessarily reflect the degree of residual disability in comparison with the normal. Thus a severely dysphasic patient might improve very considerably with speech therapy yet remain grossly disabled for practical purposes. A mild case, on the other hand, might improve relatively little yet prove to be very little handicapped in ordinary life. Our ratings therefore give no guide to absolute residual disability, and this may best be assessed from the figures for resettlement given at the end of this paper.

OUTCOME OF REEDUCATION

The results for the two groups are given in Table 33-3. This table shows the total cases in each group with defects of speech, reading, writing, and calculation classified in terms of initial severity and condition on final examination. The patients were graded separately in every field as *much improved* (M), *improved* (I), or *unchanged* (U).

It will be seen from Table 33-3 that speech in

TABLE 33-3.

		Speech			Reading			Writing			Calculation		
		M	I	U	M	I	U	M	I	U	M	I	U
Severe	Group 1	12	7	9	7	5	8	11	7	14	5	4	11
	Group 2	0	3	3	1	2	3	2	4	2	0	3	3
Moderate	Group 1	8	5	0	5	9	1	4	7	0	4	7	2
	Group 2	1	0	0	1	2	0	0	1	0	1	3	0
Mild	Group 1	6	3	0	5	5	0	4	1	0	3	6	0
	Group 2	3	3	0	2	1	1	2	1	1	0	1	1
	Total	30	21	12	21	24	13	23	21	17	13	24	17

TABLE 33-4.

	Speech			Reading			Writing			Calculation		
	M	I	U	M	I	U	M	I	U	M	I	U
Severe	40	26	34	31	31	38	33	26	41	21	29	50
Moderate	56	38	6	62	38	0	33	67	0	33	54	13
Mild	58	42	0	57	36	7	63	25	12	27	64	9

TABLE 33-5.

	Mixed			Expressive			Receptive			Amnesic		
	M	I	U	M	I	U	M	I	U	M	I	U
Group 1	2	1	3	16	4	2	5	4	5	2	5	1
Group 2	0	0	2	3	4	1	0	2	0	1	0	0
Total	2	1	5	19	8	3	5	6	5	3	5	1

over one-half of the patients in Group 1, and in nearly one-third of those in Group 2, was judged to be much improved after reeducation. The outcome in the case of reading, writing, and calculation is less satisfactory—the last in particular—but it will be noted that a minority of patients in both groups were considered to be unchanged from the point of view of these abilities.

Table 33-4 shows the outcome in percentage form for both groups combined in relation to the initial severity of the disabilities. It will be seen that speech in 40 percent of severe cases, 56 percent of moderate cases, and 58 percent of mild cases underwent a marked improvement. On the other hand, the speech condition was unchanged in 34 percent of the severely disabled patients.

The outcome in relation to the type of dysphasic syndrome is indicated in Table 33-5. The figures suggest (but do not establish statistically) that the most favorable results are given by the cases of predominantly expressive dysphasia. Thus nearly three-quarters of the cases of this type underwent a marked improvement.

Table 33-6 shows the outcome as related to the etiology of the dysphasic condition when oral speech alone is considered. It will be seen that 21 of the 35 traumatic cases were much improved in this respect and the speech condition unchanged in only two. In the vascular and neoplastic groups, on the other hand, speech was unimproved in roughly a third of the cases.

A word is in place regarding the disposal from hospital of these patients. Of the 55 adults in our series who had been formerly in economic employment, 37 were resettled in gainful occupations. Of these, one was returned to military duty, 11 to clerical work, 12 to skilled manual jobs, and 13 to unskilled work. Ten patients were totally incapacitated. Of the patients who had been formerly in skilled employment, over half were returned to skilled work, and most of the remainder to unskilled work. In a number of cases, however, the job to which the patient was returned was lighter or less exacting than his former (civilian) occupation.

It was not found possible to record any significant change in the four cases of developmental dysphasic syndrome included in our series, but in none was it possible to continue training for more than a few weeks. We were, however, in the position to offer some suggestions as to the scholastic management of three of these cases and to arrange for further special training in one.

TABLE 33-6.

	Traumatic		Vascular		Neoplastic	
	Group 1	Group 2	Group 1	Group 2	Group 1	Group 2
Much improved	18	3	4	2	3	0
Improved	10	2	2	4	3	0
Unchanged	2	0	4	3	3	0
Total	30	5	10	9	9	0

SUMMARY

(1) The problem of reeducation in aphasia is briefly considered and some practical methods of retraining described.

(2) The outcome of reeducation in a group of 70 dysphasic cases is reviewed and evaluated. Treatment in 14 of these cases was begun six months or more after the onset of the disorder, when relatively little further spontaneous improvement was to be expected.

(3) The results are considered in relation to the various aspects of language affected (speech, reading, writing, and calculation), and to the type, severity, and etiology of the dysphasic condition. Although the number of cases is too small to permit a determination of the statistical significance of the results, it is suggested that the most favorable outcome is obtained in traumatic cases and in those whose symptoms are relatively mild and predominantly on the executive side.

(4) Two-thirds of the patients given re-educational treatment were resettled in economic employment.

Acknowledgments. We wish to express our sincere gratitude to the Directors and Staff of the Brain Injuries Unit, Edinburgh, whose co-operation and help throughout made this work possible. We wish also gratefully to acknowledge the support of the Rockefeller Foundation.

REFERENCES

Franz, S. I. (1924). *J. comp. Psychol.*, **4,** 349.

Frazier, C. H., and Ingham, S. D. (1920). *Arch. Neurol. Psychiat. (Chicago)*, **3,** 17.

Froeschels, E. (1914). *Arch. Psychiat.*, **53,** 221.

—— (1915). *Ibid.*, **56,** 1.

Goldstein, K. (1919). *Die Behandlung, Fürsorge und Begutachtung der Hirnverletzten*, Leipzig, Vogel.

—— (1942). *After-Effects of Brain Injuries in War*, London, Heinemann.

Gutzmann, H. (1916). *Berlin klin. Wschr.*, **53,** 154.

Head, H. (1926). *Aphasia and Kindred Disorders of Speech*, Camb. Univ. Press.

Isserlin, M. (1941). (Unpublished).

Mills, C. K. (1904). *J. Amer. med. Ass.*, **43,** 1940.

Poppelreuter, W. (1917). *Die psychischen Schädigungen durch Kopfschuss*, Leipzig, Voss.

Reichmann, F., and Reichau, E. (1919). *Arch. Psychiat.*, **60,** 8.

Singer, H. D., and Low, A. A. (1933). *Arch. Neurol. Psychiat (Chicago)*, **29,** 162..

Weisenburg, T. H., and McBride, K. E. (1935). *Aphasia*, New York, The Commonwealth Fund.

Zangwill, O. L. (1945). *Brit. med. J.*, **2,** 248.

34

The Recovery Process in Aphasia

CHARLES M. GODFREY
ERNEST DOUGLASS

CHARLES M. GODFREY, M.D., is director of the course in speech pathology and audiology and is with the department of medicine at the University of Toronto, and with the department of veterans affairs at Sunnybrook Hospital, Toronto.

ERNEST DOUGLASS, L.C.S.T., is with the department of psychiatry of the University of Toronto and with the department of research electronics at the Massachusetts Institute of Technology, Cambridge.

The literature concerning aphasia is not only voluminous, which is an obstacle in itself to many students, but it is confusing with respect to the numerous and often diverse systems of classification, nomenclature employed, and the question of cerebral localization of language functions.

Such problems are of more than theoretical interest of course, but meantime we are faced with the necessary and somewhat formidable task of attempting to provide a realistic therapeutic service. This article will therefore deal with some of the difficulties and dynamics involved in rehabilitation of aphasic patients. Tradition has preserved the term aphasia; but we recognize that dysphasia is more frequently the more accurate term, since in actual practice the majority of cases have partial rather than total loss of language functions. For the purpose of this discussion, however, we propose to use the terms synonymously.

The question of retraining in aphasia is a controversial one. Many medical practitioners still hold to the view that attempts at language retraining have little or no value in aphasic disturbances; and this opinion seems to be based primarily upon the belief that cerebral cells, once damaged, cannot undergo restoration of function. The concept of spontaneous recovery in the sense of physiological restoration is, however, accepted generally; and whatever recovery does take place is attributed solely to this "natural" process. This is based on notions that adjacent cerebral areas or the non-dominant hemisphere take over language functions. Other investigators, however, such as Goldstein (*1*), Butfield and Zangwill (*2*), Weisenburg and McBride (*3*), Wepman (*4*), and Berry and Eisenson (*5*), claim that specific attempts at language retraining may appreciably influence not only the rate of improvement but also its extent. In contradition to conventional medical practice, which traditionally withholds speech retraining until the spontaneous recovery process is thought to have been concluded, these workers feel that speech therapy should commence as quickly as possible following trauma. This is based on the assumption that it is important to provide the aphasic with as much language stimulation as possible from the beginning.

From *Canadian Medical Association Journal* 80:618–24, 1959.

Scattered throughout the medical literature are to be found brief references to speech and language disorders, but usually only inasmuch as such disorders are concomitant with more widespread lesions. With regard to the possibility of speech and language rehabilitation procedures there is a remarkable poverty of concern. The same neglect is reflected in the medical curriculum of our universities and in the fact that patients may receive the best of physical care, only to live extended and isolated existences, still unable to function as useful members of society, because the vital modalities of communication remain limited as residual defects. This apparent indifference on the part of medicine is all the more surprising when one realizes that most speech surveys reveal that as many as 5 percent of the general population suffer from disorders of speech function, and we have every reason to believe that surveys confined to general hospital populations would show a considerably higher incidence. A recent survey at the Department of Veterans Affairs, Sunnybrook Hospital, Toronto, indicated approximately 10 percent to be suffering from speech and language defects of a disabling nature (*6*). When this omission on the part of medicine is realized, it is not surprising perhaps to learn that speech defectives have fallen easy prey to commercial organizations offering therapeutic services, not to mention being subjected to attempts at assistance by relatives, friends, and other well-meaning but misguided persons.

It is understandable therefore that such neglect should have given impetus to the development of the profession of speech pathology—first in Europe and later on this continent. In Britain particularly, professional training colleges were organized as one of the recognized medical auxiliary services, working both in hospital settings and in health clinics related to educational institutions. To some extent this now applies to the United States, but there the majority of such professionally qualified people are trained and work within educational institutions; evidently only a very small minority prefer to associate themselves with medical faculties and establishments. That the great need is now officially recognized in Canada by the medical profession is symbolized by the creation of a training course in speech pathology and audiology within the Faculty of Medicine at the University of Toronto. Particular emphasis is being given to medical orientation in the training of personnel, with an expectation that they will be enabled to make their contribution to a philosophy of therapeutic holism which is now fortunately gaining adherents in rehabilitation procedures.

The concept of totality is particulary relevant in aphasia, which "is not a disease but rather a symptom complex" (*5*). In addition to disturbance in one language process affecting another, such as visual language impairment disrupting written skills, or auditory language impairment affecting expressive verbal skills, the aphasic usually suffers concomitant defects such as hemiplegia, dysarthria, intellectual deficit, and personality reactions in response to chronic illness of this nature. This is to say nothing of other psycho-social factors related to family attitudes in response to the disaster, and vocational problems which arise in consequence. The speech therapist, by virtue of his specialized training and knowledge, should not only be well equipped to make therapeutic attempts directed towards specific language and speech disability but should also have a working knowledge and be capable of cooperating intelligently with persons in related specialities such as physical medicine, psychiatry, neurology, psychology, and social work.

The aphasia rehabilitation project to be reported was formulated originally as an emergency measure: to offer treatment facilities to aphasic patients in the absence of more adequate provision in terms of specialized personnel, technical equipment and accommodation (*7*). The experience, however, proved so worth while that it is considered worthy of fuller presentation for study and criticism. We are aware, of course, that the enquiry has many shortcomings and is open to adverse comments on methodological grounds. If the study is less than sound, it is at least subject to repetition by other workers with better experimental design, to refute or confirm our impressions.

THE GROUP REHABILITATION PROGRAM

By force of circumstances rather than by premeditation, the mechanics of speech retraining were not emphasized in this group rehabilitation program, which involved 38 aphasic patients over a period of 12 months. A typical physically orientated rehabilitation regimen was utilized including physiotherapy, exercises, gymnasium, walking and pool activities, as well as conventional occupational therapy procedures. Included, however, as a part of the day's rehabilitation activities were "social-speech" group therapy sessions utilizing two occupational therapists who had only the most elementary knowledge of speech therapy techniques. Although these therapists offered some so-called "direct" language therapy, this of necessity was of a primitive nature owing not only to lack of specialized knowledge of the subject, but also to lack of technical aids in the way of equipment designed for language reeducation. However, if the facilities available had no other effect, they did provide a focus of mutual interest and concern which obviously enhanced group cohesion and patient-therapist relationship.

With the serving of coffee and the creating of an informal setting, it became obvious that a socio-psychotherapeutic process was in fact operative. Because they were so involved and enthusiastic about the project, the two occupational therapists were anxious to learn more of aphasia-therapy principles, but it was felt that their very lack of sophistication in this respect was in fact an asset rather than a deficit, and so they were not encouraged to acquire the complex technical terminology and concepts current in the literature on aphasia and clinical psychology. Implicit within the speech-social group climate was an enthusiasm and initiative on the part of the therapists which had a "natural" and "warm" character and which might only too easily become a studied and self-conscious effort with the acquisition of technical knowledge in these matters. There could be no doubt that patient-therapist relationships were of such a nature that the patients were responding to this factor, gathering from it support and strength in consequence of which there were obvious signs of markedly reduced anxiety, lowering of defensive attitudes, less withdrawal from human relationships and lifting of depression. Although in some cases language functions themselves did not particularly improve, the patient's ability to accept the limitations of disability, and to acquire relatively objective unemotional attitudes and to relate to others, was a striking and impressive feature.

ASSESSMENT OF GROUP MEMBERS

Groups were restricted to not more than six patients, this being felt to be the optimum number for effective interpersonal contacts. An attempt was made to group patients in terms of age, extent of disabilities, and compatability of personalities. Initial investigations were made which included assessments of physical disabilities, including especially visual and auditory defects. Psychologists attempted to assess damage to the central nervous system with a view to determining changes both before and during the therapeutic period. Because of the communication difficulty inherent in aphasia, the conventional psychometric tests were felt to be inadequate. No universally acceptable and standardized psychological tests exist as yet which are applicable to persons suffering from aphasia. Furthermore, it was felt that formal tests introduced an "artificial" character, and often more accurate assessments could be made by clinical judgment.

The consulting speech therapist assessed the speech impairment, pointing up specific language modalities which remained relatively intact and by means of which communication could best be established with the patient in group therapy. If it was felt that group therapy would penalize the patient in that he would not receive specialized speech therapy, he was excluded from the group and received individual attention.

Language was reassessed for all patients after every three-month period during group therapy. Although in these ratings a standard aphasic test protocol was utilized for the sake of uniformity and later comparison, the assessments were arrived at by clinical judgment in a setting of informality. This procedure took longer perhaps than the administration of a systematized test, but it was felt that more realistic and accurate assessments were possible in this way, as opposed to the anxiety-arousing elements in formal testing where so many more variables give rise to false and inconsistent results.

The social work department interviewed the patient and family in an attempt to determine the pretraumatic personality, vocational activities, and hobbies, and gain an impression of the family constellation.

In the absence of tests giving reliable and objective measures of progress, clinical judgment, although subjective, is probably as satisfactory as any other available method, and in many instances more satisfactory. A three-point scale of progress was therefore utilized upon the basis of which ratings were made:

1. *Good results:* language ability and psycho-social adjustment improved.
2. *Fair results:* language ability showed no marked improvement, but patient better adapted to group therapy, hospital setting and home situation, together with a decrease in emotional lability and psychological reactions such as depression, withdrawal, and anxiety.
3. *Unchanged:* the ability to communicate, to participate in a program, and personality features remained unchanged.

Of the patients involved in the rehabilitation program, the initial language diagnoses were as follows:

(a) *Predominantly expressive aphasia.*—Symptoms predominant in inability to express by spoken or written symbols.

(b) *Predominantly receptive aphasia.*—Symptoms predominant in inability to comprehend spoken or written symbols.

(c) *Mixed aphasia.*—All language process equally impaired, so that no one modality might be said to be superior.

(d) *Global aphasia.*—All language processes so extensively impaired that no preceding category was applicable.

After therapy, the progress distribution was as in Table 34-1.

TABLE 34-1.

Progress	Diagnosis Type	No.	Total	Age range	Mean age
Good results	Expressive	13	14	33–83	57.0
	Receptive	1			
	Mixed	—			
	Global	—			
Fair results	Expressive	7	16	47–70	58.0
	Receptive	2			
	Mixed	7			
	Global	—			
Unchanged	Expressive	—	8	63–74	68.0
	Receptive	—			
	Mixed	5			
	Global	3			

The mean duration of the condition before therapy in 34 cases was 3.5 weeks; the remaining four cases were long-standing conditions ranging from eight months to two years. The patients ranged in age from 33 to 83 years. All patients were males who had suffered a cerebral vascular accident. None had received speech therapy before entering the group.

RESULTS

During the 12-month period of this program, seven patients died as the result of further cardio-vascular accidents, and although it was not felt that these were in any way precipitated by the rehabilitation program, their occurrence does raise the point whether practitioners should question the wisdom of intensive rehabilitation procedures when it is realized that the survival rate is approximately one to five years. However, the age range of these patients was 62 to 75 years with a mean age of 68 years, and so one may perhaps postulate an optimum age for admittance to a rehabilitation program of this kind.

It is generally believed that restoration of language function is more complete in younger than in older patients. The wide scatter in age range of our patients does not permit conclusions in this respect, although it is observed that our data tend in the expected direction.

As reported above, four of our patients had long-standing aphasic conditions, and it is interesting to note that, contrary to general medical belief, these "static" aphasics who were included in the "fair" category appeared to respond as readily, and showed improvement comparable to that in cases of more recent onset. In this connection, one wonders about current concepts of spontaneous recovery and residual defects in aphasia. The general impression within medicine seems to be that some degree of physiological restoration occurs during the initial recovery phase up to a period of approximately six months, after which the condition becomes static, and irreversible residual defects are to be found.

DISCUSSION

Current concepts regarding the recovery process appear to be based upon very meagre scientific evidence. No sufficiently comprehensive and long-term follow-up studies seem to have been published which record in any detail this process, with the possible exception of one(*9*). This was evidently concerned with traumatic aphasias, and reports: "of 394 patients, 43 percent showed 'residual signs' which would require reeducation or psychotherapy. The other patients recovered spontaneously within the 'initial' period," but no further studies are available nor are there data concerning language recovery rates in cases of vascular and neoplastic origin.

Reassessment of our cases after therapy shows that approximately 37 percent of results were classified as "good," which category, it should be noted, required the patients to achieve psycho-social as well as language adjustment, and 42 percent were classified as "fair," which required psycho-social adjustment only. It is to be observed, however, that all except one in the "good" category had expressive aphasia, which confirms the findings of other workers that expressive aphasics have the best prognosis for language recovery(*2–4*, *10*). It should be pointed out that our study was concerned with cases of vascular etiology; in the absence of basic research concerning spontaneous recovery rates in such conditions, the results reported cannot be accepted as scientific evidence for the effectiveness of therapy but may well represent only the spontaneous recovery rate. Not only is there a poverty of data in this respect, but there are few published studies concerning the effectiveness of language retraining in aphasia which offer anything approaching scientific evidence to support claims made for language restitution as the result of therapy. Three studies are available which do offer such objective evidence but they are only partially comparable to one another and to the present investigation because of numerous variables such as the etiological groups used, the age ranges involved, the duration of the condition before therapy, the duration of therapy and the rating scales employed. However, one such study(*2*), involving 63 patients, reported that speech in one-half of the patients treated less than six months after the onset of the disorder, and in nearly one-third of those treated more than six months after onset, "was judged to be much improved after reeducation." This study was concerned with traumatic, vascular and neoplastic cases, and the results reported were on the basis of oral speech alone. The results in terms of other and more general language modalities were "less satisfactory." If we refer to the data concerning the vascular cases which comprised 19 of the total group, we find that 40 percent of those treated less than six months after onset, and 22.2 percent of those treated after more than six months, were "much improved." In addition, it is perhaps significant to know that the great majority of the patients involved in this study were young adults between 20 and 45 years of age.

The second study reported(*4*) involved 68 aphasics, the vast majority traumatic, with an overall age of 19–38 years, but who did not receive language therapy until six months after trauma. The original investigation utilized previous school-grade levels and educational achievements as evidence for the effectiveness of language therapy, but in order to compare the results subsequently applied the same rating scale as in the previous study (*2*) and reported 51.5 percent "much improved."

The third and most recent study offering statistical evidence of the effects of language therapy(*10*) is perhaps the most comparable to our own as regards the rating scale utilized, in that the vast majority of cases were of vascular etiology and in persons over 50 years of age. A four-point rating scale was used and the following distribution reported: excellent, 6.9 percent; good, 22.0 percent; fair, 21.4 percent; and poor, 49.7 percent.

Admittedly, comparison of data is difficult, but making due allowance for the variables involved, such as criteria of rating scales, varying etiological factors, duration of condition before reeducation, extent and method of therapy, and age of patients, we see that claims for the percentage of patients improved by language therapy range between approximately 40 and 50 percent. Since Luria's study concerning spontaneous recovery rates(*9*) reports that 43 percent showed "residual signs," the implication is that 57 percent showed "no residual signs" and recovered completely. Such an implication suggests that it is this 57 percent which is comparable to the "most improved" categories of the reported studies related to the effectiveness of therapy, while the "improved" and lower-order categories by definition comprised patients who still had progress to make, that is, who still had residual signs. Clearly there is an imperative need for large-scale investigations to provide further data concerning spontaneous recovery rates, but meantime, on the basis of the only data available, any forms of therapy would have to demonstrate considerably more improvement than in 40 to 50 percent, in order to be considered as making a significant contribution if the spontaneous recovery rate is 57 percent.[1] In fact, on the evidence available, there appears to be an inverse relationship between recovery from aphasia and formalized reeducational language attempts!

Such conclusions are of course tentative but nevertheless may be disquietening and raise some threatening questions for those of us engaged in therapeutic endeavors. Objectivity towards the available facts however is essential, and will, we hope, only give impetus to the development of studies designed to establish base lines in recovery rates against which other data may be compared. It may be difficult to relate recovery rates for "functional" disorders to those for "organic" disorders, but it is interesting to note that roughly comparable figures have been recorded concerning neurotic disorders(*12*), of which approximately 66 percent recover. Although speculative, it is fascinating to consider the possibility that some general factors are operative throughout many disorders and that the statistics reflect a clinical law, as yet little recognized or understood because of the meagre data available at this level of enquiry. We are not saying that "spontaneous recovery" is *not* a purely physiological process, nor are we saying that language therapy in aphasia rehabilitation is *not* beneficial; but we *are* saying that observation data indicate that we presently operate upon very unsound premises. Further progress in objectively measuring degrees of language disorder in aphasia, its changes during spontaneous recovery, and hence the effectiveness of therapy, is not possible until base lines concerning recovery rates are better established.

Perhaps we may address ourselves in somewhat greater detail to some of these fundamental issues. There can be little doubt, for instance, that a process known as "spontaneous recovery" does occur in the sense that some degree of physiological restoration takes place in language and other functions. To view this as a purely physical process, however, without reference to the pretraumatic and post-traumatic personality configuration and without reference to the patient's social environment,

[1] It should be noted that Luria's cases comprised young patients with war wounds of the head in the acute period of recovery.—Personal communication, A. R. Luria, University of Moscow, March 1959.

would appear to be an obvious over-simplification. Some attention has been paid to the social and emotional aspects of aphasia(*13–15*), but these studies are related to therapeutic method rather than to the influence of these factors during spontaneous recovery. We do not know whether the spontaneous recovery process is or is not a more or less exclusively physiological event and, if it is not, then what influence psychological, social, educational and indeed economic factors play at various age levels and in various types of aphasia. Until such facts are established, any claims regarding the nature of spontaneous recovery and any claims for the effectiveness of therapy are no better than speculation and subjective judgments.

Although we realize that there may be social and ethical objections to the proposal, we suggest that it would be possible to obtain such data as outlined above by controlled experiments involving detailed observational follow-up studies of aphasic patients in the various diagnostic and psycho-socioeconomic categories during the spontaneous recovery period in a relatively impoverished environment as opposed to a stimulating social environment. Indeed, whether we like it or not, owing to lack of rehabilitation facilities, conditions such as those required for such a study already exist, but we are not taking advantage of the otherwise negative conditions by making observations in accordance with research criteria.

Another basic requirement is that for valid and reliable methods of assessing degrees of dysphasic disorder. Because of the nature of the dysphasic disturbance, this is a particularly difficult problem with regard to which some workers(*8*, *16*, *17*) are making valiant attempts. Meantime, in the absence of more objective tests, we must resort to clinical judgment; and this should not deter us from attempting to compare the effectiveness of various methods of therapy. Indeed, experiments should be designed to use control groups of patients not treated at all during the period of the investigation and compared with experimental groups receiving therapy. Comparative studies of various methods of therapy are also required in view of the fact that claims are made for numerous therapeutic approaches, while our study may indicate, among other things, that during the first 12 months of the recovery period at least, there is apparently little if any significant difference between "skilled" and "unskilled" therapeutic attempts in terms of functional recovery. Just what contribution language therapy makes in recovery from aphasia has not been unequivocally demonstrated.

Many speech therapists appear to contribute to the belief that in aphasic language therapy some phonetic and mechanical approach is usually a necessary part, at least, of the therapeutic process(*2*, *18*, *19*). Resort is made frequently to reeducational techniques for the stimulation of specific language modalities by means of auditory, visual and tactile methods employing, in a "modern" clinic, especially designed electronic equipment, such as voice recorders, amplifiers, tachistoscopic apparatus and visual aids of numerous kinds. The array of equipment is indeed often impressive, and one might wonder whether the equipment itself might not have a therapeutic effect upon the patient in terms of suggestion! However, we do not wish to depreciate the value of mechanical reeducational speech therapy techniques; perhaps such methods are of value. On the other hand, in the light of our recent experience and that of a few other workers who did not emphasize the mechanics of speech therapy(*14*), we urge that the therapeutic value of "direct" reeducational methods be not over-estimated or the reasons for their apparent effectiveness be misplaced. As clinically experienced speech therapists know, the aphasic patient during therapy often makes gains in language functions quite unrelated to the specific language modalities being stimulated. Not infrequently, when progress is being made, there is a general rather than a specific language development; and this phenomenon is difficult to explain if we adhere to the effectiveness of singular reeducational techniques or methods in therapy. Recent research, for instance, which investigated the relative effectiveness of "goal-directed" and "incidental learning" in predominantly expressive aphasics compared with a control group of non-aphasics demonstrated "that goal-directed instructions, as compared with incidental instructions, produced higher recall scores in the non-aphasics, but not in the aphasics" (*11*). The inference seems to be that direct methods of learning for aphasics are not the most effective techniques, and one might well speculate therefore about a possible therapeutic agent that is operative yet evidently implicit in the recovery process.

Empirical observations seem to point to a therapeutic variable present in the recovery process, whether this be during so-called spontaneous recovery or during formalized rehabilitation procedures. Essentially the therapeutic element appears to be a psycho-social factor, but this is seldom made explicit or thereby fully utilized to enhance the recovery process. Only too frequently indeed is the patient left more or less to his own devices in this respect during the spontaneous recovery phase, while in formal therapy it often remains an unrecognized factor giving rise to the application of only the most primitive psychotherapy through the medium of tests, direct language reeducational methods and the various "tools" used by the therapist in conventional language therapy. A few workers have attempted to study the therapeutic process at this level of enquiry(*8*, *13*, *14*), and one investigator has stated: "It is axiomatic to say that language therapy without psychotherapy is futile and often harmful in itself, for the aphasic patient who has recovered language, but has not resolved his behavioral adjustment problems, must be considered an unsuccessfully treated patient" (*4*); but the concept has actually received little real acceptance, in spite of the fact that language is generally conceded to be, for one thing if not primarily, a social activity. To state the matter concisely, the need for "milieu" therapy in the treatment of aphasics is obvious.

It would be difficult indeed to find a more multi-functional disorder than aphasia, where it is so self-evident that an interdisciplinary approach to rehabilitation is essential. A holistic approach unfortunately does not arrive merely as the result of paying lip service to the principle. The bringing together of workers in the various specialities concerned gives rise to problems of another nature, a discussion of which may best be reserved for another occasion. However, "although it is a new word, rehabilitation is an old purpose. All medical treatment has basically no other aim" (*2*). Nevertheless, we should be cognizant of the fact that the need to "do something"—to "treat the patient"—so dominates our present thinking and philosophy that it is frequently carried out only at the expense of basic research requirements. Unless the function of research is constantly subserved, we may find, as we suspect in the instance of aphasia and its therapy, some erroneous basic assumptions, false inferences and inadequately understood therapeutic methods. We may thus remain complacent in attributing effectiveness of treatment to methods of practice which are not in fact effective at all, or at least not for the reasons generally propounded.

SUMMARY

The outcome of a rehabilitation attempt in a group of 38 dysphasic cases is reviewed and compared with the only three additional studies offering statistical data to support claims made for the effectiveness of language therapy.

It is pointed out that the improvement rates claimed as the result of language therapy do not compare favorably with those reported for spontaneous recovery alone.

The concept of "spontaneous recovery" as a purely physiological process without reference to psycho-social influences is called into question. The imminent need for the establishment of recovery rate base lines in various dysphasic groups is emphasized.

Comparative studies are also advocated to assess the relative effectiveness of various therapeutic methods.

REFERENCES

1. Goldstein, K: After effects of brain injuries in war, Grune and Stratton, New York, 1942.
2. Butfield, E. and Zangwill, O. L.: *J. Neurol., Neurosurg. and Psychiat.*, **9**:75, 1946.
3. Weisenburg, T. and McBride, K. E.: Aphasia: A clinical and psychological study, Commonwealth Fund, New York, 1935.
4. Wepman, J. M.: Recovery from aphasia, Ronald Press Co., New York, 1951.
5. Berry, M. F. and Eisenson, J.: Speech disorders: Principles and practices of therapy, Appleton-Century-Crofts, Inc., New York, 1956.
6. Douglass, E.: *Bull. Acad. Med. Toronto*, **28**:246, 1955.
7. Godfrey, C. M.: *Canad. M. A. J.*, **80**:616, 1959.
8. Eisenson, J.: Examining for aphasia, Psychological Corporation, New York, 1954.
9. Luria, A.: Topical syndromes of traumatic aphasia, unpublished manuscript loaned by Helen Black, literary agent of the U.S.S.R., New York, quoted by Wepman, J.: Recovery from aphasia, Ronald Press Co., New York, 1951, p. 34.
10. Marks, M., Taylor, M. and Rusk, H. A.: *Arch. Phys. Med.*, **38**:219, 1957.
11. Katz, L.: *J. Consulting Psychology*, **22**:143, 1958.
12. Eysenck, H. J.: Scientific study of personality, Routledge and Kegan Paul Ltd., London, 1952.
13. Blackman, N.: *J. Nerv. and Ment. Dis.*, **3**:154, 1950.
14. Aronson, M., Shatin, L. and Cook, J. C.: *J. Speech and Hearing Disorders*, **21**:352, 1956.
15. Biorn-Hansen, V.: *Ibid.*, **22**:53, 1957.
16. Halstead, W. C. and Wepman, J. M.: *J. Speech and Hearing Disorders*, **14**:9, 1949.
17. Schuell, H.: *Neurology*, **7**:625, 1957.
18. ——, Carroll, V. and Street, B. S.: *J. Speech and Hearing Disorders*, **20**:43, 1955.
19. Granich, L.: Aphasia: A guide to retraining, Grune and Stratton Inc., New York, 1947.
20. Jefferson, G.: Quoted by Zangwill, O. L.: *Brit. J. Psychol.*, **37**:61, 1947.

35

Evolution of Aphasia and Language Rehabilitation: A Retrospective Exploratory Study

LUIGI A. VIGNOLO

LUIGI A. VIGNOLO, M.D., is with the Clinica delle Malattie Nervose e Mentali of the Università di Milano, Italy.

The present study is concerned with the outcome of language disturbances in a group of adult aphasic patients who were followed at the aphasia unit of the Clinic for Nervous and Mental Diseases of Milan between 1960 and 1964. Being retrospective rather than experimental in nature, its only purpose is to point out some methodological problems connected with research in this field and to advance some hypotheses to be tested with a more rigorous experimental design.

Despite the fact that the rehabilitation of aphasia is an established activity in many countries, the central question "Does specific language training and reeducation have a decisive influence on the course and outcome of aphasia?" has so far received quite unsatisfactory answers. This is due, I think, to the fact that investigators in this area are faced with a number of problems which, being difficult to solve, either have been overlooked or handled in quite different and therefore hardly comparable ways. There are, I think, three basic problems. A brief discussion of them may perhaps clarify why our knowledge on this topic is still so meager and will illustrate the present approach to the question.

1) First, an *objective evaluation* of the language defect must be made. Its purpose is twofold: *a*) assessing the degree of impairment and hence improvement, and *b*) defining the types of aphasia in view of a differential prognosis of recovery. Since aphasia is a composite disturbance and does not lend itself to quantitative and univocal measures, such objective assessment is difficult in both instances. Different criteria have been used for purpose *a*. Butfield and Zangwill (1946)[1] rated initial severity of symptoms in speech, reading, writing and calculation as severe, moderate and mild, on the basis of a clinical examination. Taylor (1964) used an original Functional Communication Profile in which 50 communication behaviors considered common language functions of everyday life were rated along an 8-point scale on the basis of informal interaction with the patient in a conversational situation. Scores in speaking, reading, understanding, movement and a miscellaneous category, including writing and calculation, were obtained, as well as an Overall Score which was considered representative of the subject's overall verbal effectiveness in everyday life. While undoubtedly the most realistic and functional, this latter approach is, like the former, largely subjective. Wepman (1951) adopted the Progressive Achievement Tests which provided more objective scores in reading, writing, spelling and arithmetic, in terms of school grades. All these methods involved in different proportions functions other

[1] These and other references in this paper are illustrative rather than exhaustive.

From *Cortex* 1:344–67, 1964.

than language alone, e.g., general intelligence; in addition, comparisons among their results are difficult because of differences in scales used and types of behavior observed. Comparisons of results among different studies are further complicated by the fact that improvement was sometimes referred both to normal standards and to pretraining defect (Wepman, 1951; Taylor, 1964) and sometimes to pretraining defect alone (Butfield and Zangwill, 1946). In other studies (Leischner, 1960), improvement was rated along a 6-point scale but initial degree of impairment was not reported. A Weisenburg-McBride expressive-receptive-global-amnesic type of clinical classification was most often adopted for purpose *b*; however, the various syndromes were seldom precisely defined.

In the present study I did not consider the whole behavioral status of the patients, but only the specific language disturbances that constitute the bulk of aphasic syndromes. I tried to assess them by giving the patients some language task, as little contaminated as possible by intellectual difficulties and as little facilitated as possible by extra-verbal situational cues. In this way, my assessment may have lost breadth but it gained precision and objectivity.

2) Second, the *spontaneous evolution* of aphasia must be studied. It is evident that if we intend to investigate the influence of reeducation on the evolution of aphasia, we need to know what happens under similar circumstances when no treatment is applied, i.e., we need to compare evolution under training with spontaneous evolution. This might be done by comparing the outcome of the disturbance in two groups of patients, of which only one was given formal reeducation. To my knowledge, such a comparison has never been made until now. All published studies involving large groups of cases (Butfield and Zangwill, 1946; Wepman, 1941; Leischner, 1960; Luria, 1963) have dealt with reeducated aphasics only, probably because the social duty to try to help all aphasics who come to a speech clinic prevented the therapists from intentionally excluding some of them from treatment. None of the preceding studies, therefore, was in a position to assess the effectiveness of language rehabilitation on the course of aphasia directly. Evidence of such effectiveness had to be indirectly inferred. Improvement made by patients who started therapy more than 6 months after onset was often ascribed—partly at least—to reeducation, on the assumption that spontaneous recovery, when it occurs, is likely to be both limited and slow after 6 months from onset.

When we started to reeducate aphasics a few years ago, we realized that personal, family or transportation problems would prevent many patients from attending therapy sessions. We have been trying ever since to take advantage of this type of unintentional selection due to extraneous factors by checking the language status of the excluded subjects whenever the opportunity arose. We were thus able to constitute a group of not reeducated aphasics, whose evolution could be compared with that of the reeducated group.

3) Third, it must be realized that reeducation is merely one of a *considerable number of variables* which may be reasonably expected to influence the process of evolution. Some of them are connected with the cerebral insult itself: nature of lesion, extent and locus of lesion, time elapsed from onset, time interval over which evolution is considered, severity and type of disorder, etc. Other variables are related to the physiological and psychological status of the patient prior to injury: age, education, profession, language skills, cerebral dominance, etc. We do not know how all these factors operate, but it is presumed that they interact differently at different levels. For example, the effect of a 3-month period on improvement might be different immediately after onset as compared to one year from onset; but this difference itself may be modified if rehabilitation takes place during this period; furthermore, this may be true for one type of aphasia and not for another, etc. Thus, even if we are primarily interested in knowing the effects of reeducation—this being the only variable which depends upon us—we cannot possibly avoid considering *all* such variables and their interaction.

Indeed, the requirement of a statistical measure of interaction constitutes the main problem of research in this field. In our studies, information about the status of most variables is conveyed in the form of nominal scales (e.g., aetiology may be either vascular or neoplastic or traumatic, etc.) or of scores in a partially ordered scale (e.g., degrees of severity). A few variables could be measured in an interval or ratio scale (age in years, evolution time in days, etc.) but such measures cannot be reasonably expected to be always normally distributed in our samples. Correct statistical treatment of this type of data requires the use of nonparametric tests, and unfortunately failure to assess interaction is a well-known limitation of such tests (Siegel, 1956). Faced with this problem, an investigator may adopt either or both of two procedures (and this is in fact what has been done thus far):

a) He can decide that, in order to assess the influence of reeducation on improvement, it will be sufficient to compare the evolution of two groups, "Reeducated" (R) and "not Reeducated" (nR) aphasics, not significantly different with respect to each of the major remaining variables. This procedure virtually ignores interactions and its results are therefore questionable. For instance, suppose one takes two groups of aphasics, R and nR, not significantly different with respect to age and initial severity, and suppose one finds that the R group improve significantly more than the nR group. We would tend to conclude that reeducation alone is responsible for the difference. However, if the effects of these two variables (age and severity) on improvement happen to interact and if the majority of young patients in one group are also mild aphasics while this is not true for the other group, any comparison as to improvement in the two groups will be biassed in the sense that results will not merely reflect the influence of reeducation—as postulated—but the combined effect of rehabilitation + age + severity on improvement.

b) On the other hand, the investigator can proceed to comparing improvement in R and nR subjects at different levels of an additional variable. For example, he can compare improvement in R and nR *old* patients, and see if there is a significant difference; and then compare improvement in R and nR *young* patients, and see if there is a significant difference. He will try to make the two groups of each comparison as similar as possible with respect to the other relevant variables (i.e., severity, etc.). And he will have to draw conclusions by comparing the significance of differences; if the difference between R and nR is significant in young patients and is not significant in old patients, he will conclude that rehabilitation is effective in young aphasics and not in old ones. Results thus obtained are biassed from a statistical point of view in many respects; in particular, this method induces one to make many independent comparisons (old vs. young in R, old vs. young in nR, etc.) among variables which presumably do interact, and this enhances the risk of finding some significant difference when in reality there are no such differences. Moreover, the number of subjects which are available for each such analytical comparison is necessarily limited, and this fact reduces the sensitivity of any statistical test. Inferences drawn from this procedure are not quite reliable, because they allow different interpretations and give hints more than established facts. Conclusions based upon them are therefore partly statistical and partly "impressionistic."

Currently this is the most frequently used procedure to treat data, and I too have adopted it, for want of any better. However, I should like to stress the point that sound conclusions about the evolution of aphasia will only be possible when statisticians provide us with nonparametric tests for evaluating interactions. The findings of our "impressionistic" study might then be used to state more accurately some hypotheses to be tested with that method.

In conclusion, the present approach to the main difficulties of research in this field can be summarized: objective testing, limited to the specific language deficits of aphasia; constant reference to spontaneous evolution; and, finally, caution in evaluating the results.

Three very broad questions guided the present inquiry:

1) Does spontaneous evolution of aphasia exist and does it show any quantitative and qualitative trends? In particular, do aphasic syndromes generally tend to improve or deteriorate spontaneously? Do the qualitative characteristics of the disorder tend to change in any particular direction?

2) What is the influence of natural factors, such as age, type of aphasia, etc., on the course of aphasia?

3) Does language rehabilitation influence evolution and, if so, under what conditions?

MATERIAL AND METHODS

I looked for the answers to the preceding questions by examining the records of 69 adult aphasic patients who were tested at least twice (with a minimum time interval of 40 days between 1st and 2nd examination) by a standard examination for aphasia.

Assessment of aphasia was made by means of one or both of two highly correlated tests which covered all modalities of language behavior, both oral and written. In the present preliminary study, however, only three language performances will be taken into consideration: oral description (D), oral naming (N), and comprehension of oral commands (C). The nature of these tasks is shown in Table 35-1.

All these tasks are simple from a linguistic standpoint, but they are more demanding than they may appear at first glance. D and N require exact speech production and their performance is aided by no situational cues. This is also true for the oral commands, which, however brief, do not fit in the usual doctor-patient relationship and have very little redundancy.

TABLE 35-1.

(D)	For men: "Please try to describe to me as accurately as you can all you do when you shave." For women: "Please try to describe to me as accurately as you can all you do when you cook spaghetti."
(N)	Naming of pictures of 20 common objects (e.g. a table, an umbrella, etc.).
(C)	Understanding of 10 oral commands (e.g. "Turn up the light," "Blow your nose," etc.).

Both the verbal and nonverbal behavior of the patient during examination was accurately recorded. Performance on all three tasks was rated on the following scale:

3 = good
2 = sufficient to serve the purpose of communication
1 = poor
0 = nil

It should be noted that score 2 represents the critical level for communication: a patient who gets a score of 2 is able to communicate, however awkwardly, through the examined language channel. A score was assigned to N and C tasks on the basis of number of correct responses, and to D task on the basis of combined judgment by two independent examiners. For D task, a scoring guide for examiners, in which possible responses were considered, was constructed in advance on the basis of responses given by 10 normal subjects.

A unified score for Expression (E) was then given to each subject by combining D and N scores in the following way: D score was increased by an additional point if N score was 2 or 3; if N score was 0 or 1, E score was represented by D score alone. This was done in order to give more weight to D with respect to N, considering that capacity to utter words in propositions, as required by description, is more important than mere capacity to find isolated words. The unified E score ranged thus from 0 to 4, and the critical level for communication was set at score 3.

Finally, an attempt to define broad aphasic "syndromes" was made by plotting C score against the unified E score, as shown in Table 35-2. It is important to point out that these by no means claim to be overall clinical definitions of aphasia. We merely adopted a simple method of grouping together aphasic subjects from one limited point of view, namely, their level of communication in D, N and C, i.e., according to their capacity to understand oral language and to make themselves understood through speech. This is a quantitative expressive-receptive classification, and does not take

TABLE 35–2.

Expression (unified E score)	Comprehension (C)	Aphasic "syndrome"	Severity
3-4	*2-3*	MAS = Mild aphasic symptoms, not affecting communication	3
1-2	*2-3*	EM = Expressive, moderate	2
0	*2-3*	ES = Expressive, severe	1
1-2	1	MS = Mixed expressive-receptive, severe	1
0	0-1	G = Global	0

N.B. 1) Scores *in italics* indicate performances above communication level.
2) A purely receptive "syndrome" was not considered, because no patient in the whole series ever showed the combination E = 3-4 and C = 0-1.

into consideration such important qualitative aspects of aphasia as, for instance, fluency or reduction of oral speech. Therefore, quite different clinical types of aphasia may fall into these categories. Thus, our ES group does not only include the typical Broca aphasics with anarthria but also those jargon aphasics (phonemic jargon in particular) who happen to understand well; and the G group includes not only global aphasics in the classic sense, with no understanding and no speech at all except perhaps for some recurring utterances, but also some conspicuous verbal jargon aphasics who would be immediately (and correctly) classified as Wernicke's aphasia by a clinician. It is true, however, that practically all subjects classified as MS showed the clinical pictures of Wernicke's aphasia and that the majority of ES were typical Broca's aphasias.

Aphasic "syndromes" also were ranked according to severity from 0 (Global) to 3 (MAS). From the point of view of general communication, MS and ES were considered on the same level, and the same score was assigned to both. This was done because differences between the two conditions are qualitative rather than quantitative, and neither syndrome is better than the other from the point of view of general oral communication.

Thus, our method of assessing aphasia provided us with different types of scores for each patient: discrete D, N and C scores; a unified E score; a definition and a score for combined levels of performance in both expression and reception. Each score provided a criterion for judging improvement and recovery. On second examination, any area of performance was considered "improved" if it showed an increase in score, while it was considered "recovered" only if it reached the level of communication.

Definition of reeducation. Subjects who had been treated with a minimum of 20 language therapy sessions over the course of not less than 40 days and with a minimum frequency of 1 session a week were considered reeducated. Our series of 69 aphasics was divided into two groups: 42 reeducated aphasics and 27 not reeducated aphasics.

The rationale and techniques of reeducation are described elsewhere in detail (Vignolo, in press) and need only be briefly mentioned here. On first examining the patient the therapist focuses his attention on the following main aspects of language behavior:

1) *Intention to communicate:* Is the patient willing to listen and make himself understood to others? If not, why? (Inertia, poor intelligence, emotional problems, etc.).

2) *Expression and reception:* How is he able to express himself through language and to understand linguistic messages? Is there a significant discrepancy between language intake and output?

3) *Structural levels of language:* Is his disturbance more at a phonemic level (anarthria, phonemic paraphasias, phonemic jargon), at a lexical level (anomia, verbal paraphasias), or at a grammatico-syntactical level (agrammatism, paragrammatism)?

4) *Control of speech rate or automatisms:* Is the patient's speech reduced or fluent? Does it show *blocking* (anarthria, anomia, agrammatism) or *lack of control* (phonemic jargon, paraphasias, paragrammatism)? To what extent is automatic speech better than voluntary speech?

5) *Reading and writing:* How do they compare with oral language?

A detailed standard examination of aphasia and the performance scale of the WAIS is given to each patient in order to assess each of the preceding points. Assessment of points 3 and 4 in particular requires a careful evaluation of the qualitative aspects of speech. Information thus obtained is used by the therapist to enhance the patient's motivation and to choose and apply therapeutic exercises correctly.

Therapeutic exercises are viewed as a S-R situation in which the therapist is expected to elicit and consolidate a language response by giving stimuli and reinforcements. The following general rules are kept in mind:

1) Responses should be as "physiological," i.e. usable in real communication, as possible. In eliciting responses, facilitation is looked for along the lines of the Jacksonian automatic-voluntary dissociation. First, an automatic way to elicit a correct response is found, and the response is then tentatively elicited in more and more voluntary ways. Sometimes the patient may be taught to employ the facilitation intentionally as a compensatory roundabout way to get to a correct response by himself. However, the habit of using such artificial roundabout ways is not encouraged if it is felt that the subject will be able eventually to give physiological verbal responses, i.e. responses which are both highly intentional and highly automatic.

2) Stimuli and responses involve the lexical and grammatico-syntactic levels of language from the very beginning of therapy. Comprehension and expression of entire and meaningful words and sentences are stressed. Among exercises rehearsing specifically the phonemic level, only those requesting the discrimination and utterance of phonemes within meaningful words and sentences are permitted. Exercises involving the use of isolated phonemes are banned unless anarthria, agraphia or alexia are so complete as to require a rebuilding of the phonemic code itself. This is commonly the case with anarthria, where articulatory and oral apraxic disorders make it necessary to start teaching the articulation movements per se. Such atomistic exercises are abandoned as soon as possible.

3) The receptive and expressive aspects are both trained together, unless expression is far worse than comprehension (as in severe anarthria). Oral and written language are also drilled together, unless the patient has a global aphasia, in which case reading and writing may be included at the beginning of therapy only if they facilitate the use of oral language.

4) Finally, emphasis is placed on appropriate use and dosage of reinforcement. Since most exercises may be used for different purposes, reinforcement should vary accordingly and consistently. Right responses are always given a positive reinforcement; wrong ones are regularly given negative reinforcement only in patients with impaired control of speech, while in patients with expressive reduction and blocking they are sometimes better overlooked.

Characteristics of patients at the time of first examination

Figs. 35-1 and 35-2 show that at the time of the first examination the two groups were not significantly different with respect to *nature of lesion* (all but a few had a cerebral vasular accident), *sex* (all but a few were male), *type of aphasia*, and *time elapsed from onset.* On the other hand nR subjects were on the whole somewhat older and less educated than R subjects.

Fig. 35-2 also shows that there was no significant difference between the two groups with respect to time interval between first and second examination.

EVOLUTION OF APHASIC DISORDERS

In examining and discussing the data on the course of our patients' aphasia let us follow the order of the questions we set on page 373.

1) *Spontaneous evolution* is represented in Fig. 35-3a. The figure shows that there is a positive association between time flow and change of type of aphasia. Of our 27 nR patients, 15 were found to have changed between the 1st and 2nd examination, while 12 had not changed. Out of the 15 who had changed, 14 improved and 6 reached communication level, while only 1 deteriorated. The significance of change in the direction of improvement is very high ($p = .0007$ by the Sign test) which means that spontaneous evolution does exist and it is in the direction of improvement and restitution of function.

Fig. 35-3a also shows that patients who on 1st examination had a severe impairment of both expression and comprehension, and were

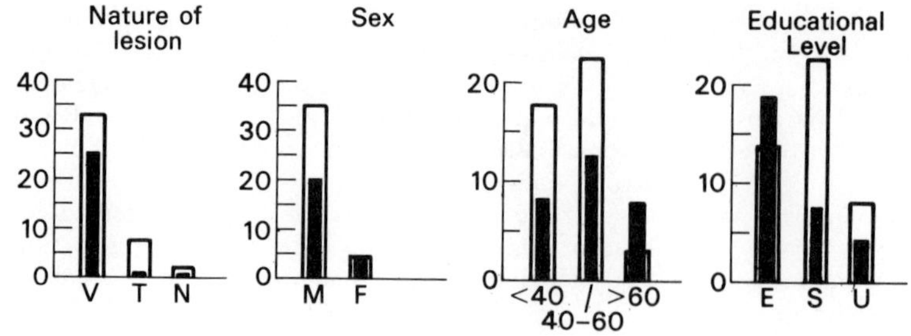

Fig. 35–1. V = vascular; T = traumatic; N = neoplastic. M = male; F = female. E = elementary (up to 6 years of school); S = secondary (7 to 13 years); U = university (over 13 years).
■ not reeducated
□ reeducated

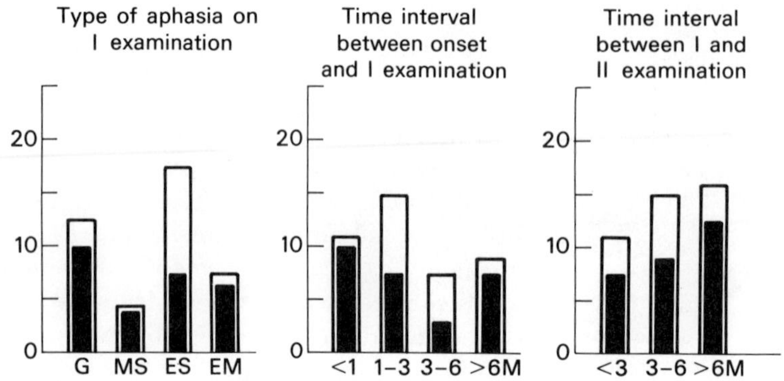

Fig. 35–2. G = global; MS = mixed, severe; ES = expressive, severe; EM = expressive, moderate. M = months.
■ not reeducated
□ reeducated

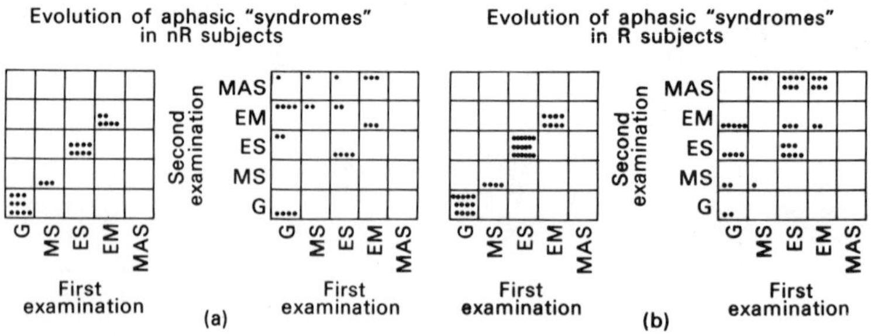

Fig. 35–3. G = global; MS = mixed, severe; ES = expressive, severe; EM = expressive, moderate; MAS = mild aphasic symptoms, not affecting communication; nR = not reeducated; R = reeducated.

therefore defined as having *global* aphasia or *mixed severe* aphasia, on 2nd examination were left with a severe impairment limited to the *expressive* side. This suggests that the receptive side clears up more than the expressive side during spontaneous evolution. In fact, a very definite trend seems to exist in the spontaneous evolution of aphasia in that the receptive side remains all the way along superior to the expressive. This trend is shown in Fig. 35-4a. On first examination, comprehension is preserved in more subjects than is expression; about 50 percent of patients are able to communicate on the receptive side, while all of them fall below communication level in expression. On second examination, overall recovery of communication appears to be more frequent on the receptive than on the expressive side.

Another interesting trend appears if the global E score is analyzed into the discrete D and N scores, as in Fig. 35-4b. The graph suggests that, within expression, naming is consistently better than description; and in fact, an examination of each individual record in the series discloses that N is always equal to or greater than D.

The evolution of oral language functions in R subjects shows a pattern which is quite similar to the pattern of spontaneous evolution (Figs. 35-3b and 35-5). Thus, the hypothesis that N would improve more (with respect to C and D) in R than in nR subjects, as a consequence of repeated naming drill involved in speech therapy, does not find confirmation in these

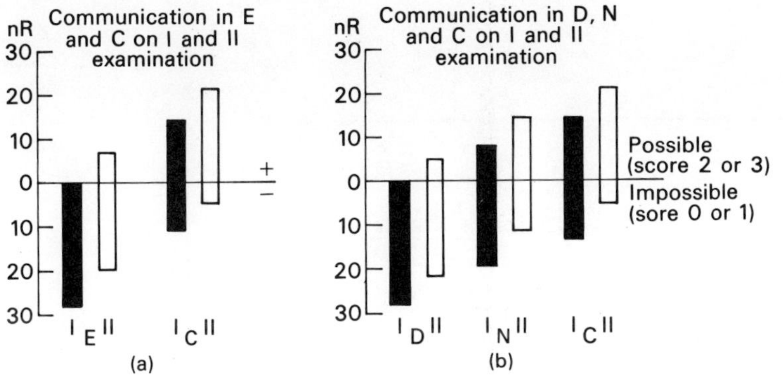

Fig. 35–4. Evolution pattern of oral language functions in not reeducated (nR) aphasics. E = oral expression (unified score); D = description; N = naming; C = auditory comprehension.
■ *1st examination*
□ *2nd examination*

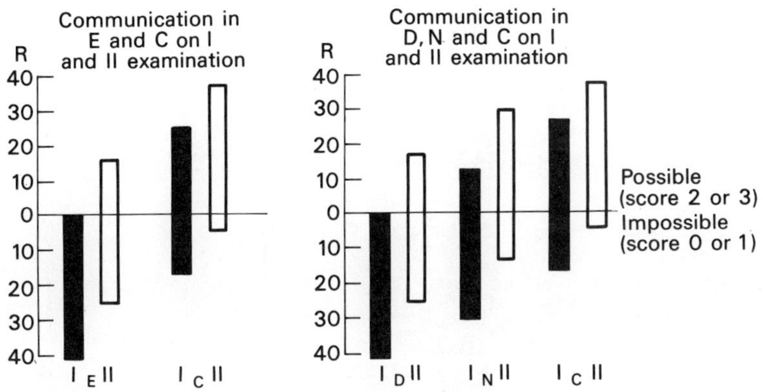

Fig. 35–5. Evolution pattern of oral language functions in reeducated (R) aphasics.
■ *1st examination*
□ *2nd examination*

data. Only one difference between R and nR patients with regard to the evolution pattern of language performance was found. The hypothesis was tested that comprehension not only recovers in more patients than does expression, but that it improves in every patient equally or more than expression. This was found to be true for nR subjects ($p=.031$ by the Sign test) but not for R subjects. This fact may perhaps suggest that reeducation tends to reduce the gap between expression and comprehension, which is maintained throughout spontaneous evolution.

It may be concluded that by and large aphasic disturbances of oral language tend to improve spontaneously and that auditory comprehension improves more than oral expression. In 1960 Leischner reported the outcome of a group of 46 reeducated aphasics, and reached the conclusion that mixed, global and sensory aphasias tend to become expressive aphasias. Our findings are strongly supportive of this view and show furthermore that the same general trend is present in the spontaneous evolution of aphasia.

2) and 3) The second and third questions concern possible effects on evolution of *a*) *factors other than reeducation,* and *b*) *reeducation itself.* They will be considered together. Limitations of our sample compel us to consider only the following five variables:

a) Age (less than 40; 40 to 60; more than 60 years old).

b) Time between onset and 1st examination (less than 2 months; from 2 to 6 months; more than 6 months).

c) Type of aphasia on 1st examination (G, MS, ES, EM).

d) Time between 1st and 2nd examination (less than 6 months, more than 6 months);

e) Reeducation (present or absent).

Table 35-3 gives a summary of the percentages of subjects who improved and of subjects who reached communication in the different classes of each variable. The information provided by this table is limited because it does

TABLE 35–3. STATUS OF APHASIC PATIENTS ON SECOND EXAMINATION

	Age (in years)			Time interval onset-1st exam. (in months)			Type of Aphasia on 1st exam.				Time 1st-2nd exam. (in months)		Reeducation (General)		Reeducation (Balanced)	
	<40	40-60	>60	<2	2-6	>6	G	MS	ES	EM	<6	>6	—	+	—	+
IMPROVED																
Reached communication level	10 *40*	11 *31.4*	1 *11.1*	16 *43.3*	4 *25*	2 *12.5*	1 *4.3*	4 *57.1*	8 *32*	9 *64.3*	10 *24.4*	12 *42.9*	6 *22.2*	16 *38.1*	6 *24*	14 *38.8*
Did not reach communication **level**	8 *32*	14 *40*	1 *11.1*	15 *40.5*	6 *37.5*	2 *12.5*	16 *69.6*	2 *28.6*	5 *20*	— —	14 *34.1*	9 *32.1*	9 *33.3*	14 *33.3*	8 *32*	11 *30.6*
Total number of improved subjects	18 *72*	25 *71.4*	2 *22.2*	31 *83.8*	10 *62.5*	4 *25*	17 *73.9*	6 *85.7*	13 *52*	9 *64.3*	24 *58.5*	21 *75*	15 *55.5*	30 *71.4*	14 *56*	25 *69.4*
UNCHANGED	7 *28*	10 *28.6*	7 *77.8*	6 *16.2*	6 *37.5*	12 *75*	6 *26.1*	1 *14.3*	12 *48*	5 *35.7*	17 *41.5*	7 *25*	12 *44.5*	12 *28.6*	11 *44*	11 *30.6*
Total number of subjects	25	35	9	37	16	16	23	7	25	14	41	28	27	42	25	36

N.B. 1) Percentages are indicated *in italics* and refer to each class.
2) The only subject who deteriorated is considered among unchanged subjects in this table.

not take into account interactions among variables. However, it may be convenient to take it as starting point for our exploration.

a) *Age.* Improvement appears to be much less frequent in old people than in young people. While more than 70 percent young patients improved and 40 percent reached communication level, out of 9 old patients only 2 (22.2 percent) improved and only 1 (11.1 percent) reached communication level. However, the two cases who did improve show that the outcome of aphasia in old age is not necessarily bad. In this connection, it is interesting to note that both of them were first examined within 2 months from onset. One was a 62-year-old MS with typical verbal paraphasias; he was not reeducated and evolved towards EM aphasia. The other one, a 70-year-old ES with anarthria, began training on the 15th day after stroke and recovered completely within 4 months, showing merely a residual dysprosodia on 2nd examination. These cases suggest that prognosis of aphasia in patients over sixty need not be pessimistic if, at the time of the examination, less than 2 months have elapsed from onset.

b) *Time interval between onset and 1st examination.* Table 35-3 shows that the percentage of subjects who improve decreases as the time interval from onset increases. Let us investigate if this influence is still apparent when the other factors are also considered. Figure 35-6 shows the combined influence of 3 factors on improvement: a) time between onset and 1st examination, b) time between 1st and 2nd examination, c) reeducation. Age and type of syndrome are not represented in the graph, but they will be taken into consideration during the discussion.

What first strikes us here is the sharp difference in improvement between nR subjects who were first examined within 2 months from onset and nR subjects who were first examined after 2 months. The overall difference between the two groups is highly significant ($p < .005$, by the Fisher exact probability test) and so it remains when the two groups are "equated" for age and types of aphasia ($p < .01$). The difference in improvement is still significant when all the patients—nR plus R—are considered, and all subjects first examined before 2 months from onset are compared to all subjects examined after 2 months from onset. (On the other hand, if the R group alone is considered, the difference between subjects examined before and after 2 months is never significant. This point will be further discussed when dealing with reeducation.)

Thus Figure 35-6 confirms that time elapsed from onset is a very important prognostic factor in aphasia. Moreover, it suggests that the end of the second month represents a turning point in the course of the disturbance. Indeed,

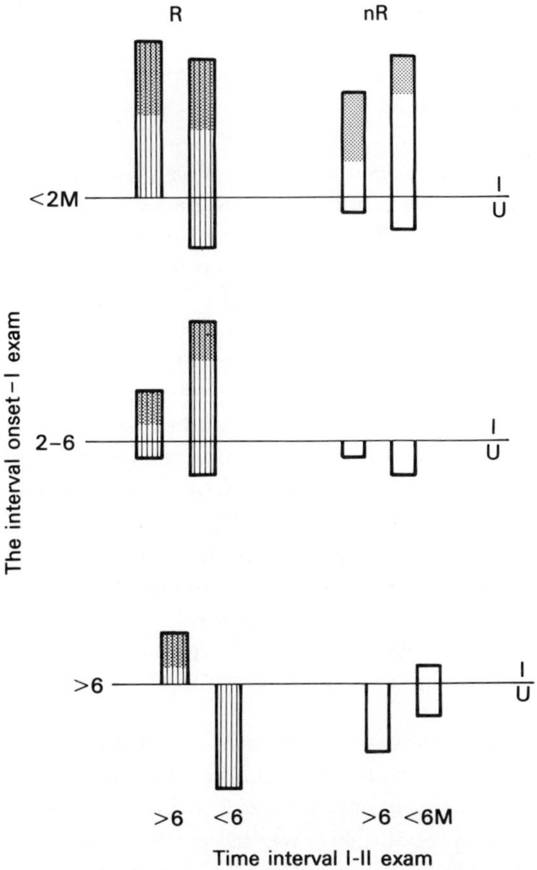

Fig. 35–6. Combined influence of a) time between onset and 1st examination, b) time between 1st and 2nd examination and c) reeducation on improvement.
U = unchanged; I = improved; × = recovered; M = months.

it appears as if any degree of spontaneous restitution could occur in subjects examined for the first time within two months from onset, no matter how severely affected they are. Some striking cases may illustrate this point. For instance, the one patient in the whole series who reached communication level starting from global aphasia with severe phonemic jargon belongs to this category. On the other hand, subjects taken after more than 2 months seem to have only limited possibilities of spontaneous recovery. It has been reported in previous work on the rehabilitation of aphasia that spontaneous evolution virtually ceases within 6 months from onset, and this is said to be particularly true for traumatic cases (Butfield and Zangwill, 1946). The above considerations, which are drawn from an almost exclusively non-traumatic series, suggest that a 2-months period be also taken into consideration in future research.

c) *Type of aphasia.* Table 35-3 shows among other things that all MS patients but one improved. This fact becomes interesting, when we recall that all MS patients were Wernicke's aphasics and that classically this syndrome is reported to have a particularly bad prognosis, because of severe impairment of the mechanism of auditory comprehension. Our data do not seem to support this view, and suggest that we further investigate the differential role of expressive and receptive deficits in evolution. The following questions may be asked:

1) Is overall recovery of oral communication limited more by impairment of expression or by impairment of comprehension?

2) Are there some specific aphasic symptoms, which have a particularly bad prognostic significance?

1) We have seen (Figure 35-4 and 35-5) that E is more frequently impaired than C on first examination and that it continues to be so during evolution; we have also seen that spontaneous improvement of C is significantly greater than spontaneous improvement of E. These facts indicate that overall recovery of oral communication is handicapped more by expressive than by receptive deficits. However, one might maintain that recovery of E is influenced by initial status of C; this contention may be expressed in the proposition that the speech of Wernicke's aphasia (with poor C) improves less than the speech of Broca's aphasia (with good C). In order to check this hypothesis, all subjects with equal level of E were considered, and improvement in E of those with poor C was compared with improvement in E of those with good C. Results shown in Figure 35-7 indicate that there is no significant difference between the two groups. In particular, there is no difference in expressive improvement between G and ES subjects, nor between MS and EM subjects. The Fisher exact probability test yields nonsignificant differences in all comparisons. The same is true with respect to number of patients who reached the level of communication in E. It is to be noted that the two groups in both comparisons are similar with respect to time elapsed from onset, so that one of the major factors probably affecting improvement is ruled out.

A provisional conclusion might be as follows: expressive disorders have poorer prognosis and much greater negative effect on overall recovery than do receptive disorders; moreover,

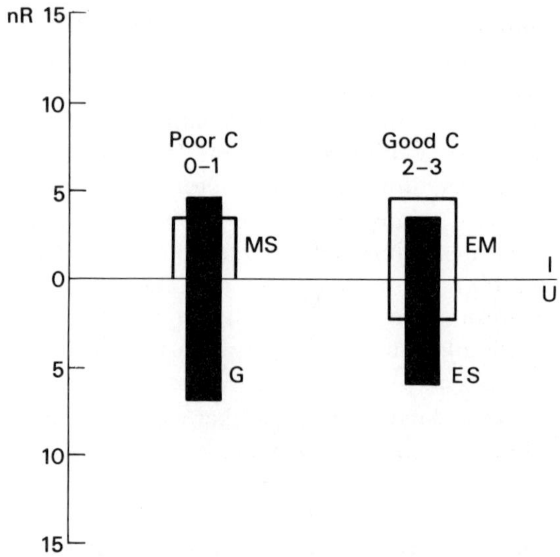

Fig. 35–7. Does initial level of C influence improvement of E?
■ E = 0 □ E = 1 or 2
I = improved U = unchanged

the initial level of comprehension does not seem to influence the evolution of expressive disorders; in particular, poor auditory comprehension does not prevent improvement of oral expression to take place. Therefore the factor limiting recovery of oral expression is to be found within expression itself.

2) Is there, then some expressive symptom specifically associated with limitation of recovery? Figure 35-7 shows that subjects with E = 0 improve significantly less frequently than subjects with E = 1 or 2. This would indicate that total inability to communicate through oral speech (on tests such as ours) is in itself a bad prognostic sign. However, the figure also shows that the prognostic value of this quantitative sign is not absolute, since about one-third of aphasics with E = 0 do show improvement in E. We recall that a score E = 0 may be obtained with different types of speech production, which only have in common absolute inadequacy for communication purposes. In particular, E = 0 may result from fluent as well as from reduced speech, and from disturbances at a phonemic level as well as at a lexical level. It is then possible that only one or some qualitative symptoms be endowed with strong negative prognostic value. On the basis of these considerations the hypothesis may be advanced that one specific expressive symptom, *anarthria*, be responsible for limiting expressive recovery. Anarthria is characterized by severe reduction in the flow of speech, marked phonemic disorders of expression—such as elisions or substitutions of phonemes—and articulatory difficulties, usually accompanied by oral apraxia. Thus defined, anarthria includes both speechlessness with recurring utterances and the "syndrome de désintégration phonétique" described by Alajouanine, Ombrédane and Durand in 1939; it leaves out, among other expressive syndromes, phonemic jargon on one side and anomia on the other.

In order to test the hypothesis, anarthric (AN) and non-anarthric (nAN) patients of the nR series are compared. As Figure 35-8 shows, the AN group shows a significantly smaller proportion of improved subjects than the nAN group, both in a general comparison (*a*) and

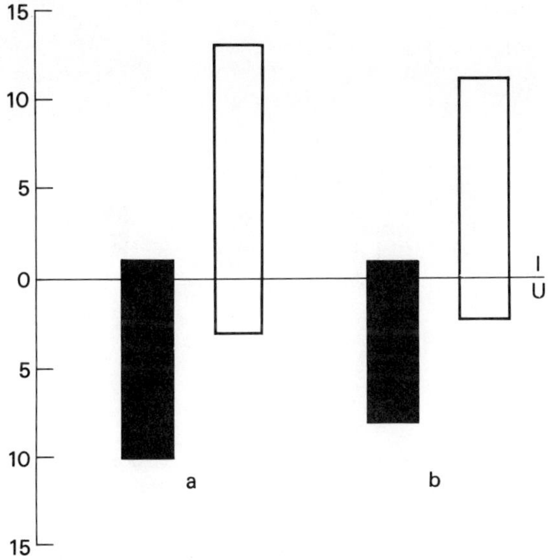

Fig. 35–8. Improvement of E and anarthria in nR Ss.
■ *anarthric patients* □ *non-anarthric patients*
I = improved U = unchanged

when the two series are equated with respect to age (*b*). The Fisher exact probability test yields a p = .005 in both instances. A similar comparison, where only subjects with E = 0 are considered, gives analogous results. The negative correlation shown by Figure 35-8 is very significant indeed, and highly supportive of the hypothesis that anarthria is a bad prognostic sign. However, the question is still open; indeed, a more careful scrutiny discloses that all nR AN patients but two were first examined after over 2 months from onset, while all nR nAN patients but one were first examined after less than 2 months from onset. This association is really unfortunate, because it leaves the question whether lack of improvement in these patients is really due to anarthria or to time elapsed from onset or to both factors. Additional information on this question is obtained by comparing AN and nAN subjects in the R group, where they are equally distributed in terms of time interval from onset. Four comparisons are made, as represented in Figure 35-9: *a* is a general comparison; in *b* subjects are matched in age, time elapsed from onset and length of therapy; in *c* only patients first seen after more than 2 months from onset

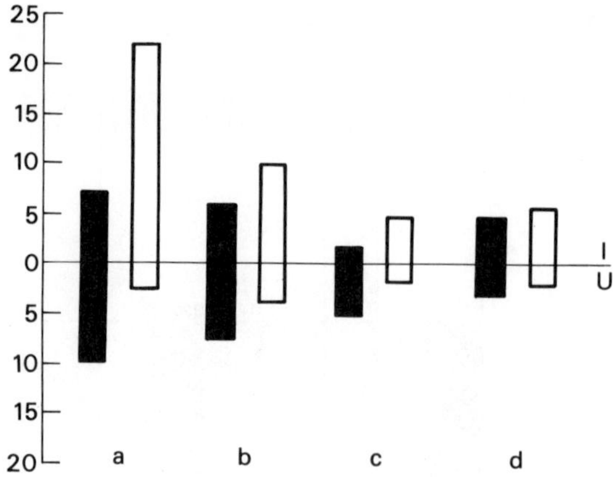

Fig. 35–9. Improvement of E and anarthria in R Ss.
■ *anarthric patients* □ *non-anarthric patients*
I = improved U = unchanged

are considered; and in *d* the patients are limited to those first seen within 2 months from onset. It is interesting to observe that a differential—although not significant—trend towards minor improvement in AN patients as compared to nAN patients is consistently present in comparisons *a, b* and *c,* but does not appear in *d.* I think that these data may be tentatively interpreted as follows: anarthria has a limiting effect on improvement of expressive oral language; however, its negative prognostic significance is great only if more than 2 months have elapsed from the date of onset, while it becomes much weaker in patients examined before that time.

Summing up, there are hints that anarthria has a negative influence on recovery of expression, but we cannot demonstrate it unequivocally because we cannot isolate anarthria from other variables (time from onset, in particular). From a practical point of view it may be interesting to add that anarthria in patients first seen more than 2 months after onset makes their prognosis significantly poorer than that of all other aphasics where such association is lacking; while absence of anarthria in patients first examined within 2 months makes their prognosis significantly more optimistic.

d) *Time between 1st and 2nd examination.* One might expect the frequency and degree of improvement to be greater in patients who are allowed more than 6 months to evolve, than in patients checked after a shorter time interval. However, the differences shown in Table 35-3 are not significant. On the other hand, Figure 35-6 clearly suggests that the length of the period of time over which evolution is considered (less or more than 6 months) has a differential effect on improvement only when more than 6 months have elapsed between the onset of aphasia and the beginning of such a period, and when reeducation takes place during it.

e) *Reeducation.* Table 35-3 shows that a general comparison between R and nR subjects with respect to improvement is not significant nor is a comparison when the two groups are balanced with respect to all other variables. However, a trend towards greater improvement and frequency of recovery in the R group is apparent in both comparisons.

Why is this difference not significant? It may be that rehabilitation has no influence on improvement or that its effects are too subtle to be assessed through our methods of examination and with our limited material. But it is also possible that our definition of reeducation is too broad and includes patients who were not actually reeducated long enough. If we take only subjects reeducated for more than 6 months and compare their evolution with that of patients reeducated for less than 6 months, we find (Figure 35-10) that frequency of improvement is significantly greater in the first group. This holds true also when the two groups are balanced in terms of time from onset and age. An overall comparison between R and nR patients checked more than 6 months after the first examination also shows a much higher frequency of improvement in the R group. Moreover, importance of length of reeducation is particularly evident in Figure 35-6, which suggests that a training period lasting more than 6 months has a decisive influence on aphasics who come for rehabilitation after more than 6 months from onset. All these data, however incomplete, seem to indicate that training extending over at least 6 months *is* effective.

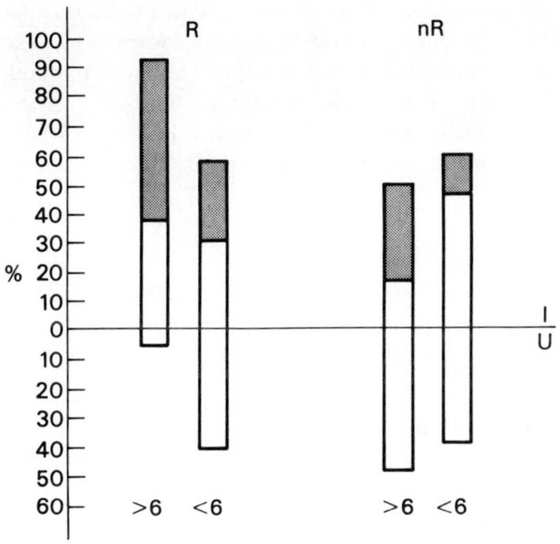

Fig. 35–10. Influence of length of reeducation on improvement.
U = unchanged I = improved ■ = recovered

Figure 35-6 also suggests that reeducation has different effects on recent and long-standing aphasia. Comparisons between R and nR patients in this figure disclose that 1) the great majority of R subjects who were first seen before 2 months do improve but so do the majority of nR patients; 2) subjects taken between 2 and 3 months do not improve unless they are reeducated; 3) subjects taken after more than 6 months do not improve unless they are reeducated for over 6 months[2]. Thus it seems that patients whose treatment starts early after onset have a better prognosis; however, the specific effects of reeducation appear more evidently in patients whose treatment starts after that date. It looks as if the potentiality for spontaneous recovery were so great in recent aphasia as to conceal the presumably positive effects of reeducation; on the contrary, so little potentiality seems to be left in old aphasia as to almost prevent reeducation from making any difference at all. Only the period which extends from 2 to 6 months after the onset of aphasia seems to provide a ground where intrinsic capacity for recovery can be highly enhanced by the intervention of planned training.

Our series gives us no hints as to a possible differential influence of reeducation on one type of aphasia rather than another. From a practical point of view it may be interesting, however, to point out one symptom which, in our experience, has a good prognostic value in R patients. This is the characteristic which French authors call "conduites d'approche," and that occurs whenever a patient with word-finding difficulties makes repeated attempts to find the right formulation of a word, and in so doing produces a series of utterances which are phonemic variations of the word he is looking for. Six of our R patients showed this sign as a major characteristic of their oral expression on 1st examination and all of them reached communication level.

[2] In the group of nR patients first examined after more than 6 months and then checked more than 6 months later, one subject did improve; it should be noted, however, that the only patient who deteriorated also belonged to this group.

SUMMARY AND CONCLUSIONS

A retrospective inquiry on the evolution of disturbances of oral communication in 69 aphasic patients suggests that the following points are worth taking into consideration as hypotheses for future research:

1) Disturbances of oral expression and comprehension in aphasia undergo spontaneous evolution in the direction of recovery of function.

2) The receptive aspect tends to improve more than the expressive aspect. Expressive disturbances are more important than receptive disturbances in preventing restitution of overall verbal communication.

3) Improvement of oral expression is not influenced by the initial level of auditory comprehension.

4) On the other hand, there are hints that anarthria has a significant retarding effect on recovery of expression.

5) Time elapsed from onset is an important prognostic factor: 2 and 6 months from onset seem to be important milestones in the progress of aphasia.

6) Reeducation has a specific effect provided that it lasts more than 6 months. Its influence seems decisive in patients examined for the first time in the period between 2 and 6 months from onset.

Acknowledgments. I am greatly indebted to Mrs. Anna Micheli Basso, whose retraining work with the patients made this study possible. I also wish to thank Dr. Gino Pizzamiglio for his participation in the collection of data and Prof. Arthur L. Benton for his valuable advice on the manuscript.

REFERENCES

Alajouanine, Th., Ombrédane, A., and Durand, M. (1939) *Le Syndrome de Désintégration Phonétique dans l'Aphasie.* Masson, Paris.

Butfield, E., and Zangwill, O. L. (1946) *Re-education in aphasia: a review of* 70 *cases*, "J. Neurol. Neurosurg. Psychiat.," **9,** 75–79.

Leischner, A. (1960) *Zur Symptomatologie und Therapie der Aphasien*, "Nervenarzt," **31,** 60–67.

Luria, A. R. (1963) *Restoration of Function after Brain Injury*, Pergamon Press, Oxford.

Siegel, S. (1956) *Non Parametric Statistics for the Behavioral Sciences.* McGraw-Hill, New York.

Taylor, M. L. (1964) *A measurement of functional communication in aphasia.* Paper presented at the American Academy of Physical Medicine and Rehabilitation, Boston, August 24, 1964 (unpublished).

Vignolo, L. A. *Afasia.* Chapter in Terapia Fisica e Riabilitazione, ed. by P. Farneti, Wassermann, Milano (in press).

Wepman, J. M. (1951) *Recovery from Aphasia.* The Ronald Press, New York.

36

The Relationship between Self-Correction and Recovery from Aphasia

JOSEPH M. WEPMAN

JOSEPH M. WEPMAN, Ph. D., is with the department of psychology and is director of the Speech and Language Clinic of the University of Chicago.

In 1937, Piotrowski (*4*) reported the isolation of various indicators of brain pathology on Rorschach protocols. Subsequently, other researchers using the same projective test failed to confirm the consistency of appearance of all of Piotrowski's indicators, while attesting to the confirmation of others (*1*, *3*). Prominent in the confirmed signs was the one Piotrowski called "impotence" (*2*, *4*). Baker (*2*) in her discussion of this sign said, "Impotence (the giving of a response in spite of the recognition of its inadequacy, together with the inability to withdraw or improve it) . . . is one of the best signs for moderate and severe damage, probably because feelings of insecurity and inferiority become complicated with appreciable intellectual deficit." Without becoming presently involved with Baker's psychological interpretation of its cause, the fact of the existence of in most brain-injured aphasic patient's language of an "impotence" factor should be recognized. It is with this factor and its implications that the present communication is concerned.

The ability to recognize and self-correct errors made in language production which is a commonplace in the behavior of the unimpaired speaker or writer is defective to some degree in almost every aphasic adult patient. The severity of the defect and its effect upon the patient is felt to be one of the last indicators of the extent of the language problem. The time it takes a particular patient to move from one level of the ability to self-correct to another is felt to be an excellent indicator of the prognosis for the patient.

Personal observations made over the past two decades on aphasic patients of all types point to the factor of self-criticism as one of the primary goals recognized by patients in language therapy. Many such patients have indicated that their difficulty in recognizing and in correcting the errors they make represents to them the aphasic difficulty they are having. They tend to look upon this problem as being the language impairment itself. Only as they see themselves improving in their capacity to be self-critical can they see themselves as functioning independently in language production. The possible usefulness of this observation in aphasia therapy will be commented upon later.

Disturbances in the ability to self-correct can be viewed along a continuum. At one extreme would be those patients who cannot recognize their own errors and cannot correct them when they are pointed out; at the other extreme would be those who can and do recognize their errors and who correct them spontaneously. It is the movement through this continuum that seems of such importance to rehabilitation. The failure to move from one level to another is thought to be a bad prognostic sign, while

From *Journal of Speech and Hearing Disorders* 23:302–05, 1958.

speed of movement should be a good sign for recovery.

As an illustration, consider two patients. One at the time of his initial evaluation makes many errors of substitution, fails to recognize them and correct them when the examiner points them out to him. After a period of time in therapy he seems able to repeat a few more words, may even substitute somewhat less often, but is still unable to recognize or correct errors as he speaks or writes. It is felt that as long as this condition exists, the chance of independent, spontaneous use of meaningful communication for this patient must be held seriously in question. A second patient who comes to therapy in essentially the same condition, but who begins to recognize his errors and who recovers some ability to make corrections when these and other errors are called to his attention must be considered a much better risk. For, in essence, this patient is approaching the behavior of the unimpaired speaker—he is able to reject errors of production—he is able to be self-critical to some degree.

While it is felt that the degree of loss in the capacity to self-correct at the time of an original evaluation of an aphasic patient is an indication of the severity of the problem faced by the patient, it has not been found that the degree of difficulty correlates with any eventual level of recovery. Rather, the degree of loss in this capacity indicates only the distance the patient must go before he can be said to be a recovered aphasic patient. The speed with which he passes through the various stages of self-correction is felt to be a better indicator of his prognosis. Thus, a patient who begins his therapy at a very low level, but who succeeds in rather rapid order in going from one stage to another is likely to be the more successful patient. While in contrast the patient who begins at a somewhat higher original level, but who fails to make much change in his ability to be self-critical is likely to plateau and reach a lower level of eventual spontaneous language.

To assist the aphasia therapist in objectifying his observations on language impotence as here described, the writer constructed the following eight-point scale:

Level 1. Fails to recognize errors made in any modality. Cannot recognize errors when they are pointed out and therefore cannot correct them.

Level 2. Fails to recognize errors in any modality. Can recognize them when they are pointed out, but cannot correct them.

Level 3. Fails to recognize errors in *either* speech or writing. Can recognize errors when pointed out, but cannot correct them.

Level 4. Fails to recognize errors in *either* speech or writing. Can recognize the errors when pointed out and can correct them with assistance.

Level 5. Recognizes errors made in *both* speech and writing. Cannot correct them without assistance.

Level 6. Recognizes errors in *both* speech and writing. Can correct errors in one without assistance, but not in both.

Level 7. Recognizes errors made in *both* speech and writing. Can correct them without assistance most of the time but only with considerable effort and even then with some mistakes.

Level 8. Recognizes errors made in both speech and writing. Corrects them easily without assistance. May subvocalize as a means of self-correction before exposing his speech efforts.

While the scale was originally intended only as a method for structuring the problem, it is readily seen that the eight levels represent a hierarchy from mild to severe disturbance. No attempt has been made to make the steps of the scale equidistant. Undoubtedly intermediate stages could be described between each level. However, most aphasic patients can be placed somewhere on the scale and notations relative to change over time are relatively easily made. Because of this, the scale seems to have a potential use as a research tool, since it provides the numerical base for consideration of change which is so necessary in comparison studies either in longitudinal studies of single cases or in patient-to-patient research designs.

This potential as a research tool was something of an unlooked for by-product of the scale. If empirical data is forthcoming which confirms the thesis of the present paper, then aphasia research should benefit. Researchers into the processes underlying recovery from aphasia will have at hand a quantifiable criterion for estimating change over time, the rapidity of such change, the tendency toward plateauing, the tendency toward regression and other important factors about which so little is presently known. The difficulty of obtaining such data because of the complexity and breadth of the language act has always been a major deterrant to obtaining such knowledge. Some of the relationships between self-correction and the stimulus-response patterns of aphasic patients are now being studied and will be reported upon completion (*5*, *6*).

Some patients have been approached in therapy almost solely from the viewpoint of improvement in self-correction. This has been possible only with patients who have some recognition of their difficulty in communication. By using this outside criterion of improvement, rather than the intermittent or uneven function of the language act itself, a greater degree of motivation and independence seems to be obtained at a much earlier time in therapy. It places the process of recovery on a self-help basis, on the patient and his efforts rather than on the therapist. This involvement of the patient in his own recovery, in gauging his own changes and in working toward language-usage goals rather than word production has been found to be extremely beneficial in many instances. Some care must be exercised in the selection of patients for the method since it may bring on a greater recognition of the extent of a language problem than a particular patient can accept. This may produce some withdrawal or more anxiety about recovery. Most such difficulties can be avoided, however, by introducing the idea of self-correction slowly and insisting on it only as the individual patient seems able to accept it.

SUMMARY

One of the more commonly seen psychological signs of brain-injury, called "impotence" by Piotrowski (*4*) from his study of Rorschach protocols, has been found to be of value in describing the language behavior of such patients. Its importance as an indicator of success in therapy and a method by which it can be objectified for use as a diagnostic and prognostic tool as well as in research has been presented. It is hoped that the research mentioned concerning the relationship of self-correction to other responses on aphasia tests will shed some empirical light on what has been up to now only a clinical observation (*5*, *6*). The writer offers the scale for anyone's use in diagnosis, therapy or research, hoping it will bring some further order to this very complex field of aphasia.

REFERENCES

1. Aita, J. A., Reitan, R. M. and Ruth, J. M., Rorschach's Test as a diagnostic aid in brain injury. *Amer. J. Psychiat.*, **103,** 1947, 770–779.
2. Baker, G., Diagnosis of organic brain damage in the adult. In Klopfer *et al.*, *Developments in the Rorschach Technique*. Yonkers, N. Y.: World Book Co., 1956.
3. Kelley, D. M. and Margulies, H., Rorschach case studies in the convulsive states. *Rorschach Res. Exch.* **4,** 1940, 157–190.
4. Piotrowski, Z., The Rorschach inkblot method in organic disturbances of the central nervous system. *J. nerv. ment. Dis.*, **86,** 1937, 527–537.
5. Wepman, J. M. and Jones, L. V., Stimulus-response relationships in the residual language of aphasic adults. Research supported in part by Neurological Diseases and Blindness Study Section, U.S. Public Health Service, Grant No. B 710.
6. Wepman, J. M. and Jones, L. V., The production and demonstration of a primary language abilities test for aphasia. Investigation supported in part by special Project Grant (S-168 A), OVR, Department of Health, Education and Welfare.

37

Electroencephalographic Findings and Recovery from Aphasia

RONALD S. TIKOFSKY
KENNETH A. KOOI
MADISON H. THOMAS

RONALD S. TIKOFSKY, M.D., is with the departments of psychology and of speech at the University of Michigan, Ann Arbor.

KENNETH A. KOOI, M.D., is chief of the EEG Laboratory of the departments of neurology and psychiatry at the University of Michigan, Ann Arbor.

MADISON H. THOMAS, M.D., is director of the EEG Department at the LDS Hospital, Salt Lake City, with the department of psychiatry at the University of Utah College of Medicine, and consultant in neurology at Utah and Wyoming State Hospitals.

Although many authors have described abnormal electroencephalographic patterns in patients with aphasia (*1–8*), the possible prognostic value of the electroencephalogram for recovery of speech has not been formally recognized. A measure to aid in estimating the ultimate prognosis of aphasic patients would be of value in planning the direction of treatment, estimating duration of treatment, and predicting the possibilities for economic and social rehabilitation of these individuals. The finding of Van Buskirk and Zarling (*9*) that electroencephalographic patterns are related to the course of rehabilitation in vascular hemiplegia permits speculation that progress in speech therapy might be similarly related.

As part of their neurologic study, many of the aphasic patients undergoing speech therapy at the Veterans Administration and Salt Lake City General hospitals were examined electroencephalographically. Preliminary evaluation of the electroencephalograms of these patients suggested that electroencephalographic patterns might relate to the patient's improvement in speech. From gross clinical observations, it appeared that the most fruitful electroencephalographic patterns to explore would be the background frequencies and the over-all delta incidence of each hemisphere.

From *Neurology* 10:154–56, 1960.

PROCEDURE

A total of 33 adult aphasic patients who had received speech therapy for periods of two months to two years was divided into "no progress" and "fair to good progress' groups. Progress was determined by an examination of the therapy records compiled by the speech therapists who had worked with the patients. Patients who demonstrated definite and consistent improvement in any of the language areas found to be impaired in the initial speech examination were placed in the "fair to good progress" group.

Patients who demonstrated either little or no improvement in the language areas found to be impaired in the initial speech examination were placed in the "no progress" group. Of the 16 patients who were in the "no progress" group, 14 had a diagnosis of cerebrovascular accident and 2, posttraumatic encephalopathy; of the 17 in the "fair to good progress" group, 10 had a diagnosis of cerebrosvascular accident, 6, posttraumatic encephalopathy, and 1, focal encephalitis. Average age of the patients in the "no progress" group was 56 with a range of 34 to 69 years; average age of the patients in the "fair to good progress" group was 42 with a range of 23 to 64.

All of the subjects were given electroencephalographic examinations before or early in the course of speech therapy. The electroencephalographic recordings were made on a Grass Model III D electroencephalograph, using both scalp to scalp and scalp to ear combinations; 8 electrodes were placed on each side of the head in the frontal, lower premotor, anterior temporal, midtemporal, posterior temporal, central, lateral parietal, and occipital positions.

The analysis of the electroencephalographic records was based on the frequency of cerebral patterns and their relative incidence and location. The dominant occipital frequency for each hemisphere was determined from epochs characterized by well developed rhythmic activity. This was recorded to the nearest 0.5 cps. Frequencies above 8.5 cps and below 13 cps were considered to fall within the normal alpha range.

A delta incidence score for each of the electrodes was obtained in the following manner: a score of "3" was given for a particular electrode if episodic slow wave activity within the frequency range of 0.5 to 3 cps occurred more than 66 percent of the time, "2" if this type of episodic activity occurred 33 to 66 percent of the time; and "1" if this activity occurred 33 percent of the time or less or if only 4- to 7-cps slow wave activity was present. The sum of the scores for all 8 electrodes for the right or left hemisphere was considered as the subject's over-all delta incidence for that hemisphere. Electroencephalograms and speech therapy records were evaluated independently.

RESULTS

The number of patients with dominant patterns above and below 8.5 cps in the 2 therapy progress groups are indicated in Table 37-1. Patterns below 8.5 cps were usual in those aphasic patients who made no significant progress during therapy. The prognosis was very poor in those patients with an abnormally slow pattern over the *right* hemisphere, as well as the left. The differences between the average basic frequencies over each hemisphere for the "no" and "fair to good" progress groups were highly significant (right hemisphere, $t = 4.2$, $p < 0.01$; left hemisphere, $t = 2.8$, $p < 0.01$). Similar "t" values were obtained when only those patients in the 2 groups with cerebral vascular accidents were compared (right hemisphere, $t = 4.1$, $p < 0.01$; left hemisphere, $t = 2.3$, $p < 0.05$).

The 2 groups of patients were also compared with regard to the degree of over-all hemispheric delta incidence. The "t's" were not significant at the 0.05 level of confidence for either hemisphere (right hemisphere, $t = 0.41$; left hemisphere, $t = 1.75$).

TABLE 37-1. PROGRESS IN SPEECH THERAPY RELATED TO ELECTROENCEPHALOGRAPHIC BASIC FREQUENCY

	No progress		*Fair to good progress*	
Dominant frequency	*Hemisphere Left*	*Right*	*Hemisphere Left*	*Right*
8.5 cps and above	3	4	11	16
Below 8.5 cps	13	11	6	1
Totals	16	15*	17	17

*Pattern on right not classifiable in 1 case.

DISCUSSION

The results presented above suggest that the electroencephalogram may give information of predictive value relative to recovery from aphasia. The basic frequency appears to be an important prognostic index, good recovery being the rule (12 of 13 cases) with frequencies within the alpha range and rare (1 of 12 cases) with frequencies below the alpha range over both hemispheres. When the basic frequency was below 8.5 cps over the left hemisphere only, partial recovery was frequent (5 of 7 cases). Lesser delta incidence and areal spread over the left hemisphere were also correlated with good recovery from aphasia, although the relationship was not high. Thus, left hemisphere delta activity should receive only minor weight as an indication of poor prognosis, occasional patients being seen who do well in therapy even in the face of a moderate to marked delta wave hemispheric abnormality. The higher correlation between relearning speech and right hemisphere basic frequency is intriguing and suggests the possibility of an as yet undefined role for the non-dominant hemisphere in recovery from aphasia.

Perhaps these findings also require a re-evaluation of the functional or behavioral criteria of prognosis. It is essential to recognize that aphasia is, by definition, a symptom of brain damage. Up to the time of the present study, no measures of physiologic function of the brains of aphasics have been employed as a prognostic device. The present findings suggest that certain characteristics of the brain damage, as reflected in the electroencephalogram, are important variables that partially determine the course of recovery. It is desirable to utilize this information, in addition to evaluation of the "premorbid personality," and other qualitative means of evaluating the patient's history and test results. The electroencephalographic data do not supplant other means of predicting the success of therapy but constitute an integral part of the overall evaluation of the patient.

SUMMARY AND CONCLUSIONS

A sample of 33 adult aphasic subjects who had received speech therapy for a period ranging from two months to two years was divided into 2 groups, those who made no progress and those who made fair to good progress in therapy. Electroencephalographic recordings for each of the subjects were made before or early in the course of the subject's therapy. Their recordings were analyzed in terms of the background frequencies for each hemisphere and delta distribution and incidence over the left and right hemispheres. The results of the statistical analyses indicated relationships between the elctroencephalographic variables and recovery. Poor progress was usual when patients exhibited abnormally slow electroencephalographic patterns. A comparison of the basic frequencies of the right hemispheres differentiated the "no progress" and "fair to good progress" groups better than those of the left hemisphere, although both were highly statistically significant.

It is concluded that there is strong evidence to suggest that subjects with slow background electroencephalographic frequencies may do poorly in speech therapy, particularly if both hemispheres are involved. A left hemisphere delta focus, however, is not inconsistent with a good prognosis.

REFERENCES

1. Marinesco, G., Sager, O., and Kreindler, A.: Etudes électroencéphalographiques; électroencéphalogrammes dans l'aphasie. Bull. Acad. de Méd., Paris, **116**:182, 1936.
2. ——, ——, ——, L'électroencéphalogramme dans certain états pathologiques. Presse méd., **46**:650, 1938.
3. Sager, O., and Kreindler, A.: L'électroencéphalogramme dans l'aphasie. Bull. Acad. méd. Roumanie, **29**:569, 1947.
4. Cohn, R., Raines, G. N., Mulder, D. W., and Neumann, M. A.: Cerebral vascular lesions; electroencephalographic and neuropathologic correlations. Arch. Neurol. & Psychiat., **60**:165, 1948.
5. Strauss, H., and Greentstein, L.: The electro-

encephalogram in cerebrovascular disease. Arch. Neurol. & Psychiat., **59**:395, 1948.

6. Weinstein, E. A., Kahn, R. L., and Strauss, H.: Correlation of clinical and EEG abnormalities in tumors and vascular disease of the brain. Tr. Am. Neurol. A., **75**:277, 1950.
7. Jones, E. V., Jr., and Bagchi, B. K.: Electroencephalographic findings in verified thrombosis of major cerebral arteries (14 cases). Univ. Michigan M. Bull., **17**:295, 1951.
8. Roseman, E., Schmidt, R. P., and Foltz, E. L.: Serial electroencephalography in vascular lesions of the brain. Neurology, **2**:311, 1952.
9. Van Buskirk, C., and Zarling, V. R.: EEG prognosis in vascular hemiplegia rehabilitation. Arch. Neurol. & Psychiat., **65**:732, 1951.

38

Long-Term Assessment of Language Function in Aphasia Due to Stroke

ELAINE S. SANDS
MARTHA TAYLOR SARNO
DONALD P. SHANKWEILER

ELAINE S. SANDS, M.S., is with the department of speech pathology and audiology at Adelphi University, Garden City.
MARTHA TAYLOR SARNO, M.A., is director of the speech pathology service of the Institute of Rehabilitation Medicine, New York University Medical Center, and is with the department of rehabilitation medicine of the New York University School of Medicine.
DONALD P. SHANKWEILER, Ph.D., is with the department of linguistics of the University of Connecticut.
The work reported in this paper was supported in part by the Social and Rehabilitation Service, Department of Health, Education, and Welfare, under the designation of New York University as a Rehabilitation Research and Training Center.

Careful study of the course of language recovery following stroke or traumatic injury to the brain is an important requirement for assessing the effects of treatment and ought to be a primary concern of the rehabilitation center dealing with aphasic patients. Speech pathologists must frequently make the decision to accept or reject an aphasic patient for treatment (*1*). At present adequate guidelines do not exist for making such a decision, because, except in extreme cases, we do not know enough to predict which patients will recover significantly and which ones will improve little. Although some studies report the language changes observed during the course of therapy (*2, 3*), few investigators have extended their observations over a long period of time. Few have examined the changes, if any, which occur following discharge (*4*), so little can be said about the changes that might reasonably be anticipated in the second and third year following the occurrence of the damage.

It is widely assumed that little further gain can be expected after the first year, and some rehabilitation workers suspect that aphasic patients may not even retain their achieved level of language function following the termination of therapy. In our experience, however, the patient and his family often report gradual improvement over a period of several years. Obviously this question must be submitted to a carefully controlled inquiry (*3, 5*). The problems of accurately describing the course of recovery in relation to whether therapy is given, when it is begun, and how long it is continued are too important to be left to casual observation and hearsay.

This paper will present the findings in 30 aphasic patients who received speech therapy daily and were followed from 4 months to 1 year after treatment was terminated. The duration of treatment ranged from 2 weeks to 2 years and 8 months. We realize that this study of so few

From *Archives of Physical Medicine and Rehabilitation* 50:202-07, 1969.

cases cannot answer the questions we have raised. However, we believe that the questions themselves need analysis and discussion and that our tentative findings are of interest to those concerned with stroke.

MEASUREMENT OF LANGUAGE FUNCTION

One of the major obstacles to the systematic study of the recovery of language has been the lack of means of measuring language function with adequate sensitivity to small changes (*3*). One of us (M. T. S.) has developed a measure which seems to sample skills most significant for daily living and is sufficiently sensitive to detect even small changes in function. The Functional Communication Profile (*6*), which we will call the FCP, was used for measuring residual language function in this study.

The FCP (Figure 38-1) consists of 45 nine-point rating scales, which yield part-scores for five broad language and language-related categories: movement, speaking, understanding, reading, and a miscellaneous category which includes writing and calculation. An overall score reflects the sum of the weighted part scores[1] and can be used as a single measure of an individual's communicative effectiveness, where 100 percent represents the estimated premorbid communication proficiency which, of course, varies from person to person. Therefore, an overall score of 62 percent for example, indicates that a given aphasic patient is performing at 62 percent of his estimated premorbid communication level.

Since the FCP is intended to assess functional language by informal interaction with the patient and his family in a conversational situation, its rationale differs markedly from tests which elicit verbal responses to standard tasks. FCP scores, may therefore, more directly reflect actual functional capacities than measures obtained through test responses. However, there is a high degree of statistical agreement between FCP scores and standard aphasia test batteries (*8*). A recent study that examined the interexaminer reliability of the FCP concluded that when used in a setting where the frame of reference is similar, the FCP possesses a high degree of reliability. The FCP scale forces examiners to relate the realities of daily language requirements to observed residual language function.

Many variables had to be considered which might influence the recovery outcome (*1, 5*). The relationship of overall language progress to age, time elapsed before beginning treatment, time in treatment, amount of treatment, and severity of impairment at onset, were considered important variables. In the group of patients studied nearly half had passed the most dramatic phase of spontaneous recovery —or, the first 3 months, before therapy was begun.

FCP scores were collected on at least three occasions including the initial evaluation prior to beginning treatment, at discharge, and at subsequent reevaluation. These scores were examined in relation to the variables mentioned above.

RESULTS

The median length of speech therapy for the 30 patients was 7.5 months. The median overall gain in language function for the whole group as measured by the FCP, was 10 percentage points. In the interval between the discharge from treatment and reevaluation (median 13 months), the group gained an average of 5 percent. Thus from the time of beginning treatment to the follow-up reevaluation, there was a gain of 15 percent, modest, but surely significant. Examining the upper and lower sixths of the total group, we find that those who improved most achieved an average gain of 36 percent whereas those who experienced the least change gained an average of 4 percent on the FCP (Figure 38-2). Of the total group of 30 patients, 27 showed some measured improvement whereas 3 remained the samc or regressed.

[1] The weights are proportional to factor loadings on a single common factor which accounted for 95 percent of the total variance in the total set of items (*6, 7*).

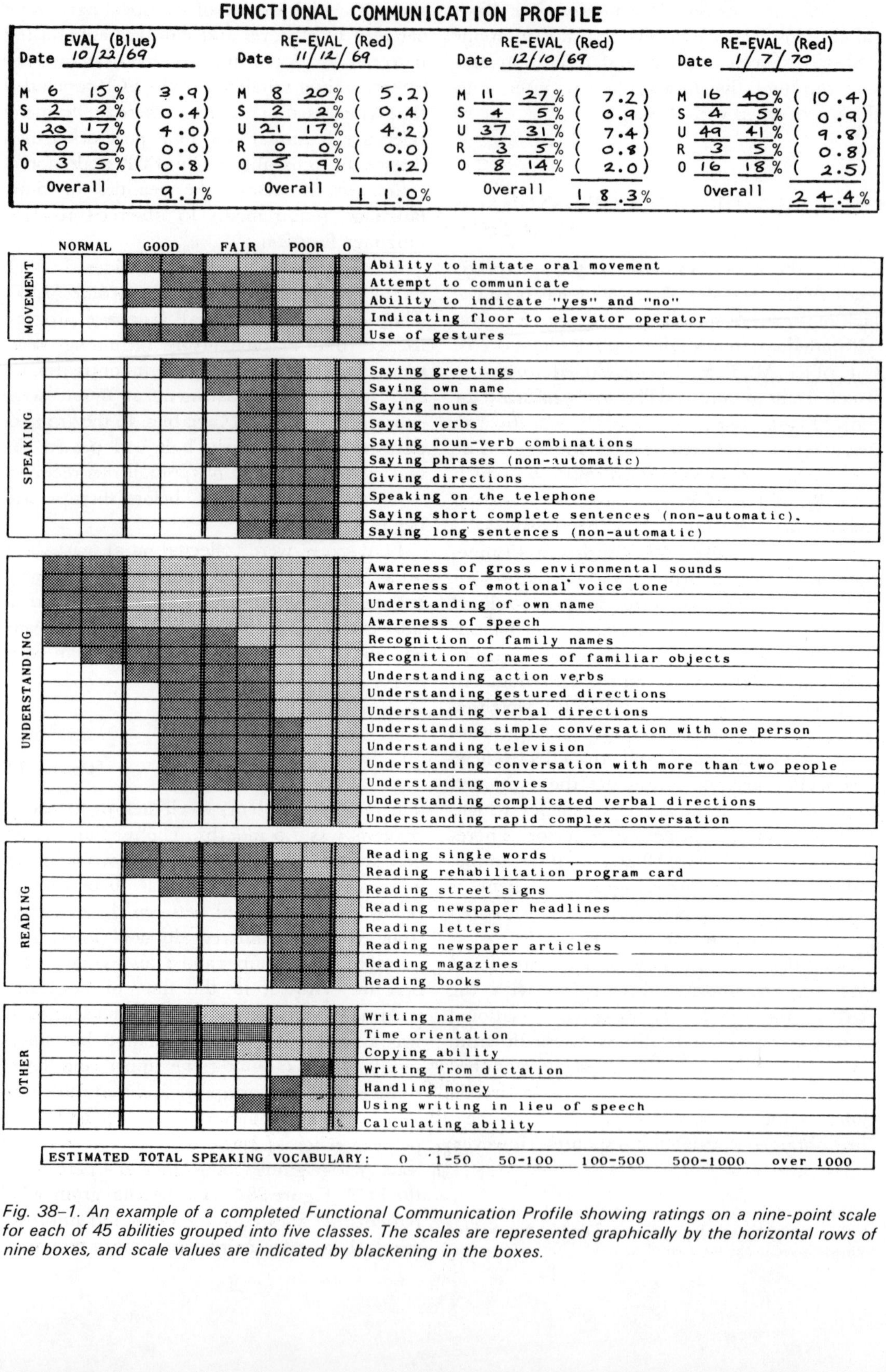

Fig. 38–1. An example of a completed Functional Communication Profile showing ratings on a nine-point scale for each of 45 abilities grouped into five classes. The scales are represented graphically by the horizontal rows of nine boxes, and scale values are indicated by blackening in the boxes.

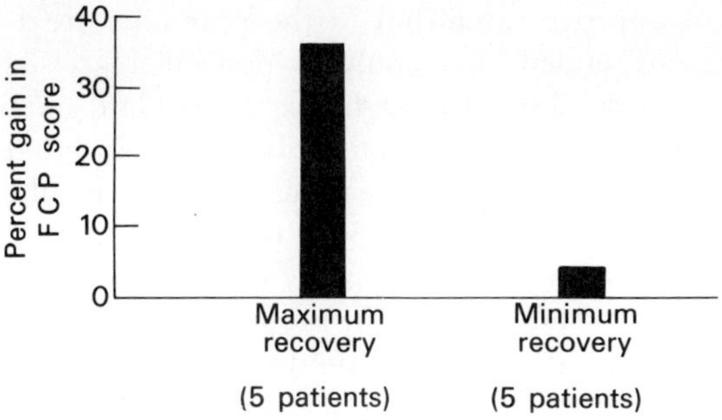

Fig. 38–2. Average gains in FCP scores for patients showing maximum and minimum recovery from aphasia.

It is generally agreed that there is a negative correlation between severity of aphasia in the early recovery period and the amount of improvement which occurs during the recovery process whether or not speech therapy is given (*2, 4*). Our data indicate that the higher intake score predicts a higher outcome score. Conversely, the lower the intake score, the poorer is the prognosis for recovery. In the high-gain group the average intake FCP score was 38.3 percent. In the low-gain group the average intake score was 17.2 percent (Figure 38-3). Thus, the severity of language impairment at initial evaluation is a moderately good predictor of the amount of recovery that may be expected.

Our group consists on the whole, of middle-aged and elderly patients. The average age was 56.5 years. Age appeared to be the most potent variable influencing recovery. We assessed the contribution of age by examining the extremes in our group. When we considered the sixth which showed the greatest improvement, we found these patients to be the youngest in our series, having an average age of only 47. Whereas those (that is, the sixth) who recovered least averaged 61 years. Figure 38-4 illustrates this relationship. This finding agrees with a number of other reports in the literature on aphasia (*1, 5, 7*).

We do not yet have the necessary data to make a definite statement concerning whether a given treatment helped this or that group of patients. A control group is needed to determine categorically the question that a given treatment is or is not superior to no treatment. Our findings did indicate that the average length of treatment for the sixth of our group who changed most between initial and final evaluation was 15 months, and for the sixth who gained least it was 8 months. These figures cannot simply be taken to mean that treatment is more effective if it is continued more than 8 months. Patients were in fact, retained in therapy only as long as they continued to show measurable gains so that the comparison is not simply between two randomly selected groups of patients arbitrarily assigned to different lengths of treatment. Such a procedure is nearly as difficult to carry out in a clinical setting as a no-treatment control group (*3*). Both of these

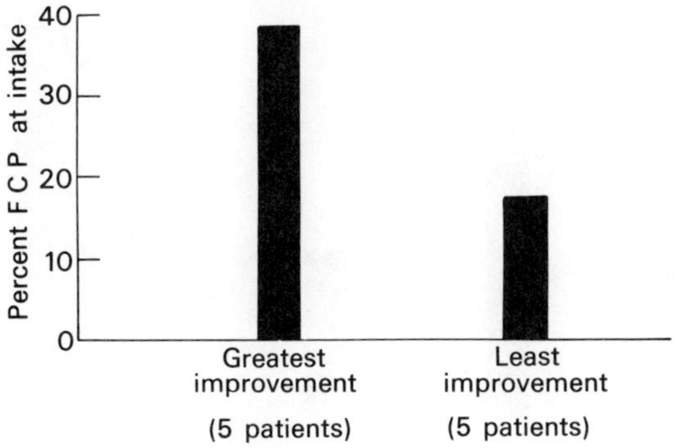

Fig. 38–3. FCP level at intake as a predictor of amount of improvement.

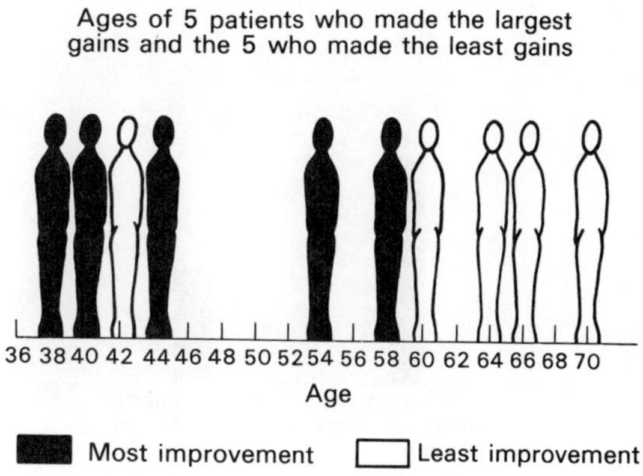

Fig. 38–4. Prognosis for improvement in relation to age.

steps must be taken if we are to have unequivocal answers to questions about the effect of treatment.

A related question is: when should therapy begin? To approach this question we considered separately those of our 30 patients whose treatment had begun no later than 2 months after the occurrence of the stroke, and those whose treatment was begun after 4 months. As it turned out the numbers for this comparison were nearly equal (Figure 38-5). There appears to be a definite advantage for the early treatment group. The interpretation of this finding is equivocal, however, since, other things being equal, we may expect that the "early" group had more still to gain from spontaneous recovery than the "late" group. Therefore, we wish to stress the point that the greater improvement of the "early" group cannot necessarily be attributed to therapeutic intervention. Neither can we exclude the possibility that early treatment is advantageous. The finding, in any case is consistent with a number of reports in the literature on aphasia (*3*, *5*, *9–12*). This suggestion needs to be explored further and clarified by the study of comparable groups, one of which receives no treatment. This is a matter of great importance on which there is no general agreement, since some have argued that formal speech therapy should be delayed until the period of spontaneous recovery has passed (*13*).

Finally, we return to a finding we noted earlier: most patients with stroke did continue to improve somewhat in the year after treatment ended, and only 7 percent regressed (Figure 38-6). Although few of these late gains are dramatic, it ought to be borne in mind that significant improvement may occur in the second and third year. So, if in language as well as in motor and sensory function, stroke patients often have a prolonged period of recovery, much more attention should be paid to the shape of the recovery curve in relation to a variety of neurologic variables.

CONCLUSION

At the beginning of this paper we pointed out the general lack of guide-lines for deciding who among aphasic patients is likely to benefit from treatment. We have begun to take steps toward gaining the understanding needed to make rational decisions in this difficult matter, and in gaining the necessary information about the recovery process in cases of language disturbances due to a stroke. In view of our increasing commitment to the care of the aged, it appears that the questions we have raised have not yet received sufficient consideration and study.

The following tentative suggestions are made on the basis of our work so far:

(1) Significant improvement often occurs after the first year following a stroke.

(2) The prognosis for good recovery is much better for patients less than 50 years of age than in those more than 60.

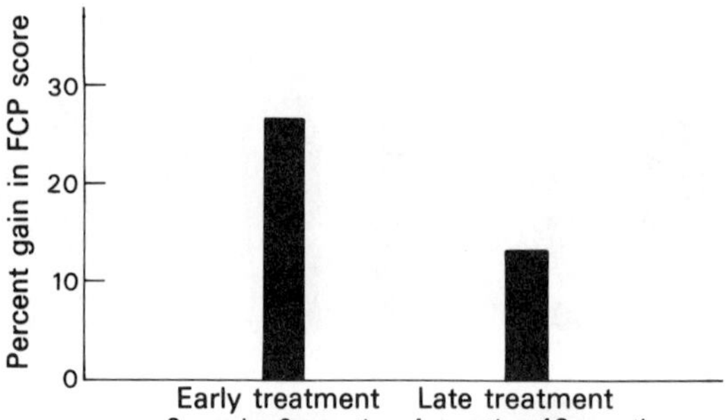

Fig. 38–5. Improvement in FCP scores in relation to time elapsed before beginning treatment.

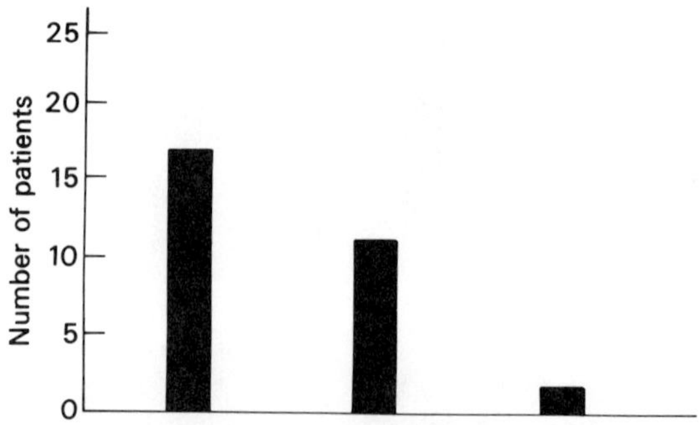

Fig. 38–6. Change in FCP scores after termination of treatment.

(3) The study which conclusively demonstrates the efficacy of speech therapy in aphasia has not been done. However, there is some reason to believe that if therapy is to succeed it must be initiated early.

REFERENCES

1. Eisenson, J.: Prognostic Factors Related to Language Rehabilitation in Aphasic Patients. *J. Speech Hearing Dis.,* **14**:262–264 (Sept.) 1949.
2. Buttfield, E., and Zangwill, O. L.: Re-education in Aphasia: A Review of 70 Cases. J. Neurol Neurosurg. Psychiat., **9**:75–79 (Apr.) 1946.
3. Marks, M.; Taylor, M., and Rusk, H. A.: Rehabilitation of the Aphasic Patient: A Survey of Three Years Experience in a Rehabilitation Setting. Arch. Phys. Med., **38**:219–226 (Apr.) 1957.
4. Schuell, H.: Diagnosis and Prognosis in Aphasia. Arch. Neurol. Psychiat., **74**:308–315 (Sept.) 1955.
5. Vignolo, L. A.: Evolution of Aphasia and Language Rehabilitation: A Retrospective Exploratory Study. Cortex 1: 344–367 (Dec.) 1964.
6. Taylor, M.: A Measurement of Functional Communication in Aphasia. Arch. Phys. Med., **46**:101–107 (Jan.) 1965.
7. Gerstman, L., and Woodbury, M.: Computer Prediction of Language Recovery After Stroke. Digest of the 6th International Conference on Medical Electronics and Biological Engineering. Tokyo, 1965.
8. Greenberg, F.: Functional Communication Ability and Responses to a Structured Language Test in Dysphasic Adults. Unpublished data.
9. Berry, M. F., and Eisenson, J.: Speech Disorders: Principles and Practices of Therapy. New York, Appleton-Century-Crofts, Inc., 1956.
10. Eisenson, J.: Aphasia: A Point of View as to the Nature of the Disorder and Factors That Determine Prognosis for Recovery. Int. J. Neurol., **4**: 287–295, 1964.
11. Lowman, E. W., and Rusk, H. A.: Self Help Devices: Aphasia Therapy, Part I. Postgrad. Med., **32**:79–185 (July) 1962.
12. Weisenburg, T., and McBride, K. E.: Aphasia. The Commonwealth Fund. New York, 1935.
13. Boone, D. R.: Relationship of Progress in Speech Therapy to Progress in Physical Therapy. Arch. Phys. Med., **42**:30–32 (Jan.) 1961.

39

On Learning Characteristics of the Adult Aphasic

DANIEL H. CARSON
FLORENCE E. CARSON
RONALD S. TIKOFSKY

DANIEL H. CARSON, Ph.D., is with the College of Human Development, Pennsylvania State University.

FLORENCE E. CARSON, B.A., was formerly with the Mental Health Research Institute, University of Michigan.

RONALD S. TIKOFSKY, Ph.D., is with the departments of psychology and of speech at the University of Michigan, Ann Arbor.

This research was supported in part by Grant NIH-5-R01-NB05374 from the National Institute of Neurological Diseases and Blindness, U.S. Public Health Service, and in part by a grant from the Edwin S. George Foundation.

Conventional approaches to the psychological study of aphasia typically relate behavioral measures to neurological findings and to type and severity of language deficit. Of particular concern to theorists is the relationship between language deficit and general intellectual functioning. The advantages and limitations of these approaches are well known and documented (Piercy, 1964; Tikofsky, 1966).

Another general approach to research in aphasia, one taken in this paper, attempts to supplement more conventional explorations. This approach seeks to gain greater latitude in experimentation by temporarily setting aside classifications based on neurological information and analysis of aphasic language. It begins with an analysis of learning behavior. Specifically, changes in both verbal and nonverbal performance may be assessed.

With this general approach, aphasic subjects (*S*s) are not viewed as different from one another or from other populations *except* as they differentiate themselves by changes in performance on the tasks being investigated. The aims are: first, to determine broad learning characteristics of the aphasic population, and second, to establish stable differences in learning among subgroups.

Classifications of the population according to this procedure will not be in complete agreement with more conventional classifications based on diagnostic instruments. But new information deriving from the partial correlations can aid in the structure of future research and rehabilitation. However, before any correlations are made, stable normative data must be obtained using the learning materials. Because of the small populations used in the present studies, precise statistical relationship with other classification schemes are deferred for the present time.

In this paper, interest is limited to a selected group of learning tasks, all of which examine changes in perceptual and cognitive functions. Emphasis is on analyzing performance change as a result of practice rather than comparing single isolated measures. Variables such as speed, accuracy and amount of information are used to assess consistencies and variations in aphasics' performance. Initial emphasis has

From *Cortex* 4:92–112, 1968.

been on the average range of performance change to be found in a group of aphasics, whether or not the properties of this performance change prove to be unique to aphasia. Because of small samples, statistical comparison of these changes with language deficits has not been made. Finally, no effort has been made to utilize nonaphasic brain damaged control subjects or carefully matched normals at this time, although normal *S*s were used for incidental comparison in some experiments.

EXPERIMENTAL PROCEDURES AND RESULTS

The experimental population. Subjects were patients enrolled in an intensive residential language rehabilitation program at the University of Michigan. They were all beyond the acute stages of illness, the majority having been aphasic from six months to two years at the time of the experiments. The nature of the rehabilitation program eliminated *both* minimally impaired aphasics and chronic deteriorated patients. Table 39-1 contains more detailed clinical and biographical data.

Experiments. Four experimental topics of the current research program are described below. Since the purpose of this paper is to outline an approach to the experimental study of aphasia, complete experimental details and statistical analysis are not reported here.

The research described is still in progress and the number of *S*s studied to date is small. The several experiments each examine a different type of performance. Taken singly, they offer only isolated facts. Taken together, they leave strong impressions about various behavioral characteristics of aphasics and suggest further directions for research.

Stimulus uncertainty and response time

The basic task is a variation of the classical simple and choice reaction time experiments (Woodworth and Schlosberg, 1954). Studies using a variety of stimulus and response modes have shown that brain damaged *S*s show longer response time than normals (Blackburn and Benton, 1957; Costa, 1962; De Renzi and Faglioni, 1965). In this experiment, effects of increasing uncertainty and practice on speed and accuracy of response were examined. Different stimulus sets tested transfer. Eighteen normal and 18 aphasic adult *S*s were used.

Stimuli. The stimuli employed were highly discriminable black geometric forms on a white

TABLE 39-1. DESCRIPTION OF APHASIC POPULATION

Language Classification[1]	Hand Used[2]	Age: 30 and below			31-45			46-60			61 and above		
		Education[3]											
		G	H	C	G	H	C	G	H	C	G	H	C
Semantic	R			1*			2	2	1	10	1		
	L			1*		1	1*	1	1	6			1
Syntactic	R												
	L						2		2				
Sem-Syn	R				1				3*	3			2
	L		2*					1					
Global	R		1*						1*		3		1
	L			1*		1	1	3		2			1

Total: 62

[1] 2 other *S*s were in Jargon category.
[2] Only 2 of 64 *S*s were premorbidly left-handed.
[3] G = Grade school; H = High school; C = College.
* Patient with traumatic or other cause of damage. All other *S*s had vascular lesions.

background. Three different sets were used in order to control for effects of stimulus shape on response time. Each set contained seven forms to provide 1, 2 and 4 different stimuli for 0-, 1- and 2-bit uncertainty conditions, respectively.

Procedures. *S*s matched a stimulus presented on a display panel with a corresponding stimulus on a response board, and registered their responses by pressing the appropriate button.

Following a brief training period, *S*s were given five experimental sessions, one on each of five consecutive days. Each session had all three uncertainty conditions, a daily total of 168 separate responses. The size of the stimulus set was always equal to that of the response set. Individual stimuli were presented in a random order with 1- and 2-bit conditions. Orders of all three uncertainty conditions were balanced.

To ensure that variations in performance were not due to special characteristics of a particular stimulus set, three separate sets of figures were constructed, and presented to the same group of *S*s in the following manner: Subjects were given three experimental sessions with one set, which provided a measure of the effects of practice on performance. On the fourth and fifth sessions *S*s were given the second and third sets, respectively, which provided a measure of transfer. Three orders of presentation of the three stimulus sets were balanced across *S*s. Since results indicate that differences were not significant, the data from the three stimulus sets were pooled. However, introducing new sets of stimuli on the fourth and fifth days, regardless of set used, did make a difference. Errors of both aphasics and normals were so rare, analysis of errors was not performed.

Results. The effects of practice on aphasic performance are shown by the first three curves labeled *A* in Figure 39-1. Aphasics show statistically significant improvement in performance over the first three days under *all* uncertainty conditions.

For the 0-bit condition, where *S* must respond to a single stimulus pattern, no choice is involved. The different patterns presented on days 4 and 5 have no influence on the task, and aphasics continue to show improvement. For the 1-bit condition, where choices are involved, there is even greater improvement over the first three days, perhaps because initial performance is worse. However, this steady improvement is not sustained over days 4 and 5. For the 2-bit condition, the same trends occur, but are more pronounced. If the experiment had been extended over more practice sessions, aphasics might be expected to show improvement on the new stimulus sets. Therefore, *S*s failure to improve on days 4 and 5 is primarily the result of their having to readjust the new stimulus materials. But such readjustment does not reduce performance to original levels and some learning is retained.

If these data are compared with data from a group of normals matched for age and sex, two consistent differences appear. First, aphasics are significantly slower than normals in response time on all tasks. Second, normals have flatter curves than aphasics, their better initial performance leaving little room for improvement. Since the type of activity in these

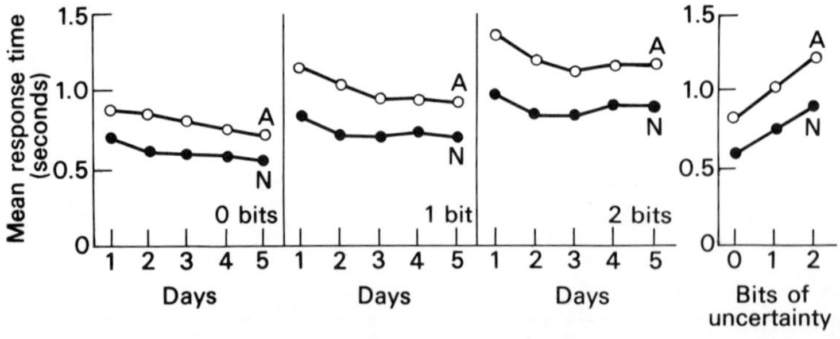

Fig. 39–1. Effects of stimulus uncertainty on response time. Means of data from 18 aphasics (A) and 18 normals (N) for each of 5 days are plotted in the first three graphs. Overall means for each uncertainty condition are plotted to the right.

tasks is familiar to normals, most of their improvement occurs very early in practice.

Despite these differences, curves for aphasics are remarkably similar to the corresponding curves for normals in overall shape, suggesting that aphasics exhibit similar but slower information handling processes.

On a variety of stimulus materials, normals exhibit a nearly linear increase in response time with increasing stimulus uncertainty (Hick, 1952; Hyman, 1953). That is, as the number of alternative stimuli increases, *S* handles information at nearly a constant rate. The fourth set of curves in Figure 39-1 shows average response time for each uncertainty condition. Clearly, the relationships reflect constant rate of information handling by both groups of *S*s. An examination of this relationship was made for individual *S*s and for individual sessions. The pattern is stable. Aphasic and normal *S*s exhibit the same lawful and orderly behavior on this information handling task.

Rote serial learning

The basic task required *S*s to learn two different lists of words in the order of their presentation. The purpose was to find out if aphasics could use word associations known to exist in the normal population to facilitate learning of the serial lists. Stimuli and responses were both verbal. Ten aphasics, who could repeat single words, and 14 normals were used as *S*s.

Stimuli. Two 10-word lists were constructed, each having different degrees of association between adjacent items. Words in the high associates (HA) list were arranged so that each word was followed by its most frequently given associate in the Palermo and Jenkins lists (1964). The same words were used in the low associates (LA) list, but were arranged to minimize associations between adjacent items[1].

Procedures. Cards with single words on them were shown to *S*s one at a time while the words were pronounced. One exposure of the full list constituted a *trial*. On all trials after the first, *S*s were asked to anticipate serially each word in the list. Only 10 trials were given on each of four consecutive days whether *S*s learned the list perfectly or not. Half the *S*s in both aphasic and normal groups were given two days of practice on the HA list followed by two days on the LA list. Remaining *S*s received the lists in reverse order. Only verbal responses were accepted.

Results. Data to the left in Figure 39-2 are plotted in terms of half-sessions (5 trials each) over four consecutive days. Aphasics show improvement on both lists of words within each day. They also show consistent improvement

[1] HA list: School, Work, Hard, Soft, Bed, Sleep, Eat, Drink, Water, Wet. LA list: Hard, Eat, Bed, Work, Water, Sleep, Wet, Soft, School, Drink.

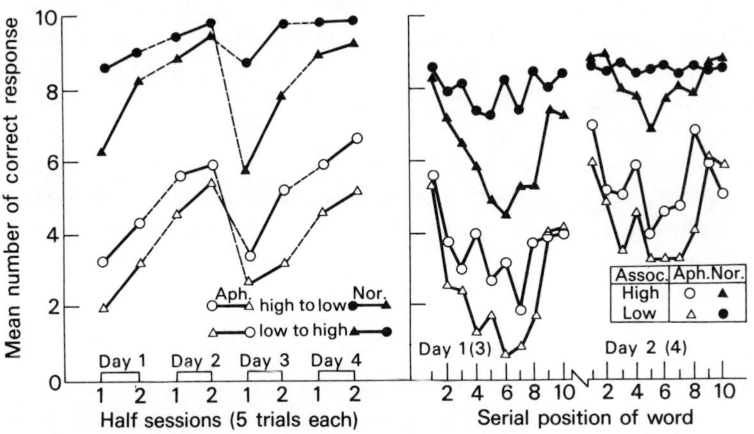

Fig. 39–2. Learning and serial position curves in rote serial learning. Curves on the left show effects of list reversal on learning over half sessions for 4 consecutive days. Curves on the right show the effect of serial position of words in each list on each population averaged over 2-day periods. Insets explain symbols.

across *pairs* of days. But their performance taken across *four* days does not show steady improvement. Rather, it reflects the effect of introducing a different list of words on the third day. At all points, performance on the HA list is superior to that on the LA list, indicating that aphasics do retain some use of common associations.

The subgroup getting the LA list first did as well as the subgroup getting the LA list second. This result obtained for the HA list also. If it were not known which subgroup had which list first, it would be impossible to sort them out. Words in both lists were not only identical, but were also very common words, therefore familiarity through practice may be assumed. But practice on individual words in either order had no influence on learning a different order, or structure, of the list. Each list was treated as independent without any transfer from one to the other. Normals reproduced these results exactly, except that they reached a significantly higher level of performance than aphasics. Average gains were about the same for both populations.

The difference between the HA and LA curves is accounted for by the previous learning with which each *S* entered the experiment. The higher probability of getting a correct response on the HA list is a function of the amount of experience with common associations. Aphasics retained some of this learning. However, they did not use these common associations as well as normals.

Another way to demonstrate that aphasics did not make as effective use of strong associations is illustrated to the right in Figure 39-2. Unlike the normal population, aphasics were still showing about as much serial position effect on the HA list as on the LA list after two days of practice. Of course, aphasics' impaired ability to make use of highly probable verbal structures merely reflects their aphasia. This point is clear because we cannot assume that their premorbid learning of associations was any worse than normal learning. But it is equally clear that certain arbitrary contingencies between words can be learned with practice by aphasics.

Repeated Digit Symbol task

The basic task required that *S*s respond rapidly to a series of digits by drawing a specific symbol for each. This task is given for one 90-second trial as the Digit Symbol subtest of the Wechsler Adult Intelligence Scale (WAIS), and a more complete description of it may be found in Wechsler (1958). By repeating the task several times, it was possible to assess aphasics' improvement as a result of practice.

Aphasics typically show impairment on this subtest even though they may be superior on other performance subtests during the standard administration of the Wechsler Scale. Achievement is low for all types and degrees of aphasia, for aphasics without measurable visual or motor defects, and for aphasics with no evidence of motor apraxia. Finally, aphasics typically do not make errors, and their lower scores are exclusively because of their slow rate of responding (Alajouanine and Lhermitte, 1964; Carson and Tikofsky, 1964).

Impairment in handling this task is not limited to aphasics. The task is sensitive to a variety of disturbances of the central nervous system (Wechsler, 1958). However, it is valuable as a means of studying aphasic learning behavior because it is a nonverbal, symbolic task on which aphasics show much room for improvement. Moreover, it has been used as a learning task with normals who show improvement with practice (Burik, 1950). In addition, this task has much in common with the more complex parts of the response time task described above. They are both information handling tasks which emphasize processing time.

Procedures. Twenty-seven aphasics, all premorbidly righthanded, were given the standard Wechsler instructions for the Digit Symbol subtest, but the test was administered for 5 90-second trials on each of 2 consecutive days. No rest periods intervened between trials. Following a week of no practice, 9 of the 27 *S*s were given 2 additional days of practice. On each of these additional days, the 9 *S*s were given 10 90-second trials without intervening rest periods. This subgroup had been incorporated into a later experiment on massed practice, but their additional data are so consistent with their previous data that they are plotted in their entirety in Figure 39-3.

Results. Performance was measured in terms of standard Scale scores, corrected for age according to the normative data in Wechsler (1955). The upper part of Figure 39-3 shows that mean group performance (circles) improved consistently within each practice period and retention was high across practice periods. It is also apparent from the data that *S*s who used their unimpaired right hand, the righthand group, were significantly superior to those who were forced to use their nondominant hand. Normals also show this difference between hands on this task (Briggs, 1960).

Since all aphasics improved with practice over 2 days, it might be expected that continued practice would result in further improvement. Data for the subgroup over 4 days (x's) support this expectation. But the righthand group approaches normal levels after 2 days and is continuing to improve after 4 days, while the lefthand group appears to be reaching an upper limit much sooner. Even after an indefinite amount of practice, this group may not be capable of reaching normal performance.

The data in the lower part of Figure 39-3 show that those individuals who had both higher initial and higher average performance also made proportionally greater gains. But it should be noted that all members of the subgroup except S_7 retain their original gains after a period of no practice, so that their mean scores on day 3 are the same or higher than those on day 2, a week earlier.

Rule learning tasks

The basic task required *S*s to sort a group of stimuli into two categories according to some rule. Stimuli shared several variables (attributes) but were discriminably different, and stimuli always outnumbered response. See Garner (1962) for descriptions of the general rule (concept) learning task.

Stimulus sets. The 32 stimuli in the master set were generated by taking all possible combinations of 5 dichotomous variables. These

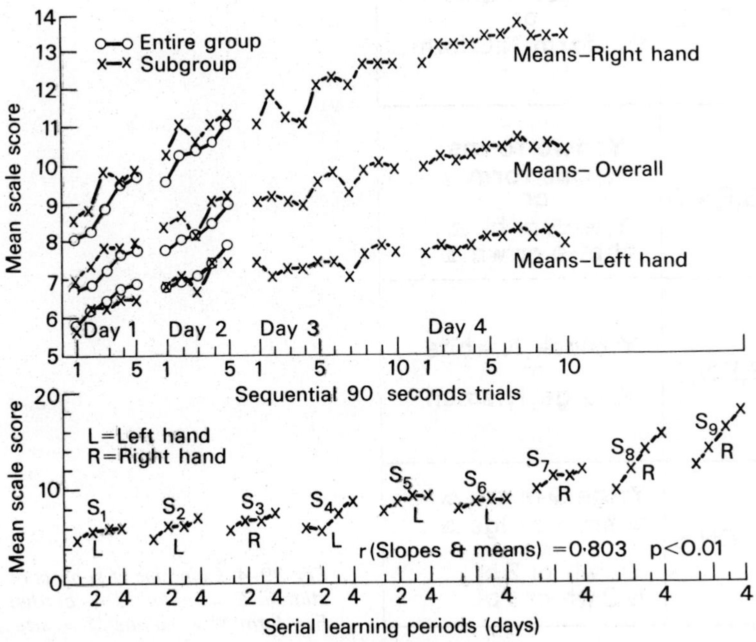

Fig. 39–3. Aphasic performance on repeated digit-symbol test. The upper set of curves shows the learning over trials on two consecutive days for a group of 27 aphasics, and the learning over trials on four consecutive days for a subgroup of 9 aphasics. The two groups are also separated by the hand used in the test. All Ss were premorbidly right-handed. The lower set of curves shows individual performance over days for the subgroup.

variables were: color (black-white), border (circular-triangular), form (circles-triangles), number (one form-two forms) and size (small forms-large forms). Sub-master sets of 16 stimuli were also used in some cases. Learning subsets were selected for particular tasks. Examples of subsets, grouped by response class, are illustrated to the left in Figure 39-4.

Two closely related observations guided the choice of such abstract stimuli. First, familiar objects vary in an uncontrollable number of different ways. Not having these variables under control limits the usefulness of interpretations. Second, familiar objects have different strengths of association which may place undue bias on particular variables (Higgins, Mednick and Taylor, 1963; Deese, 1964). Since rules are constructed in terms of the variables, this procedure of avoiding familiar objects provides a better control for ease or difficulty of the tasks.

Stimulus Sets		*Variables	Rules
YES Class	NO Class		
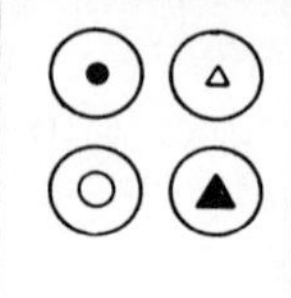	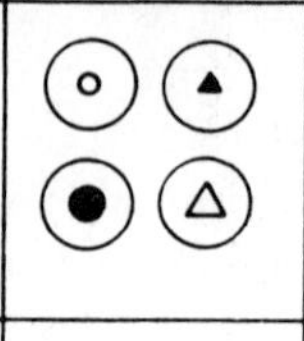	C,–,F,–,S	No rule (rote task)
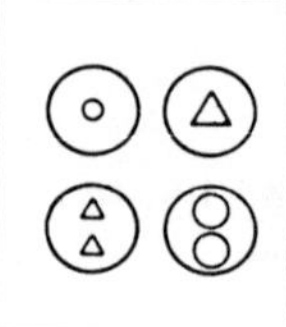	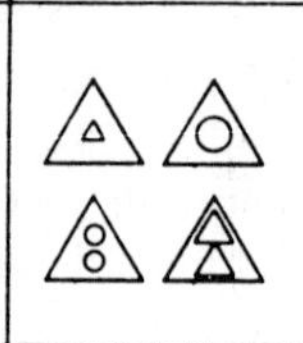	–,B,F,N,S	Y: ○ border; N: △ border
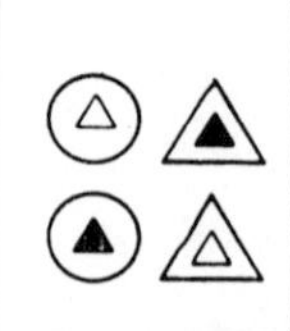	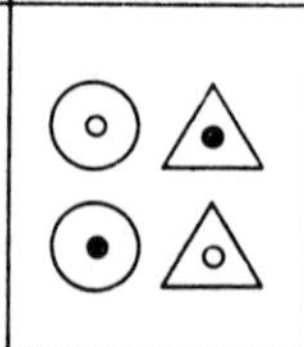	C,B,F,–,S	Y: large; N: small or Y: △ form; N: ○ form
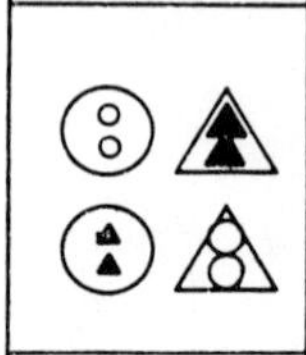	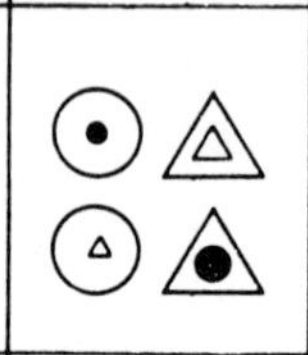	C,B,F,N,S	Y: two forms N: one form or Y: wh. Ⓢ or bl. △ N: bl. Ⓢ or wh. △
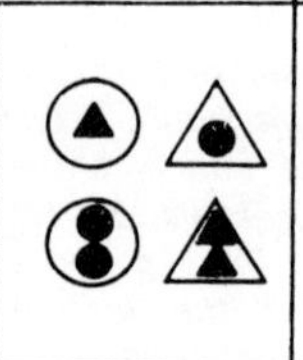	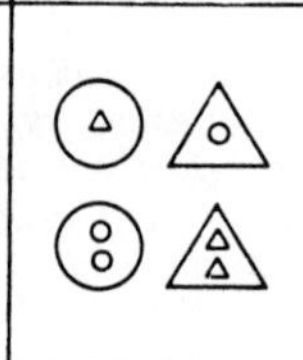	C,B,F,N,S	Y: black; N: white or Y: large; N: small
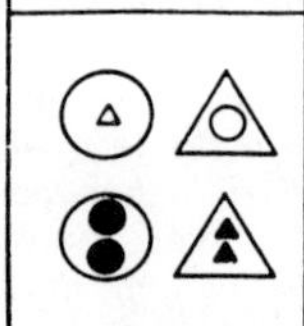	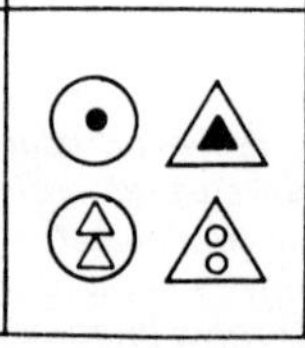	C,B,F,N,S	Y: lge. Ⓢ or sm. △ N: sm. Ⓢ or lge △ or Y: 1 wh. or 2 bl. N: 2 wh. or 1 bl.

Fig. 39–4. Examples of subsets of stimuli. C = color; B = border; F = form; N = number; S = size.

Method of presentation. For these tasks, a method which would enhance differences among *S*s was desired, and the method chosen is considered cognitively difficult (Whitman and Garner, 1963; Peterson, 1962). It served this purpose, without being so difficult that solutions were precluded.

Stimuli were presented in repeated random series. The complete subset of stimuli, say 8, were shown to *S*s singly, and the response category to which each belonged was identified. Showing the whole subset in this way constituted the first *trial*. Then followed a series of trials, each of which contained a different random order of the subset, and *S*s had to sort the stimuli into the appropriate response classes, either "yes" or "no." *S*s were told whether they were correct or incorrect after each response. Trials continued until *S*s had achieved two completely correct trials or until 45 minutes had expired.

Following each learning task a nonverbal transfer task was given. After rule tasks, *S*s were required to sort the master set into two categories according to the rule just learned. After rote tasks, *S*s selected the subset from the master set and then sorted the subset into the appropriate categories.

Rules. All tasks demanded of the *S* that he learn only one rule, although there may have been more than one possible rule available to learn. Other rule learning situations of a similar type (cf. Hull, 1920; Heidbreder, 1948) have used a multivariate response where several rules had to be learned simultaneously. Such problems, being quite difficult, are often solved by normals by rote alone and the rules are frequently not learned at all. Hence, such situations were avoided.

Rules for sorting the subsets of stimuli into the two response classes were in terms of one or more of the variables used to generate the stimuli. In Figure 39-4, the six rows illustrate several types of tasks used. In the first column to the left are illustrations of the actual stimulus subsets sorted into the two response classes. In the second column, particular variables appearing in these learning subsets are abbreviated. In the third column, the specific rule or rules associated with that subset are given. Note that any rule which could be used in the rote case must involve all variables and reduces to a specific description of each stimulus.

Four separate experiments were performed, each using different combinations and types of rules and different numbers of stimuli in the learning subsets. For convenience, these different experiments are merely labelled I, II, III and IV, with the subscripts 4 and 8 referring to the number of stimuli used. All results are reported using the measure of percent correct.

Rote vs. rule learning. In any rule learning situation where a number of discriminably different stimuli must be sorted without error into two or more different response classes, two kinds of performance are required. At least during the initial stages of learning there is the element of rote learning as well as that of rule learning. Other things being equal, the rote task should show higher average percent correct scores than the rule task, since only one kind of performance is required in the former. The summary of data from the several experiments plotted in Figure 39-5 does not support this conclusion.

Two kinds of data are plotted in Figure 39-5, one by circles and the other by crosses. Circles refer to the differences between rote and rule tasks. Data are mean differences across all rule tasks for each *S*. Neglecting experiment III_4 which is discussed below, the other data show that rule learning is superior to rote learning for normal and aphasics alike, as indicated by the first row of significance levels (P's) below the data plots.

The crosses are corresponding plots of mean differences for those rule tasks in which stimuli were *not* learned by *S*s. In all but one experiment, differences between rote and unsolved rule tasks are not significantly different as indicated by the second row of P's below the data plots. Even in this one experiment, IV_8, the mean difference is reduced.

Although two kinds of performance are

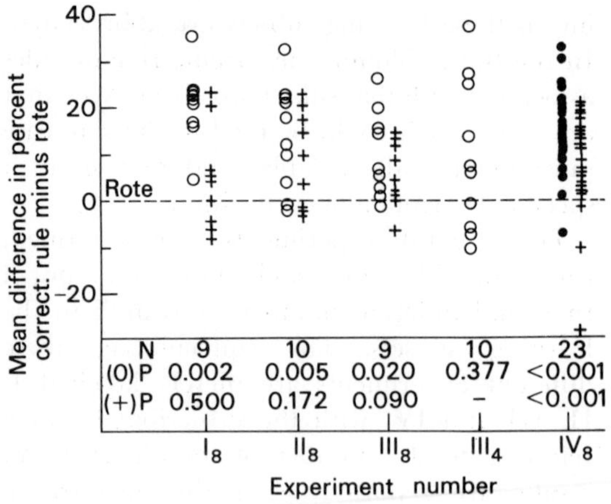

Fig. 39–5. Rote vs. rule learning in classification tasks. Plot shows mean differences in percent correct scores between rote and rule tasks for each S averaged over the several tasks in each of 4 experiments. Circles are means for all tasks and crosses are means only for tasks on which stimuli were not learned. Number of Ss is given below each plot. Experiment IV contains data from normals only. The other 3 experiments contain data from aphasics only.

required in the rule tasks, what *S* gets from each stimulus in the rule task is of more general help than what is gotten in the rote task. Another way of putting this is to say that when concentrating on rules, each stimulus, since it contains some aspect of each of the variables which could be used in a rule, gives some information about *each* of all possible rules. Each stimulus in the rote task gives only information about itself and hence has to be memorized singly. It appears that *S*s take advantage of the greater efficiency of learning rules and this is reflected in their better average scores on rule tasks.

In those taks where the best strategy was to use rules rather than perform the task by rote, it is clear that aphasics were using rules to help them in their classification. In tasks which were entirely comparable in kind and number of stimuli (being drawn from the same master set) but which had to be memorized by rote, aphasics performed less well. Normals also follow this pattern.

Of course, if the rote task has fewer stimuli so that the overall task load is smaller, as in experiment III_4, results from rote and rule tasks should be more nearly alike. The data from III_4 plotted in Figure 39-5 fail to show a difference between rote and rule tasks when only 4 stimuli are used in each.

Effects of repeated stimuli. In all but experiment I_8, certain stimulus pictures were repeated in nearly all of the tasks of a given experiment. This procedure made it possible to assess learning across tasks in a highly controlled fashion by measuring performance on specific stimuli. Control was achieved by selecting 3 particular stimuli and repeating one with a constant "yes" response, one with a constant "no" response, and a third with alternating "yes" and "no" responses.

Results in mean percent correct on each of these cards in each task where they were used are plotted in Figure 39-6. The data there are plotted by consecutive task sessions but each task session is an average of several different rule tasks since *S*s did not all receive the same order of tasks. The plot shows how much improvement there was on these specific constant cards as *S*s saw them repeated in the same or in alternating response categories.

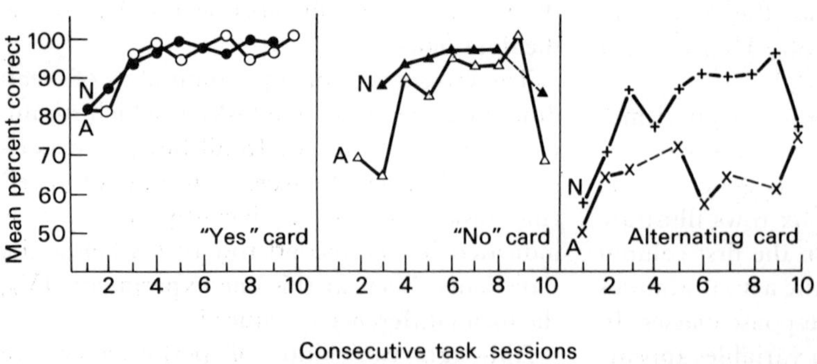

Fig. 39–6. Learning of repeated single stimuli in classification tasks by aphasic (A) and normal (N) subjects. Plots show mean percent correct on the selected stimuli averaged across subjects and tasks as a function of consecutive task sessions. Curves from left to right show performance on constant "yes" stimulus, constant "no" stimulus, and stimulus which alternated serially between "yes" and "no" response classes, respectively.

It is clear from Figure 39-6 that there is no difference between normals and aphasics for the "yes" card. And although normals appear to be higher than aphasics on the "no" card, the difference is not significant. However, on the alternating card, there is a clear and significant difference between the normals and aphasics. Casual questioning of both groups suggest that the normals were no more aware of this card being repeated than were the aphasics. Yet, it would appear, from Figure 39-6, that the normals were learning more than the aphasics on the alternating cards.

More detailed analysis which compared differences in learning on the repeated stimuli with that on specific subsets of other stimuli, shows another important difference between aphasics and normals. Aphasics improve relatively more on "yes" and "no" stimuli than on the alternating stimuli. The reverse is true for normals.

Aphasics are diverging from their own average learning, becoming more attentive to the simple presentation of "yes" and "no" cards and less attentive to the alternating card (or to the other cards in the subset), while the normals are converging toward average learning, and are paying attention to all cards about equally. A simple task (learning consistently repeated stimuli) interferes with a complex task (learning rules) more for aphasics than for normals.

Transfer of rules. Three kinds of results support the conclusion that aphasics learned rules and applied them in the transfer task. First, learning and transfer scores were consistently higher in rule than in rote tasks having the same number and kind of stimuli. Second, even with the interference of using simple and complex rules and small and large transfer sets in experiment III (III_8 and III_4), aphasics correctly transferred 36 percent of the rules. Third, aphasics achieved some perfect rule transfers to the 32-stimulus master set.

These results were obtained in spite of a stringent criterion on the number of stimuli incorrectly sorted, which left the probability of an inferred correct sorting by chance at .01. The probability of a perfect sorting by chance is vanishingly small for either the 16- or 32-stimulus set.

Aphasics correctly sorted in 34 percent of all cases when transferring to the 32-stimulus set and in 79 percent of all cases when transferring to the 16-stimulus set, an overall average of 56 percent correct sortings. They also sorted correctly on 29 percent of the complex rules and on 70 percent of the simple rules. Normals, who were given practice on complex rules and 32-stimulus master sets only, achieved 79 percent correct sortings.

Simple rules require less language processing, and therefore smaller memory load, than complex rules which require statements of contingencies between pairs of variables. Smaller transfer sets have greater similarity to fixed learning sets because a larger proportion of the transfer set has already been seen and learned in the learning set. It is clear that using simple rules and small transfer sets, aphasics were approaching the performance of normals who were using complex rules and larger transfer sets. Providing memory load for learning and number of transfer items are not too great, aphasics can learn and transfer rules constructed from the abstract properties of the stimuli.

It should be emphasized that despite the nonverbal stimuli and responses used in the rule learning situations, the overall task has only a very small perceptual factor. There is little in the way of immediate apprehension of the stimuli which can aid in performance. Rather, there is a large amount of what would normally be called conceptual, or language, behavior in that substitution, equivalence, abstraction of properties, and symbolic coding are required. In short, the task is an information handling task with a large element of internal language manipulation required for good performance (Zangwill, 1964).

Support for this conclusion is given in Table 39-2, which shows intercorrelations between three of four experiments mentioned in this report, together with other tests, for a subgroup of 23 aphasics only. Correlations in Table 39-2 are arranged so that an emphasis is

TABLE 39-2. CORRELATIONS BETWEEN TESTS AND EXPERIMENTS

	Rote Verbal Learning	Rule Learning Tasks	Raven Matrices (1938 edition)	WAIS[1]
Rule Learning Tasks	.52*	—	.27	.18
Rote Verbal Learning Tasks	—	—	—	.08
Raven Matrices (1938 edition)	.23	—	—	.47*
Digit Symbol Subtest	.05	.26	.28	.57*

[1] Performance scores only
*$p < .05$

placed on the perceptual and cognitive differences among the tasks. The rule learning tasks show much higher relationship to the verbal tasks than to the nonverbal or performance tasks. The response time study was not included because *S*s in that study did not participate in other experiments.

Summary of rule learning. When experimental conditions eliminate some of the uncontrollable effects of familiarity, aphasics can manipulate quite abstract and complicated rules. Their performance is entirely comparable to normals on several variables, though their overall level of accomplishment is lower. In learning rules, aphasics do not learn first by rote. Rather they concentrate on the task of abstracting properties of the stimuli. In fact, rote learning performance is not as good as rule learning performance for either group of *S*s, other things being equal, and it is particularly bad for aphasics.

Only 2 of the 35 aphasics ever reached the rote criterion of two correct trials on any rote task with 8 stimuli. Of the normals, 6 of the 24 *S*s reached criterion on the first rote task and 7 reached it on the second. Normals are clearly superior to aphasics in handling information in the rote situation. In the sense that rule learning was logically easier than rote learning in these tasks, aphasic performance reflected this difference in difficulty. Judging from performance on the constant cards, aphasics concentrated on the easier part of the overall task. Given limited capacity, their approach is quite rational.

It can be said that some structural properties of aphasics' rule learning ability are virtually the same as that of the normals, but that two factors handicap the aphasic. First, the sheer number of stimuli he can apprehend simultaneously, rather than any abstract properties of these stimuli, limit his performance. Second, a simple task will interfere with his performance on a more complicated task by diverting his attention away from the latter task. This interference is in contrast with normal performance on comparable tasks, where it is taken in stride and the simpler task incorporated into the more complicated one.

SUMMARY AND DISCUSSION

The performance of 64 aphasics and 64 normals in four kinds of experiments was investigated. The experiments were: 1) stimulus uncertainty and response time, 2) Rote serial learning, 3) Repeated Digit Symbol task, and 4) Rule learning tasks.

Aphasics showed significant regularities in their ability to learn new tasks, to retain their skill over time, and to handle a wide range of complexity in stimulus material. Characteristics which distinguished them from normals were their slower speed and frequently their lower level of attainment. They did not distinguish themselves as a group from normals by inability to perform on any of the difficult experimental tasks.

In particular, consistent improvement as manifested by decreased times in the Response Time experiment, by increased number of correct anticipation in the Rote Serial Learning experiment, and by faster rates of responding in the Digit Symbol experiment. Increases in correct classification of single, repeated stimuli across rule learning tasks were evident in the Rule Learning experiment.

When compared with normals, aphasics showed a greater effect of increasing uncertainty in the Response Time experiment, less facility in using serial associations in the Rote Serial Learning experiment, and greater interference from repeated stimuli in the Rule Learning experiment. When subgroups of aphasics were compared, those who retained use of their right hand in the Digit Symbol experiment were initially better and improved more than aphasics who had to use their left hand.

Despite the fact that aphasics demonstrated limited retention and transfer of learning in general, virtually every aphasic improved with practice in a specific stimulus-response situation. For example, where they might have called upon old learning in a specific routine task, they seemed to treat the task as totally new. However, given sufficient practice, they were able to approach normal levels of performance. Finally, while variability between aphasics remained high compared with normals, individual variability was reduced with practice; aphasics' data were consistent and dependable.

These results point to the value of an experimental approach to the study of nonverbal learning by aphasics and its relationship to some problems in the evaluation of progress during therapy.

We have a great deal of analytic information from diagnostic instruments which use language or neurological evaluation. But we have very little general and specific experimental information about crucial learning variables, such as absolute levels of performance, rates of acquisition, and ability to transfer, particularly with nonverbal materials. Recent literature emphasizes the importance of examining nonverbal variables in aphasics to determine their relationship to language deficits (cf. de Reuck and O'Connor, 1964).

While a variety of diagnostic tests can predict learning ability in extreme cases, those at the ends of the distribution, they typically fail to discriminate among the rest of the individuals. For example, specific measures of learning performance on verbal and nonverbal materials may have little correlation with measured language deficits. Therefore, they may provide additional diagnostic and theoretical information.

In the present experiments, it was observed that severe language deficit was sometimes associated with high levels of acquisition, and that low levels of acquisition were sometimes associated with relatively intact language. These relationships obtained when the ostensibly nonverbal task required some internal language processing for effective performance.

Attention in the present studies was directed toward finding out if aphasics are able to learn and transfer specific new materials rapidly or to relearn specific old materials. Although indefinitely long retention was not examined, it was clear that aphasics learned some specific skills and retained them over relatively long periods without practice, up to a week in some cases.

Experimental studies on learning can be applied to the problem of testing for progress during therapy, insofar as the studies measure specific learning and transfer abilities. Aphasia therapy is aimed at practical goals. Clinicians frequently report that patients show progress during therapy, but that this progress is not reflected in improved scores on standard tests of language impairment (J. Simonson, Director of Aphasia Therapy, University of Michigan, personal communication).

In order for aphasics to show improvements on standard tests, they must transfer learning from specific materials used in therapy to the criterion materials in the test. They are limited in this ability. In addition, standard diagnostic instruments, designed for high reliability, are insensitive to the small changes of practical significance due to therapy. Clinicians have discovered through experience that more precise measurement of change can be made by using materials actually employed in therapy. The present studies support this practice.

REFERENCES

Alajouanine, T., and Lhermitte, F. (1964) *Non-verbal communication in aphasia,* in Disorders of Language, ed. by de Reuck, A. V. S., and O'Connor, M., CIBA Foundation Symposium, Little, Brown and Co., Boston.

Blackburn, H. E., and Benton, A. L. (1957) *Practice effects in reaction time tasks in brain injured patients,* "J. Abnorm. Soc. Psychol.," **54,** 109–113.

Briggs, P. F. (1960) *The validity of WAIS performance subtests completed with one hand,* "J. clin. Psychol.," **16,** 318–320.

Bruner, J. S., Goodnow, J. J., and Austin, G. A. (1954) *A Study of Thinking,* Wiley, New York.

Burik, T. E. (1950) *Relative roles of the learning and motor factors involved in the Digit Symbol task,* "J. Psychol.," **30,** 33–42.

Carson, F. E., and Tikofsky, R. S. (1964) *Adult aphasic solutions of performance subtest on the Wechsler adult intelligence scale,* "ASHA," **6,** 393.

Costa, L. D. (1962) *Visual reaction time of patients with cerebral disease as a function of length and constancy of preparatory interval,* "Percept. Mot. Skills," **14,** 391–397.

Deese, J. (1964) *Principles of Psychology,* Allyn and Bacon, Boston.

De Renzi, E., and Faglioni, P. (1965) *The comparative efficiency of intelligence and vigilance tests in detecting hemispheric cerebral damage,* "Cortex," **1,** 410–433.

De Reuck, A. V. S., and O'Connor, M., eds. (1964) *Disorders of Language* (CIBA Foundation Symposium), Little, Brown and Co., Boston.

Garner, W. R. (1962) *Uncertainty and Structure as Psychological Concepts,* Wiley, New York.

Heidbreder, E. (1948) *The attainment of concepts. VI Exploratory experiments on conceptualization at perceptual levels,* "J. Psychol.," **26,** 193–216.

Hick, W. E. (1952) *On the rate of gain of information,* "Quart. J. Exp. Psychol.," **4,** 11–26.

Higgins, J., Mednick, S. A., and Taylor, S. L. (1963) *A replication of facilitation of concept formation through mediated generalization,* "J. Exp. Psychol.," **65,** 421–422.

Hull, C. L. (1920) *Quantitative aspects of the evolution of concepts,* "Psychol. Monogr.," **28,** 161.

Hyman, R. (1953) *Stimulus information as a determinant of reaction time,* "J. Exp. Psychol., **45,** 188–196.

Palermo, R. S. and Jenkins, J. J. (1964) *Word Association Norms Grade School Through College,* University of Minnesota Press, Minneapolis.

Peterson, M. J. (1962) *Some effects of the percentage of recent cues and presentation methods on concept identification,* "J. Exp. Psychol.," **64,** 623–627.

Piercy, M. (1964) *The effects of cerebral lesions on intellectual function: A review of current research trends,* "Brit. J. Psychiat.," **110,** 310–352.

Tikofsky, R. S. (1966) *Approaches to the study of aphasia in adults,* in Speech Pathology, ed. by Rieber, R. W., and Brubaker, R. S., North-Holland Publishing Co., Amsterdam.

Wechsler, D. (1958) *The Measurement and Appraisal of Adult Intelligence,* Williams and Wilkins, Baltimore.

Wepman, J. M., and Jones, L. V. (1961) *Studies in Aphasia: An Approach to Testing,* "Educ.-Indus. Serv.," Chicago.

Whitman, J. R., and Garner, W. R. (1963) *Concept learning as a function of form of internal structure,* "J. of Verb. Learn. Verb. Behav.," **2,** 195–202.

Woodworth, R. S., and Schlosberg, H. (1954) *Experimental Psychology,* Holt and Winston, New York.

Zangwill, O. L. (1964) *Intelligence in aphasia,* in Disorders of Language (CIBA Foundation Symposium) ed. by de Reuck, A.V.S., and O'Connor, M., Little, Brown and Co., Boston.

Writing in Aphasia: A Learning Study

LUIGI R. PIZZAMIGLIO
MARGARET M. ROBERTS

LUIGI R. PIZZAMIGLIO, M.D., is with the department of psychology of the Faculty of Medicine, Università Cattolica del S. Cuore, Rome.

MARGARET M. ROBERTS, Ph.D., is chief of the speech pathology for children and youth project at Children's Hospital, Columbus.

This study was supported by a grant to the Ohio State University Research Foundation from the Vocational Rehabilitation Administration, RD 1184.

This study was conducted in the course of language therapy with adult aphasic patients. An increasing number of investigations have dealt with the rate of learning of linguistic and motor activities among aphasic patients: the effect of goal-directed activity (Katz, 1958); the learning rate of aphasic individuals relative to normal ones (Tikofsky and Reynolds, 1962); the perseveration of errors in successive trials of a task (Zangwill, 1946: Rocheford and Williams, 1962; Lopatkiewicz, 1961); discrimination among geometric figures (Rosenberg and Edwards, 1964; Edwards, 1965); learning and transferring of classification rules (Carson and Smith, 1965); the effect of the associative content of word lists in rote learning (Tikofsky and Berman, 1965). Several studies emphasize the weakness of short-term memory among aphasics (Isserlin, 1922; Zangwill, 1946). The present study has both theoretical and practical implications since it is based on a comparison of the learning achieved in therapy sessions of two frequencies of occurrence.

Two hypotheses were tested:

1) There is no difference in the rate of learning to "write" verbal materials between those aphasic patients who practice the task every 24 hours and those who practice it every 48 hours.

2) There is no difference in the level of performance of these two groups of patients at the end of their period of training and at a subsequent testing period one week later.

EXPERIMENTAL SUBJECTS

Twenty adult aphasics, predominantly expressive type, participated in the experiment. Nineteen had experienced cerebrovascular accidents, and one cerebral trauma; of the 19 CVA patients, one had suffered hemorrage and the others thrombosis. One-half of the patients were males, one-half females.

The 20 cases were arbitrarily divided into two equal groups, designated Group 1 and Group 2. Both ranged from 33 to 65 years of age; the mean age of Group 1 was 42.0, S.D. = 10.4, and that of Group 2, 48.9, S.D. = 8.33 ($t = 1.32$, $p > 0.20$); the means in school achievement were 12.4, S.D. = 1.43, and 13.2, S.D. = 1.99 respectively ($t = 0.98$, $p > 0.30$). The scores of the two groups on the Progressive Matrices (1938) were 23.4, S.D. = 5.58, and 21.3 S.D. = 5.57 ($t = 0.77$, $p > 0.40$).

The subjects were under treatment in three hospitals; hence the available measures of

From *Cortex* 3:250–57, 1967.

language skills were not uniform. Clinical observation suggested, however, that the two groups were quite similar. Three aphasics in Group 1 and three in Group 2 had a speech production extremely reduced, and limited to very few intelligible words. Five patients in Group 1 and four in Group 2, showed difficulties mainly in word-formulation and articulation. Two aphasics in Group 1 and three in Group 2 had grammatical disturbances.

PROCEDURE

The subjects were asked to master tasks: *a*) to supply the final word in each of eight written sentences, and *b*) to provide the names of single objects represented in ten pictures.

Sentences: 1) We eat at the *table*. 2) Are lemons sweet or *sour*? 3) Do you like to drink coffee that is strong or *weak*? 4) I bought a loaf of *bread*. 5) I turned on the light because it was *dark*. 6) They went with their mother and *father*. 7) The baby cries all day and *night*. 8) Cut the meat with a *knife*.

Pictures: hammer, squirrel, church, key, elephant, toothbrush, bed, scissors, umbrella, safety pin.

A unique feature of the experimental situation was the use of the Language Retrieval Unit in both the presentation of the sentences and as the instrument on which all responses were made. This unit, shown in Figure 40-1, provides the patient with a typewritten output and an external keyboard for registering the input. Controlled by punch tape, the typewriter (Teletype) provides automatically any material that the experimenter has stored. Thus, in the present instance, the machine typed each of the eight sentences except for the final word. The patient was expected to provide the final word of each sentence by means of the external keyboard, which is made up of translucent keys for each of the letters of the alphabet, plus the space. Each time an incorrect key is punched, the correct one is illuminated, guiding the patient through the word with a minimum of frustration. The maximum number of errors is equal to the number of letters in the text.

For the second task, the experimenter showed the patients a picture and the patient was required to type the name by means of the external keyboard. The subject was free to speak (i.e., to say the sentences aloud, spell the words, etc.) or to remain silent. At the conclusion of each item, the experimenter spoke the test word aloud. Each subject was given one trial per experimental day on each task.

The score of a subject for each part of the experimental task (sentence completion or picture naming) was the number of correct responses that he made on the external keyboard. He was assumed to have mastered the task when he responded with 90 percent accuracy on three successive repetitions of the task. He was retested one week later for assessment of retention.

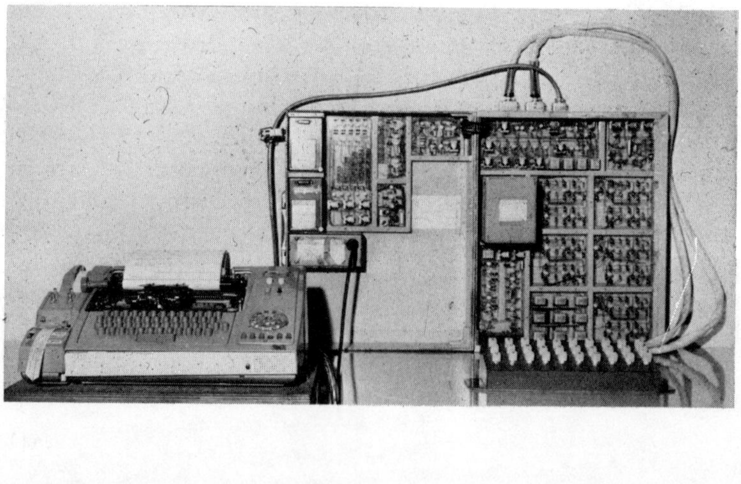

Fig. 40–1. The Language Retrieval Unit, showing control circuitry, Teletype typewriter, and external keyboard.

The members of Group 1 were tested daily, and the members of Group 2, on alternative days.

RESULTS

Sentences. There are 38 letters in the final words of the eight stimulus sentences. On Trial 1 the mean number of correct responses of Group 1 was 22.5, S.D. = 3.9; and that of Group 2 was 23.2, S.D. = 4.5. This difference is not statistically significant: $t=1.13$, $p>0.20$. The subsequent results are summarized in Table 40-1.

TABLE 40-1. SESSIONS REQUIRED BY THE TWO EXPERIMENTAL GROUPS IN LEARNING TO REPRODUCE THE SUCCESSIVE LETTERS OF THE TERMINAL WORDS OF EIGHT SENTENCES

Groups	Number of Patients	Average Number of Sessions Required to Meet Criterion	S. D.
Group 1 (Working daily)	10	4.8	0.60
Group 2 (Working every other day)	10	7.9	1.89

The average number of experimental trials required to reach the criterion score (90 percent correct on three successive trials) was 4.8 sessions for Group 1, i.e., the experiment required an average of approximately five days for each of these patients. For Group 2, which underwent the experimental task every other day, an average of 7.9 sessions was required per subject. The difference between the two groups, shown in Table 40-1, was statistically significant ($t=3.22$, $p<0.001$). Since the two groups started at the same level and attained the same criterion of success in different numbers of sessions, the mean amount of improvement per sessions differed from one group to the other. These data were obtained as follows: the total increment reached by each subject in the experiment was divided by the number of sessions required. Then, the average increment in correct responses per sessions was computed within each group.

The final results are shown in Table 40-2. The subjects who worked with the experimental task daily achieved a mean of 2.7 additional correct responses in each successive session; those who worked on alternate days, 1.2 additional correct responses. As indicated by the standard deviation of the average increment in correct responses, there was considerable variability in improvement from patient to patient. The difference between the two groups was statistically significant ($t=2.103$, $p<0.05$).

TABLE 40-2. PERFORMANCES OF THE TWO EXPERIMENTAL GROUPS IN LEARNING TO REPRODUCE THE SUCCESSIVE LETTERS OF THE TERMINAL WORDS OF EIGHT SENTENCES

Groups	Number of Patients	Mean Increment in Correct Responses per Session	S. D.
Group 1 (Working daily)	10	2.7	4.2
Group 2 (Working every other day)	10	1.2	3.6

Naming Pictures. The names of the ten pictures included 70 letters. On Trial 1, the mean numbers of correct responses of the two groups were 36.3, S.D. = 14.2, and 37.5, S.D. = 9.9, not significantly different ($t=0.48$, $p>0.6$). The record of the two groups' progress toward the criterion of success (90 percent correct on three successive trials) is summarized in Tables 40-3 and 40-4. The differences between the two groups were similar to those of Tables 40-1 and 40-2: patients who were confronted with the experimental task daily mastered it in an average of 4.4 sessions, S.D. = 1.02; on alternate days, 7.8 sessions, S.D. = 1.94. The difference is statistically significant ($t=2.94$, $p>0.01$). The mean increment in correct responses per sessions was 5.0, S.D. = 6.3, and 1.8, S.D. = 3.8, respectively. The difference is statistically significant: $t=3.10$, $p>0.01$.

TABLE 40-3. SESSIONS REQUIRED BY THE TWO EXPERIMENTAL GROUPS IN LEARNING TO REPRODUCE THE SUCCESSIVE LETTERS OF THE NAME OF TEN PICTURES

Groups	Number of Patients	Number of Sessions Required to Meet Criterion	
		Mean	S. D.
Group 1 (Working daily)	10	4.4	1.02
Group 2 (Working every other day)	10	7.8	1.94

TABLE 40-4. PERFORMANCES OF THE TWO EXPERIMENTAL GROUPS IN LEARNING TO REPRODUCE THE SUCCESSIVE LETTERS OF THE NAMES OF TEN PICTURES

Groups	Number of Patients	Increment in Correct Responses per Session	
		Mean	S. D.
Group 1 (Working daily)	10	5.0	6.3
Group 2 (Working every other day)	10	1.8	3.8

Retention. Fourteen of the twenty subjects were available for retesting one week after the conclusion of the experiment. The mean scores of the final experimental session and of the post-session test are summarized in Table 40-5. The 14 patients included persons from both experimental groups, 1 and 2. In neither task, providing the terminal word or naming a picture, did the subjects forget during the post-session week the material that they had learned during the experimental sessions. The mean correct responses to terminal words in the final test and in a post-session test are respectively: 36.0, S.D. = 2.57, and 34.6, S.D. = 3.08. The differences between the scores on the two sessions were not statistically significant: $t = 1.32$, $p > 0.2$. The mean correct responses to naming pictures in the final and post session tests are respectively: 63.0 S.D. = 6.8, and 59.4, S.D. = 7.6. The differences between the two sessions were not statistically significant: $t = 1.44$, $p > 0.1$.

DISCUSSION AND CONCLUSIONS

Two practical results emerge from this study: in working with adult aphasic patients, daily sessions are more fruitful than sessions on alternative days; and verbal tasks that have been mastered by aphasic patients are retained for at least a week.

The first of these supports experimentally the clinical suggestion to use massed therapy with adult aphasics (Longerich and Bordeaux, 1954).

The second is in keeping with the work of Hull (1917) who suggested that brain-damaged non aphasic individuals, although disturbed in their fixation processes, are capable of retaining the task that they have mastered. The different performances in fixation and retention processes are discussed also by Zangwill (1946)

TABLE 40-5. THE MEAN NUMBER OF CORRECT RESPONSES IN THE FINAL EXPERIMENTAL TESTING SESSION AND IN A POST-SESSION TEST

	Number of Patients	Correct Responses in Terminal Words		Correct Responses in Naming Pictures	
		Mean	S. D.	Mean	S. D.
Final Test	14	36.0	2.57	63.0	6.8
Post-session Test	14	34.6	3.08	59.4	7.6

and Meyer (1961), and fit in with the hypothesis that different neurophysiological processes underlie these performances (Chauchard, 1963).

Although the Language Retrieval Unit was not fully exploited in its intended functions as a teaching machine, it proved to be a convenient, stimulating and unbiased device for presenting some of the stimuli and for collecting all of the responses of the experiment.

SUMMARY

Two groups of adult aphasic individuals mastered two letter-prediction tasks. One group worked at the tasks daily; the other, on alternate days. The former made much faster progress than the latter. When retested a week after the terminal experimental session, the subjects were found to have retained the tasks they had learned.

Acknowledgments. The authors are grateful to the V.A. Hospitals of Cleveland and Dayton, Ohio, to the Speech and Hearing Center in Dayton, Ohio, and the Highland View Hospital in Cleveland, Ohio, for their kind permission to work with their patients in experimental sessions. The authors wish to express their gratitude to Dr. J. W. Black who supervised the work and revised the paper.

REFERENCES

Abnett, A. C. (1966) *Design, Operation and Circuitry of the Language Retrieval Unit.* The Ohio State University Research Foundation Report, Columbus, Ohio 43212.

Chauchard, P. (1963) *Les mécanismes cérébraux de la mémoire,* "Civiltà delle Macchine," **21,** 55–61.

Carson, D. H., and Smith, E. (1965) *Aphasic performance on a complex classification task.* Paper presented at the ASHA Convention, Chicago.

Edwards, A. (1965) *Automated training for a "Matching-to-Sample" task in aphasia,* "J. Speech Hearing Res.," **8,** 39–42.

Hull, C. L. (1917) *The formation and retention of association among insane,* "Am. J. Psychol.," **28,** 419–435.

Katz, L. (1958) *Learning in aphasic patients,* "J. Consult. Psychol.," **22,** 143–146.

Isserlin, A. (1922) *Über Störugen im Extrapyramidalen System mit besonder Berücksichtigung der postencephalitischen,* "Dtsch. Zeitschr. Nervenheilk.," **74,** 319–342.

Longerich, M. C., and Bordeaux, J. (1954) *Aphasia Therapeutics.* MacMillan, New York.

Lopatkiewicz, P. (1961) *Analysis of nomination disorders in aphasic patients,* "Rozpr. Wyds. Nauk. Med. Pol. Akad. Nauk.," **2/6,** 129–144.

Meyer, V. (1961) *Psychological effects of brain damage,* in Handbook of Abnormal Psychology, ed. by Eysenck. Basic Books, New York.

Rocheford, V., and Williams, M. (1962) *Relationship between nominal dysphasia and the acquisition of vocabulary in childhood,* "J. Neurol. Neurosurg. Psychiat.," **25,** 222–227.

Rosenberg, B., and Edwards, A. (1964) *The performance of aphasia in three automated perceptual discrimination programs,* "J. Speech Hearing Res.," **7,** 295–298.

Tikofsky, R. S., and Berman, M. (1965) *Rote learning by adult aphasics.* Paper presented at the ASHA Convention, Chicago.

——, and Reynolds, G. (1962) *Preliminary study: non-verbal learning and aphasia,* "J. Speech Hearing Res.," **5,** 133–143.

——, —— (1963) *Further study of non-verbal learning and aphasia,* "J. Speech Hearing Res.," **6,** 329–337.

Zangwill, O. (1946) *Some qualitative observation on verbal memory in cases of cerebral lesions,* "British J. Psychol.," **37,** 8–19.

41

Clinical Treatment of Aphasia

HILDRED M. SCHUELL
VIRGINIA CARROLL
BARBARA S. STREET

HILDRED M. SCHUELL, Ph.D., (deceased) was director of the aphasia section of the neurology service of the Minneapolis Veterans Administration Hospital, and was with the department of neurology of the Graduate School of Medicine, University of Minnesota.

VIRGINIA B. CARROLL, B.A., is a speech pathologist in private practice, St. Paul, Minnesota.

BARBARA S. STREET, M.A., is a speech pathologist in private practice, Hopkins, Minnesota.

It is the purpose of this paper to cite certain significant clinical findings in aphasia, present a meaningful framework in which these may be considered, state principles underlying treatment, and describe specific techniques which have been found effective.

It is beyond the scope of this paper to discuss psychological problems of brain-injured patients, or to review methods in family counseling, and group therapy. These are omitted not because they are considered unimportant, but because this paper is written to meet expressed needs for clinically-tested methods and materials.

Principles and techniques for the treatment of involvement of auditory processes, sensorimotor processes, and visual processes in aphasia will be presented. A list of clinical materials is appended. Techniques are presented not to be followed unquestioningly, but to be evaluated and adapted to the needs of individual patients. The authors themselves are constantly engaged in critical examination and revision of their own methods.

From *Journal of Speech and Hearing Disorders* 20:43–53, 1955.

AUDITORY INVOLVEMENT

Test findings for more than 250 aphasic patients examined on the Neurology Service of the Minneapolis Veterans Administration Hospital, have shown that all aphasic patients are impaired in the retention and recall of sound patterns; the problem of impairment of auditory recognition has been discussed in another paper (*1*). Clinical findings indicate that impairment of auditory retention and recall are reversible to a considerable degree; and that improvement of articulation, word-finding, reading, and writing often results from the use of a single therapeutic principle: strong, controlled, intensive auditory stimulation. The aphasic patient needs to hear and grasp meaningful sound patterns over and over, day after day, month after month, as long as even minimal aphasic symptoms exist. Auditory stimulation may well be considered the foundation of all aphasia therapy.

There are six important principles involved in the use of effective auditory stimulation. These are:

1. *Material used should be meaningful to the patient and relevant to the context in which it is used.* The

clinician usually begins by naming objects directly at hand, objects on the desk, objects in the room, to which the patient's attention is directed. Test responses have proved that it is possible to use pictures effectively from the beginning, thus enlarging the scope of materials. It is obviously impossible to bring a barn, a cow, or a tractor into the clinic; but a patient from a farm may respond far more to pictures of these than to a comb, a cup, or a spoon placed in his hand.

2. *Length of each auditory unit presented must be carefully controlled.* This means that the clinician must use language units short enough for the patient to grasp. This varies from patient to patient, and the length of unit which can be effectively used increases steadily as therapy progresses. Means of determining auditory retention span have been described in a previous study (*2*). Most patients do not receive effective auditory stimulation from the ordinary environment, because people talk too fast, and say too much at a time for them to grasp.

3. *The patient should make a specific response to each language unit presented.* The clinician must wait for this response and reinforce it with repetition of the stimulus, timing this repetition to coincide with the patient's response. Van Riper (*3*) considers timing of primary importance: the clinician attempts to say the word at the exact moment the patient is groping for it.

When the patient has no speech, the required response may be pointing to an object or picture named by the clinician, following a direction, or performing a series of actions with the clinician. The clinician gives the direction and repeats it as the patient carries it out. Almost all patients begin to verbalize spontaneously with the clinician during this process.

When this response, the patient verbalizing with the clinician, is well-established, there are two variations which help the patient move from talking with the clinician to more voluntary speech. The first is asking the patient to repeat what he has just said, with an immediate *Say it again.* As a further step, before a set of objects or pictures are presented, the patient is instructed casually, *Say it if you can. If it doesn't come, listen, think it, say it with me.* This procedure is not used until the patient has been observed to initiate some responses. No pressure is placed on the patient to initiate the word; he is merely given an opportunity to do so if he can. If the word does not come, the clinician pronounces it; if it does, additional stimulation is given anyway, by using the word in short, common phrases (for example: *door; open the door; close the door; lock the door; go to the door*). Usually both the number and length of spontaneous responses tend to increase gradually.

In more advanced stages of therapy, patients are asked to repeat words, phrases, and sentences of controlled length, and to write these units from dictation. Length of words and length of units presented should be slowly but progressively increased. The patient's ability to formulate sentences of his own, both in speech and in writing, improves with his ability to retain language patterns; and techniques are varied to permit this as soon as it is feasible. The transition from repeating and writing from dictation to independent formulation is probably best accomplished by giving the patient a few additional easier words each day, to try on his own. Materials change from pictures of familiar objects to pictures of a single activity (man cutting grass), and then to more complex situational pictures in which the patient describes what is happening, adding more and more details as language increases. Printed materials are used to an increasing extent.

4. *Abundant and varied materials should be used during each clinical period.* This principle is based on the assumption that the aphasic patient does not need to be taught words as does, for example an adult learning a foreign language. The aphasic patient has words; they are not readily available to him. The process of therapy is not teaching words but stimulating damaged processes to function again. It is further based on the clinical observation that giving the patient a great deal of auditory

stimulation in controlled units, and giving him time to respond to each unit produces a good deal of language in a relatively short time, while drilling on five or six words produces frustration and tends to inhibit progress.

5. *The maximal number of verbal attempts should be made by the patient during each clinical period.* This would seem obvious. The fact that he has spoken a hundred or more times during the clinical hour gives the patient confidence in his ability to talk, as well as more reinforcement of language processes. Because of this experience, he is more apt to try to talk when he goes back to the ward than he would if he had spent the hour trying to learn a few words he could not be sure of having available when he wanted them.

6. *Defective responses should not usually be corrected.* The patient talks as well as he is able to talk at a given time. Early correction is frustrating, and consumes time which should be spent more productively. Errors tend to decrease and disappear as more language becomes available. When the patient begins to monitor his speech for himself, and ask for help, it should be given.

CLINICAL TECHNIQUES FOR AUDITORY STIMULATION

Among the techniques for auditory stimulation which follow, it will be noted that many involve reading and writing. This is recommended procedure, for one language modality serves to reinforce another, and similar recovery curves are seen in all modalities. Exceptions exist but are rare: a completely illiterate patient; a patient whose visual involvement is so severe that he cannot see a whole word (these may spell orally and learn to write); a patient whose sensori-motor system is so impaired he cannot trace or copy (these patients sometimes enjoy reading). Techniques must always be adapted to the patient's interests, level of performance, and pattern of impairment.

1. Present a group of objects or a group of pictures, ask patient to point to object or picture named and then attempt to say it with clinician, who repeats it as patient identifies correctly.

2. Place picture before patient, repeat word in common phrase, and ask patient to listen, think it, then say it with clinician. Examples: *bed: go to bed; in bed; make the bed.* Increase length gradually.

3. Ask patient to carry out simple directions; patient verbalizes actions with clinician, as he performs them. Examples: *Close the door; pick up the pencil; put the money in the box.*

4. Have patient count, say the days of the week, the months, and the alphabet, in unison with clinician. (These activities are aided by strongly-established previous associations, and are useful for giving the patient early success, and demonstrating that he can talk.)

5. Ask patient to point to objects, using phrases, such as *the man smoking a pipe.* Repeat after clinician, as in 1.

6. Present phrases and sentences using common associations and ask patient to complete phrase. (This is easier than naming objects and patients have earlier success with it.) Examples: *a cup of________; I go to bed at________.*

7. Have patient read with clinician. (This may be used with all patients who are able to match simple words to pictures.) The clinician selects a short paragraph with vocabulary somewhat above patient's word recognition level. The paragraph is read in unison four or five times; the clinician points or asks the patient to point to each word as it is spoken. The paragraph is read slowly the first time, but with normal inflection and phrasing. On successive readings, rate is gradually increased as long as the patient is able to follow. On the final reading the clinician attempts to follow the patient, and to drop out whenever possible, until the patient is able to read unassisted. Lastly, the clinician asks questions about the material read. Difficulty of material should be gradually increased.

On the first reading, the patient may speak no words intelligibly. He is told this doesn't matter. Percentage of intelligible words tends to increase on each re-reading, sometimes slowly, sometimes dramatically, and to rise from week to week. When questions are asked, most patients are first able to respond only by pointing to the desired word, which is then spoken by the clinician; next they respond with a single word. As therapy progresses, patients become able to make more numerous and more adequate responses. For example, a patient who had progressed from no speech to ability to use two or three word responses, answered the question, *How large is Sweden?* with a fluent, *About two hundred miles wide and a thousand miles long*, and was amazed at what he had said. This is a frequent occurrence with this technique.

8. Ask the patient to repeat words, progressing from one-syllable, to words of two, three, four, and five syllables. Direct patient's attention to listening to end of word, then listening to each syllable.

9. Ask the patient to repeat sentences, gradually increasing length. Conversational usage should be stressed, and material should be structured towards daily situations, or patient's special interests. Examples: *Pass the cream and sugar; Has the paper come? Someone called you this morning, but I don't know who it was.*

10. Give an ordinary message. Ask patient to listen to get the main ideas, then answer question in his own words. Examples:

a. *Get a loaf of bread, a dozen eggs, and a pound of butter.* Question: *What did I ask you to get?*
b. *Paul called last night, and said he and Mary were going to California Friday. They want to have us over when they get back.* Questions: *Who called? Where are he and Mary going? When are they leaving? What do they want to do when they get back?*

11. Have the patient write letters of alphabet from dictation. Use random order.

12. Employ spelling aloud.

13. Have the patient write from dictation. Dictate 30 or 40 words at a time, beginning at patient's spelling level, and gradually increasing difficulty. Give patient misspelled words to study for next day. Ask him to write a sentence using each word, as soon as he is able to do so.

14. Ask the patient to write sentences from dictation. Adapt vocabulary to spelling level. Dictate entire sentence, have patient repeat, then write.

15. Ask the patient to write names, addresses, and telephone numbers from dictation. (This is especially necessary for patients who will return to an occupation requiring them to take telephone messages.)

16. Ask patient to listen to a short radio newscast and report it.

17. Have patient use recorded sentences or paragraphs for extra practice. Include questions for patient to answer in writing.

18. Ask the patient to read aloud and retell. Use materials of progressive length and difficulty.

19. Read factual material aloud to patient, ask him to write down essential facts on what has been read, and retell. (This is necessary for patients who wish to go on to further vocational or educational training.)

TECHNIQUES FOR INCREASING VOCABULARY AND LANGUAGE USAGE

All the techniques described for auditory stimulation increase the patient's vocabulary, but as he acquires more language, additional techniques should be introduced to place increasing responsibility for speech on the patient. These are listed in the order of the patient's ability to perform them.

1. Carry on simple conversations, involving greetings, patient's name and address, names of members of his family, and daily activities.

2. Have the patient name objects and describe pictures.

3. Have the patient answer questions related to a situation, or materials being used.

4. Use word-association. The clinician speaks a word and asks patient to respond with a different word that comes into his mind. Start with easy associations, such as opposites, colors, common categories such as clothing, furniture, etc. As vocabulary increases more general words may be used.

5. Use word-associations. The clinician speaks a word and asks patient to name as many things as he can that the given word makes him think of. (Stimulus words should reflect patient's special interests and may range from farm crops to plays by Shakespeare.)

6. Have patient formulate sentences using

given words. At first this may be used with pictures as a further development of 2 under auditory stimulation. Example: *Now you give me a sentence using bed. What could you say?* (At first patients tend to repeat phrases the clinician has used and this is acceptable.)

7. Have the patient define words. (This requires more precision in the use of language, but may be started simply.) The patient is asked *What is an orange? Just tell me in your own words.* At one stage of therapy *eat* may be an acceptable response. At a later stage a response may be obtained such as *A citrus fruit. It grows on trees in the tropics.*

8. Ask the patient to explain techniques or processes with which he is familiar, such as how to fix a tire, fill a tooth, or make a will.

9. Read and retell, using materials of progressive difficulty.

10. Use word games for advanced patients. The clinician says *I am thinking of a word that rhymes with air.* Instead of naming word patient defines it, as *Is it something you sit on?* and the clinician replies *No, it is not chair.* Roles reverse if patient guesses correctly, or if clinician fails to identify the correct word.

SENSORI-MOTOR INVOLVEMENT

Almost all aphasic patients have some expressive aphasia; that is, vocabulary is limited, word-finding errors and mispronunciations occur; speech may be partially intelligible, or unintelligible. In most patients the defective speech is a reflection of impairment of ability to reauditorize language sequences. In a few, a specific sensori-motor disability coexists with impairment of auditory processes. Criteria for discriminating between the two kinds of involvement, either of which may result in defective speech, have already been published (*2*).

For patients with specific sensori-motor involvement, it is considered advisable to use additional techniques for obtaining voluntary control of the speech musculature. As auditory techniques are chiefly stimulation techniques, motor techniques may be regarded chiefly as facilitation techniches (*4*). Some clinicians consider sensori-motor techniques unnecessary, and auditory stimulation through which speech is normally acquired is used exclusively. The authors tend to believe that if sensori-motor techniques are used, speech is facilitated, emerges sooner, and is more accurate—thus shortening the initial period of frustration, and insuring a better end result. Sensori-motor techniques should always be used in addition to auditory stimulation, except in the following circumstances:

1. When the patient says some short phrases with normal articulation and inflection.

2. When it is possible to get the patient to count to 10, name the days of the week, or repeat short words, with adequate auditory stimulation; or when some words are spoken normally on these attempts.

Sensori-motor techniques are usually required when the following conditions obtain:

1. The patient has difficulty imitating gross movements such as opening and closing mouth, protruding tongue, blowing out a match, or initiating phonation.

2. When alternating movements, such as protruding and retracting tongue and moving tongue laterally and vertically, are markedly hesitant and uncertain, and speech is markedly impaired.

The lower facial paralysis seen in hemiplegia commonly has little observable effect on speech. Patients often compensate extremely well for a mild paresis of the tongue and palate, and speech is well within normal range. It is probably patients with most severe sensory involvement who have most trouble with movement patterns.

Techniques may be divided into techniques for general facilitation of movement patterns, techniques for obtaining specific sounds, and techniques for reinforcing and facilitating learned patterns.

TECHNIQUES FOR FACILITATION OF MOVEMENT PATTERNS

Vocal cord paralysis has not been reported or observed in hemiplegic patients. However, differences probably exist in the amount of bilateral innervation among individuals, and conditions which suggest mild sensori-motor involvement are found. What is observed, in order of frequency, is impairment of ability to alter pitch voluntarily, irregular pitch intervals, impairment of ability to sustain phonation, decrease in volume, and impairment of ability to initiate phonation.

Phonation can usually be secured if the clinician places his hand on the patient's throat at the level of the larynx, and then asks the patient to take a deep breath and push forward against the clinician's hand as he expells it. The deep breath apparently offers some facilitation, and is possible for hemiplegic patients. Pressing with the hand simply helps the patient to know where to start.

Valuable techniques include asking the patient to:

1. Say *ah* with prolonged phonation. Timing the phonation obtained increases interest.
2. Vocalize up and down the scale.
3. Open and close jaw on rhythmic count.
4. Open and close jaws with phonation *(mamamamama)*. Vary rate and rhythm.
5. Protrude and retract tongue on command; *Out, in.*
6. Move tongue laterally on rhythmic count.
7. Move tongue vertically inside mouth on count or command; *Up, down.*
8. Sing familiar tune with *lalalalala.*
9. Sing familiar song in unison with clinician. Ask patient to sing words as well as he can.
10. Blow out a match.
11. Draw water (as in siphoning) from one bottle to another with glass tubes. (This technique is useful when there is some paresis of soft palate.)
12. Blow in spirometer.

TECHNIQUES FOR OBTAINING SPECIFIC SOUNDS

With aphasic patients the most effective way to produce specific sounds seems to be to use a minimal placement cue, combined with a visual and an auditory one. It is usually sufficient to tell the patient, in non-technical language, what to do to start. Watching the clinician and watching himself in a mirror helps, in the beginning, to compensate for reduced proprioceptive and kinesthetic cues. The auditory cue is important. The patient needs to hear the sound. At the beginning this is not enough to enable him to reproduce it, but as therapy progresses it becomes so, and placement and visual cues can gradually be eliminated. It is almost never necessary to teach the formation of each speech sound. As sensori-motor processes begin to function more efficiently new sounds tend to emerge. For this reason, exploration, through auditory stimulation, should be a part of each clinical period.

The following minimal placement cues are found effective:

[m] Close lips. Hum.
[b] Press lips. Say sound.
[p] Press lips. Whisper.
[l] Press tongue up. Sing. Try *lalalalala.*
[d] Press tongue up. Say sound.
[t] Press tongue up. Whisper.
[g] Press with back of tongue. Say sound.
[k] Press with back of tongue. Whisper.
[r] Say *ah.* Now raise tongue gradually. (When patient can produce at will, ask him to omit the *ah.*)
[ð] Bite tongue. Say sound.
[θ] Bite tongue. Whisper.
[z] Close teeth. Say sound.
[s] Close teeth. Whisper.
[ʃ] Close teeth, blow. Like [s], but make it bigger. (Sometimes helps to have patient think, "Sh, be quiet.")
[w] Lips round. Say sound.
[ʍ] Lips round. Whisper.
[j] Press tongue down. Say sound.
[dʒ] Close teeth. Press tongue up. Say sound.
[tʃ] Close teeth. Press tongue up. Whisper.
[ŋ] Press with back of tongue. Hum.
[ɑ] Open mouth wide. Say vowel.
[oʊ] Say *ah.* Now make lips round. Now, alone.
[u] Say [oʊ]. Make it smaller.
[i] Say *ah.* Now smile. Now the [i] alone. (It is usually not necessary to ask

patient to elevate tongue-tip. He may be told to do this if necessary.)

[ɑɪ] Say *ah*. Now close mouth slowly.

[eɪ] Say [i]. Now open mouth a little.

[ɔ] Say *ah*. Now round lips a little.

[ɔɪ] Say [ɔ]. Now smile. (Or put an [i] on the end of it.)

Consonants can usually be secured in a syllable followed by [ɑ] before they can be isolated. Front vowels usually come first in common words, and are the last speech sounds to emerge for these patients. It is sometimes possible to move from the long sound of a vowel to its short sound, however, when the long ones are well established.

2. Ask the patient to count in unison with clinician. Use groups of three, giving strong rhythmic auditory stimulation.

3. Have patient say alphabet as above. Give placement cue when necessary.

4. Have him give the days of week, names of months with the above procedure.

5. Have him read in unison with clinician. Begin with short conversational sentences.

6. When these patients are able to repeat, they tend to produce words simultaneously with clinician. As a step towards voluntary speech, ask patient to say word or phrase twice, then three times. Finally ask him to wait and pronounce the word at a signal from clinician.

7. Use all techniques for auditory stimulation where possible.

TECHNIQUES FOR REINFORCING SOUNDS AND FACILITATING SPEECH MOVEMENTS

1. For each obtained sound:

a. Combine immediately with *ah*. Repeat, (as mamamamama) increasing rate, and varying rate and thythm.
b. Combine consonant with other vowels patients can make.
c. Repeat short familiar words beginning with desired consonant. Accept as correct if initial consonant is correct, but record other sounds which appear.
d. Associate learned sound with printed symbol. Write and say.
e. Place cards with learned sound on desk. Ask patient to indicate sound produced by clinician.
f. Place cards with learned sounds on table. Pronounce words beginning with these sounds. Ask patient to indicate the initial sound. Later he may be asked to point to the final sound.
g. Have patient imitate learned sounds daily with only auditory stimulation. Explore for new sounds in the same manner.
h. Present learned sounds on individual cards; give patient opportunity to initiate sound on presentation of symbol. Give patient set of cards with learned sound for practice.
i. Using words which start with learned sound in *Golden Dictionary*, read word with clinician. Give patient opportunity to initiate word when he can. Before patient is able to read sentences, present word in short familiar phrase (as *across the street*); have patient try to repeat.

VISUAL INVOLVEMENT

Suggestions for treatment of visual disturbances will be confined to those affecting reading and writing.

It must be remembered that a patient who cannot reauditorize a word, who cannot say it to himself, remains unable to do this when presented with a printed word. As a result, reading is defective when there is no visual involvement. A patient is usually unable to write a word unless he can say it to himself, and sometimes he needs to be able to spell it to himself. Thus writing is often impaired also, with no direct visual involvement.

The patients who need special techniques for reading and writing impairment, beyond those of auditory stimulation, are those with the following difficulties:

1. Confusion of letters with similar visual configurations, such as *EF, CG, PBR, WM, hnru, VAN, pdbq*, etc. (Patients with auditory involvement tend to confuse letters whose names sound alike, such as *BCDE, SF, AHJ, IY*, etc.) Confusions appear on reading and writing when not present on discrimination.

2. Reversals of letter sequences in words.

3. Confusion of words which look alike, such as *watch* and *match, dark* and *pink*.

4. Special difficulty with ends of words.

5. Slowness of word recognition.

6. Confusion of upper and lower case letters in writing.

7. Special difficulty with double letters in spelling (sounding does not help).

8. Tendency to spell phonetically.

9. Difficulty in keeping place and in following a line.

Unless auditory processes are severely impaired, most of these patients will be able to spell aloud better than they can write. In fact, they frequently spell a word correctly and write it incorrectly, because of impaired revisualization of symbols or symbol sequences.

The impairment may be so severe that the patient can read or write nothing when first seen. At the end of four of five months he may be able to write an acceptable letter, and read at his former level, but with marked reduction in rate of both performances.

TECHNIQUES FOR VISUAL INVOLVEMENT

The patient must relearn visual symbols, both to recognize and to recall them. In severe cases, begin with upper case print. When upper case forms are learned, combine each upper case symbol with the same symbol in lower case. Do not introduce script until reading rate is close to normal. Effective devices are the following:

1. Writing and naming individual symbol simultaneously.

2. Writing and saying letters in alphabetical order, in groups of five or six; combine learned groups.

3. Pointing to letter named by clinician. Use groups of letters, then alphabet.

4. Naming letters presented in random order.

5. Writing letters from dictation, presented in random order.

6. Writing words from dictation. Begin with two and three letter words; gradually increase length.

7. Reading single words; use Dolch cards. Time.

8. Reading phrases; use Dolch cards.

9. Writing sentences to dictation and reading them back.

10. Pointing to word spoken by clinician. Use a picture dictionary or word list.

11. Reading short paragraph material aloud. Assignment; writing answers to printed questions.

12. Reading aloud; timing.

13. Daily spelling. Dictate thirty or forty words below patient's oral spelling level. Give misspelled words for study, and writing practice; use them in sentences when possible. Always have patient read back.

It will be seen that most of these techniques combine auditory and visual stimulation.

CLINICAL MATERIALS

All tests cited are from the Psychological Corporation, 552 Fifth Avenue, New York 18, New York, unless otherwise indicated.

1. A set of common objects used in daily life.
2. A set of pictures of common objects, including houses, rooms, furniture, toilet articles, articles of clothing, cigarettes, foods, dishes, eating utensils, car, garage, people, animals, etc. Pictures should be clear and vivid, but mounted on cards small enough for several to be presented simultaneously.
3. A set of action pictures, showing one activity: man cutting grass, raking leaves, washing dishes, fixing a tire, throwing a ball, etc.
4. A set of situational pictures, such as appear on the covers of the *Saturday Evening Post.*
5. A list of sentences (about 100) using common expressions, with a word omitted, for sentence completion. (Example: *Will you pour me a cup of . . . . . . ; I want a drink of . . . . . . ; I get up early in the . . . . . . ; it is time to go to . . . . . .*
6. *Ammons Full-Range Picture Vocabulary Test,* Southern Universities Press, Box 91 AA, Route 3, Valley Station, Kentucky.
7. *Dolch Picture Word Cards,* Garrard Press, Champaign, Illinois.
8. *Dolch Basic Sight Cards,* Garrard Press.
9. *Dolch Sight Phrase Cards,* Garrard Press.
10. *Gates Primary Word Recognition Test,* Forms 1, 2, 3, 4.
11. *Gates Advanced Primary Word Recognition Test,* Forms 1, 2, 3.
12. *Iowa Silent Reading Test* (Primary and Advanced). Vocabulary and sentence reading tests are particularly good for aphasic patients.
13. *Gray's Standardized Oral Reading Test.*

14. *Gate's Basic Reading Tests,* Types A, B, C, D, four forms for each test.
15. *Wide-Range Achievement Test,* Jastak.
16. *Directed Spelling Activities, Grades 2 to 8,* Betts and Arey, American Book Company, 88 Lexington Avenue, New York.
17. *Basic Reading Skills for High School Use,* Gray, Horseman, and Monroe, Scott Foresman Company, Chicago, Illinois.
18. *Reader's Digest Reading Skill Builders,* Reader's Digest Educational Service Incorporated, 353 Fourth Avenue, New York 10, New York.
19. Lists of common phrases, and conversational sentences: four and five word units; six and seven word units; eight, nine and ten word units.
20. *The Ellamac Pronunciary,* with materials for aphasia, published by Ellmac Inc., Evanston, Illinois. A graduated series of cards containing both visible and audible material. They have been designed specifically for the auditory stimulation of aphasic patients. The cards are recorded and are played in a viewing position which allows the user to see and hear the material simultaneously. The cards are kept in files for easy selection. They may be immediately replayed as often as is desired, and in any sequence. The sound is reproduced by an electromagnetic Pronunciary machine which is very simple to operate and can be managed by most aphasics.

SUMMARY

All aphasic patients are impaired in auditory retention and recall. In addition, specific sensori-motor involvement, specific visual involvement, or both, may coexist as complicating factors. Treatment for the individual patient is determined by the kinds of impairment which are present, as well as the degree of existing impairment, but auditory stimulation is essential for all aphasic patients. Techniques have been described for treating each kind of impairment, and materials cited.

REFERENCES

1. Schuell, H. M. Aphasic difficulties understanding spoken language. Neurology **3,** 1953, 176–184.
2. ——, Clinical observations on aphasia. *Neurology* **4,** 1954, 179–189.
3. Van Riper, C. Personal communication, 1954.
4. Wepman, J. M. A conceptual model for the processes involved in recovery from aphasia, *JSHD,* **18,** 1953, 4–13.

Socio-Psychotherapeutic Approach to the Treatment of Aphasic Patients

MANUEL ARONSON
LEO SHATIN
JEANNE C. COOK

MANUEL ARONSON, Ph.D., is a consulting psychologist in private practice, and is with the department of psychiatry of Albany Medical College.
LEO SHATIN, Ph.D., is with the department of psychiatry, New Jersey College of Medicine and Dentistry, Newark.
JEANNE C. COOK, M.A., was with the Albany Veterans Hospital.

This is a report of a group socialization and psychotherapeutic program conducted for male aphasic patients during the past twelve months at the Albany Veterans Hospital. The program was conducted under the joint auspices of Clinical Psychology (Psychiatry and Neurology Service) and Educational Therapy (Physical Medicine and Rehabilitation Service). The mechanics of speech re-training were de-emphasized in this group program, for the patients were already receiving individual speech instruction. The primary orientation was toward the patients as a group experiencing emotional difficulties in adjusting to their environment—emotional difficulties associated with the presence of a severe speech disorder.

This report describes fully the program as developed and implemented at a general medical and surgical hospital. It has a threefold purpose: (1) To describe the procedures employed in sufficient detail to permit their consideration for use by other workers in appropriate settings; (2) to evaluate such a program as it appears to patient participants and professional hospital staff; and (3) to indicate the function and applicability of such a program in a general hospital which is not a special speech center and which is not *uniquely* equipped to undertake the re-training of aphasics.

The term aphasia was defined as a defect in the power to communicate expressively through speech, writing, or other symbols, or to comprehend spoken or written language, due to injury or disease of the brain.

Although the program at Albany Veterans Hospital was conceived as a group psychotherapeutic program which in addition offered the patients an increased opportunity for socialization and communication, it soon became apparent that this medium also provided a closer liaison with the patient's physician and with ward personnel. The integration of the several treatment modalities generated an holistic approach to the patient.

Group re-education procedures in dysphasia are not new, but the group approach as social and psychological therapy for dysphasic patients is of rather recent origin. Zangwill (*16*) discussed the psychological state of the aphasic patient in the early and later stages of recovery from brain injury. He noted certain general principles associated with efforts at rehabilita-

From *Journal of Speech and Hearing Disorders* 21:352–64, 1956.

tion: compensation for injury to the central nervous system, the substitution of new responses, the use of direct training, and the need for vocational rehabilitation. Backus and Dunn (*3*) described their experiences with groups of patients in the clinical practice of speech rehabilitation, including aphasics. Although the classes were directed towards re-education of speech, they provided some opportunities for psychological treatment. Among the advantages cited were the opportunity to study the individual patient's needs, to gain insight into the nature of speech as social communication, and to observe the carry-over of new speech patterns into daily life. Social experiences were provided to assist in the acquisition of social techniques, while dramatic activities aided in the treatment of attitudes.

Backus (*1*) indicated the importance of the speech group's psychological climate and emphasized the need for activities which strengthened group cohesion. Backus (*2*) also described the need for an holistic approach to rehabilitation. She concluded that the individual's definition of the situation, his motivations and frustrations, and his course of life should be considered in the treatment program and its rationale. She pointed out that the aphasic patient's need for oral communication is most strongly felt within the group situation, and that interpersonal demands of the group may therefore facilitate social rehabilitation.

Shames (*10*) analyzed the relation between degree of homogeneity of the patients participating in group speech therapy and success in that therapy. He obtained sufficient evidence of the relationship between patient homogeneity and successful group treatment to warrant further exploration of his hypothesis.

Nielson *et al.* (*8*) described the model treatment program for traumatic aphasics at Birmingham Veterans Hospital. It was a comprehensive approach which employed the specialized techniques of Neurology, Psychology, Social Services, and Speech Pathology. Recreational activities were encouraged, together with "mental hygiene" and "psychological conditioning." Within this milieu, the language instruction attained a high level of success. Similarly oriented treatment programs have been conducted under the auspices of the United States Army (*7, 9, 11*). Wepman (*13*) discussed a model in-patient program for the treatment of aphasic adults, including full programs of social and psychological therapies. He has presented the many personal-psychologic desiderata (*14, 15*).

Corbin (*6*) analyzed her experiences with group instructional and treatment methods for veterans attending an aphasic clinic over a period of two and one-half years. The patients were designated as "motor-aphasic" or as having "dysarthric speech." Although the emphasis was upon speech rather than upon social and psychotherapeutic influences, the latter assumed an important role in the training procedure. Corbin sought to raise group morale and felt that group speech therapy gave increased carry-over of re-learned language and adjustment to the world of normal speech. Turnblom and Myers (*12*), observing the importance of patient-family interactions in determining the patient's motivations for speech rehabilitation, organized a group discussion program with families of aphasic patients. They concluded that their program did indeed aid the family to adjust emotionally to the problems of the aphasic.

Blackman and Tureen (*5*), impressed with the importance of staff and patient attitudes in attaining recovery of speech, instituted a series of group meetings designed to bolster the ego-strength of their aphasic patients. Nine patients aged 20 to 30 with head injuries dating back two to four years met at weekly intervals. In these meetings the patients expressed their inner feelings and resentments, later discussing more intimate problems after the group had become unified. The authors felt that associated disciplines such as teaching and social service were brought closer to the needs of the aphasic through this technique, thereby scting to reduce permanent invalidism. Blackman (*4*) discussed the socio-psychological situation of aphasics and described the group psychotherapeutic approach developed to meet their needs.

PROCEDURE

Subjects

All patients in the Albany Veterans Hospital with the diagnosis of aphasia, expressive or receptive, were drawn into the program. They came from both chronic and acute medical wards. Since the beginning of the program over a year ago, the group has met at weekly intervals for a period of one hour. The group has been fluid in the sense that new patients are added as previous members are discharged from the hospital. In spite of this movement, the presence of a number of long-term patients added a basic stability to the group. This core facilitated the integration of new members into the group.

The patient group membership was stabilized approximately at ten. The size of attendance at meetings varied somewhat depending upon the hospital discharge and admission rates. A total of 35 patients participated in the group program. Fourteen of this number attended only three meetings or less while 21 met with the group five or more times. The major content of the present report is concerned with the 21 patients who attended five or more times. Their mean attendance was 14.2 meetings, range 5 to 34. They are referred to as the "aphasic group" and constitute the source from which were derived the majority of the impressions reported. Table 42-1 summarizes some background data for the aphasic group.

Except for one younger patient of 29, the members of the aphasic group ranged in age from 40 to 67 years with a mean age level of 57.5 years. Thirteen had no more than a grammar school education, five attended high school, and three were college graduates. Analysis of the occupational distribution revealed that fifteen members of the group were unskilled or semi-skilled laborers, one was a farm-hand, and five came from the engineering-managerial-professional levels. Nineteen of the patients were white and two were negro. Eighteen were native born and three of foreign extraction. Three patients were widowed, nine were single, and nine married.

The cause of aphasia for nineteen of the patients was cerebral vascular accident. One had skull fracture and one a post-operative aneurysm. Seven patients were capable of free ambulation, ten were incapable of ambulation without a wheelchair, and four were classified as having limited ambulation, *i.e.*, ambulatory only in the clinic. The severity of illness was further reflected in terms of degree of self-care. Nine patients were capable of full self-care, (feed self, care for personal hygiene, and bathroom needs), nine were capable of limited self-care (feed self but unable to care for other personal needs), and three were incapable of any self-care. The classification of degree of speech impairment was as follows: five extreme, five severe, four moderate, and seven mild.

TABLE 42-1. APHASIC GROUP BACKGROUND (N = 21)

Variable	*Mean*	*Range*
Age	57.5	29–67
Educational grade level	8.9	3–16
Months since last employment	33.0	12–108
Number of hospitalizations (Prior to current one)	1.9	1–6
Total months of current hospitalization	13.9	2–96

Treating methods

At the start of the program, patients showed overt signs of frustration whenever they attempted to speak in the group. They employed several defensive mechanisms on this account, but most commonly they tended to withdraw from this situation which made demands upon speech. More and more, they relied upon non-verbal techniques to make known their wants. Initial efforts to develop a group speaking program therefore met with considerable resistance and it was necessary to resort to a variety of activities in order to achieve some degree of intragroup cohesiveness. These activities constituted a continuum from the non-verbal at one pole (*e.g.*, rhythm group) to the completely verbal at the other (*e.g.*, group-centered discussion). Seldom was interest sustained in any single activity, especially at first. It was therefore necessary to shift techniques and activities from time to time in order to maintain the necessary interest and group cohesion. The techniques are described below, in sequence from the least verbal to the most verbal.

A. Music rhythm group.[1] Music is a universal language in the sense that there are few people incapable of responding to it on some level. The use of rhythm instruments by the patients played to the accompaniment of well-known marches, waltzes, and popular songs was quite helpful during the initial phase of this program in the attainment of a feeling of group unity. So reluctant were patients to talk in the beginning that the very matter of simple introductions was a difficult task for the group. Rhythm band activity served several purposes: (1) It was a group activity; and each man was therefore given the opportunity to work with others; (2) it was a vehicle whereby the individual patient released pent-up feelings through motor action; and (3) it emphasized rhythm, an essential aspect of speech.

B. Group singing. The rationale for the use of rhythm instruments is also applicable to group singing, with the additional advantage that group singing utilizes the voice and speech. All patients participated despite their speech limitations, even when this meant only to hum along with the group. Old and familiar tunes occasioned difficulty only for the most severely disabled, but more recently popular songs caused difficulty for a majority of the patients.

C. Story time. As the patients became more comfortable in the verbal situation, stories by well-known writers such as O. Henry and Sinclair Lewis were read to them. Discussion of the content and meaning of the tale always ensued. One short mystery by S. S. Van Dine was particularly successful. After hearing the story and all essential clues, the group became quite active in its analysis of the tale and in its attempt to ascertain the villain.

[1] Rhythm group facilities were provided through the courtesy of the Hospitalized Veterans Music Service of the Musicians Emergency Fund, Inc., New York.

D. Speech games. These helped the patients to utilize their verbal abilities and permitted the leaders to observe patients' reasoning power. A form of "Lotto" permitted direct concentration upon vocabulary. The interpretation of proverbs helped the leaders to estimate the abstractive levels of the various members. Responses to proverbs often yielded clues pertaining to the personality structure. Speech games often gave rise spontaneously to emotionally charged discussions.

E. Puppets. Opportunity was provided the groups to engage in unstructured but dramatic situations involving puppets. This medium was less structured than the speech games. Male and female puppet characters of varying roles and age levels were used, and informal participation was encouraged.

F. Tape recordings. The tape recorder was used both diagnostically and therapeutically. It permitted the patient to evaluate changes in his speech from time to time by comparing recordings of his voice. The opportunity to record and hear their own speech was a new experience for all the men. Each man approached the recorder with some apprehension, and several times the recording session constituted a near-catastrophic experience. The latter does *not* constitute contra-indication for the use of this equipment. Reactions to playbacks varied. Two patients became depressed and cried, several were fairly elated because they felt their speech was not as bad as they had suspected. The frustration of inability to say all that one wishes to was observed in every instance. Each man was recorded individually, but in the presence of the whole group. The group was always attentive to this procedure. The efforts of each man touched off considerable discussion in every instance. The discussion was primarily of a supportive type. Words of encouragement and praise were given sincerely and spontaneously even by the most hostile members of the group. This, more than any other activity, invariably led to sympathetic display among the members of the group.

G. Group-centered discussions. As self-confidence increased and as relationships among the members of the group solidified, group discussions became possible without the aids previously described. A variety of feelings were explored, including attitudes toward each other, toward group leaders, and toward hospital personnel and routine. Discharge was discussed, with its implications for economic and/or social dependence upon others. The patients evaluated their physical limitations, as well as their problems of interpersonal and intra-familial relationships. Gradually they became more capable of perceiving themselves against the background of family and society. There was movement from fixation upon speech *per se* to a consideration of self as a person confronted with the problem of adjusting to everyday living.

Refreshments[2] were served at all meetings and successfully enhanced the informal social atmosphere. The methods described above were presented in varied sequence, according to the developing needs of the patients. During the initial meetings there was greater emphasis upon non-verbal techniques. This gave way slowly to the verbal methods of later meetings, but considerable variety was necessarily employed to maintain the group at a high level of stimulation and interest. Complete reliance upon group discussion alone was not feasible. Occasionally the group carried on spontaneously for several sessions, but invariably a retrogression would set in. When this occurred it became essential to introduce a planned activity in order to help the group reestablish integration and unity. Hence, this pool of varied techniques was held available and employed with flexibility in order to maintain maximum motivation.

[2] These, together with the services of two volunteers, were provided through the courtesy of the American Red Cross. The Albany Veterans Hospital Special Services Department made possible this assistance.

Methods of observation

This program was conceived from the standpoint of treatment rather than research, hence no formal experimental design was projected. For the purpose of reporting these experiences, several types of observations were made and survey data gathered. These are described below.

A. Patient reactions. The patients' reactions to the speech program were evaluated by three separate approaches: rating, interview, and qualitative analysis of group behavior. The patient ratings and interviews were conducted during the months of May and June 1955, with all patients in the treatment group who had received five or more treatments. There were eleven such patients. A twelfth was excluded because he was unable to comprehend the questions.

1. Ratings. A seven-item, five-point check list was constructed for the purpose of eliciting the patients' impressions of the aphasie program. The items were geared to reflect feelings toward the group meetings and the group leaders, toward own speech, and finally toward relationships with others. The patients were also asked to rank, in order of preference, the various activities employed. The scale was administered to each of the patients by an experienced psychological examiner in an individual interview situation. Each item was read aloud by the psychologist, and, when necessary, explanations were given until the patient understood the question satisfactorily. It was then rated by the patient on a 5-point scale (1 through 5), with 1 indicating the most favorable or satisfied response for that item and 5 indicating the least so (most rejecting).

2. Interview. This was structured so as to clarify the responses to the check list. It also enabled the patient to express significant feelings and attitudes not otherwise covered by the items. Since the interview was held after the check list had been administered, it made possible a qualitative exploration of the patient's responses without contaminating his

answers to the items on the check list.

3. Analysis of group behavior. Complete notes were kept for each of the group meetings. These were analyzed from the standpoint of the members' individual reactions and intragroup dynamics.

B. Observations by hospital personnel. Hospital personnel working closely with the patients were interviewed to determine whether the group program affected patient behavior in day-by-day routine. These included ward physicians, nurses, and a variety of rehabilitation therapists, including corrective therapy, educational therapy, manual arts therapy, occupational therapy, and physiotherapy.

The interview was standardized, and based upon a ten-item questionnaire. The interviewee responded to each item with "yes" or "no" or "cannot say," and was then encouraged to elaborate upon his replies. The items were designed to elicit the staff's observations and opinions concerning the effect of the program on the patient's speech, feeling of well-being, and interpersonal relationships. The respondent was provided opportunity to air his satisfaction or dissatisfaction with the results of the program.

C. Observations by group leaders. As a final step, the group leaders held periodic conferences in which they analyzed their subjective impressions of the group program. In these sessions they integrated and coordinated their judgments concerning the meaning of this program to the patients. They pinpointed the main difficulties encountered in establishing such a program and discussed methods which might be employed to meet these difficulties.

ANALYSIS OF FINDINGS

A. Patient reactions.

1. Ratings. These were elicited from all patients in treatment at the time of this report, eleven in number. Table 42-2 presents the group mean self-ratings and range for each of the 7 items. It will be recalled that each item was ratable 1 to 5, and a low rating was in the favorable direction. The rank order number of the mean rating for each of the 7 items is listed in the final column of Table 42-2. Rank order number 1 indicates most favorable response, rank order number 7 least favorable.

The data reflected in Table 42-2 are suggestive rather than definitive, for they are too sparse to justify further statistical treatment or significance tests. They do suggest that the patients responded most favorably to those items reflecting attitudes toward the group procedures, while items concerned specifically with the patients' perception of change in speech or feelings about speech received the lowest ratings. In summary, the group responded quite favorably toward the program as a whole and toward the manner in which it was conducted, and expressed a need to continue with it.

At the end of the check list, the patients were asked to rank the several group activities in order of preference. Only two of the eleven

TABLE 42-2. PATIENT RATINGS OF SPEECH PROGRAM (N = 11)

Item	*Mean Rating*	*Range*	*Rank Number**
1. Satisfaction with meetings	1.73	1–3	2.5
2. Meetings relaxing vs tensional	1.82	1–4	4
3. Effect on own speech	2.27	1–5	6
4. Effect on *feelings* about own speech	2.44	1–5	7
5. Desire to continue with group	1.73	1–4	2.5
6. Value of group leaders in solving speech problems	1.54	1–3	1
7. Meetings as aids to social interaction	2.09	1–5	5

* Lowest score constitutes highest degree of acceptance and highest rank.

patients were able completely to rank all eight activities in order of preference. Four listed two to four preferences, four others were able to list but a single preference, and one patient could not designate any preference.

The activity which seemed to impress itself most on the minds of the patients was that of recording and listening to one's voice. Although only two patients could give complete rankings, nine of the eleven patients did include this activity in their rankings. More significantly, seven patients gave it an extreme rank (upper *or* lower). Five members of the group gave it a number one ranking, one patient a number two ranking, and one patient ranked it last in order of preference. Hence, it appears that this activity elicited a more clear-cut reaction than did any of the others. It is reasonable to hypothesize that attitudes and emotional reactions aroused by self recordings are intense, whether positive *or* negative. Inspection of the rankings further indicated that rhythm band activity and group singing were also high in order of preference, but not to the extent of tape recordings.

2. Interview. All patients but two expressed a positive attitude toward the program. One of the two exceptions voiced dissatisfaction with his speech progress, and the other criticized the general intellectual level of the group. The interviews revealed the definite existence of a generalized "halo" reaction to the sessions. The majority of patients expressed a favorable attitude toward the group program. Where this was found, generally positive attitudes were also expressed toward one's own speech, group leaders, ward physicians, and hospital care. Only the two patients of high educational level and with mild impairment were capable of independently variable positive or negative opinions depending upon the item or phase of the program under consideration.

3. Analysis of group behavior. An outstanding feature of the notes on the weekly meetings was the gradual change which they indicated in the patients from strong resistance to almost complete acceptance of the *idea* of group psychotherapy. Resistance seemed to result from two factors: the usual self-absorption of the physically damaged or ill and an ingrained belief that psychology is for "crackpots." It was necessary in the beginning to introduce every activity primarily as an aid to speech, since all were willing to admit some speech disability but none wished to admit any need for psychotherapy. As an example, it is of interest to record the changes in attitudes observed in one of the patients:

Mr. R., alone in the world as were the majority of these patients, exemplified those who found a circle of friends in the group. His initial apprehension and resistance ('They're working me too hard already; I don't need it.') cleared as the hospital schedule fell into place and his attendance at the group meetings became the high point of his week. Beginning with a wholehearted enjoyment of the refreshments, he progressed to an interest in every group activity, followed conversations closely, and began to enter into them spontaneously—if not pertinently. For example, at the end of a lively political discussion wherein even one totally speechless patient had participated by drawings and by gestures, Mr. R. declared himself: 'I'm in favor of the whole Salvation Army!' Nor did he resent or misinterpret the ensuing laughter; he realized that it was with him rather than at him.

The ability to laugh at one's self and to laugh with others has been an obvious achievement of interpersonal action within the group. Rigidity, tension, and self-pity have been seen to disappear in the laughter of a group drawn together by a common disability. The gradually developing group integration was accompanied by change in group attitude from distrust of psychotherapy to a feeling of welcome relief at the weekly opportunity offered for the expression and exchange of personal problems.

B. Observations by personnel.

These were obtained in a structured interview through the administration of a personnel questionnaire. The 21 patients of the source group received a total of 68 ratings from three professional staff groups. Eighteen of these ratings were made by seven physicians, fifteen were made by eight nurses, and thirty-five by eleven rehabilitation therapists of the Physical Medicine and Rehabilitation Service.

Table 42-3 tabulates the percentage of "yes" responses of each professional group to each item of the personnel questionnaire. A "yes" reply was in the favorable direction for all items except items 6 and 9. A "no" response to item 6 (Did disturbance increase?) was considered a positive reply and therefore a *low* "yes" percent score would be in the favorable direction. A "yes" reply to item 9 was not necessarily favorable or unfavorable.

The "yes" percent score was derived by the formula:

$$\text{yes } \% = \frac{\text{yes responses}}{\text{yes + no + cannot say responses}}$$

Therefore, "cannot say" responses were treated as negative responses for purposes of this analysis.

Inspection of Table 42-3, especially column 4, reveals that all personnel respondents expressed a favorable attitude toward the group program. This was well reflected in their recommendations of such a program for other aphasic patients (item 10A). In only 1 percent of the ratings was there any feeling that disturbance resulted from the program (item 6). Although 83 percent of the replies stated that the general effects were beneficial (item 5), the favorableness of response dropped considerably when specific benefits and effects were individually considered: speech benefits, 65 percent favorable, relationships with other patients, 58 percent favorable, and relationships with personnel, 58 percent favorable (items 2, 3, 4). Eighty-eight percent believed the program helped to prevent further deterioration in speech and 91 percent were of the opinion that it helped to prevent further deterioration in social relationships (item 8B). There was also fairly general agreement (81 percent) that the program increased the patients' motivation to communicate with others (item 7).

In 24 percent of the ratings, the staff indicated a desire to receive more information concerning the program's progress than was actually received from the group leaders (item 9). This desire for information pertained to the progress the patient was making in the group and to information the group leaders might transmit which could be applied to the daily ward management of patients. The remaining 76 percent of the ratings indicated that further information was not required, the staff having been kept sufficiently well informed. Finally, 88 percent of the replies were in the affirmative direction with respect to the question of recommending a similar program for other disabled patients including geriatric and chronic medical problems (item 10B).

The extent to which the three rating groups (doctors, nurses, rehabilitation therapists) agreed on the order or rank of the benefits (items covered by personnel questionnaire)

TABLE 42-3. PERCENT 'YES' RESPONSES TO GROUP SPEECH PROGRAM IN PERSONNEL QUESTIONNAIRE RATINGS

Item	*Physicians*	*Nurses*	*Rehabilitation Therapists*	*Combined*
1. Knowledge of patient attendance	100	100	100	100
2. Program's effect on patient speech	50	80	65	65
3. Program's effect on patient rehabilitation	67	54	54	58
4. Program's effect on patient relationships with nurses and attendants	55	60	57	58
5. Were general effects beneficial?	76	88	85	83
6. Disturbances increased	6	0	0	1
7. Increased patient motivation for speech	83	94	74	81
8. Program helps prevent patient speech deterioration				
A. Speech	88	100	88	91
B. Interpersonal relationships	88	100	85	88
9. More information and progress notes desired	33	40	12	24
10. Interest in recommending				
A. Aphasics	100	100	100	100
B. Other disabled	100	54	100	88

derived from the program was evaluated. The mean rating score for each of the items for each of the three groups was determined. The mean scores for each of the items were then ranked from high to low for each group and rank order correlations between groups were calculated.

TABLE 42-4. AGREEMENT AMONG PERSONNEL GROUPINGS IN RATINGS OF BENEFITS TO PATIENTS

Groups Correlated	*Rho*	*Significance Level*
Physicians with rehabilitation therapists	.94	.01
Nurses with rehabilitation therapists	.71	.05
Physicians with nurses	.69	.05

Table 42-4 reports these correlations together with their significance levels. A review of the mean score for each of the items for each of the three groups indicates that the nurses have a somewhat different perspective than do the physicians or rehabilitation therapists. This perhaps is due to the nature of their contacts, which are more continuous and include a broader segment of the patient's life span. The nurses are relatively more enthusiastic about the program's favorable effect upon patient speech and motivation for speech. They also concur more fully with the view that this program decelerated deterioration of speech and of interpersonal relationships.

OBSERVATIONS

These comments were derived from observations made by the group leaders. Several conferences were held in which these observations were evaluated and their implications for this and similar programs analyzed. It is emphasized that they are qualitative in nature and made from a clinical viewpoint. They do not come from controlled experiments or statistical tests of significance.

The aphasic patient's identification with the group is achieved slowly. In addition to the usual adjustments necessary for adequate group relationships, the aphasic patient has the further handicap of limited expressive and receptive communication. This, together with his initial self-absorption and the strangeness of the new situation, constitutes a formidable barrier to interaction. However, once the patient discovers that all present have speech difficulty he shows greater evidence of striving toward group identification. Where total inattention continues beyond several meetings, it may predicate general progressive deterioration. It is a definite indication for discontinuance from the group.

Since group therapy helps to reduce anxiety in aphasic patients, it assumes practical importance from the standpoint of speech re-training. With the concomitant aid of group psychotherapy, more time in individual speech sessions can be given to instruction and less to support of the patient's ego.

Periods in group therapy where the tape recorder was employed were productive in two ways. First, members of the group gave support and encouragement to inexpressive patients by praising them for their effort, and this practice resulted in more persistent effort in individual speech re-training. Secondly, it increased the ability for self-criticism. This was important for patients who tended to be overactive or euphoric and did not "hear" their own defective speech.

The speech instructor also noted a carry-over from individual lessons to group sessions. Rapport with the speech instructor can be rather quickly established and communication may go well in individual treatments, but the instructor has few means of knowing how well instructions are being carried out in group situations. Group therapy provides a social speech situation wherein the speech instructor can observe the patient's ability to translate into actual communication the skills he has been learning.

The aphasic feels extremely threatened by the very notion of damage to his brain. He often attempts to blame his difficulties on a variety of other, less threatening, conditions. Repeatedly, patients blamed their communication difficulties upon their teeth, their hearing, and similar disabilities. However, the patients did come to accept a simple, carefully phrased explanation of their defect when this was given in an atmosphere of support and reassurance.

The aphasic patient finds it difficult to maintain sustained interest in any single activity. It is therefore necessary to shift techniques frequently in order to maintain maximum group cohesion. The patient, however, must be prepared carefully for shifts and for new programs. Although he may lose interest in the on-going activity, it remains the known and familiar, and he is unwilling to shift over to another. Careful preparation and structuring must be given to every shift of program. The patients were told why an activity was recommended. The group leader's attitude is also significant. Only insofar as he takes the new venture seriously does the patient view it so.

Although it was markedly heterogeneous in degree of illness and in background, the group derived profit from the program. However, it is suggested that homogeneous groupings are desirable when this is feasible. Grouping together of patients with the same general degree of communication impairment leads to more group movement and progress than does a heterogeneous grouping.

The group leaders had the extensive use of an excellent volunteer service. It was found that such personnel could make a fine contribution in a variety of areas. In addition to providing and assuming responsibility for the refreshments served at each meeting, they also contributed to specific programs by leading group singing and playing the piano for rhythm band sessions. Their mere presence gave a sympathetic and informal atmosphere to the meeting. This was important to all patients and especially to those who had limited contacts outside of the hospital environment.

The efforts of the several rehabilitative disciplines are indeed effective when the workers plan an integrated approach. In this project, the educational (speech) therapist was a co-leader for the group and gave individual speech lessons to group members. She could observe her patients in social settings not available to her before, and she utilized information thus gained in speech retraining. Furthermore, she brought interesting activities and content into the group meetings at times when verbal discussion *per se* was rejected by the patients. The clinical psychologist heightened the patients' motivation to interact socially, lessened the ever-present threat of general apathy, and served as psychological consultant to the educational therapist. The Chief of the Physical Medicine and Rehabilitation Service made available his complete facilities to assist in this program. The several hospital sections and services concerned with the welfare of these aphasic patients were gradually forged into a more close-knit and integrated treatment unit —or more accurately, treatment complex.

SUMMARY

A group socialization and psychotherapeutic program conducted with 21 male aphasic patients in a general hospital is described. The primary orientation was toward emotional difficulties and interpersonal relationships of the patients rather than correction of speech *per se*. Various observations were made including psychological interview and ratings by patients, qualitative analysis of group behavior, and questionnaires administered to hospital personnel (doctors, nurses, rehabilitation therapists). The reactions of the patients and personnel were quite favorable to this program. General observations and comments were presented concerning the group program.

REFERENCES

1. Backus, O. L. The use of a group structure in speech therapy. *JSHD,* **17,** 1952, 116–122.
2. ——, The rehabilitation of persons with aphasia. In West, R., Kennedy, L., and Carr, A., *The Rehabilitation of Speech.* New York: Harper & Brothers, 1947.
3. ——, and Dunn, H. M. Intensive group therapy in speech rehabilitation. *JSD,* **12,** 1947, 39–60.
4. Blackman, N. Group psychotherapy with aphasics *J. nerv. ment. Dis.,* **111,** 1950, 154–163.
5. ——, and Tureen, L. L. Aphasia—A psychosomatic approach in rehabilitation. *Trans. Amer. neurol. Ass.,* **73,** 1948, 193–196.
6. Corbin, M. L. Group speech therapy for motor aphasia and dysarthria. *JSHD,* **16,** 1951, 21–34.
7. Huber, M. Linguistic problems of brain-injured servicemen. *JSD,* **11,** 1946, 143–147.
8. Nielsen, J. M., Schultz, D. A., Corbin, M. A., and Crittsinger, B. A. The treatment of traumatic aphasics of World War II at Birmingham General VA Hospital, Van Nuys, California. *Milit. Surg.,* **102,** 1948, 351–364.
9. Peacher, W. G. Speech disorders in World War II: V. Organization of a speech clinic in an army general hospital. *JSD,* **11,** 1946, 233–239.
10. Shames, G. H. An exploration of group homogeneity in group speech therapy. *JSHD,* **18,** 1953, 267–272.
11. Sheehan, V. M. Rehabilitation of aphasics in an army hospital. *JSD,* **11,** 1946, 149–157.
12. Turnblom, M. and Myers, J. S. A. group discussion program with the families of aphasic patients. *JSHD,* **17,** 1952, 393–396.
13. Wepman, J. M. The organization of therapy for aphasia: I. The in-patient treatment center. *JSD,* **12,** 1947, 405–409.
14. ——, *Recovery from Aphasia.* New York: Ronald Press Co., 1951.
15. ——, A conceptual model for the processes involved in recovery from aphasia. *JSHD,* **18,** 1953, 4–13.
16. Zangwill, O. L. Psychological aspects of rehabilitation in cases of brain injury. *Brit. J. Psychol.,* **37,** 1947, 60–69.

Aphasia Therapy: Some "Relative" Comments and Some Purely Personal Prejudices

JOSEPH M. WEPMAN

JOSEPH M. WEPMAN, Ph.D., is with the department of psychology and is director of the Speech and Language Clinic of the University of Chicago.

In research on the psycholinguistic nature of the language deficit (Wepman and Jones, 1964, 1966) in aphasia, some part of which has been reported in the literature, a classification of the parts-of-speech categories of English was elaborated. One of these was the category called "relatives" which included "all those forms which may introduce both subordinate and interrogative constructions, e.g., who, which, what, why, where, how, etc. (Jones, Goodman, and Wepman, 1963). The use of such "relative" words in the speech of aphasic adults can be shown to differentiate aphasic patients one from the other.

The interrogatives listed also serve to introduce questions of extreme relevance to aphasia therapy, such as: *who* should do the therapy; *of what* should therapy consist or *how* should it be done; *when* should it be instituted, *when* discontinued. This meaning of relativity shall also be explored.

In the former, the parts-of-speech analysis, we deal with certain rather hard, objective data. In the latter, however, the purely personal prejudices of the writer are seen—not as a report of data collected but of observations and clinical experiences interpreted within the framework of the writer's background and his concepts of aphasia.

From *Proceedings of Conference on Language Retraining for Aphasics*, Ohio State University.

To set the stage for my personal biases let me redefine aphasia in terms which have become meaningful to me over the years. Aphasia is viewed broadly as an impairment in the use of verbal symbols—the decoding, integration and encoding of messages—due to neurological insult. The condition of ill-being is therefore describable as a neurological problem with all of the behavioral after-effects consequent to any disturbance demonstrated by central nervous system dysfunction, or the consequential effects of the organism readjusting to its lesser capacities, including language comprehension, formulation and use, but not necessarily limited to it.

The language impairment itself is seen as one, but only one, vital pattern of behavior affected by the CNS disturbance. While the use of verbal symbols is a species-common behavior it is not seen as a primary behavior in that man can exist without speech, reading, or writing. He can exist, but he is less a man for having to exist in that way since communication between man is viewed as the common bread of their interpersonal existence. Thus, aphasia which is due to a neurological insult demonstrated in part by a linguistic disability affects the individual's relationship with his environment in a truly social sense. The over-all behavior of the aphasic patient has its counterparts due to the neurological event which caused it, the linguistic event it caused, and the social event or environment in which it exists. Aphasia is therefore best described as a psychoneurological, psycholinguistic, and psychosocial problem. It is only when all three aspects are considered that we believe one can obtain a clear picture of the aphasic patient and his problems, as Goldstein so cogently recognized (Goldstein, 1948).

Some distinction must be made here between aphasia, the verbal symbol impairment, and common neurologically based speech and hearing problems, the apraxias and agnosias. These "kindred disorders," to use Head's terms, are seen as relating specifically to input and output transmission of signals and play only a subsidiary role in verbal symbolic formulation, comprehension or use (Head, 1920). Thus, Kreindler and Fradis, in a most excellent work on aphasia which I heartily recommend to you, differentiate a variety of agnosic and apraxic disorders which can be seen as dysfunctions below the level of thought and language, but by their fundamental nature affecting the transmission of necessary input and output signals (Kreindler and Fradis, 1968). This they find in keeping (as does Grewel, 1967), with the Pavlovian concept of levels of function. The differentiation between first and second order signalling systems has been widely reported in other terms by the present writer (1960).

To complete our picture, the concept of aphasia therapy also needs definition, in keeping with the construct proposed above. Since recovery in one sense or another can be said to be the basic goal of therapy, we must plan for procedures which are in keeping with the neurological event and its immediate physiological, as well as behavioral, counterparts. Thus, for the hemiplegic patient, handwriting with the previously nondominant hand may be paramount; while the onset of therapy should be delayed until the common post-traumatic state of euphoria has been overcome, etc. The attack upon the linguistic problem should reflect the patient's present level of linguistic behavior, thus, "naming" would be contraindicated for a patient whose essential problem was unintelligibility due to jargon usage. But, most importantly, the societal environment of the patient, the attitude of those around him, his own approach to external events . . . are essential. Language is the common tool of interpersonal relations—the interpersonal needs, the climate of recovery, the motivation to continue—such truly interpersonal and intrapsychic events require our most heartfelt attention.

Rogers has pointed out in many different reports the value of interpersonal relations in counseling therapy (Rogers, 1942). In a quite recent reprint of his, "Learning to be Free" (Rogers, 1968), which I would also recommend to you, he said in part: "It is thus necessary . . . that the student (patient) of whatever level be confronted by issues which have meaning and relevance for him. In our culture we tend to insulate the student (patient) from too many of the actual problems of life. . . . If we desire to have students (patients) learn to be free and responsible individuals, we must be willing for them to confront life, to face problems" (p. 428). For our purposes the word *patient* can be substituted for *student* wherever the word occurs.

Aphasia therapy, like any therapy, is designed to help change behavior. Not in the confines of a therapeutic setting alone, but in life. It must be tailored to the neurological, linguistic, and social needs of the patient. It should not be confused with therapy for the agnosias and apraxias which need to be and can be attacked directly. Recovery from aphasia is a global event; the neurological component adapted to, the linguistic progression enhanced, the social events both inter- and intra-personal exposed and adjusted to. This over-all goal may need to be achieved in small, partial increments, but each aspect must be related to each other and not seen or treated as a separate condition.

With aphasia defined and the therapeutic design seen as a reflection of the definition, let us turn to some of the more prosaic "relative" concepts which research as well as observation has brought forward. We have reported on the tendency for "talking aphasic patients" to fall into one of three categories defined as "pragmatic," "semantic," and "syntactic," (Wepman and Jones, 1964) following the semiotic constructs of Morris (1938). Review of their spontaneous use of language (telling stories to TAT pictures) shows that a significant difference occurs in their noun pronoun ratio—the pragmatic aphasic using approximately the same number of each of the nominals, the semantic aphasic under-using nouns and over-using pronouns, the syntactic aphasic over-using nouns and under-using pronouns, the unimpaired adult using almost the identical number of nouns and pronouns (Wepman and Jones, 1966). Looking at the use of "relatives," the words which indicate a questioning nature, a seeking for information, the following interesting ratios are seen. The pragmatic aphasic (whose speech consists of words but of little substantive communication value and with no apparent feedback or self-correction) under-uses the "relatives"; only 1.8 percent of their total output fell in this category. The semantic patient (whose major difficulty lies in his inability to express specifics) uses approximately the same number of "relatives" found in a group of selected normal speakers (2.3 percent of their total verbal product). The syntactic patient (whose speech is specific but often agrammatical or paraphasic; whose feedback is excellent; whose search is for a normalcy which is just beyond his grasp) over-uses the "relative" questioning words (3.8 percent of his speech is involved in this category). As has been indicated, the over- and under-use of categories is determined by the mean use of each category by unimpaired speakers (2.4 percent of their total output being classified as "relatives").

This type of data points up the advantage of a psycholinguistic evaluation of the retained language. The interpretation has been made that a given patient uses those linguistic parameters (in this instance the "relative" words) which are available to him in his impaired state. As he becomes better in the sense of being more efficient in the function of his neurophysiological mechanism for speech, he will be able to utilize more complete linguistic forms; his needs will change and the words he uses will be a reflection again of his recovering and, therefore, more elaborate language status.

Some time ago it was postulated that aphasia might be looked upon as a regressive phenomenon with recovery as a reversal of this regression (Wepman and Jones, 1964). The linguistic data reported, when coupled with the psychological meaning to the individual, seems a confirmation of this concept. A patient's language doesn't improve—he improves, and his language reflects it.

Turning to other "relative" matters where research data is less available, the prejudice of the writer becomes even more apparent. I believe from what I have seen clinically that aphasic patients do not recover because they are taught to speak again. No learning in the sense of reinforcement, reduction of frustration, repetition or practice, plays anything but the most minor role if, indeed, it plays any role at all.

I have seen aphasic patients whose language usage seemed to have plateaued for from three to six months suddenly and dramatically begin to speak fluently. Not sufficient time elapsed between total failure and total success to account for the change on any external basis. Confirmation of this type of change of a non-learned pattern is seen in the patients who apparently recover almost overnight when the neurological deficit was impermanent as in the case of cerebral edema following trauma or stroke. Certainly here no specific learning process is involved. The brain, at one moment incapable of the high level integration necessary for language, finds the task simple when the nervous system becomes functionally intact.

The foregoing has led to a number of generalizations about therapy—"relative" generalizations. First, do not do therapy while the patient is in the early post-traumatic period—permit time for restabilization to occur. How much time? A rule of thumb says: fortunately man is euphoric in the immediate post-traumatic period . . . change can only occur due to frustration . . . if the patient is euphoric he can't be frustrated unless you force it on him . . . begin direct therapy when the euphoria subsides.

A second common observation about when to start therapy is almost the opposite side of the "euphoria." As many patients come out of their state of well-being, they are overwhelmed by what has happened to them, by the state they are in, by the inability to communicate even though they have something to say (Hodgins, 1964). This produces marked emotional lability. It is not a good time for direct language therapy, but may be an excellent time to reassure and support the patient.

When should one cease doing therapy? When the patient continually denies his therapeutic effort and no change in language usage occurs for a given period. Such patients should still be seen periodically to avoid having discontinued during a period of self-deprecation.

How far can a therapist go in stimulating a patient? . . . To the outer reaches of the moon if necessary. *Illustration:* some of the best (most successful) therapy I have seen was built around a daily poker game. The reward was the opportunity to play cards openly where it was forbidden by army rule. A whole therapeutic regimen was built around the poker table. These men were engaged in a man's activity, an act of ordinary existence, far from an artificial clinical situation.

Another illustration is the patient who struggled with individual and group direct therapy for two years without notable success and was sent (at his request) on a trip to Japan by boat—a bridge-playing cruise—where every passenger was a successful bridge player at the masters level. The pre-traumatic avocation of the patient was bridge at this level. He returned to talking.

A final example—when our tri-level concept with differential modality functions (Wepman, Bock, Jones, and Van Pelt, 1956) was being developed—a patient was seen on consultation over a thousand miles from Chicago. The routine aphasia examination revealed a global aphasia in a hemiplegic patient completely nonambulatory and able to take nourishment only when fed. She had not been heard to make an attempted sound since her "stroke" two years previously. To those of you who have found yourself in this position the situation will be familiar. You are being consulted on language in a non-language-using person. My bag of examining tricks was soon exhausted, but I was too far from home to just turn around and go back after saying "uh huh," the previous diagnosis is confirmed, she can't talk.

At this time my super-ego took over and said in effect, "perhaps she needs a more forceful single modality stimulation, perhaps the multiple-stimuli of the "busy" bedroom was too dispersed, too distracting for her." We darkened the room, put ear phones on her, increased the volume of speech to a 40 dB level through the recorder/amplifier. She turned toward the source of the sound, then toward the examiner who had asked her to say her name and said as clearly as I could have said it, "My name is Mrs. John Doe." Explanations for this behavior are evident—when sound reached her level of transmissibility (her threshold for hearing pure tones was later found to be down by about 50 dB at each of the speech frequencies) she evidenced no aphasia, nor indeed any language problem. When the opposite modality was tested—by masking both ears and presenting visual stimuli—she was able to make only the most minimal response. Our conclusion was that she had had a stroke and secondary to it, 1) visual agnosia, severe, with 2) deafness, bilateral conductive type. This of course paved the way for therapy to be designed appropriate to her disability.

From examples such as these comes my conviction that recovery from aphasia should be thought of in terms of an expanded use of previously learned behavior. Not the learning how to talk, but the re-establishment of language usage. Not stimulus-response behavior, but spontaneous use of verbal expressions.

Still another bias of mine relates to the manner in which therapists in general tend to overlook the psychosocial aspects of aphasia, especially in patients whose recovery programs are limited to the artificiality of the clinic. We have commented previously on the need to understand a patient's pre-traumatic vocational and avocational drives to foster a therapy in keeping with his life expectation (Wepman, 1958). I recall the patient who rather violently attacked a therapist when he was introduced to a pre-primer as his source material for a day's word-finding. The patient is entitled to be treated other than as a deficient child. If programs for recovery are to be used they should be rather carefully constructed to meet not only the therapist's concern but the patient's.

Yet even more than our imperfect knowledge of, and reference to, the patient's personality is the attempt to treat a patient as though he lived alone—in a nonspeaking, nonthinking, nonacting world. Yet some patients seen recently illustrate this situation, and the effect of the personality of the people in their environment on therapy will be readily seen.

One patient, for example, following his stroke had a severe, global type of aphasia. Over time his understanding of what was said to him improved as did his ability to secure some meaning from the printed page. He could copy most things he saw, but could not write spontaneously. These conditions all improved while he was hospitalized during the first three post-stroke months. His home environment changed, however. His most amenable and accepting wife (while he was hospitalized) became completely over-protective of every act he attempted as soon as he came home. She resented the therapist's provision of material of increased difficulty. She infantilized the patient to such a degree that he fell back upon gesture rather than attempt verbalization when she stressed the need for him to be "perfect" in whatever he tried. She acted as though she had lost a husband but gained a baby son. Her maternalism became the source of his succorance and his behavior relapsed into complete infant-like withdrawal. No ordinary, directed therapy could cope with this situation. It took the combined psychotherapeutic efforts of a team of therapists including a psychologist to reduce the burden of parent-child relationship before language therapy, as such, could be reinstated.

This case not only illustrates the environmental aspects but introduces the concept that aphasia, while the direct product of neurological impairment, evidences its linguistic process alteration by alteration of the stages of dependency and can through this means so easily become a psychosocial problem. Most patients return to their homes from relatively brief absences in the hospital during the acute stages of their neurological and linguistic disturbances. In those instances where physical recovery is necessary some rehabilitative efforts are made just as when speech and reading, etc., are still affected some language therapy is or can be provided. At least this is true in many communities today. What is so often overlooked, however, is the role of the patient as a convalescent in his family endeavor, the attitudes and personality of the people closest to him and their ability to turn the world, not just their homes, into a therapeutic agency. For alcoholics we have an Alcoholics Anonymous, for mental health patients a half-way house, a restoration center, a bridge to independent living. For the sufferers from aphasia —nothing.

A common expression of affect on the part of hemiplegic adult aphasic patients is their demand for dependency. Too often they become autocratic manipulators of home and hearth. Their latent dominant needs having been suppressed pre-traumatically become evident as they "rule" their associated wives or husbands. They demand attention, show little inner resources for self-care, and demonstrate their inadequate emotional control by utilizing every means to obtain their regressed needs. The therapist in such a situation must be cautious about becoming "involved" in the domestic inequities that are evident, yet must work toward the establishment of an equitable relationship. Otherwise therapy for language will be meaningless. It will exist in the vacuum of therapist-patient, stimulus-response behavior, out of context with the reality of the patient's life pattern.

The behavior of a wife toward her husband who had suffered a stroke from which he was recovering is one example as shown above. It is only fair to point out that husbands of wives who are aphasic most often err in even more gross manners. Almost invariably they try to do too much for the patient. Their guilt for needing to leave them each day becomes overbearing so when they are at home they outdo themselves. They not only offer their assistance, they insist on their right to provide it. While they may not infantilize their wives they quite openly increase their dependency. They keep them as patients, not convalescents. They almost openly refuse to let them get better.

Language therapy when offered via the husband or the wife of the types illustrated is usually resolved by being reduced to childlike repetition. They run their lives and their spouses' lives entirely from the heart and almost never from the head. There is a great danger that outside direct language therapy will feed into this type of situation. The materials of therapy—the vocabulary, the pictures, the books, etc.—are so often selected for their utter simplicity. The patient is rarely provided with the stuff of which abstractions are made.

To overcome this climate of good will the patient must develop outgoing behavior almost in spite of good will meaning but misguided mates. The therapist in this situation who is limited to educational learning techniques is often helpless. His basic role should be to create a climate for recovery, one in which change and frustration can provide the opportunity for the restoration of function. What is done in such therapy is less important than the fact of its being done. The family's role in recovery must be turned into an active, seeking, mutual program. Most of all it is up to the language therapist to create this role with the family. The group dynamics is more important than the individual's use of verbal symbols.

In one case a misdirected concentration upon the patient proved quite improper. This man in his early fifties was a successful businessman in a small Ohio town. His store was the leading emporium for all merchandise. His children had grown up and moved away. His wife was apparently content as a housewife and member of the local bridge club, the garden club, and the town betterment committees. She had played no role in the economics of the family's life.

When her husband suffered his stroke and lost his ability to communicate, his personality remained, as she reported it, very much the same. He was a warm, soft, accepting man who was loved by everyone. Her personality, however, seemed to change almost at once. While the family's business was in good hands, she assumed its total management. She enjoyed every phase of it, the buying, the selling, the merchandising, the personal work, even the maintenance. She became a driving, unaccepting, harsh businesswoman. She managed within six months to antagonize most of the good people who worked for the business. At home, her new personality became more apparent. She insisted that therapy was of no value, but kept it up only because it wouldn't look right if she didn't. She derided every attempt her husband made to improve. She actively discouraged his efforts to improve. However, since she was busy now with her own active outlets she permitted other people to see her husband and work with him until one day he was well enough to make his way to the family store. While still far from being capable of running the business, she saw his return even as a visitor as a threat to her new-found role in life. She brought all therapy and even social visits to a halt, sold the family car so that her husband could not move readily and announced that no changes in her present status could be considered.

Their children in their vists now saw these changes occurring and finally with the assistance of a local psychologist were able to reduce her tension states, and finally to induce her to accept psychotherapy.

I submit that more attention must be paid to the psychosocial environment, the inter- and intra-psychic life of the patient: that he not only does not or cannot be expected to redevelop verbal communication in the vacuum of therapy, but must readjust to life and to its changing processes. Admittedly, the cases here presented are somewhat unusual, not every individual changes personality in the face of opportunity, but enough do to make the psychological aspects of aphasia as important as the physiological or the psycholinguistic aspects wherever it occurs.

Finally let me discuss my attitude toward the machine and all that goes with it. As is evident from the foregoing, my tendencies are humanistic. To me that is not a pejorative word. I believe in the worth of people and their self-expression. Verbal therapy is made up of a communication dyad, the establishment of rapport between patient and therapist leading to acceptance of each other as worthwhile human beings. Anything that would come between these two would tend to disrupt this relationship. The teaching machine is a devil's box which does just that. It comes between the therapist and the patient. It provides a situational stimulation outside reality, artificially constructed to satisfy a generalized process which the therapist believes will be in line with the needs of "any" aphasic patient. In my experience aphasic patients rarely need the same thing as other aphasic patients. Even though the dyad be broken by the insertion of an intervening machine, many aphasic patients, being nice people for the most part, will go along to satisfy the therapist. When they don't see the need, conceive of the machine and its programs as childlike, their frustration behavior will soon be apparent.

Why, then, I ask myself, do people turn to teaching machines? Grant they look, as I do not, upon aphasia therapy as a learning problem; grant they see no need for interpersonal direct relations with the patient but feel a machine, programmed for naming or phrases or reading or what have you is all ready and at hand. The only rationale I see is that the therapists fear immediate contact with the patient—fear in the sense of being afraid to face the multi-dimensional psychological, neurological, linguistic and social problems presented by the patient. They place an obstacle between them. The flow of the dyad is directed toward the machine: the therapist provides the program, the patient relates to it and not to the therapist. True, no need will then be seen for working through the commonly found depression of the patient, his impatience, his struggle for self-expression. True, the social variety of the environment can be pushed aside, the future of the patient left to his own or others' devices. The problem is made unidimensional: if a man cannot talk, teach him to talk. But a man is not unidimensional. He is the confluence of his background, his training, and his motivation.

One of the questions I would raise is, is it really therapy to use a previously tailored yet generalized program for aphasics or is it all an escape mechanism for the fearful therapist?

No one should be under the impression that I believe aphasia therapy to be easy. In fact, having been engaged in a variety of psychotherapies, speech therapies, and aphasia therapies most of my life, I believe aphasia therapy to be the equal in difficulty of all forms of therapy and certainly the most challenging.

I would restate my conviction that recovery from aphasia is a matter of recapturing one's previously held ability, that what is lost is process, not function; that what must be recovered is the ability one previously possessed. Only to this limit can aphasia therapy be beneficial within the constraining limits of the impaired cortex to function in the manner of the previously unimpaired cortex and the degree of personal motivation of the patient. Not new learning but use of old learning should be the basis of treatment. This viewpoint has been expressed previously in the tripartite approach to therapy subtended under the terms "stimulation," "facilitation," and "motivation" (Wepman, 1956). Stimulation is what the therapist does, facilitation is what the impaired cortex is capable of doing when properly stimulated. Motivation is the internal state of the patient enhanced by the climate of his environment.

Because I state this as a personal opinion I would not like to have it thought that I disclaim the value of direct therapy nor the processes of rehabilitation. I favor both. Over the years situations have occurred where we have been able to judge the effects of therapy by the apathetic, lethargic, unstimulating condition that develops when aphasia patients are left to their own resources. The back wards of many state mental hospitals, and I'm afraid the private and semi-private rooms of nursing homes, still hold populations of aphasic patients who because of their incapacity to communicate, their evident dependency and their lack of a stimulating climate for recovery seem doomed to be forgotten men.

Aphasia, as has been pointed out, requires an environmental attitude in which to change. The aphasic patient is not just a person impaired in a communication skill but a living, adapting organism who like the flora of the countryside requires a fitting climate to enhance his growth and re-establish his identity. The attitudes of those around him, the materials used in his therapy, the family he lives with, the therapist involved—his "lebensraum"—must be appropriate to him as a person and to his needs.

If, as has been suggested in another context, there is an aspect of linguistic regression about the processes of communication impairment in aphasia, there might also be thought of a corollary regression (Wepman, 1964). Severe aphasia, the type 5 described by Schuell and her co-workers (1964), or the global aphasia described by Wepman and Jones (1964), is the most dependent of all aphasics. Only slightly better off is the full jargon aphasic who verbalizes, but whose language attempts are unintelligible. Both such patients suffer not only in language but in the behavioral areas where language as the inter-personal code is vital. There is a tendency for infantile behavior, for frustration or even for Goldstein's catastrophic reaction pattern, which I have long thought of as additive frustration. Along with the behavior itself comes the tendency of others to infantilize the patient, to treat him as he acts, as though this were his developmental level.

The pragmatic aphasic—he who can talk in understandable words for the most part but who makes little sense to his listener—is less dependent. He is able to carry out only one-half of the dyad of inter-personal communication. Most often he has or uses no apparent feedback and continues to verbalize despite the failure to communicate or the rewards which are said to follow. Much doubt must be cast in any case on the use of automated programs on these three types of aphasic patients, the global, jargon or pragmatic types. In such patients by the very nature of their total problem, their situational dependency and their apparent inability to utilize feedback from the environment in the specifics of verbal forms, conditioning practices would therefore be literally impossible to assess. Reinforcement without an adequate input system becomes repetitive noise.

I believe in aphasia therapy. I think it does good to understand a patient's neurological problem, his linguistic problem, and his social problem. The aphasic patient is challenging because his problems are complex, because it takes so much effort to understand and to support the patient. I can even go so far as to say that for some carefully selected aphasic patients even teaching machines may be stimulating . . . perhaps more stimulating than therapists who use them. Recovery from aphasia, however, is the spontaneous use of intentful behavior, not the muttering of a new word or two as a light flashes. At least there are my personal prejudices, and they are all "relative" to aphasia.

REFERENCES

1. Goldstein, K., *Language and Language Disturbances.* New York: Grune and Stratton (1948).
2. Grewel, F., Principles in the psychological examination of oligophrenics, *Folia Psychiatrica, Neurologica et Neurochirurgica Neerlandica,* **60,** 475–492 (1957).
3. Head, H., Aphasia and kindred disorders of speech, *Brain,* **43,** 87–165 (1920).
4. Hodgins, E., *Episode.* New York: Atheneum (1964).
5. Jones. L. V., M. F. Goodman, and J. M. Wepman, The classification of parts of speech for the characterization of aphasia, *Language and Speech,* **6,** 97–107 (1963).
6. Kreindler, A. and A. Fradis, *Performances in Aphasia.* Paris: Gauthier-Villars (1968).

7. Morris, C., Foundation of the Theory of Signs. *In* Neurath, M. (ed.) *International Encyclopedia of Unified Science.* Chicago: University of Chicago Press (1938).
8. Rogers, C., *Counseling and Psychotherapy.* Cambridge: The Riverside Press (1942).
9. ——, Learning to be Free, chapter 41. *In* Natchez, G. (ed.) *Children with Learning Problems.* New York: Basic Books (1968).
10. Schuell, Hildred, J. J. Jenkins, E. Jimenez-Pabón, *Aphasia in Adults.* New York: Harper and Row (1964).
11. Wepman, J. M., A conceptual model for the processes involved in recovery from aphasia, *Journal of Speech and Hearing Disorders,* **18,** 4–13 (1953).
12. ——, R. Bock, L. V. Jones, and Doris Van Pelt, Psycholinguistic study of aphasia, *Journal of Speech and Hearing Disorders,* **21,** 468–477 (1956).
13. ——, Aphasia and the "whole person" concept, *American Archives of Rehabilitation Therapy,* **6,** 1–8 (1958).
14. Wepman, J. M., L. V. Jones, R. D. Bock, and Doris Van Pelt, Studies in aphasia: background and theoretical formulations. *Journal of Speech and Hearing Disorders,* **25,** 323–332 (1960).
15. Wepman, J. M., and L. V. Jones, Five Aphasias: a commentary on aphasia as a regressive linguistic phenomenon. *In* Rioch, M. and Weinstein, E. A. (eds.) *Disorders of Communication.* Baltimore: Williams and Wilkins Co., (1964).
16. ——, ——, Studies in aphasia: clarification of aphasic speech by the noun-pronoun ratio, *British Journal of Disorders of Communication,* **1,** 46–54 (1966).

44

Speech Therapy and Language Recovery in Severe Aphasia

MARTHA TAYLOR SARNO
MARLA G. SILVERMAN
ELAINE S. SANDS

MARTHA TAYLOR SARNO, M.A., is director of the speech pathology service of the Institute of Rehabilitation Medicine, New York University Medical Center, and is with the department of rehabilitation medicine of the New York University School of Medicine.

MARLA G. SILVERMAN, M.A., is a speech pathologist in private practice in New York City.

ELAINE S. SANDS, M.S., is with the department of speech pathology and audiology at Adelphi University, Garden City.

This investigation was supported in part by the Social and Rehabilitation Service, Department of Health, Education and Welfare under the designation of New York University as a Rehabilitation Research and Training Center and by Research Grant # RD-2131-S-68-01 from the Division of Research and Demonstration Grants, Social and Rehabilitation Service, Department of Health, Education and Welfare.

Recovery from aphasia has been an area of interest and speculation among neurologists, psychologists, speech pathologists, and others for many years. As early as 1890, Bateman (1890) suggested that "reeducation" might be a means of restoring language in aphasia. Since that time, and particularly since World War II, a substantial number of aphasic patients have been treated by speech pathologists in a variety of settings. The majority of these patients have sustained cerebrovascular accidents.

There are diverse points of view concerning the process of recovery in aphasia and the effects of speech therapy, ranging from a confidence in the effectiveness of speech rehabilitation to the belief that language recovery is a function of physiological restitution (Lenneberg, 1967). As Lenneberg states:

> ". . . the adult patient does not relearn language. Neither training nor conditioning are guarantees for the restoration of language . . . . there are reasons to believe that this is due to physiological restoration of function rather than a learning process."

In contrast to this view, Butfield and Zangwill (1946), Godfrey (1959), Godfrey and Douglass (1959), Marks, Taylor, and Rusk (1957), and Vignolo (1964), have reported studies which support the hypothesis that speech therapy enhances language recovery in aphasia. For the most part these investigators based their conclusions on clinical ratings of improvement rather than objective data. Since patient samples were not well specified and therefore may be vastly different with respect to type and degree of aphasia, it is difficult to determine whether the reported outcomes are in fact similar.

It has often been said that there are as many methods of treating aphasia as there are

From *Journal of Speech and Hearing Research* 13:607–23, 1970.

aphasics (Wepman, 1953; Taylor, 1964). A variety of therapeutic techniques have been reported as effective language rehabilitation methods. Perhaps the most commonly used approach utilizes auditory stimulation as a primary technique. This is based on Schuell's view that impairments of auditory processing underlie aphasia (Schuell, 1955). Wepman (1953) also suggests a "stimulation" approach, advocating any technique which stimulates the patient to use language.

A great variety of techniques including drug therapy, sociotherapeutic techniques, group therapy and role-playing have also been reported in the literature as effective (Linn, 1947; Aaronson and Shatin et al., 1956; Bloom, 1962; Backus and Henry, 1947).

The most recent attempts to modify aphasic residuals have focused on operant conditioning (Tikofsky and Reynolds, 1963; Goodkin, 1966; Jacobs and Taylor, 1966) and programmed instruction (Rosenberg and Edwards, 1965; Taylor and Sands, 1966). Since aphasic patients have been said to require smaller steps, more than an average number of repetitions, and a more systematically structured teaching procedure—techniques fundamental to programmed instruction—this method lends itself to experimentation with these patients.

Studies employing programmed instruction techniques indicate that some aphasics have learned to match visual configurations, to perform visual oddity tasks, and to write their names under a programmed approach (Filby and Edwards et al., 1963; Rosenberg and Edwards, 1965).

This study was an outgrowth of a pilot study in programmed instruction for severely impaired aphasic patients (Taylor and Sands, 1966).

PROBLEM

Despite reports of the efficacy of speech therapy, there have been, to date, no controlled studies testing this hypothesis. Many investigators have stressed the need for such a study (Eisenson, 1949; Marks, Taylor and Rusk, 1957; Godfrey and Douglass, 1959; Vignolo, 1964).

It was our intent to investigate whether speech therapy enhances language recovery in severe expressive-receptive aphasics. The results of our pilot experience suggested that programmed instruction might be more effective than any "conventional" method of therapy, and it was, therefore, adopted as one of the therapeutic methods.

We were interested in the following issues:

1. The effect of speech therapy on language recovery in severe aphasia.
2. The effect of speech therapy on the retention of learned language behaviors.
3. A comparison of the effectiveness of nonprogrammed and programmed instruction on language recovery.

METHOD

Subjects

Patients were at least 18 years old, had suffered a CVA with right hemiplegia, were premorbidly right handed, and spoke fluent American English. There was no upper age limit. All patients exhibited severe aphasic symptomatology of at least three months duration. This cutoff point was chosen to avoid biasing the results with the possible effects of spontaneous recovery (Eisenson, 1964; Lenneberg, 1967). There was no upper limit on duration of symptoms. Severe aphasia was operationally defined as an Overall Functional Communication Profile (see Materials section) score of below 31 percent. For the most part patients in this category had no speech function and little understanding of speech. At best, some were able to say a few words and understand some simple commands. Despite the severity of their language impairment, the majority of the patients were alert.

Those who did not have adequate motor and sensory function in at least one hand, and vision and hearing adequate for the task requirements, were excluded, as were those who were heavily medicated or had a premorbid language impairment. The presence of a right homonymous hemianopsia was not considered sufficiently incapacitating to preclude participation

TABLE 44-1. RANGE, MEDIAN, AND MEANS FOR AGE, OVERALL FCP SCORES, DURATION OF SYMPTOMS FOR ALL TREATMENT GROUPS

Treatment Group	*Age*			*Duration of Symptoms*			*FCP Overall Scores*		
	Range	*Mean*	*Median*	*Range*	*Mean*	*Median*	*Range*	*Mean*	*Median*
Programmed Instruction	46-80	63.81	63.50	3-144 months	33.69	19.50	5-31	17.06	18.00
	$n = 16$	$n = 16$	$n = 16$	$n = 16$	$n = 16$	$n = 16$	$n = 15$	$n = 16$	$n = 16$
Non-programmed	54-83	66.86	64.00	3-72 months	27.00	18.00	11-27	16.29	14.00
	$n = 7$	$n = 7$	$n = 7$	$n = 7$	$n = 7$	$n = 7$	$n = 7$	$n = 7$	$n = 7$
Control	54-70	63.71	65.00	18-72 months	41.14	45.00	5-29	17.75	20.00
	$n = 7$	$n = 8$	$n = 8$	$n = 7$	$n = 8$	$n = 8$	$n = 8$	$n = 8$	$n = 8$

in the study. All study candidates were examined by a neurologist to exclude patients who showed signs of bilateral brain damage.

Patients with aphasia secondary to brain trauma or tumor were excluded since their recovery process is known to be different from that of the post-CVA patient.

A total of 31 patients were assigned to three groups: programmed instruction, nonprogrammed speech therapy, and an untreated control group. It was virtually impossible to balance the treatment groups by random assignment due to the varied location of the patients, limitations in the availability of a programmed-instruction clinician and/or a nonprogrammed clinician. However, all groups were found to be equivalent with regard to age. symptom duration, Functional Communication Profile (FCP) scores, previous speech therapy, total time on program, and number of treatment sessions (See Tables 44-1 and 44-2).

Materials

The examinations fell into two major areas: (1) Language Testing, and (2) Pre- and Posttesting.

Language testing

The functional Communication Profile (FCP) is a clinical tool which attempts to measure spontaneous language usage based on an estimate of the patient's premorbid language level. It is a list of 48 communication behaviors considered common language functions of everyday life. On the basis of informal interaction with the patient in a conversational

TABLE 44-2. COMPARISONS BETWEEN SUBJECTS ASSIGNED TO PROGRAMMED INSTRUCTION, NONPROGRAMMED INSTRUCTION AND CONTROL GROUPS

Groups	*Age*		*Symptom Duration*		*FCP*		*Previous Speech Therapy*		*Time in Therapy (Weeks)*		*Therapy Sessions*	
	t	df	t	df	t	df	t	df	t	df	df	df
PI-NPI	0.70	21	0.41	21	0.23	20	0.75	19	0.53	20	0.91	19
PI-C	0.03	21	0.47	21	0.19	21	0.90	20	—	—	—	—
NPI-C	0.66	12	1.13	12	0.36	13	0.26	13	—	—	—	—

Note: None of the *t*-values were significant at the 0.05 level.

TABLE 44–3. SUMMARY CHART OF PROGRAMS

Code	*Modality*	*Frames Per Program*	*Goal*	*Terminal Behavior*
IM-I	Imitation		To condition the patient to perform gross movements in response to clinician modeling cues.	Imitation with or after clinician.
VR-I	Visual Recognition—Matching and Selection	108	To improve (1) awareness of identical (pictorial) stimuli; (2) the ability to match and select visual (pictorial) stimuli; (3) consistency of performance.	Selecting two identical pictures out of three choices.
VR-II	Visual Recognition—Matching and Selection	500	To improve (1) awareness of conceptually and related visual stimuli (pictorial and graphic); (2) the ability to match and select related visual stimuli (pictorial and graphic); (3) consistency of performance.	Selecting word and appropriate picture. 2 out of 3 and 3 out of 4 choices.
VR-III	Visual Recognition—Matching and Selection	106	To improve recognition of selected vocabulary.	Selecting 2 identical words out of 3, then 4 choices.
WR-I	Writing-Copying, Filling-in and Fading	66	To improve (1) accuracy of performance in writing skills; (2) increased consistency of performance in writing skills; (3) increased ability to use unaffected hand for writing purposes.	Copying, filling in incomplete geometric forms.
WR-II	Writing	350	To improve (1) ability to use unaffected hand for writing purposes; (2) writing of content items upon presentation of picture cues.	Copying, filling in missing letters of single words and phrases. Spontaneous production to picture cue.
AU-I	Auditory Comprehension	588	To improve (1) awareness of verbal stimuli (auditorily presented); (2) discrimination among single words and short phrases (auditorily presented).	Selection of 1 out of 2 to auditory stimulus.
AU-II	Auditory Comprehension	220	To improve (1) awareness of verbal stimuli (auditorily presented); (2) discrimination among single words and short phrases (auditorily presented).	Writing words and phrases from dictation.
OR-I	Oral Production		To condition the patient to perform oral movements in response to clinician modeling cues.	Imitation of sound with or after clinician.
OR-II*	Oral Production	36	To improve the oral imitation of the selected vocabulary in response to clinician's production.	Imitation of words and phrases with or after clinician.
OR-III	Oral Production	189	To improve the oral production of the selected vocabulary in response to verbal (auditorily presented), pictorial and graphic stimuli.	Spontaneous oral production to picture, word cues.

*OR-II and OR-III were considered as two parts of one program to teach spontaneous oral production. The separation was for our convenience as OR-II and OR-III

situation, ratings of each behavior are made on an eight-point scale. These ratings are totalled, and percentages are derived in each of five areas: speaking, reading, understanding, movement, and a miscellaneous category which includes writing and calculation (Taylor, 1965). An overall score of 31% for example, indicates that a patient's overall verbal effectiveness is rated at 31% of his estimated premorbid level.

Pretests

Pretests were designed to assess the pretreatment level of the patient's language residuals corresponding to the experimental tasks i.e., terminal behaviors. There were 10 pretests. The OR III pretest corresponded to programs OR II and OR III combined where OR refers to oral production and the numerals refer to increasing complexity. The pretests ranged from 6 to 48 items, averaging 16 items per test. A score of 1 was given for a correct response and a 0 for an incorrect response. The sum of scores constituted the total score. In general, the items were presented in order of difficulty (pretesting for oral production of words began with single words followed by two-and then three-word phrases). The directions for pretest administration were specific. Each pretest consisted of items selected from the corresponding program and was representative of its range of complexity.

Posttests

Items on posttests were identical to pretests and were administered after treatment.

Programmed instruction regimen

The programs were designed on the basis of a presumed hierarchy of skills which we thought representative of the order of acquisition of skills in the recovery process. The hierarchy began with the imitation of body movements and proceeded to visual recognition, writing, auditory comprehension, and finally oral production (See Table 44-3. The programmed instruction vocabulary consisted of two nouns (*pen, book*), two numbers (*1, 2*), and two adjectives (*red, blue*).

The sequence of vocabulary presentation that ran through the programs was: single words, with nouns (*pen, book*) first; followed by numbers (*1, 2*); then colors (*red, blue*); combinations of numbers and nouns (*2 books*); and last the combination of number, color, and noun into three-word phrases (*2 red books*). The same vocabulary was used in all programs, except IM I and OR I which were imitation of body movements and sounds, respectively. There were 11 programs in all (See Figure 44-1 for program samples).

Nonprogrammed regimen

All clinicians received printed instructions which included the vocabulary to be taught in each modality (auditory comprehension, imitation, oral production, etc.) and an explanation of the behaviors to be learned. These were the same terminal behaviors which the programmed instruction materials were designed to teach.

Equipment

A teaching machine was designed to present all of the programs except body imitation and two of the oral production programs. It was a device which did nothing more than expose teaching and reinforcement frames by electric and manual means and present a light, a bell, and a sliding frame which revealed the correct response as reinforcement for correct responses. In addition to these methods of reinforcement, clinicians at times smiled and said "good" for correct responses. The light was discontinued shortly after the study began, because it was found that patients were not attending to it. When responses were incorrect, the patient was shown the reinforcement frame. Either the experimenter or patient could operate the machine. However, none of the patients in the study group were able to do so consistently or adequately.

A Sony Videocorder (Model CV 2000) was used for OR II. The videotape presented via a television monitor, a man saying the vocabulary and showing graphic and picture cues.

A Bell and Howell Language Master was used for the OR III program in order to keep

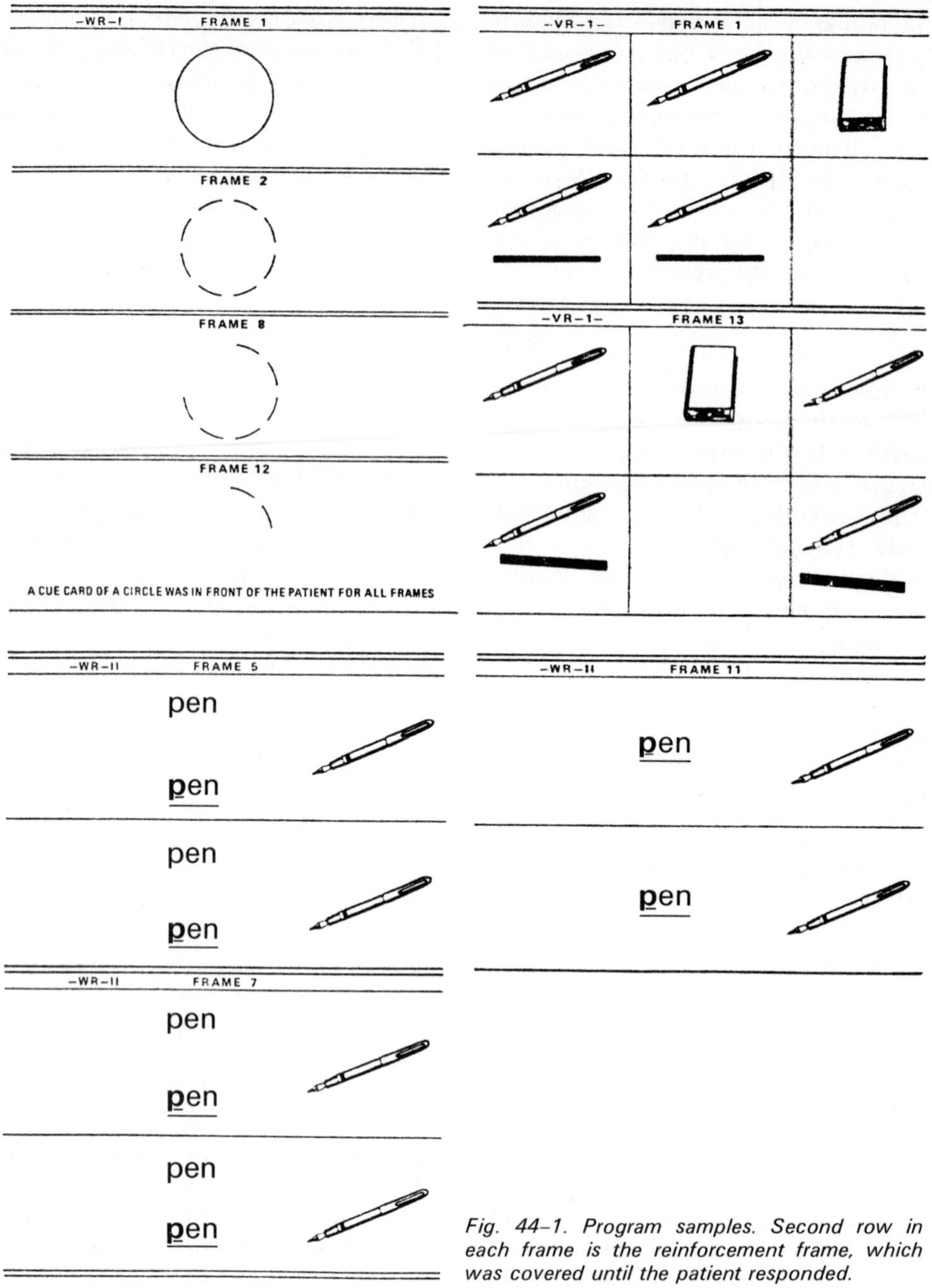

Fig. 44–1. Program samples. Second row in each frame is the reinforcement frame, which was covered until the patient responded.

the stimuli constant. It was initially used in the two auditory comprehension programs, but was discontinued because it was distracting to the patients. The clinician's live voice was substituted in those programs.

PROCEDURE

All patients were initially assessed through pretests to determine whether they were able to perform the terminal behaviors which constituted the goals of the speech therapy programs. Patients involved in the experimental treatment conditions were given either programmed or nonprogrammed therapy; control patients did not receive treatment.

Pretest items were scored pass or fail on the basis of one trial per item. When a subject failed a predetermined number of items on a pretest, it established his residual level of function in that modality, thus indicating the terminal behaviors to be learned. If a patient passed the pretest items, the corresponding program was not administered. Success on the oral production pretests (OR I and OR III) was determined according to number of correct responses. In addition, responses were examined for extraneous productions (additions or substitutions of phonemes or words).

The first posttest (Post 1) was given to the patients receiving programmed instruction, immediately upon conclusion of a program. For the nonprogrammed group, it was administered after the patient had learned the desired behavior, or after the clinician concluded, based on her clinical judgment, that the patient was unable to learn the task.

Failure on Post 1 led to teaching the succeeding terminal behavior in the same or different modality, except in four terminal behaviors (IM I, VR I, WR I, and the beginning of OR II for the programmed group and the equivalent tasks for the nonprogrammed group). Failure on Post 1 resulted in readministration of the relevant program for the programmed group, and continued practice for the nonprogrammed group.

The second posttest (Post 2) was administered at the termination of all treatment which occurred after all terminal behaviors had been taught, or, after the equivalent of 80 half-hour therapy sessions, whichever came first.

A month later, a third posttest (Post 3) was administered to measure retention.

In the case of the no-treatment group, follow-up tests were given approximately three months after initial testing. This posttest corresponded to Post 2 tests in the treatment groups.

Nonprogrammed treatment was conducted by five clinicians at three institutions. In all, eight patients were seen under this regime. The nonprogrammed clinicians were instructed to teach the terminal behaviors in any way they felt most expedient and to notify the Project Coordinator when a specific terminal behavior was reached, or when they felt continued treatment for a terminal behavior was contraindicated. Posttesting was then administered. Each clinician was free to use clinical judgment regarding the order of teaching tasks, and was permitted to work in as many modalities as he felt necessary during the course of each session.

It is of interest that all of the nonprogrammed clinicians chose to work on several different tasks within each session and to teach the vocabulary in pairs (*red-blue, pen-book*) rather than at random. Also, each clinician began with single words and proceeded to two-, and then to three-word phrases. In order to teach two-word phrases, one clinician combined color and noun (*red book*) as well as the number and noun combinations (*1 book*) presented in the programs. Another clinician chose to include vocabulary apart from that specified, in the hope that it would enhance learning of the specified vocabulary.

The two treatment groups were treated for 80 half-hour sessions (or the equivalent, 40 one-hour sessions) or until all of the programs were completed—whichever criterion was met first. Patients who were near completion of a program at the 80th session were allowed to finish that program. Whenever possible, treatment sessions were given in the morning hours and always before 4 p.m. to eliminate possible effects of fatigue.

Patients were seen in two settings: nursing homes, and as in- or outpatients at hospitals or rehabilitation clinics. In the nonprogrammed group, three patients were treated in nursing homes, two were outpatients and two inpatients. In the programmed group one patient was treated at a nursing home. There were four outpatients and eleven inpatients. In the no-treatment control group three of the subjects were living at home, two were in a nursing home, and three were in a hospital setting.

RESULTS

Treatment ranged from 4 to 36 weeks with a mean of 17.1 weeks, while the number of sessions ranged from 13 to 91 with a mean of 55.95 sessions (1 session = 30 minutes). This broad range was due to the number of terminal behaviors to be taught, inability of some patients to complete the series (due to illness, refusal to continue, discharge from hospital, death, etc.) and number of sessions per week.

Independent Variables

A. Groups
   1. Programmed Instruction
   2. Nonprogrammed Instruction
   3. Control Group.
B. Repeated Measurements
   1. Pretest: Administered as a battery of 10 tests before treatment.
   2. Posttest 1: Administered for each terminal behavior immediately after completion of teaching of that terminal behavior.
   3. Posttest 2: Administered as a battery of 10 tests after the completion of all terminal behaviors.
   4. Posttest 3: Administered as a battery to the 2 treatment groups one month after the completion of all treatments (i.e. Post 2).

Dependent Variables

1. Change scores from Pretest to Post 2 for the 3 groups to determine the effects of treatment methods.
2. Change scores from Pretest to Post 1 for the 2 treatment groups to determine the effects of the treatment methods immediately after treatment.
3. Change scores from Post 2 to Post 3 for the 2 treatment groups to determine the effects of the treatment methods on retention of material taught.
4. Programmed Group: Comparisons between Post 1 and Post 2 scores to determine the effects of repetition of the experimental vocabulary in different modalities.
5. Nonprogrammed Group: Comparisons between Post 1 and Post 2 scores to determine the effects of repetition of the experimental vocabulary in different modalities.
6. Change scores from Pretest to Post 2 for patients with (1) initial FCP overall scores of 0–15%, and (2) initial FCP scores of 16–31% to investigate the homogeneity of the patients.

Kruskal-Wallis nonparametric one-way analyses of variance (Siegel, 1956), were used to determine whether there were any group differences in improvement from Pretest (initial level before treatment) to Post 2 (given at the completion of all terminal behaviors). Change scores for each group in each terminal behavior were derived according to the following expression:

$$\frac{\text{Post 2 minus Pretest}}{\text{Pretest}}$$

to make the changes independent of initial performance level (the Pretest scores of any patient). Analyses were carried out for each terminal behavior, including two analyses each for OR I and OR III based on correct responses and extraneous responses. Of these analyses (see Table 44-4) only four yielded significant results at the 0.05 level: VR I, VR II, VR III, and OR III (words extraneous). It should be noted that these analyses across all 3 groups could be carried out only for Pre- to Post-2 changes, since only these data were available for subjects in all 3 conditions (the control group did not receive Post 1 or Post 3).

TABLE 44–4. KRUSKAL-WALLIS ANALYSES OF VARIANCE BASED ON PROGRAMMED INSTRUCTION, NONPROGRAMMED INSTRUCTION AND CONTROL GROUPS FOR $\frac{\text{POST 2 SCORES MINUS PRESCORES}}{\text{PRESCORES}}$

Programs	*H*
IM I	1.41
VR I	6.89*
VR II	8.76**
VR III	10.00***
WR I	2.91
WR II	5.79
AU I	4.96
AU II	1.13
OR I (correct)	4.57
OR I (extraneous)	2.56
OR III (words correct)	1.56
OR III (words extraneous)	6.43*

* Significant beyond 0.05 level, two-tailed test.
** Significant beyond 0.02 level, two-tailed test.
*** Significant beyond 0.01 level, two-tailed test.

TABLE 44–5. MANN-WHITNEY *U* TESTS FOR TERMINAL BEHAVIORS WHERE GROUP DIFFERENCES WERE INDICATED THROUGH KRUSKAL-WALLIS ANALYSES

Terminal Behavior	*Programmed vs Non-Programmed Instruction*	*Programmed Instruction vs No Treatment*	*Nonprogrammed Instruction vs No Treatment*
VR I	6.5($n_1 = 4, n_2 = 8$)	15.0($n_1 = 5, n_2 = 8$)	2.5($n_1 = 4, n_2 = 5$)
VR II	19.0($n_1 = 5, n_2 = 10$)	16.0($n_1 = 8, n_2 = 10$)	0***($n_1 = 5, n_2 = 8$)
VR III	0**($n_1 = 4, n_2 = 8$)	25.0($n_1 = 7, n_2 = 8$)	0*($n_1 = 4, n_2 = 7$)
OR III -words extraneous	4.5($n_1 = 4, n_2 = 7$)	7.5($n_1 = 7, n_2 = 7$)	3.5($n_1 = 4, n_2 = 7$)

*$p < 0.006$
**$p < 0.004$
***$p < 0.002$

Mann-Whitney *U* tests (Siegel, 1956) were computed to compare each pair of groups where significant Kruskal-Wallis *H* values were obtained (see Table 44-5). Of the 12 *U* values, 3 reached significance, i.e., in VR II (matching words and pictures) nonprogrammed instruction seemed superior to the absence of treatment (control group). In VR III (matching words) nonprogrammed treatment was superior to both programmed instruction and the absence of treatment. Since 36 Mann-Whitney *U* tests were employed, the significance level of 0.02 was used to decrease the possibility of significant findings based on chance.

Comparisons based on the difference between Post 1 (testing immediately after treatment for each terminal behavior) and Pretest performance, were carried out only for the nonprogrammed instruction and programmed instruction groups, as Post 1 scores were not available for the control group. Differences in initial levels were accounted for by the use of the expression:

$$\frac{\text{Post 1 minus Pretest}}{\text{Pretest}}.$$

Only one of 12 Mann-Whitney *U* tests reached significance at the 0.02 level. In IM I (gross body imitation) the programmed group was superior to the nonprogrammed ($U = 3$, $p < 0.02$). This *U* value may be primarily attributed to lack of changes for the nonprogrammed group, in contrast to the programmed instruction group. Thus extreme limitation in variability may maximize the statistical difference between programmed and nonprogrammed groups. In essence, these results suggest that there were no group differences in immediate learning as a function of treatment.

Retention of vocabulary as a function of method of therapy was analyzed for the nonprogrammed and programmed groups using the expression:

$$\frac{\text{Post 3 minus Post 2}}{\text{Post 2}}$$

for change scores, and Mann-Whitney *U* tests at the 0.02 level for significance of the difference in change between groups. Post 3 refers to testing one month after the completion of treatment.

Because differences in the effects of nonprogrammed and programmed instruction were found only for VR III after the completion of treatment (i.e., nonprogrammed instruction showed significantly greater improvement; see Table 44-4), the issue of retention is most pertinent to this task. No significant difference was found in the level of retention of VR III for the two groups.

Although no significant differences in retention were found for the other terminal behaviors (where no differences in therapy effects were obtained) further discussion of retention in the absence of learning (as indicated by comparisons of Post 2 minus Pretest scores) is not fruitful. Post 1 to Post 2 changes were examined for the programmed group to determine whether practice of the same tasks in different modalities would reinforce the initial tasks. Initial level (pretest level) was accounted for by the method utilized above. Wilcoxon Matched-Pairs Signed-Ranks tests (Siegel, 1956) were used for each terminal behavior. Of 10 Wilcoxon T values, none were significant at the 0.05 level. In the case of the oral programs for correct responses, limitations in sample size precluded statistical analyses. However, no salient changes were apparent. For OR I (correct responses) improvement occurred in three cases; decrease in performance and no changes were seen in two and one cases respectively, whereas for OR III (words correct) three cases improved and two decreased in level of performance.

Statistical analysis of Post 1 to Post 2 changes of subjects in the nonprogrammed group was precluded by limitations in sample size. However, no trend was apparent in the number of patients whose scores improved, remained the same, or decreased for each terminal behavior. (See Table 44-6.) To determine whether the group was homogeneous in severity, change from Pretest to Post 2 (after completion of treatment for the programmed and nonprogrammed groups, and three months after pretesting for the no treatment group) was compared as a function of initial FCP overall scores, regardless of treatment condition. Subjects were assigned to a higher group (16–31 percent overall FCP scores) and a lower group (0–15 percent overall FCP scores). Comparison between changes of the high and low FCP groups were assessed by means of 12 Mann-Whitney U tests. No significant differences were obtained between groups for any of the terminal behaviors at the 0.05 level. For these analyses the 0.05 level was used since the occurrence of significance by chance would, in this case, be very small at this level.

In summary, it was found that the nonprogrammed group was significantly better than the control group in VR II and VR III, and that the nonprogrammed group was significantly better than the programmed group in VR III.

No significant differences were found in the following comparisons:

1. Nonprogrammed and programmed groups on eight terminal behaviors.
2. Initial overall FCP scores of 0–15 percent were compared with scores of 16–31 percent on improvement on terminal behaviors regardless of treatment conditions.
3. Programmed and nonprogrammed groups were compared on learning immediately after therapy for each terminal behavior (Post 1).
4. Programmed and nonprogrammed groups were compared for 1 terminal behavior on retention one month after completion of therapy (Post 3).

TABLE 44-6. CHANGES FOR NONPROGRAMMED INSTRUCTION GROUPS BETWEEN POST 2 AND POST 1 SCORES*

Post 2–Post 1 Nonprogrammed Instruction (NPI) Subject Change Scores	*Improved*	*Unchanged*	*Decreased*
IM I: 0; −1.0; −0.17	0	1	2
VR I: 0; 0; −7; 0.11	1	2	1
VR II: −1; 10; −0.50; 20.0	2	0	2
VR III: 2.0; −1.0; 0; 0	1	2	1
WR I: −0.20; −1.66; −38; −0.15	0	0	4
WR II: −7.0; −2.0; 0.57; 2.34	2	0	2
AU I: −4.0; −8.0; 3.0; −0.06	1	0	3
AU II: 4.0; 0; −0.25	1	1	1
OR I: Correct: −1.0; −0.14; −0.30; −2	0	0	4
Extraneous: −1.0; −0.14; −0.50; 1.0	1	0	3
OR III: Words Correct: 0; −1.0; 0; −1.0	0	2	2
Words Extraneous: 0; 0; 0; −0.50	0	3	1

* Post 1 = Testing after each terminal behavior.
Post 2 = Testing after completion of all terminal behaviors.

DISCUSSION

This study was concerned with two hypotheses about the treatment of severe aphasia: (1) that severe aphasics can learn, and (2) that programmed instruction is an effective method for teaching them. Our results did not support either of these hypotheses.

Our findings demonstrated significant differences in learning between the treatment groups for only two of the ten terminal behaviors. These were in visual recognition tasks requiring matching words and pictures. In these two behaviors the nonprogrammed group improved more than the control group as expected. We had predicted that the programmed group would perform better than the nonprogrammed group, since programmed therapy was so carefully structured. We further expected that the two treatment groups would do better than the control group because of the effects of practice. However, programmed instruction was not more effective than either of the other groups. The flexibility of the nonprogrammed group which allowed for a greater number of trials when needed may have accounted for this difference. In the majority of tasks, the groups did not change significantly, even with practice.

The similarity of the results between the two treatment groups might be accounted for by two factors: (1) the restricted range of difficulty of the terminal behaviors may have precluded differentiation among treatment methods, or (2) the majority of the nonprogrammed instruction was administered by our own speech pathology service. We do not know to what degree these clinicians might have been influenced by exposure, in the IRM clinical program, to the rationales and materials used in our programmed instruction.

A modality hierarchy of complexity was assumed in constructing the treatment design for programmed instruction. Using the same vocabulary, imitative tasks were presented first, followed by tasks we thought to be more difficult, culminating in oral production. We would have expected that mastering imitation would aid in learning visual recognition, and these in turn would aid in writing tasks, and eventually in the acquisition of auditory comprehension and oral production skills. These assumptions were not supported in our findings since some patients demonstrated their poorest performance in what we had considered the simplest tasks, and did best in tasks we considered more difficult.

Repetition of the same vocabulary in different modalities did not appear to improve learning in new modalities. This can be seen by lack of significant gains from pretesting to posttesting after the completion of therapy for all terminal behaviors for both therapy groups. These patients had to be reintroduced to the vocabulary with each new modality. In this regard, patients did not appear to have the capacity necessary to transfer or generalize information.

Although gains were small and similar for all groups, many of the study patients showed at least minimal gains. What is surprising is that this was true for the untreated patients as well. Since the untreated patients were only seen once for pretesting and several months later for posttesting, their improvement cannot be attributed to the possible placebo effect of receiving attention. These gains may be due to the day-to-day performance inconsistencies observed in aphasics. Or, it may be, that aphasic patients, no matter how severe, make subtle changes for long periods after a stroke, sometimes for years (Sands, Sarno et al., 1969). This may also explain why so many aphasic patients and their families describe continual improvement even when it is not noticeable to the supposedly sophisticated observer.

The fact that speech therapy, of either type, did not affect language recovery in this study is no doubt related to the severity of their aphasia.

This study supports the clinical impression that severe aphasic stroke patients do not benefit from speech therapy. Further studies using other methods of treatment and a larger group of patients are indicated.

Since patients with less than 20 percent overall scores on the FCP have been reported as representing 41 percent of cases in a typical rehabilitation center speech program (Sarno, 1968), these findings have serious clinical implications. It might be more appropriate, with severe patients, for the speech pathologist to assume the role of consultant and educator to those involved in aiding the patient in adjustment, than to continue in the role of language clinician. Further, the speech pathologist might make more profitable use of his time attempting to refine the techniques for patient selection for speech therapy and improve methods of treatment for those more amenable to treatment.

Acknowledgement. The authors are indebted to the staff of the Department of Rehabilitation Medicine of Goldwater Memorial Hospital and Morristown Memorial Hospital, the Kessler Institute for Rehabilitation, the nursing homes of New York City for their participation in patient recruitment and treatment, and our own speech pathology staff.

REFERENCES

Aaronson, M., Shatin, L., and Cook, J. C., Sociopsychotherapeutic approach to the treatment of aphasic patients. *J. Speech Hearing Dis.*, **21,** 352–364 (1956).

Backus, O. L., and Henry, L., *Aphasia in Adults.* Ann Arbor, Michigan: Univ. Michigan Press (1947).

Bateman, F., *On Aphasia and the Localization of the Faculty of Speech*, 2nd Edition. London: Churchill (1890).

Bloom, L. M., A rationale for group treatment of aphasic patients. *J. Speech Hearing Dis.*, **27,** 11–16 (1962).

Butfield, E., and Zangwill, O. L., Re-education in aphasia: a review of 70 cases. *J. Neurol. Neurosurg. Psychiat.*, **9,** 75–79 (1946).

Eisenson, J., Prognostic factors related to language rehabilitation in aphasic patients. *J. Speech Hearing Dis.*, **14,** 262–264 (1949).

——, Aphasia: a point of view as to the nature of the disorder and factors that determine prognosis for recovery. *Int. J. Neurol.* **4,** 287–295 (1964).

Filby, Y., Edwards, A. E., and Seacat, G. F., Word length, frequency and similarity in the discrimination behavior of aphasics. *J. Speech Hearing Res.*, **6,** 255–261 (1963).

Godfrey, C. M., A dysphasia rehabilitation clinic. *Canad. Med. Ass. J.*, **80,** 616–618 (1959).

——, and Douglas, E., The recovery process in aphasia. *Canad. Med. Ass. J.*, **80,** 618–624 (1959).

Goodkin, R., Case studies in behavioral research in rehabilitation. *Percept. Motor Skills*, **23,** 171–182 (1966).

Jacobs, C., and Taylor, M., The application of operant conditioning techniques to aphasia therapy. Paper presented at the Annual Meeting of the American Speech and Hearing Association, Washington, D.C. (1966).

Lenneberg, E. H., *Biological Foundations of Language.* New York: J. Wiley (1967).

Linn, L., Sodium amytal in treatment of aphasia. *AMA Arch. Neurol. Psychiat.*, **58,** 357–358 (1947).

Marks, M. M., Taylor, M. L., and Rusk, H. A., Rehabilitation of the aphasic patient: a survey of three years' experience in a rehabilitation setting. *Neurology*, **7,** 837–843 (1957).

Rosenberg, B., and Edwards, A. E., An automated multiple response alternative training program for use with aphasics. *J. Speech Hearing Res.*, **8,** 415–419 (1965).

Sands, E., Sarno, M., Shankweiler, D., Long-term assessment of language function in aphasia due to *stroke. Arch. Med.*, **50,** 203–207 (1969).

Sarno, M. T., Method for multivariant analysis of aphasia based on studies of 235 patients in a rehabilitation setting. *Arch. Phys. Med.*, **49,** 210–216 (1968).

Schuell, H., Diagnosis and prognosis in aphasia. *AMA Arch. Neurol. Psychiat.*, **74,** 308–315 (1955).

Siegel, S., *Nonparametric Statistics.* New York: McGraw-Hill, 75–79, 83, 116–120, 184–194 (1956).

Taylor, M. L., A measurement of functional communication in aphasia. *Arch. Phys. Med.*, **46,** 101–107 (1965).

——, Language therapy. In Burr, H. G., (Ed.): *The Aphasic Adult: Evaluation and Rehabilitation.* Proceedings of the Short Course in Aphasia. Charlottesville; Wayside Press, 139–160 (1964).

——, and Sands, E., Application of programmed instruction techniques to the language rehabilitation of severely impaired aphasic patients. *Nat. Soc. Prog. Inst. J.*, **5,** 10–11 (1966).

Tikofsky, R. S., and Reynolds, G. L., Further studies of nonverbal learning and aphasia. *J. Speech Hearing Res.*, **6,** 329–337 (1963).

Vignolo, L. A., Evolution of aphasia and language rehabilitation: a retrospective exploratory study. *Cortex*, **1,** 344–367 (1964).

Wepman, J. M., A conceptual model for the processes involved in recovery from aphasia. *J. Speech Hearing Dis.*, **18,** 4–13 (1953).

ADDITIONAL SUGGESTED READINGS ON: RECOVERY AND REHABILITATION

1. Bergman, P. S., Green, M. Aphasia: Effect of Intravenous Sodium Amytal. *Neurology* **1**:471–475, 1951.
2. Billow, B. W. Observation of the Use of Sodium Amytal in the Treatment of Aphasia. *Med. Rec.*, **162**:12–13, 1949.
3. Blackman, N. Group Psychotherapy with Aphasics. *J. Nerv. Ment. Dis.*, **111**:154–163, 1950.
4. ——, Tureen, L. L. Aphasia—A Psychosomatic Approach in Rehabilitation. *Trans. Amer. Neurol. Ass.*, **73**:193–196, 1948.
5. Bloom, L. M. A Rationale for Group Treatment of Aphasic Patients. *J. Speech Hearing Dis.*, **27**:11–16, 1962.
6. Boone, D. R. A Plan for Rehabilitation of Aphasic Patients. *Arch. Phys. Med.*, **48**:410–414, 1967.
7. Critchley, M. Articulatory Defects in Aphasia. *J. Laryng.*, **66**:1–17, 1952.
8. Eisenson, J. Prognostic Factors Related to Language Rehabilitation in Aphasic Patients. *J. Speech Hearing Dis.*, **14**:262–264, 1949.
9. Filby, Y., Edwards, A. E. An Application of Automated Teaching Methods to Test and Teach Form Discrimination to Aphasics. *J. Prog. Inst.*, **2**:25–33, 1963.
10. Goodkin, R. Case Studies in Behavioral Research in Rehabilitation. *Percept. Motor Skills*, **23**:171–182, 1966.
11. Hemphill, R. E. Restoration of Speech in Severe Aphasia by Intravenous and Oral Priscol. *Brit. Med. J.*, **2**:891–892, 1951.
12. Kaplan, L. T. A Descriptive Continuum of Language Responses in Aphasia. *J. Speech Hearing Dis.*, **24**:410–412, 1959.
13. Katz, L. Learning in Aphasic Patients. *J. Consult. Psychol.*, **22**:143–146, 1958.
14. Keenan, J. S. Method for Eliciting Naming Behavior from Aphasic Patients. *J. Speech Hearing Dis.*, **31**:261–266, 1966.
15. Keith, R. L., Darley, F. L. The Use of a Specific Electric Board in Rehabilitation of the Aphasic Patient. *J. Speech Hearing Dis.*, **32:**148–153, 1967.
16. Kirkner, F. J., Dorcus, R. M., et al. Hypnotic Motivation of Vocalization in an Organic Motor Aphasic Case. *J. Clin. Exper. Hypn.*, **1**:47–49, 1953.
17. Lane, H. L., Moore, D. J. Reconditioning a Consonant Discrimination in an Aphasic: An Experimental Case History. *J. Speech Hearing Dis.*, **27**:232–243, 1962.
18. Linn, L. Sodium Amytal in Treatment of Aphasia. *AMA Arch. Neurol. Psychiat.*, **58**:357–358, 1947.
19. Marks, M. M., Taylor, M. L., et al. Rehabilitation of the Aphasic Patient. A Survey of Three Years' Experience in a Rehabilitation Setting. *Neurology*, **7**:837–843, 1957.
20. Mason, C. F. Hypnotic Motivation of Aphasics. *Int. J. Clin. Exper. Hypn.*, **9**:297–301, 1961.
21. Mills, C. K. Treatment of Aphasia by Training. *JAMA.* **43**:1940–1949, 1904.
22. Montgomery, J. A Case for the Lowly Alphabet. *J. Speech Hearing Dis.*, **32**:297–298, 1967.
23. Morley, H. J. Applying Linguistics to Speech and Language Therapy for Aphasics. *Lang. Learn.*, **10**:135–149, 1960.
24. Scargill, M. H. Modern Linguistics and Recovery from Aphasia. *J. Speech Hearing Dis.*, **19**:507–513, 1954.
25. Schuell, H. M. Auditory Impairment in Aphasia:

Significance and Retraining Techniques. *J. Speech Hearing Dis.*, **18**:14–21, 1953.

26. Stoicheff, M. L. Motivating Instructions and Language Performance of Dysphasic Subjects. *J. Speech Hearing Res.*, **3**:75–85, 1960.
27. Weinstein, S. Experimental Analysis of an Attempt to Improve Speech in Cases of Expressive Aphasia. *Neurology*, **9**:632–635, 1959.
28. Wepman, J. M., Morency, A. Filmstrips as an Adjunct to Language Therapy for Aphasia. *J. Speech Hearing Dis.*, **28**:191–194, 1963.
29. ——, Van Pelt, D. A. A Theory of Cerebral Language Disorders Based on Therapy. *Folia Phoniat.*, **7**:233–235, 1955.
30. West, R., Stockel, S. The Effect of Meprobamate on Recovery from Aphasia. *J. Speech Hearing Res.*, **8**:57–62, 1965.

Appendix 1

SELECTED BIBLIOGRAPHY

Aita, J. A. Modern Considerations of the Man With Brain Injury. *J. Neurosurg.*, **4**:240–254, 1947.

Alajouanine, T. Aphasia and Artistic Realization. *Brain,* **71**:229–241, 1948.

—— Verbal Realization in Aphasia. *Brain,* **79**: 1–28, 1956.

—— Baillarger and Jackson: The Principle of Baillarger-Jackson in Aphasia. *J. Neurol. Neurosurg. Psychiat.*, **23**: 191–193, 1960.

——, Lhermitte, F. Aphasia and Physiology of Speech. In: Rioch, D. M., Weinstein, E. A., (eds.), *Disorders of Communication.* Baltimore, Williams and Wilkins, 1964. Pp. 204–219.

Allan, C. M., Turner, J. W., et al. Investigations into Speech Disturbances Following Stereotaxic Surgery for Parkinsonism. *Brit. J. Disord. Commun.*, **1**: 55–59, 1966.

Allison, R. S. *The Senile Brain.* London, Arnold, 1962.

——, Hurwitz, L. J. On Perseveration in Aphasics. *Brain,* **90**:429–448, 1967.

American Heart Association. *Aphasia and the Family.* New York, American Heart Association, 1965.

Anastasopoulos, C. K. Aphasic Disorders and Verbal Hallucinations. *J. Neurol. Sci.*, **4**:83–93, 1966.

Anastasopoulos, G., Kokkini, D. Cerebral Dominance and Localization of the Language Functions. *Psychiat. Neurol.*, **143**:6–19, 1962.

Arbuse, D. The Gerstmann Syndrome. *J. Nerv. Ment. Dis.*, **105**:359–371, 1947.

Archibald, Y. M., Wepman, J. M. Language Disturbance and Nonverbal Cognitive Performance in Eight Patients Following Injury to the Right Hemisphere. *Brain,* **91**:117–130, 1968.

——, ——, et al. Nonverbal Cognitive Performance in Aphasic and Nonaphasic Brain Damaged Patients. *Cortex,* **3**:275–298, 1967.

——, ——, et al. Performance on Nonverbal Cognitive Tests Following Unilateral Cortical Injury to the Right and Left Hemisphere. *J. Nerv. Ment. Dis.*, **145**:25–36, 1967.

Aring, C. D. Supranuclear (Pseudobulbar) Palsy. *Arch. Intern. Med.*, **115**:198–199, 1965.

Aronson, M., Shatin, L., et al. Socio-Psychotherapeutic Approach to the Treatment of Aphasic Patients. *J. Speech Hearing Dis.*, **21**: 352–364, 1956.

Assal, G., Chapuis, G., et al. Isolated Writing Disorders in a Patient with Stenosis of the Left Internal Carotid Artery. *Cortex,* **6**:241–248, 1970.

Backus, O. L. The Rehabilitation of Aphasic Veterans. *J. Speech Hearing Dis.*, **10**:149–153, 1945.

——, Dunn, H. M. Intensive Group Therapy in Speech Rehabilitation. *J. Speech Hearing Dis.*, **12**:39–60, 1947.

——, Henry, L. D. *Aphasia in Adults.* Ann Arbor, University of Michigan, 1947.

Bakker, D. J. Ear-Asymmetry With Monoaural Stimulation: Relations to Lateral Dominance and Lateral Awareness. *Neuropsychol.*, **8**:103–117, 1970.

Barton, M. Perception of the Mueller-Lyer Illusion

in Normal and Aphasic Adults. *Percept. Motor Skills,* **28**:403–406, 1969.
—— Recall of Generic Properties of Words in Aphasic Patients. *Cortex,* **7**:73–82, 1971.
——, Maruszewski, M., et al. Variation of Stimulus Context and its Effect on Word-Finding Ability in Aphasics. *Cortex,* **5**:351–365, 1969.
Bastian, H. C. *A Treatise on Aphasia and Other Speech Defects.* London, Lewis, 1898.
Bateman, F. *On Aphasia, or Loss of Speech and the Localization of the Faculty of Articulate Language,* 2nd Edition. London, Churchill, 1890.
Battersby, W. S., Bender, M. B., et al. Unilateral "Spatial Agnosia" ("Inattention") in Patients With Cerebral Lesions. *Brain,* **79**:68–93, 1956.
Bauer, R. W., Becka, D. M. Intellect after Cerebro-Vascular Accident. *J. Nerv. Ment. Dis.,* **120**: 379–384, 1954.
——, Wepman, J. M. Lateralization of Cerebral Functions. *J. Speech Hearing Dis.,* **20**:171–177, 1955.
Bay, E. Aphasia and Non-Verbal Disorders of Language. *Brain,* **85**: 411–426, 1962.
—— Aphasia and Intelligence. *Int. J. Neurol.,* **4**:252–264, 1964.
—— The Classification of Disorders of Speech. *Cortex,* **3**:26–31, 1967.
——The Lordat Case and Its Import on the Theory of Aphasia. *Cortex,* **5**:302–308, 1969.
Bell, E., Jr., Karnosh, L. J. Cerebral Hemispherectomy: Report of a Case Ten Years after Operation. *J. Neurosurg.,* **6**:285–293, 1949.
Bender, M. B., Diamond, S. P. An Analysis of Auditory Perceptual Defects with Observations on the Localization of Dysfunction. *Brain,* **88**: 675–686, 1965.
Benson, D. F. Fluency in Aphasia: Correlation with Radioactive Scan Localization. *Cortex,* **3**:373–394, 1967.
——, Barton, M. I. Disturbances in Constructional Ability. *Cortex,* **6**:19–46, 1970.
——, Geschwind, N. Shrinking Retrograde Amnesia. *J. Neurol. Neurosurg. Psychiat.,* **30**:539–544, 1967.
——, Patten, D. H. The Use of Radioactive Isotopes in the Localization of Aphasia-Producing Lesions. *Cortex,* **3**: 258–271, 1967.
Benton, A. L. The Fiction of the "Gerstmann Syndrome." *J. Neurol. Neurosurg. Psychiat.,* **24**: 176–181, 1961.
—— Developmental Aphasia and Brain Damage. *Cortex,* **1**:40–52, 1964.
—— Contributions to Aphasia before Broca. *Cortex,* **1**:314–326, 1964.
—— Problems of Test Construction in the Field of Aphasia. *Cortex,* **3**:32–58, 1967.
—— Development of a Multilingual Aphasia Battery: Progress and Problems. *J. Neurol. Sci.,* **9**:39–48, 1969.
——, Johann, A. P. Gesner on Aphasia. *Med. Hist.,* **9**:54–60, 1965.
——, Joynt, R. J. Early Descriptions of Aphasia. *Arch. Neurol.,* **3**:205–222, 1960.
——, et al. Three Pioneers in the Study of Aphasia. *J. Hist. Med.,* **18**:381–384, 1963.
——, Van Allen, M. W. Impairment in Facial Recognition in Patients With Cerebral Disease. *Cortex,* **4**:344–358, 1968.
Bergman, P. S., Green, M. Aphasia: Effect of Intravenous Sodium Amytal. *Neurology,* **1**:471–475, 1951.
Berman, M., Peelle, L. M. Self-Generated Cues: A Method for Aiding Aphasic and Apractic Patients. *J. Speech Hearing Dis.,* **32**:372–376, 1967.
Berry, M. F., Eisenson, J. *Speech Disorders.* New York, Appleton, 1956. Pp. 387–419.
Beyn, E. S. Peculiarities of Thought in Patients With Sensory Aphasia. *Lang. Speech,* **1**:233–249, 1958.
——, Shokhor-Trotskaya, M. K. The Preventive Method of Speech Rehabilitation in Aphasia. *Cortex,* **2**:96–108, 1966.
Billow, B. W. Observation of the Use of Sodium Amytal in the Treatment of Aphasia. *Med. Rec.,* **162**:12–13, 1949.
Biorn-Hansen, V. Social and Emotional Aspects of Aphasia. *J. Speech Hearing Dis.,* **22**:53–59, 1957.
Birch, H. G. Experimental Investigations in Expressive Aphasia. *New York J. Med.,* **56**: 3849–3852, 1956.
——, Lee, J. Cortical Inhibition in Expressive Aphasia. *AMA Arch. Neurol. Psychiat.,* **74**: 514–517, 1955.
Bisiach, E. Perceptual Factors in the Pathogenesis of Anomia. *Cortex,* **2**:90–95, 1966.
Black, J. W., Pizzamiglio, L. The Oral Reading of Aphasic Individuals. *J. Commun. Disord.,* **1**: 236–245, 1968.
Blackman, N. Group Psychotherapy With Aphasics. *J. Nerv. Ment. Dis.,* **111**:154–163, 1950.
——, Tureen, L. L. Aphasia: A Psychosomatic Approach in Rehabilitation. *Trans. Amer. Neurol. Ass.,* **73**:193–196, 1948.
Bloom, L. M. A Rationale for Group Treatment of Aphasic Patients. *J. Speech Hearing Dis.,* **27**:11–16, 1962.
Bocca, E. Clinical Aspects of Cortical Deafness. *Laryngoscope,* **68**:301–309, 1958.
Bogen, J. E. The Other Side of the Brain. I: Dys-

graphia and Dyscopia Following Cerebral Commissurotomy. *Bull. L.A. Neurol. Soc.*, **34**:73–105, 1969.

Boller, F. Latent Aphasia: Right and Left "Non-Aphasic" Brain-Damaged Patients Compared. *Cortex*, **4**:245–256, 1968.

——, Spinnler, H. Visual Memory for Colors in Patients With Unilateral Brain Damage. *Cortex*, **3**:395–405, 1967.

——, Vignolo, L. A. Latent Sensory Aphasia in Hemisphere-Damaged Patients: An Experimental Study With the Token Test. *Brain*, **89**:815–830, 1966.

Bonkowski, R. J. Verbal and Extra-Verbal Components of Language as Related to Lateralized Brain Damage. *J. Speech Hearing Res.*, **10**:558–564, 1967.

Boone, D. R. Communication Skills and Intelligence in Right and Left Hemiplegics. *J. Speech Hearing Dis.*, **24**:241–248, 1959.

—— Relationship of Progress in Speech Therapy to Progress in Physical Therapy. *Arch. Phys. Med.*, **42**:30–32, 1961.

—— *An Adult Has Aphasia*. Danville, Illinois, Interstate, 1965.

—— A Plan for Rehabilitation of Aphasic Patients. *Arch. Phys. Med.*, **48**:410–414, 1967.

Borkowski, J. G., Benton, A. L., et al. Word Fluency and Brain Damage. *Neuropsychol.*, **5**:135–140, 1967.

Boshes, B., Wachs, H., et al. Studies of Tone, Tremor, and Speech in Normal Persons and Parkinsonian Patients. *Neurology*, **10**:805–813, 1960.

Botez, M. I., Wertheim, N. Expressive Aphasia and Amusia Following Right Frontal Lesion in a Right-Handed Man. *Brain*, **82**:186–202, 1959.

Brain, R. *Speech Disorders*, 2nd Edition. Washington, D.C., Butterworth, 1965. Pp. 30–51, 92–111, 131–132.

—— The Neurology of Language. *Brain*, **84**:147–166. 1961.

Branch, O., Milner, B., et al. Intracarotid Sodium Amytal for the Lateralization of Cerebral Speech Dominance. *J. Neurosurg.*, **21**:399–405, 1964.

Brewer, W. F. Visual Memory, Verbal Encoding and Hemispheric Localization. *Cortex*, **5**:145–151, 1969.

Bricker, A. L., Schuell, H. M., et al. Effect of Word Frequency and Word Length on Aphasic Spelling Errors. *J. Speech Hearing Res.*, **7**:183–192, 1964.

Brookshire, R. H. Visual Discrimination and Response Reversal Learning by Aphasic Subjects. *J. Speech Hearing Res.*, **11**:677–692, 1968.

—— Probability Learning by Aphasic Subjects. *J. Speech Hearing Res.*, **12**:857–864, 1969.

Brown, I. Abstract and Concrete Behavior of Dysphasic Patients and Normal Subjects. *J. Speech Hearing Dis.*, **20**:35–42, 1955.

Brown, J. R. Management of Patients With Brain Damage. *Neurology*, **2**:273–283, 1952.

—— Some Clinical Aspects of Aphasia. *Ann. Otol.*, **69**:1214–1222, 1960.

——, Schuell, H. M. A Preliminary Report of a Diagnostic Test for Aphasia. *J. Speech Hearing Dis.*, **15**:21–28, 1950.

——, Simonson, J. A Clinical Study of 100 Aphasic Patients. *Neurology*, **7**:777–783, 1957.

Brown, L. G. Practical Hints Concerning Diagnosis and Management of the Aphasic Patient in the General Hospital and Rehabilitation Center. *Ala. J. Med. Sci.*, **5**:56–61, 1968.

Bryden, M. P., Zurif, E. B. Dichotic Listening Performance in a Case of Agenesis of the Corpus Callosum. *Neuropsychol.*, **8**:371–377, 1970.

Buck, J. F., Cooper, I. S. Speech Problems in Parkinsonian Patients Undergoing Anterior Choroidal Artery Occlusion of Chemopallidectomy. *J. Amer. Geriat. Soc.*, **4**:1285–1290, 1956.

Buck, M. *Dysphasia: Professional Guidance for Family and Patient*. Englewood Cliffs, Prentice-Hall, 1968.

Butfield, E., Zangwill, O. L. Re-Education in Aphasia: A Review of 70 Cases. *J. Neurol. Neurosurg. Psychiat.*, **9**:75–79, 1946.

Canter, G. J. Neuromotor Pathologies of Speech. *Amer. J. Phys. Med.*, **46**:659–666, 1967.

Carmon, A., Gombos, G. M. A Physiological Vascular Correlate of Hand Preference: Possible Implications With Respect to Hemispheric Cerebral Dominance. *Neuropsychol.*, **8**:119–128, 1970.

Carr, B. M. Ear Effect Variables and Order of Report in Dichotic Listening. *Cortex*, **5**:63–68, 1969.

Carson, D. H., Carson, F. E., et al. On Learning Characteristics of the Adult Aphasic. *Cortex*, **4**:92–112, 1968.

Casey, T., Ettlinger, G. The Occasional "Independence" of Dyslexia and Dysgraphia from Dysphasia. *J. Neurol. Neurosurg. Psychiat.*, **23**:228–236, 1960.

Charlton, M. H. Aphasia: A Review. *Amer. J. Psychiat.*, **119**:872–874, 1963.

—— Aphasia in Bilingual and Polyglot Patients: A Neurological and Psychological Study. *J. Speech Hearing Dis.*, **29**:307–311, 1964.

—— Reading Difficulty and Language Type. *Folia Phoniat.*, **16**:297–303, 1964.

Cherry, C. *On Human Communication*. Cambridge, Technology Press; and New York, Wiley, 1957.

Chesher, E. C. Some Observations Concerning the Relation of Handedness to the Language Mechanism. *Bull. Neurol. Inst. N.Y.*, **4**:556–562, 1936.

—— Aphasia: Technique of Clinical Examinations. *Bull. Neurol. Inst. N.Y.*, **6**:134–144, 1937.

Clarke, B., Smith, N. V. Lexical and Grammatical Impairment in Dysphasia. *Lang. Speech*, **9**:28–45, 1966.

Cohen, J. G., Edwards, A. E. Word Length and Discrimination Behavior of Aphasics. *J. Speech Hearing Res.*, **7**:343–348, 1964.

Cohen, P., Hannigan, H. M. "Aphasia" in Cerebral Palsy. *Amer. J. Phys. Med.*, **35**:218–222, 1956.

Cohn, R. A Study of Jargon Verbalizations. *Trans. Amer. Neurol. Ass.*, **79**:180–182, 1954.

—— Dyscalculia: A Clinical Study With Some Neuropathological Correlations. *Trans. Amer. Neurol. Ass.*, **84**:118–121, 1959.

—— A Study of Aphasia. *Trans. Amer. Neurol. Ass.*, **87**:187–189, 1962.

——, Neumann, M. Jargon Aphasia. *J. Nerv. Ment. Dis.*, **127**:381–399, 1958.

Cole, M. The Anatomical Basis of Aphasia as Seen by Pierre Marie. *Cortex*, **4**:172–183, 1968.

——, Kraft, M. B. Specific Learning Disability. *Cortex*, **1**:302–313, 1964.

Conrad, K. New Problems of Aphasia. *Brain*, **77**: 491–509, 1954.

Corbin, M. L. Group Speech Therapy for Motor Aphasia and Dysarthria. *J. Speech Hearing Dis.*, **16**:21–34, 1951.

Critchley, M. "Aphasia" in a Partial Deaf-Mute. *Brain*, **61**:163–169, 1938.

—— Aphasic Disorders of Signalling (Constitutional and Acquired) Occurring in Naval Signalmen. *J. Mount Sinai Hosp. N.Y.*, **9**:363–375, 1942.

—— Speech Iterations ("Ting a Ling" Phenomenon). *Postgrad. Med.*, **24**:19–24, 1948.

—— Articulatory Defects in Aphasia. *J. Laryng.*, **66**:1–17, 1952.

—— *The Parietal Lobes*. London, Edward Arnold, 1953.

—— Premorbid Literacy and the Pattern of Subsequent Aphasia. *Proc. Roy. Soc. Med.*, **49**: 335–336, 1956.

—— The Study of Language Disorder: Past, Present and Future. *The Centennial Lectures*. New York, Putnam, 1959.

—— Jacksonian Ideas and the Future, With Special Reference to Aphasia. *Brit. Med. J.*, **2**:6–12, 1960.

—— Head's Contribution to Aphasia. *Brain*, **84**: 551–560, 1961.

—— Dr. Samuel Johnson's Aphasia. *Med. Hist.*, **6**:27–46, 1962.

—— Speech and Speech-Loss in Relation to the Duality of the Brain. In: Mountcastle, V. B. (ed.), *Interhemispheric Relations and Cerebral Dominance*. Baltimore, John Hopkins, 1962. Pp. 208–213.

—— The Origins of Aphasiology. *Scot. Med. J.*, **1**:274–290, 1964.

—— The Drift and Dissolution of Language. *Proc. Roy. Soc. Med.*, **57**:1189–1198, 1964.

—— Symposium: Dyslexia: VI. Is Developmental Dyslexia the Expression of Minor Cerebral Damage? *Slow Learn. Child*, **13**:9–19, 1966.

—— Aphasiological Nomenclature and Definitions. *Cortex*, **3**:3–25, 1967.

Croskey, C. S., Adams, M. R. A Rationale and Clinical Methodology for Selecting Vocabulary Stimulus Material for Individual Aphasic Patients. *J. Commun. Disord.*, **2**:340–343, 1969.

Culton, G. L. Spontaneous Recovery from Aphasia. *J. Speech Hearing Res.*, **12**:825–832, 1969.

Cumming, W. J. K. An Anatomical Review of the Corpus Callosum. *Cortex*, **6**:1–18, 1970.

Darley, F. L. Speech Problems in the Aging. *Postgrad. Med.*, **33**:294–300, 1963.

—— *Diagnosis and Appraisal of Communication Disorders*. New York, Prentice-Hall, 1964.

—— Impairment of Communication Ability in Patients With Cerebrovascular Accidents. *Mayo Clin. Proc.*, **42**:648–652, 1967.

——, Aronson, A. E., et al. Motor Speech Signs in Neurologic Disease. *Med. Clin. N. Amer.*, **52**: 835–844, 1968.

——, ——, et al. Differential Diagnostic Patterns of Dysarthria. *J. Speech Hearing Res.*, **12**:246–269, 1969.

——, ——, et al. Clusters of Deviant Speech Dimensions in the Dysarthrias. *J. Speech Hearing Res.*, **12**:462–496, 1969.

Denny-Brown, D. The Nature of Apraxia. *J. Nerv. Ment. Dis.*, **126**:9–32, 1958.

De Renzi, E., Faglioni, P., et al. The Influence of Aphasia and of the Hemispheric Side of the Cerebral Lesion on Abstract Thinking. *Cortex*, **2**:399–420, 1966.

——, ——, et al. The Performance of Patients with Unilateral Brain Damage on Face Recognition Tasks. *Cortex*, **4**:17–34, 1968.

——, ——, et al. Tactile Spatial Impairment and Unilateral Cerebral Damage. *J. Nerv. Ment. Dis.*, **146**:468–475, 1968.

——, ——, et al. Impairment of Memory for Position Following Brain Damage. *Cortex*, **5**:274–284, 1969.

——, Pieczuro, A., et al. Oral Apraxia and Aphasia. *Cortex*, **2**:50–73, 1966.

——, Scotti, G. The Influence of Spatial Disorders

in Impairing Tactual Discrimination of Shapes. *Cortex,* **5**:53–62, 1969.

——, Vignolo, L. A. The Token Test: A Sensitive Test to Detect Receptive Disturbances in Aphasics. *Brain,* **85**:665–678, 1962.

De Reuck, A. V. S., O'Connor, M. (eds.), Ciba Foundation Symposium, *Disorders of Language.* Boston, Little, Brown, 1964.

Diller, L., Weinberg, J. Attention in Brain-Damaged People. *J. Education,* **150**:20–27, 1968.

Doehring, D. G., Reitan, R. M. MMPI Performance of Aphasic and Non-Aphasic Brain-Damaged Patients. *J. Clin. Psychol.,* **16**:307–309, 1960.

Dooley, J. E., Doehring, D. G., et al. Speed of Visual Perception in Aphasic and Non-Aphasic Patients With Hemiplegia. *Cortex,* **4**:389–402, 1967.

Dottner, B., Davis, V. T., et al. A Case of Subcortical Visual Verbal Agnosia. *J. Nerv. Ment. Dis.,* **116**:808–811, 1952.

Douglass, E. Diagnostic Classification and Re-Education in Aphasia. *Canad. Med. Ass. J.,* **69**: 376–381, 1953.

——, Richardson, J. C. Aphasia in a Congenital Deaf-Mute. *Brain,* **82**:68–80, 1959.

Dudley, J. G., Doehring, D. G., et al. Speed of Visual Perception in Aphasic and Non-Aphasic Patients with Hemiplegia. *Cortex,* **4**:389–402, 1968.

Ebbin, J. B., Edwards, A. E. Speech Sound Discrimination of Aphasics When Intersound Interval is Varied. *J. Speech Hearing Res.,* **10**:120–125, 1967.

Edwards, A. E. Automated Training for a "Matching-to-Sample" Task in Aphasia. *J. Speech Hearing Res.,* **8**:39–42, 1965.

Efron, R. Temporal Perception, Aphasia and Déjà Vu. *Brain,* **86**:403–424, 1963.

Eisenson, J. Aphasics: Observations and Tentative Conclusions. *J. Speech Hearing Dis.,* **12**:290–292, 1947.

—— Prognostic Factors Related to Language Rehabilitation in Aphasic Patients. *J. Speech Hearing Dis.,* **14**:262–264, 1949.

—— *Examining for Aphasia: A Manual for the Examination of Aphasia and Related Disturbances.* New York, Psychological Corporation, 1954.

—— Aphasia in Adults. In: Travis, L. E. (ed.), *Handbook of Speech Pathology.* New York, Appleton-Century-Crofts, 1957. Pp. 436–502.

—— Aphasia. In: Levin, N. (ed.), *Voice and Speech Disorders: Medical Aspects.* Springfield, Ill., Thomas, 1962. Pp. 851–873.

—— Language and Intellectual Modifications Associated With Right Cerebral Damage. *Lang. Speech,* **5**:49–53, 1962.

—— Aphasic Language Modifications Considered as a Disruption of Cultural Verbal Habits. *ASHA,* **5**:503–506, 1963.

—— Aphasia: A Point of View as to the Nature of the Disorder and Factors that Determine Prognosis for Recovery. *Int. J. Neurol.,* **4**:287–295, 1964.

—— Developmental Aphasia: A Speculative View With Therapeutic Implications. *J. Speech Hearing Dis.,* **33**:3–13, 1968.

—— Developmental Aphasia (Dyslogia): A Postulation of a Unitary Concept of the Disorder. *Cortex,* **4**:184–200, 1968.

Eliasberg, W. G. The Social Implications of Dysphasia. *J. Nerv. Ment. Dis.,* **105**:469–476, 1947.

—— Contribution to Prehistory of Aphasia. *J. Hist. Med.,* **5**:96–101, 1950.

Elvin, M. B., Oldfield, R. C. Disability and Progress in a Dysphasic University Student. *J. Neurol. Psychiat.,* **14**:118–128, 1951.

Engmann, D. L., Brookshire, R. H. Effects of Simultaneous and Successive Stimulus Presentation on Visual Discriminations by Aphasic Patients. *J. Speech Hearing Res.,* **13**:369–381, 1970.

Epstein, A. G. Auditory Memory Span for Language. *Folia. Phoniat.,* **16**:271–289, 1964.

Ettlinger, G. Sensory Deficits in Visual Agnosia. *J. Neurol. Neurosurg. Psychiat.,* **19**: 297–307, 1956.

—— Apraxia Considered as a Disorder of Movements That Are Language-Dependent: Evidence from Cases of Brain Bi-Section. *Cortex,* **5**:285–289, 1969.

——, Jackson, C. V., et al. Dysphasia Following Right Temporal Lobectomy in a Right-Handed Man. *J. Neurol. Neurosurg. Psychiat.,* **18**:214–217, 1955.

——, ——, et al. Cerebral Dominance in Sinistrals. *Brain,* **79**:569–588, 1956.

——, Moffett, A. M. Learning in Dysphasia. *Neuropsychol.,* **8**:465–474, 1970.

Faglioni, P., Scotti, G., et al. Impaired Recognition of Written Letters Following Unilateral Hemispheric Damage. *Cortex,* **5**:120–133, 1969.

——, Spinnler, H., et al. Contrasting Behavior of Right and Left Hemisphere-Damaged Patients on a Discriminative and a Semantic Task of Auditory Recognition. *Cortex,* **5**:366–389, 1969.

Fields, F. R. J., Whitmyer, J. W. Verbal and Performance Relationships With Respect to Laterality of Cerebral Involvement. *Dis. Nerv. Syst.,* **30**:177–179, 1969.

Filby, Y., Edwards, A. E. An Application of Automated Teaching Methods to Test and Teach Form Discrimination to Aphasics. *J. Prog. Inst.,* **2**:25–33, 1963.

——, ——, et al. Word Length, Frequency and

Similarity in the Discrimination Behavior of Aphasics. *J. Speech Hearing Res.*, **6**:255–261, 1963.
Fillenbaum, S., Jones, L. V. An Application of "Cloze" Technique to the Study of Aphasic Speech. *J. Abnorm. Soc. Psychol.*, **65**:183–189, 1962.
——, ——, et al. Some Linguistic Features of Speech from Aphasic Patients. *Lang. Speech*, **4**:92–108, 1961.
Fischer, R. A., Ellison, G. W., et al. Esophageal Motility in Neuromuscular Disorders. *Ann. Intern. Med.*, **63**:229–248, 1965.
Fleiss, A. Mental Symptoms and Phenomena of Agnosia, Apraxia and Aphasia. *Amer. J. Psychiat.*, **115**:340–342, 1958.
Fleming, M. Aphasic Factors in a Case of Stammering. *Acta Otorinolaring. Iber. Amer.*, **8**:164–166, 1957.
Fogel, M. L. The Gerstmann Syndrome and the Parietal Symptom-Complex. *Psychol. Rec.*, **12**:85–99, 1962.
Freud, E. D. Recent Trends in Aphasic Research. *Amer. J. Psychiat.*, **110**:186–193, 1953.
—— The Sociology of Aphasic Research. An Investigation into the Sociology of Knowledge. *Acta Otorinolaring. Iber. Amer.*, **8**:166–174, 1957.
Freud, S. *On Aphasia*. New York, International University, 1953.
Friedlander, W. J. Anosognosia and Perception. *Amer. J. Phys. Med.*, **46**:1394–1408, 1967.
Friedman, M. H. On the Nature of Regression in Aphasia. *Arch. Gen. Psychiat.*, **5**:252–255, 1961.
Froeschels, E. A Contribution to the Pathology and Therapy of Dysarthria Due to Certain Cerebral Lesions. *J. Speech Dis.*, **8**:301–321, 1943.
—— Some Voice Problems in Aphasia. In: *Selected Papers of Emil Froeschels*. Amsterdam, North-Holland, 1964. Pp. 164–173.
—— Observations on Aphasia and Ideational Type. *J. Commun. Disord.*, **3**:65–67, 1970.
——, Kastein, S., et al. A Method of Therapy for Paralytic Conditions of the Mechanisms of Phonation Respiration and Glutination. *J. Speech Hearing Dis.*, **20**:365–370, 1955.
Fry, D. B. Phonemic Substitutions in an Aphasic Patient. *Lang. Speech*, **2**:52–61, 1959.
Fry, F. R. Loss of Comprehension of Proper Names. *J. Nerv. Ment. Dis.*, **35**:617–623, 1907.
Gainotti, G., Tiacci, C. Patterns of Drawing Disability in Right and Left Hemispheric Patients. *Neuropsychol.*, **8**:379–384, 1970.
Gardner, W. J. Injection of Procaine into the Brain to Locate Speech Area in Left-Handed Persons. *AMA. Arch. Neurol. Psychiat.*, **46**:1035–1038, 1941.
Gazzaniga, M. S., Sperry, R. W. Language after Section of the Cerebal Commissures. *Brain*, **90**:131–148, 1967.
Gerstmann, J. Syndrome of Finger Agnosia, Disorientation for Right and Left, Agraphia and Acalculia. *AMA Arch. Neurol. Psychiat.*, **44**:398–408, 1940.
Geschwind, N. Non-Aphasic Disorders of Speech. *Int. J. Neurol.*, **4**:207–214, 1964.
—— The Paradoxical Position of Kurt Goldstein in the History of Aphasia. *Cortex*, **1**:214–224, 1964.
—— Disconnexion Syndromes in Animals and Man. *Brain*, **88**: (Part I) 237–294; (Part II) 585–644, 1965.
—— The Varieties of Naming Errors. *Cortex* **3**:97–112, 1967.
—— Wernicke's Contribution to the Study of Aphasia. *Cortex*, **3**:449–463, 1967.
—— The Organization of Language and the Brain. *Science*, **170**:940–944, 1970.
—— Current Concepts: Aphasia. *New Eng. J. Med.*, **284**:654–656, 1971.
——, Fusillo, M. Color-Naming Defects in Association with Alexia. *Arch. Neurol.*, **15**:137–146, 1966.
——, Quadfasel, F. A., et al. Isolation of the Speech Area. *Neuropsychol.*, **6**:327–340, 1968.
Gloning, I., Gloning, K., et al. Comparison of Verbal Behavior in Right-Handed and Nonright-Handed Patients with Anatomically Verified Lesion of One Hemisphere. *Cortex*, **5**:43–52, 1969.
——, ——, et al. A Case of Prosopagnosia With Necropsy Findings. *Neuropsychol.*, **8**:199–204, 1970.
Gloning, K., Quatember, R. Some Classification of Aphasia Disturbances with Special Reference to Rehabilitation. *Int. J. Neurol.*, **4**:296–304, 1964.
——, —— Statistical Evidence of Neuropsychological Syndromes in Left-Handed and Ambidextrous Patients. *Cortex*, **2**:484–488, 1966.
Goda, S. Spontaneous Speech, A Primary Source of Therapy Material. *J. Speech Hearing Dis.*, **27**:190–192, 1962.
Godfrey, C. M. A Dysphasia Rehabilitation Clinic. *Canad. Med. Ass. J.*, **80**:616–618, 1959.
——, Douglass, E. The Recovery Process in Aphasia. *Canad. Med. Ass. J.*, **80**:618–624, 1959.
Goldhamer, H. Use of Language in Dreams in Analysis of Aphasic Deficits. *AMA Arch. Neurol. Psychiat.*, **62**:725–727, 1949.
Goldstein, G., Neuringer, C., et al. Impairment of Abstract Reasoning in the Brain-Damaged: Qualitative or Quantitative? *Cortex*, **4**:372–387, 1968.
Goldstein, H., Cameron, H. New Method of Communication for the Aphasic Patient. *Arizona Med.*, **9**:17–21, 1952.
Goldstein, K. The Problem of the Meaning of

Words Based upon Observation of Aphasic Patients. *J. Psychol.*, **2**:301–316, 1936.
—— *After-Effects of Brain Injuries in War, Their Evaluation and Treatment.* New York, Grune and Stratton, 1942.
—— *Language and Language Disturbances.* New York, Grune and Stratton, 1948, 2nd Edition, 1965.
Goodglass, H. Examination of Purposeful Movement. In: Burr, H. G. (ed.), *The Aphasic Adult: Evaluation and Rehabilitation.* Proceedings of a Short Course in Aphasia, University of Virginia. Charlottesville, Wayside, 1964. Pp. 103–110.
—— Linguistic Changes in Aphasic Speech. In: Burr, H. G. (ed.), *The Aphasic Adult: Evaluation and Rehabilitation.* Proceedings of a Short Course in Aphasia, University of Virginia. Charlottesville, Wayside, 1964. Pp. 35–42.
—— Studies on the Grammar of Aphasics. In: Rosenberg, S., Koplin, J. E. (eds.), *Developments in Applied Psycholinguistics Research.* New York, Macmillan, 1968.
—— *Assessment of Aphasia and Related Disorders.* Philadelphia, Lea and Febiger, 1972.
——, Barton, M. I., et al. Sensory Modality and Object-Naming in Aphasia. *J. Speech Hearing Res.*, **11**:488–496, 1968.
——, Berko, J. Agrammatism and Inflectional Morphology in English. *J. Speech Hearing Res.*, **3**:257–267, 1960.
——, Fodor, I. G., et al. Prosodic Factors in Grammar—Evidence from Aphasia. *J. Speech Hearing Res.*, **10**:5–20, 1967.
——, Gleason, J. B., et al. Some Dimensions of Auditory Language Comprehension in Aphasia. *J. Speech Hearing Res.*, **13**:595–606, 1970.
——, Hunt, J. Grammatical Complexity and Aphasic Speech. *Word,* **14**:197–207, 1958.
——, Hunter, M. A Linguistic Comparison of Speech and Writing in Two Types of Aphasia. *J. Commun. Disord.*, **3**:28–35, 1970.
——, Hyde, M. R., et al. Frequency, Picturability and Availability of Nouns in Aphasia. *Cortex,* **5**:104–119, 1969.
——, Kaplan, E. Disturbance of Gesture and Pantomime in Aphasia. *Brain,* **86**:703–720, 1963.
——, Klein, B., et al. Specific Semantic Word Categories in Aphasia. *Cortex,* **2**:74–89, 1966.
——, Mayer, J. Agrammatism in Aphasia. *J. Speech Hearing Dis.*, **23**:99–111, 1958.
——, Quadfasel, F. A. Language Laterality in Left-Handed Aphasics. *Brain,* **77**:521–548, 1954.
——, ——, et al. Phrase Length and the Type and Severity of Aphasia. *Cortex,* **1**:133–153, 1964.
Goodkin, R. Case Studies in Behavioral Research in Rehabilitation. *Percept. Motor Skills,* **23**:171–182, 1966.
—— Use of Concurrent Response Categories in Evaluating Talking Behavior in Aphasic Patients. *Percept. Motor Skills,* **26**:1035–1040, 1968.
Gordon, H. W. Hemispheric Asymmetries in the Perception of Musical Chords. *Cortex,* **6**:387–398, 1970.
Granich, L., Prangle, G. *Aphasia, A Guide to Retraining.* New York, Grune and Stratton, 1947.
Green, E. Phonological and Grammatical Aspects of Jargon in an Aphasic Patient: A Case Study. *Lang. Speech,* **12**:103–118, 1969.
—— On the Contribution of Studies in Aphasia to Psycholinguistics. *Cortex,* **6**:216–235, 1970.
Greenberg, R., Dewan, E. Aphasia and Dreaming: A Test of the P-Hypothesis. *Psychophysiol.,* **5**:203–204, 1968.
Grewel, F. Aphasia and Linguistics. *Folia Phoniat.,* **3**:100–105, 1951.
—— Acalculia. *Brain,* **75**:397–407, 1952.
—— Classification of Dysarthrias. *Acta Psychiat. Neurol. Scand.,* **32**:325–337, 1957.
—— Dysarthria in Post-Encephalitic Parkinsonism. *Acta Psychiat. Neurol. Scand.,* **32**:440–449, 1957.
—— Speech, Language and Hearing Disorders in Encephalopathy. *Folia Phoniat.,* **12**:281–291, 1960.
Halpern, H. Effect of Stimulus Variables on Dysphasic Verbal Errors. *Percept. Motor Skills,* **21**:291–298, 1965.
Halstead, W. C., Wepman, J. M. The Halstead-Wepman Aphasia Screening Test. *J. Speech Hearing Dis.*, **14**:9–15, 1949.
Hardy, J. C. Suggestions for Physiological Research in Dysarthria. *Cortex,* **3**:128–156, 1967.
Harper, A. K. Aphasia as a Symptom of Otogenic Brain Abscess. *J. Laryng.*, **65**:89–101, 1951.
Hartocollis, P. The Syndrome of Minimal Brain Dysfunction in Young Adult Patients. *Bull. Menninger Clin.*, **32**:102–144, 1968.
Hawk, S. S., Froeschels, E., et al. Selected Bibliography from Current Books and Periodicals on Speech Disorders in Time of War. *J. Speech Hearing Dis.*, **8**:198–204, 1943.
Head, H. Hughlings-Jackson on Aphasia and Kindred Affections of Speech. *Brain,* **38**:1–27, 1915.
—— *Aphasia and Kindred Disorders of Speech,* Volumes I and II. New York, Hafner, 1963.
Hebb, D. O. *The Organization of Behavior.* New York, Wiley. 1949.
Hécaen, H. Clinical Symptomatology in Right and Left Hemispheric Lesions. In: Mountcastle, V. B. (ed.), *Interhemispheric Relations and Cerebral Domi-*

nance. Baltimore, Johns Hopkins, 1962. Pp. 215-243.

——, Penfield, W., et al. The Syndrome of Apractognosia Due to Lesions of the Minor Cerebral Hemisphere. *AMA Arch. Neurol. Psychiat.*, **75**:400-434, 1956.

——, Piercy, M. Paroxysmal Dysphasia and the Problem of Cerebral Dominance. *J. Neurol. Neurosurg. Psychiat.*, **19**:194-201, 1956.

Heilbrun, A. B. Vocabulary Responses as Related to Lateralization of Cerebral Lesion: An Investigation of Latent Aphasia. *J. Abnorm. Psychol.*, **57**:237-239, 1958.

Heilman, K. M., Pandya, D. N., et al. Auditory Inattention. *Arch. Neurol.*, **24**:323-325, 1971.

Hemphill, R. E. Restoration of Speech in Severe Aphasia by Intravenous and Oral Priscol. *Brit. Med. J.*, **2**:891-892, 1951.

——, Stengel, E. A Study on Pure Word Deafness. *J. Neurol. Psychiat.*, **3**:251-262, 1940.

Henschen, S. E. On the Function of the Right Hemisphere of the Brain in Relation to the Left in Speech, Music and Calculation. *Brain*, **49**:110-123, 1926.

Hirschenfang, S. A Comparison of W.A.I.S. Scores of Hemiplegic Patients With and Without Aphasia. *J. Clin. Psychol.*, **16**:351-352, 1960.

——, Shulman, L., et al. Psychosocial Factors Influencing the Rehabilitation of the Hemiplegia Patient. *Dis. Nerv. Syst.*, **29**:373-379, 1968.

Hodgins, E. *Episode*. New York, Atheneum, 1964.

Hoff, H. E., Guillemin, R., et al. An 18th Century Scientist's Observation of His Own Aphasia. *Bull. Hist. Med.*, **32**:446-450, 1958.

Holmes, J. E., Sadoff, R. L. Aphasia Due to a Right Hemisphere Tumor in a Right-Handed Man. *Neurology*, **16**:392-397, 1966.

Howes, D. Comments on the So-Called Acquiescence Set in Aphasia. *J. Abnorm. Psychol.*, **71**:151-154, 1966.

——, Geschwind, N. Quantitative Studies of Aphasic Language. In: Rioch, D. M., Weinstein, E. A. (eds.), *Disorders of Communication*. Baltimore, Williams and Wilkins, 1964. Pp. 229-244.

Huber, M. Re-Education of Aphasics. *J. Speech Hearing Dis.*, **7**:289-292, 1942.

—— A Phonetic Approach to the Problem of Perception in a Case of Wernicke's Aphasia. *J. Speech Hearing Dis.*, **9**:227-237, 1944.

—— Linguistic Problems of Brain Injured Servicemen. *J. Speech Hearing Dis.*, **11**:143-147, 1946.

—— Paragnosia and Paraphasia. *J. Speech Hearing Dis.*, **11**:321-327, 1946.

Hudson, A. J. Perseveration. *Brain*, **91**:571-582, 1968.

Hughlings-Jackson, J. Remarks on Non-Protrusion of the Tongue in Some Cases of Aphasia. *Lancet* **1**:716:717, 1878.

—— On Aphasia, With Left Hemiplegia. *Lancet*, **1**:637-638, 1880.

—— Loss of Speech: Its Association With Valvular Disease of the Heart and With Hemiplegia on the Right Side. *Brain*, **38**:28-42, 1915.

—— *Selected Writings of J. Hughlings-Jackson*. (Taylor, J., ed.) New York, Basic, 1958.

—— Defect of Intellectual Expression (Aphasia) With Left Hemiplegia. *Lancet*, **1**:457, 1868.

Humphrey, M. E., Zangwill, O. L. Dysphasia in Left-Handed Patients With Unilateral Brain Lesions. *J. Neurol. Neurosurg. Psychiat.*, **15**:184-193, 1952.

Jakobson, R. Aphasia as a Linguistic Problem. In: Werner, H. (ed.), *On Expressive Language*. Worcester, Clark University, 1955. Pp. 69-81.

—— Two Aspects of Language and Two Types of Aphasic Disturbances. In: Jakobson, R., Halle, M. (eds.), *Fundamentals of Language*. The Hague, Mouton, 1956. Pp. 55-82.

—— Aphasia as a Linguistic Problem. In: Saporta, S., Bastian, J. R. (eds.), *Psycholinguistics: A Book of Readings*. New York, Holt, Rinehart and Winston, 1961. Pp. 419-427.

—— Towards a Linguistic Typology of Aphasic Impairments. In: de Reuck, A. V. S., O'Connor, M. (eds.), *Disorders of Language*. Boston, Little, Brown, 1964. Pp. 21-46.

—— Linguistic Types of Aphasia. In: Carterette, E. C. (ed.), *Brain Function Vol. III Speech, Language and Communication*. Los Angeles, University of California, 1966.

—— *Child Language, Aphasia and Phonological Universals*. The Hague, Mouton, 1968.

Jellinek, A. Amusia: On the Phenomenology and Investigation of Central Disorders of the Musical Functions. *Folia Phoniat.*, **8**:124-149, 1956.

Jenkins, J. J., Schuell, H. M. Further Work on Language Deficit in Aphasia. *Psychol. Rev.*, **71**:87-93, 1964.

——, —— Acquiescence Response Set in Aphasics. *J. Abnorm. Psychol.*, **70**:111-113, 1965.

Johns, D. F., Darley, F. L. Phonemic Variability in Apraxia of Speech. *J. Speech Hearing Res.*, **13**:556-583, 1970.

Jones, J., Dinolt, R. Pure Word Deafness. *Laryngoscope*, **62**:194-203, 1952.

Jones, L. V., Goodman, M. F., et al. The Classification of Parts of Speech for the Characterization of Aphasia. *Lang. Speech*, **6**:94-107, 1963.

——, Wepman, J. M. Dimensions of Language Performance in Aphasia. *J. Speech Hearing Res.*, **4**: 220-232, 1961.

——, —— *A Spoken Word Count.* Chicago, Language Research Associates, 1966.

Joy, H. H. Agnosia, Alexia Without Agraphia following Trauma. *Amer. J. Ophthal.*, **31**:811-820, 1948.

Joynt, R. J. Centenary of Patient "Tan". *Arch. Intern. Med.*, **108**:953-956, 1961.

—— Paul Pierre Broca: His Contribution to the Knowledge of Aphasia. *Cortex*, **1**:206-213, 1964.

——, Benton, A. L. The Memoir of Marc Dax on Aphasia. *Neurology*, **14**:851-854, 1964.

Kann, J. A Translation of Broca's Original Article on the Location of the Speech Center. *J. Speech Hearing Dis.*, **15**:16-20, 1950.

Kaplan, L. T. A Descriptive Continuum of Language Responses in Aphasia. *J. Speech Hearing Dis.*, **24**:410-412, 1959.

Karlin, I. W., Eisenson, J., et al. A Multi-Evaluational Study of Aphasic and Non-Aphasic Right Hemiplegic Patients. *J. Speech Hearing Dis.*, **24**: 369-379, 1959.

——, Hirschenfang, S. Evaluation of Language and Intellectual Disturbances in Patients With Space Occupying Brain Lesions. *Logos*, **6**:33-40, 1963.

Katz, L. Learning in Aphasic Patients. *J. Consult. Psychol.*, **22**:143-146, 1958.

Keenan, J. S. A Method for Eliciting Naming Behavior from Aphasic Patients. *J. Speech Hearing Dis.*, **31**:261-266, 1966.

—— The Nature of Receptive and Expressive Impairments in Aphasia. *J. Speech Hearing Dis.*, **33**: 20-25, 1968.

Keith, R. L., Darley, F. L. The Use of a Specific Electric Board in Rehabilitation of the Aphasic Patient. *J. Speech Hearing Dis.*, **32**:148-153, 1967.

Kennedy, F., Wolf, A. The Relationship of Intellect to Speech Defect in Aphasic Patients. *J. Nerv. Ment. Dis.*, **84**:125-145, 293-311, 1936.

Kennedy, L. Remedial Procedures for Handling Aphasic Patients. *AMA Arch. Neurol. Psychiat.*, **57**:646-649, 1947.

Kertesz, A., Benson, D. F. Neologistic Jargon: A Clinicopathological Study. *Cortex*, **6**:362-386, 1970.

Kimura, D. Cerebral Dominance and the Perception of Verbal Stimuli. *Canad. J. Psychol.*, **15**: 166-171, 1961.

Kinsbourne, M., Warrington, E. K. Disorders of Spelling. *J. Neurol. Neurosurg. Psychiat.*, **27**:224-228, 1964.

Kirkner, F. J., Dorcus, R. M., et al. Hypnotic Motivation of Vocalization in an Organic Motor Aphasic Case. *J. Clin. Exper. Hypn.*, **1**:47-49, 1953.

Klein, R. Loss of Written Language Due to Dissolution of the Phonetic Structure of the Word in Brain Abscess. *J. Ment. Sci.*, **97**:328-339, 1951.

Kleist, K. *Sensory Aphasia and Amusia: The Myeloarchitectonic Basis.* New York, Pergamon, 1962.

Klove, H., Reitan, R. M. Effect of Dysphasia and Spatial Distortion on Wechsler-Bellevue Results. *AMA Arch. Neurol. Psychiat.*, **80**:708-713, 1958.

Kreindler, A., Fradis, A. A Study on Changes in the Latency Period of Verbal and Nonverbal Performances in Aphasics. *Int. J. Neurol.*, **4**:265-276, 1964.

——, —— *Performances in Aphasia: A Neurodynamical, Diagnostic and Psychological Study.* Paris, Gauthier-Villars, 1968.

——, Milhailescu, L. Operational Words in Aphasics. *J. Neurol. Sci.*, **11**:275-284, 1970.

Lambert, W. E., Fillenbaum, S. A Pilot Study of Aphasia among Bilinguals. *Canad. J. Psychol.*, **13**:28-34, 1959.

Lane, H. L., Moore, D. J. Reconditioning a Consonant Discrimination in an Aphasic: An Experimental Case History. *J. Speech Hearing Dis.*, **27**:232-243, 1962.

Lansdell, H. Laterality of Verbal Intelligence in the Brain. *Science*, **135**:922-923, 1962.

Lansdell, H., Purnell, J. K., et al. The Relation of Induced Dysnomia to Phoneme Frequency. *Lang. Speech*, **6**:88-93, 1963.

LaPointe, L. L., Culton, G. L. Visual-Spatial Neglect Subsequent to Brain Injury. *J. Speech Hearing Dis.*, **34**:82-86, 1969.

Lashley, K. S. *Brain Mechanisms and Intelligence.* Chicago, University of Chicago, 1929.

—— Factors Limiting Recovery after Central Nervous Lesions. *J. Nerv. Ment. Dis.*, **88**:733-755, 1938.

Lecours, A. R., Lhermitte, F. Phonemic Paraphasias: Linguistic Structures and Tentative Hypotheses. *Cortex*, **5**:193-228, 1969.

Lehiste, I. *Some Acoustic Characteristics of Dysarthric Speech.* Basel, S. Karger, 1965.

Leicester, J., Sidman, M., et al. The Nature of Aphasic Responses. *Neuropsychol.*, **9**:141-155, 1971.

Leischner, A. Disorders of Stenographers: Contribution to Agraphia in Shorthand. *Arch. Psychiat.*, **185**:271-290, 1950.

Lenneberg, E. H. Understanding Language Without Ability to Speak: A Case Report. *J. Abnorm. Soc. Psychol.*, **65**:419-425, 1962.

—— *Biological Foundations of Language.* New York, Wiley, 1967.

Leutenegger, R. R. A Bibliography on Aphasia. *J. Speech Hearing Dis.*, **16**:280–292, 1951.

Levinsohn, J. The Investigation of the Disintegration of Phonemic Discrimination on a Perceptual and Production Level in Adults With Aphasia. *J. S. Afr. Logoped. Soc.*, **16**:49–62, 1969.

Levita, E., Riklan, M., et al. Verbal and Perceptual Function after Surgery of Subcortical Structures. *Percept. Motor Skills*, **18**:195–202, 1964.

Lhermitte, F., Lecours, A. R., et al. Activation of Linguistic Units in Aphasic Transformations. In: Proctor, D. (ed.), *Biocybernetics of the Central Nervous System.* Proceedings of an International Symposium. Boston, Little, Brown, 1969. Pp. 389–417.

Liberson, W. T. Study of Evoked Potentials in Aphasics. *Amer. J. Phys. Med.*, **45**:135–142, 1966.

Liepmann, D. Motor Aphasia, Anarthria, and Apraxia. *XVIIth International Congress of Medicine Sect. XI Neuropathology.* London, 1913. Pp. 97–115.

Linn, L. Sodium Amytal in Treatment of Aphasia. *AMA Arch. Neurol. Psychiat.*, **58**:357–358, 1947.

——, Stein, M. Sodium Amytal in Treatment of Aphasia: Preliminary Report. *Bull. U.S. Army Med. Dept.*, **5**:705–708, 1946.

Longerich, M. C. *Manual for the Aphasia Patient.* New York, Macmillan, 1958.

——, Bordeaux, J. *Aphasia Therapeutics.* New York, Macmillan, 1954.

Lowman, E. W., Rusk, H. A. Self-Help Devices: Aphasia Therapy. *Postgrad. Med.*, **32**:79–81, 182–185, 1962.

Luchsinger, R., Arnold, G. E. *Voice-Speech-Language; Clinical Communicology: Its Physiology and Pathology.* Belmont, California, Wadsworth, 1965. Pp. 706–738.

Luria, A. R. Brain Disorders and Language Analysis. *Lang. Speech*, **1**:14–34, 1958.

—— The Directive Function of Speech in Development and Dissolution: Part II. Dissolution of the Regulative Function of Speech in Pathological States of the Brain. *Word*, **15**:453–464, 1959.

—— *The Role of Speech in the Regulation of Normal and Abnormal Behavior.* New York, Liveright, 1961.

——*Restoration of Function after Brain Injury.* New York, Macmillan, 1963.

—— Neuropsychology in the Local Diagnosis of Brain Damage. *Cortex*, **1**:3–18, 1964.

—— Factors and Forms of Aphasia: In: de Reuck, A. V. S.,. O'Connor, M. (eds.), *Disorders of Language.* Boston, Little, Brown, 1964. Pp. 143–161.

—— *Human Brain and Psychological Processes.* New York, Harper & Row, 1966.

—— *Traumatic Aphasia; Its Syndromes, Psychology and Treatment.* The Hague, Mouton; New York, Humanities Press, 1970.

——, Tsvetkova, L. S. Towards the Mechanisms of "Dynamic Aphasia". *Acta Neurol. Psychiat. Belg.*, **67,** 1969.

MacNeilage, P. F., Rootes, T. P. et al. Speech Production and Perception in a Patient With Severe Impairment of Somesthetic Perception and Motor Control. *J. Speech Hearing Res.*, **10**:449–467, 1967.

McFie, J., Piercy, M. F., et al. Visual Spatial Agnosia Associated With Lesions of the Right Cerebral Hemisphere. *Brain*, **73**:167–190, 1950.

——, Zangwill, O. L. Visual Constructive Disabilities Associated With Lesions of the Left Cerebral Hemispheres. *Brain*, **83**:243–260, 1960.

Malone, R. L. Expressed Attitudes of Families of Aphasics. *J. Speech Hearing Dis.*, **34**:146–151, 1969.

——, Ptacek, P. H., et al. Attitudes Expressed by Families of Aphasics. *Brit. J. Disord. Commun.*, **5**: 174–179, 1970.

Marks, M. M., Taylor, M. L., et al. Rehabilitation of the Aphasic Patient: A Survey of Three Years' Experience in a Rehabilitation Setting. *Neurology*, **7**:837–843, 1957.

Marx, O. M. Freud and Aphasia: An Historical Analysis. *Amer. J. Psychiat.*, **124**:815-825, 1967.

Mason, C. F. Hypnotic Motivation of Aphasics. *Int. J. Clin. Exper. Hypn.*, **9**:297–301, 1961.

Meyers, R. Relation of "Thinking" and Language: An Experimental Approach Using Dysphasic Patients. *AMA Arch. Neurol. Psychiat.*, **60**:119–139, 1948.

Millikan, C. H., Darley, F. L. *Brain Mechanisms Underlying Speech and Language.* New York, Grune & Stratton, 1967.

Mills, C. K. Treatment of Aphasia by Training. *JAMA*, **43**:1940–1949, 1904.

—— Cerebral Localization and Failures in Written Language. *AMA Arch. Neurol. Psychiat.*, **22**: 1127–1134, 1929.

Monrad-Krohn, G. H. Altered Melody of Language, ("Dysprosody") as an Element of Aphasia. *Acta Psychiat. Kbh. Suppl.*, **46**:204–212, 1947.

—— Dysprosody or Altered Melody of Language. *Brain*, **70**:405–415, 1947.

—— The Third Element of Speech: Prosody in the Neuro-Psychiatric Clinic. *J. Ment. Sci.*, **103**: 326–331, 1957.

Montgomery, J. A Case for the Lowly Alphabet. *J. Speech Hearing Dis.*, **32**:297–298, 1967.

Morley, D. E. The Rehabilitation of Adults With

Dysarthric Speech. *J. Speech Hearing Dis.*, **20**: 58–64, 1955.

Morley, H. J. Applying Linguistics to Speech and Language Therapy for Aphasics. *Lang. Learn.*, **10**:135–149, 1960.

Mountcastle, V. B. (ed.). *Interhemispheric Relations and Cerebral Dominance.* Baltimore, Johns Hopkins, 1962.

Mullendore, J. M., Stoudt, R. J. Speech Patterns of Muscular Dystrophic Individuals. *J. Speech Hearing Dis.*, **26**:252–257, 1961.

Nathan, P. W. Facial Apraxia and Apraxic Dysarthria. *Brain*, **70**:449–478, 1947.

Needham, E. C., Black, J. W. The Relative Ability of Aphasic Persons to Judge the Duration and Intensity of Pure Tones. *J. Speech Hearing Res.*, **13**:725–730, 1970.

Nielsen, J. M. The Possibility of Pure Motor Aphasia. *Bull. L. A. Neurol. Soc.*, 1936(b). p. 210.

—— Aphasia. *Oxford Loose-Leaf Medicine.* New York, Oxford, 1945.

—— Cerebral Localization in Aphasia and Agnosia. *AMA Arch. Neurol. Psychiat.*, **64**:748–751, 1950.

—— Spontaneous Recovery from Aphasia: Autopsy. *Bull. L. A. Neurol. Soc.*, **18**:147–151, 1953.

—— Motor Aphasia with Recovery: Report of a Case With Autopsy Verification. *Bull. L. A. Neurol. Soc.*, **22**:148–149, 1957.

—— *Agnosia, Apraxia, Aphasia: Their Value in Cerebral Localization*, 2nd Edition. New York, Hafner, 1962.

——, Friedman, A. P. Fundamental Principles in Aphasia Based on Autopsy Material of Crucial Cases. *Bull. L. A. Neurol. Soc.*, **7**:77–87, 1942.

——, Schultz, D. A., et al. The Treatment of Traumatic Aphasics of World War II at Birmingham General VA Hospital, Van Nuys, California. *Milit. Surg.*, **102**:351–364, 1948.

Noll, J. D., Hoops, H. R. Aphasic Grammatical Involvement as Indicated by Spelling Ability. *Cortex*, **3**:419–432, 1967.

Odom, G. L., Lyman, R. S. Speech Disorders Following Excision of Postcentral Gyrus. *Trans. Amer. Neurol. Ass.*, **71**:67–70, 1946.

Ojemann, G. A., Fedio, P., et al. Anomia from Pulvinar and Subcortical Parietal Stimulation. *Brain*, **91**:99–115, 1968.

Orgass, B., Poeck, K. Assessment of Aphasia by Psychometric Methods. *Cortex*, **5**:317–330, 1969.

——, —— Clinical Validation of a New Test for Aphasia: An Experimental Study on the Token Test. *Cortex*, **2**:222–243, 1966.

Osgood, C. E., Miron, M. S. (eds.). *Approaches to the Study of Aphasia.* Urbana, University of Illinois, 1963.

Oxbury, J. M., Oxbury, S. Effects of Temporal Lobectomy on the Report of Dichotically Presented Digits. *Cortex*, **5**:3–14, 1969.

Panse, F., Shimoyama, T. Aphasic Disorders in Japanese: Writing and Reading Disorders. *Arch. Psychiat.*, **193**:139–145, 1955.

Parisi, D., Pizzamiglio, L. Syntactic Comprehension in Aphasia. *Cortex*, **6**:204–215, 1970.

Peacher, W. G. Speech Disorders in World War II. *J. Speech Hearing Dis.*, **10**:155–161, 287–291, 1945.

—— The Etiology and Differential Diagnosis of Dysarthria. *J. Speech Hearing Dis.*, **15**:252–265, 1950.

—— Dysarthria. In: Levin, N. (ed.). *Voice and Speech Disorders: Medical Aspects.* Springfield, Ill., Thomas, 1962.

——, Peacher, G. M. Management of Speech Disorders in a Hospital Clinic. *Dis. Nerv. Syst.*, **9**:3–9, 1948.

Penfield, W. Conditioning the Uncommitted Cortex for Language Learning. *Brain*, **88**:787–798, 1965.

—— Speech, Perception and the Uncommitted Cortex. In: Eccles, J. C. (ed.). *Brain and Conscious Experience.* New York, Springer-Verlag, 1966. Pp. 217–237.

——, Rasmussen, T. Vocalization and Arrest of Speech. *AMA Arch. Neurol. Psychiat.*, **61**:21–27, 1949.

——, Roberts, L. *Speech and Brain-Mechanisms.* Princeton, Princeton University, 1959.

Pichot, P. Language Disturbances in Cerebral Disease: Concept of Latent Aphasia. *AMA Arch. Neurol. Psychiat.*, **74**:92–96, 1955.

Piercy, M. The Effects of Cerebral Lesions on Intellectual Function: A Review of Current Research Trends. *Brit. J. Psychiat.*, **110**:310–352, 1964.

——, Hécaen, H., et al. Constructional Apraxia Associated With Unilateral Cerebral Lesions—Left and Right Sided Cases Compared. *Brain*, **83**:225–242, 1960.

Pincas, A. Linguistics and Aphasia. *J. Aust. Coll. Speech Ther.*, **15**:20–28, 1965.

Pizzamiglio, L., Black, J. W. Phonic Trends in the Writing of Aphasic Patients. *J. Speech Hearing Res.*, **11**:77–84, 1968.

——, Roberts, M. M. Writing in Aphasia: A Learning Study. *Cortex*, **3**:250–257, 1967.

Poeck, K., Orgass, B. Gerstmann's Syndrome and Aphasia. *Cortex*, **2**:421–437, 1966.

Porch, B. E. *Porch Index of Communicative Ability.* Palo Alto, Consulting Psychologists, 1967.

Quadfasel, F. A. Aspects of the Life and Work of Kurt Goldstein. *Cortex*, **4**:113–124, 1968.

——, Goodglass, H. Language Laterality in Left-Handed Aphasics. *Brain,* **77**:521–548, 1954.

Raney, A. A., Friedman, A. P., et al. Aphasia after Major Temporal Lobectomy. *Bull. L. A. Neurol. Soc.,* **7**:154–156, 1942.

Reichstein, J. Auditory Threshold Consistency in Differential Diagnosis of Aphasia in Children. *J. Speech Hearing Dis.,* **29**:147–155, 1964.

Reinhold, M. A Case of Auditory Agnosia. *Brain,* **73**:203–223, 1950.

——, An Analysis of Agnosia. *Neurology,* **4**:128–136, 1954.

Reitan, R. M. Intellectual Functions in Aphasic and Non-Aphasic Brain Injured Subjects. *Neurology,* **3**:202–212, 1953.

—— Intelligence and Language Functions in Dysphasic Patients. *Dis. Nerv. Syst.,* **15**:131–137, 1954.

——The Performance of Aphasic, Non-Aphasic, and Control Subjects on the Rorschach Test. *J. Gen. Psychol.,* **51**:199–212, 1954.

—— The Significance of Dysphasia for Intelligence and Adaptive Abilities. *J. Psychol.,* **50**:355–376, 1960.

Richat, P. Language Disturbances in Cerebral Disease. *AMA Arch. Neurol. Psychiat.,* **74**:92–96, 1955.

Riese, W. The Early History of Aphasia. *Bull. Hist. Med.,* **21**:322–334, 1947.

—— Hughlings-Jackson's Doctrine of Aphasia and Its Significance Today. *J. Nerv. Ment. Dis.,* **122**: 1–13, 1955.

—— Semantic Aphasia. *J. Nerv. Ment. Dis.,* **123**: 18–22, 1956.

—— Dynamics in Brain Lesions. *J. Nerv. Ment. Dis.,* **127**:291–301, 1960.

—— Historical Perspective: Pioneers in Aphasia. In: Burr, H. G. (ed.), *The Aphasic Adult: Evaluation and Rehabilitation.* Proceedings of a Short Course in Aphasia, University of Virginia. Charlottesville, Wayside, 1964. Pp. 59–77.

—— The Sources of Hughlings-Jackson's View on Aphasia. *Brain,* **88**:811–822, 1965.

——, Hoff, E. C. The History of Aphasia. *J. Hist. Med.,* **6**:457–470, 1951.

Roberts, L. Alterations in Speech Produced by Cerebral Stimulation. *Trans. Amer. Neurol. Ass.,* **76**:43–47, 1951.

—— Functional Plasticity in Cortical Speech Areas and Integration of Speech. *Research Publications of the Association for Research in Nervous and Mental Disease,* **36**:449–466, 1956; and *AMA Arch. Neurol. Pyschiat.,* **79**:275–283, 1958.

—— Dysphasias from the Neurological Standpoint. In: Levin, M. (ed.), *Speech Pathology and Therapy.* Baltimore, Williams and Wilkins, 1958.

Rollin, W. J. Oral Responses of Aphasics under Different Syntactical Conditions. *Lang. Speech,* **7**:167–175, 1964.

Rolnick, M., Hoops, H. R. Aphasia as Seen by the Aphasic. *J. Speech Hearing Dis.,* **34**:48–53, 1969.

Rose, R. H. A Physician's Account of His Own Aphasia. *J. Speech Hearing Dis.,* **13**:294–305, 1948.

Rosenberg, B. The Performance of Aphasics on Automated Visuo-Perceptual Discrimination, Training, and Transfer Tasks. *J. Speech Hearing Res.,* **8**:165–181, 1965.

——, Edwards, A. E. The Performance of Aphasics on Three Automated Perceptual Discrimination Programs. *J. Speech Hearing Res.,* **7**:295–298, 1964.

——, —— An Automated Multiple Response Alternative Training Program for Use With Aphasics. *J. Speech Hearing Res.,* **8**:415–419, 1965.

Rubens, A. B., Benson, D. F. Associative Visual Agnosia. *Arch. Neurol.,* **24**:305–316, 1971.

Rusk, H. A. Aphasia. *J. Chronic Dis.,* **2**:352–358, 1955.

Russell, W. R. *Brain, Memory, Learning: A Neurologist's View.* London, Oxford University, 1959.

—— Some Anatomical Aspects of Aphasia. *Lancet,* **1**:1173–1177, 1963.

——, Espir, M. L. E. *Traumatic Aphasia: A Study of Aphasia in War Wounds of the Brain.* London, Oxford University, 1961.

Russo, M., Vignolo, L. A. Visual Figure-Ground Discrimination in Patients With Unilateral Cerebral Disease. *Cortex,* **3**:113–127, 1967.

St. Onge, K. R., Calvert, J. J. The Brain Stem Damage Syndrome: Speech and Psychological Factors. *J. Speech Hearing Dis.,* **24**:43–50, 1959.

Salibi, B. S. Speech and Aphasia (Speechlessness). *Med. Trial Techn. Quart.,* **11**:11–30, 1965.

Sands, E., Sarno, M. T., et al. Long-Term Assessment of Language Function in Aphasia Due to Stroke. *Arch. Phys. Med.,* **50**:203–207, 1969.

Sarno, J. E., Sarno, M. T. *Stroke: The Condition and the Patient.* New York, McGraw-Hill, 1969.

——, ——, et al. Evaluating Language Improvement after Completed Stroke. *Arch. Phys. Med.,* **52**:73–78, 1971.

——, Swisher, L. P., et al. Aphasia in a Congenitally Deaf Man. *Cortex,* **5**:398–414, 1969.

Sarno, M. T. Verbal Impairment Related to Stroke. *Actas del Primer Congreso del Caribe sobre Medicina Física y Rehabilitación.* First Caribbean Congress on Physical Medicine and Rehabilitation, 1966. Pp. 105–112.

—— Method for Multivariant Analysis of Aphasia

Based on Studies of 235 Patients in a Rehabilitation Setting. *Arch. Phys. Med.*, **49**:210–216, 1968.

—— *The Functional Communication Profile Manual of Directions.* Rehabilitation Monograph 42. New York, Institute of Rehabilitation Medicine, New York University Medical Center, 1969.

—— A Survey of 100 Aphasic Medicare Patients in a Speech Pathology Program. *J. Amer. Geriat. Soc.*, **18**:471–480, 1970.

——, Levita, E. Natural Course of Recovery in Severe Aphasia. *Arch. Phys. Med.*, **52**:175–179, 1971.

——, Sands, E. S. *A Selected Bibliography of Acquired Verbal Impairment Secondary to Brain Damage.* New York, New York University Medical Center, 1967.

——, Silverman, M., et al. Psychosocial Factors and Recovery in Geriatric Patients with Severe Aphasia. *J. Amer. Geriat. Soc.*, **18**:405–409, 1970.

——, ——, et al. Speech Therapy and Language Recovery in Severe Aphasia. *J. Speech Hearing Res.*, **13**:607–623, 1970.

Sasanuma, S., Fujimura, O. Selective Impairment of Phonetic and Non-Phonetic Transcription of Words in Japanese Aphasic Patients: Kana vs. Kanji in Visual Recognition and Writing. *Cortex*, **7**:1–18, 1971.

Scarff, J. E. Recovery of Speech Following Evacuation of Subcortical Haematoma. *Proc. Roy. Soc. Med.*, **36**:405–406, 1943.

Scargill, M. H. Modern Linguistics and Recovery from Aphasia. *J. Speech Hearing Dis.*, **19**:507–513, 1954.

Schiller, F. Aphasia Studied in Patients With Missile Wounds. *J. Neurol. Psychiat.*, **10**:183–197, 1947.

Schlanger, P. H., Schlanger, B. B. Adapting Role-Playing Activities With Aphasic Patients. *J. Speech Hearing Dis.*, **35**:229–235, 1970.

Schuell, H. M. Paraphasia and Paralexia. *J. Speech Hearing Dis.*, **15**:291–306, 1950.

—— Aphasic Difficulties Understanding Spoken Language. *Neurology*, **3**:176–184, 1953.

—— Auditory Impairment in Aphasia: Significance and Retraining Techniques. *J. Speech Hearing Dis.*, **18**:14–21, 1953.

—— Clinical Observations on Aphasia. *Neurology*, **4**:179–189, 1954.

——Diagnosis and Prognosis in Aphasia. *AMA Arch. Neurol. Psychiat.*, **74**:308–315, 1955.

—— *Minnesota Test for Differential Diagnosis of Aphasia*, Research ed. Minneapolis, University of Minnesota, 1955.

—— A Short Examination for Aphasia. *Neurology*, **17**:625–634, 1957.

—— Reading and Writing Disturbances in Adult Aphasics. *Education*, **79**:438–443, 1959.

—— Review of the Month: Speech and Brain Mechanisms. *Rehab. Lit.*, **21**:3–6, 1960.

—— Clinical Findings in Aphasia. *Lancet*, **80**: 482–490, 1960.

—— *Differential Diagnosis of Aphasia with the Minnesota Test.* Minneapolis, University of Minnesota, 1966.

—— A Re-Evaluation of the Short Examination for Aphasia. *J. Speech Hearing Dis.*, **31**:137–147, 1966.

—— Some Dimensions of Aphasic Impairment in Adults Considered in Relationship to Investigation of Language Disturbances in Children. *Brit. J. Disord. Commun.*, **1**:33–45, 1966.

——, Carroll, V. A., et al. Clinical Treatment of Aphasia. *J. Speech Hearing Dis.*, **20**:43–53, 1955.

——, Jenkins, J. J. The Nature of Language Deficit in Aphasia. *Psychol. Rev.*, **66**:45–67, 1959.

——, —— Comment on "Dimensions of Language Performance in Aphasia." *J. Speech Hearing Res.*, **4**:295–299, 1961.

——, —— Reduction of Vocabulary in Aphasia. *Brain*, **84**:243–261, 1961.

——, —— The Nature of Language Deficit in Aphasia. In: Saporta, S., Bastian, J. R. (eds.), *Psycholinguistics: A Book of Readings.* New York, Holt, Rinehart and Winston, 1961. Pp. 427–448.

——, ——, et al. Relationship between Auditory Comprehension and Word Frequency in Aphasia. *J. Speech Hearing Res.*, **4**:30–36, 1961.

——, ——, et al. A Factor Analysis of the Minnesota Test for Differential Diagnosis of Aphasia. *J. Speech Hearing Res.*, **5**:349–369, 1962.

——, ——, et al. *Aphasia in Adults.* New York, Harper & Row, 1964.

——, Shaw, R., et al. A Psycholinguistic Approach to Study of the Language Deficit in Aphasia. *J. Speech Hearing Res.*, **12**:794–806, 1969.

Schulhoff, C., Goodglass, H. Dichotic Listening, Side of Brain Injury and Cerebral Dominance. *Neuropsychol.*, **7**:149–160, 1969.

Scripture, E. W. Records of Speech in Disseminated Sclerosis. *Brain*, **39**:455–477, 1916.

Sefer, J. W., Henrikson, E. H. The Relationship between Word Association and Grammatical Classes in Aphasia. *J. Speech Hearing Res.*, **9**: 529–541, 1966.

Semmes, J. Agnosia in Animal and Man. *Psychol. Rev.*, **60**:140–147, 1953.

Serafetinides, E. A. Auditory Recall and Visual Recognition Following Intracarotid Sodium Amytal Injections. *Cortex*, **2**:367–372, 1966.

—— Speech Findings in Epilepsy and Electro-Cortical Stimulation: An Overview. *Cortex*,

2:463–473, 1966.

Shankweiler, D. P., Harris, K. S. An Experimental Approach to the Problem of Articulation in Aphasia. *Cortex,* **2**:277–292, 1966.

——, ——, et al. Electromyographic Studies of Articulation in Aphasia. *Arch. Phys. Med.,* **49**: 1–8, 1968.

Sheehan, V. M. Rehabilitation of Aphasics in an Army Hospital. *J. Speech Hearing Dis.,* **11**:149–157, 1946.

—— Techniques in the Management of Aphasics. *J. Speech Hearing Dis.,* **13**:241–246, 1948.

Shenk, V. W. D. Phonetic Disorders in Sensory Aphasia. *Encephale,* **42**:158–169, 1953.

Sherwood, M., McNamee, H. B. Psychological Study of the Amnesic Syndrome: Effects of Interference on Recall. *Cortex,* **4**:359–371, 1968.

Sidman, M., Stoddard, L. T., et al. Behavioral Studies of Aphasia: Methods of Investigation and Analysis. *Neuropsychol.,* **9**:119–140, 1971.

Siegel, G. M. Dysphasic Speech Responses to Visual Word Stimuli. *J. Speech Hearing Res.,* **2**:152–160, 1959.

Siegenthaler, B. M., Goldstein, J. Auditory and Visual Figure-Background Perception by Adult Aphasics. *J. Commun. Disord.,* **1**:152–158, 1967.

Singer, H. D., Low, A. A. The Brain in a Case of Motor Aphasia in which Improvement Occurred With Training. *AMA Arch. Neurol. Psychiat.,* **29**:162–165, 1933.

Sklar, M. Relation of Psychological and Language Test Scores and Autopsy Findings in Aphasia. *J. Speech Hearing Res.,* **6**:84–90, 1963.

—— *Aphasia and Rehabilitation.* Beverly Hills, Western Psychological Services, 1965.

Smith, A. Certain Hypothesized Hemispheric Differences in Language and Visual Functions in Human Adults. *Cortex,* **2**:109–126, 1966.

—— Intellectual Functions in Patients with Lateralized Frontal Tumors. *J. Neurol. Neurosurg. Psychiat.,* **29**:52–59, 1966.

—— Verbal and Nonverbal Test Performances of Patients with "Acute" Lateralized Brain Lesions (Tumors). *J. Nerv. Ment. Dis.,* **141**:517–523, 1966.

Smith, R. P. Aphasia in Relation to Mental Disease. *Proc. Roy. Soc. Med. (Neurology),* **11**:1–20, 1917–1918.

Snidecor, J. C. A Method of Disparities for Evaluating Aphasic Disturbances. *J. Nerv. Ment. Dis.,* **122**:92–93, 1955.

Solomon, A. An Unusual Receptive Aphasia as a Manifestation of Temporal Lobe Epilepsy: Report of a Case Treated by Surgery. *New Eng. J. Med.,* **257**:313–317, 1957.

Sparks, R., Geschwind, N. Dichotic Listening in Man After Section of Neocortical Commissures. *Cortex,* **4**:3–16, 1968.

——, Goodglass, H., et al. Ipsilateral Versus Contralateral Extinction in Dichotic Listening Resulting From Hemisphere Lesions. *Cortex,* **6**:249–260, 1970.

Spellacy, F., Blumstein, S. The Influence of Language Set on Ear Preference in Phoneme Recognition. *Cortex,* **6**:430–439, 1970.

——, and Spreen, O. A Short Form of the Token Test. *Cortex,* **5**:390–397, 1969.

Sperry, R. W. Neurology and the Mind-Brain Problem. *Amer. Sci.,* **40**:291–312, 1952.

Spiegel, D. K., Jones, L. V., et al. Test Responses as Predictors of Free-Speech Characteristics in Aphasia Patients. *J. Speech Hearing Res.,* **8**:349–362, 1965.

Spinnler, H., Vignolo, L. A. Impaired Recognition of Meaningful Sounds in Aphasia. *Cortex,* **2**:337–348, 1966.

Spreen, O. Psycholinguistic Aspects of Aphasia. *J. Speech Hearing Res.,* **11**:467–480, 1968.

——, Benton, A. L., et al. Auditory Agnosia Without Aphasia. *Arch. Neurol.,* **13**:84–92, 1965.

——, ——, et al. Dissociation of Visual and Tactile Naming in Amnesic Aphasia. *Neurology,* **16**:807–814, 1966.

Stamm, C. Nominal Aphasia Due to Extradural Temporal Lobe Abscess. *Confin. Neurol.,* **13**:10–16, 1953.

—— The Significance of Aphasia in Otology. *Laryngoscope,* **63**:44–60, 1953.

Starr, M. A. The Pathology of Sensory Aphasia, With an Analysis of Fifty Cases in Which Broca's Center Was Not Diseased. *Brain,* **12**:82–101, 1889.

Stengel, E., Patch, I. Central Aphasia Associated With Parietal Symptoms. *Brain,* **78**:401–416, 1955.

Stewart, F. J. A Nucleus Vocabulary in the Therapy of Dysphasia: Word Finding, Naming and Recall: Case Report. *J. Amer. Geriat. Soc.,* **14**:768–771, 1966.

Stoicheff, M. L. Motivating Instructions and Language Performance of Dysphasic Subjects. *J. Speech Hearing Res.,* **3**:75–85, 1960.

Stookey, B. Jean-Baptiste Bouillaud and Ernest Auburtin: Early Studies on Cerebral Localization and the Speech Center. *JAMA,* **184**:1024–1029, 1963.

Stoudt, R. Linguistic Considerations in Language Therapy. In: Burr, H. G., (ed.), *The Aphasic Adult: Evaluation and Rehabilitation.* Proceedings of a Short Course in Aphasia, University of Virginia. Charlottesville, Wayside, 1964. Pp. 161–171.

Street, B. S. Hearing Loss in Aphasia. *J. Speech Hearing Dis.*, **22**:60–67, 1957.

Subirana, A. The Prognosis in Aphasia in Relation to Cerebral Dominance and Handedness. *Brain*, **81**:415–425, 1958.

—— The Relationship between Handedness and Language Function. *Int. J. Neurol.*, **4**:215–234, 1964.

Suter, C. Anomic Aphasia. *JAMA*, **151**:462–468, 1953.

Swisher, L. P., Sarno, M. T. Token Test Scores of Three Matched Patient Groups: Left Brain-Damaged With Aphasia; Right Brain-Damaged Without Aphasia; Non-Brain-Damaged. *Cortex*, **5**:264–273, 1969.

Symonds, L. Aphasia. *J. Neurol. Neurosurg. Psychiat.*, **16**:1–6, 1953.

Taylor, M. L. *Understanding Aphasia: A Guide for Families and Friends.* New York, Institute of Physical Medicine and Rehabilitation, 1958. (Portuguese translation ed., 1957; Japanese translation ed., 1958; Spanish translation ed., 1959; Arabic translation ed., 1963; Danish translation ed., 1965; Urdu translation ed., 1968).

—— Aphasia. In: Rothenberg, E., (ed.), *Dynamic Living for the Long Term Patient.* Dubuque, Brown, 1964. Pp. 42–46.

—— Language Therapy. In: Burr, H. G., (ed.), *The Aphasic Adult: Evaluation and Rehabilitation.* Proceedings of a Short Course in Aphasia, University of Virginia. Charlottesville, Wayside, 1964. Pp. 139–160.

—— Linguistic Considerations in the Verbal Behavior of the Brain-Damaged Adult. In: *Selected Conference Papers of the NAFSA English Language Section, 1962,* NAFSA Studies and Papers, English Language Series, No. 8. New York, National Association for Foreign Student Affairs, 1964.

—— Linguistic Considerations of the Verbal Behavior of the Brain-Damaged Adult. *Ling. Rep.*, **6**:1–2, 1964.

—— Principles in the Management of Communication Impairment. In: Rusk, H. A. (ed.), *Rehabilitation Medicine* (Third Ed.). St. Louis, Mosby, 1971. Pp. 238–250.

—— A Measurement of Functional Communication in Aphasia. *Arch. Phys. Med.*, **46**:101–107, 1965.

—— Programmed Instruction and Speech Rehabilitation. *N.Y. Speech Hearing Ass. Newsl.*, **5**: 1966.

—— Programmed Instruction-Therapy in Aphasia. *N. J. Speech Hearing Ass. J.*, **5**:7–10, 1967.

——, Marks, M. M. *Aphasia Rehabilitation Manual and Therapy Kit.* New York, McGraw-Hill, 1959.

——, Rusk, H. A. Speech Problems of Hemiplegics. *Pub. Health Rep.*, **72**:832–835, 1957.

——, Sands, E. S. Application of Programmed Instruction to the Language Training of Severely Impaired Aphasic Patients. *Nat. Soc. Prog. Inst. J.*, **5**:10–11, 1966.

Teitelbaum, H. A. An Analysis of the Disturbances of the Higher Cortical Functions, Agnosia, Apraxia and Aphasia. *J. Nerv. Ment, Dis.*, **97**:44–61, 1943.

Teuber, H. L. The Premorbid Personality and Reaction to Brain Damage. *Amer. J. Orthopsychiat.*, **30**:322–329, 1960.

Thurston, J. R. An Empirical Investigation of the Loss of Spelling Ability in Dysphasics. *J. Speech Hearing Dis.*, **19**:344–349, 1954.

Tikofsky, R. S. Language Problems in Adults. In: Rieber, R. W., Brubaker, R. S. (eds.), *Speech Pathology.* Philadelphia, Lippincott, 1966. Pp. 261–284.

—— Two Studies of Verbal Learning by Adult Aphasics. *Cortex*, **7**:106–125, 1971.

—— *Phonetic Characteristics of Dysarthria.* Ann Arbor, University of Michigan, 1965.

——, Kooi, K. A., et al. Electroencephalographic Findings and Recovery from Aphasia. *Neurology*, **10**:154–156, 1960.

——, Reynolds, G. L. Preliminary Study: Nonverbal Learning and Aphasia. *J. Speech Hearing Res.*, **5**:133–143, 1962.

——, —— Further Studies of Nonverbal Learning and Aphasia. *J. Speech Hearing Res.*, **6**:329–337, 1963.

——, Tikofsky, R. P. Intelligibility Measures of Dysarthric Speech. *J. Speech Hearing Res.*, **7**:325–333, 1964.

Tobis, J. S. Physical Medicine and Rehabilitation Management in Aphasa. *JAMA*, **171**:393–395, 1959.

Tureen, L. L., Smolik, E. A., et al. Aphasia in a Deaf Mute. *Neurology*, **1**:237–249, 1951.

Turnblom, M. L., Myers, J. S. A Group Discussion Program With Families of Aphasic Patients. *J. Speech Hearing Dis.*, **17**:393–396, 1952.

Ullman, M. Behavioral Changes in Patients Following Strokes. Springfield, Ill., Thomas, 1962.

U.S. Dept. of Health, Education, and Welfare, Social and Rehabilitation Service, Rehabilitation Services Administration. *The Vocational Rehabilitation Problems of the Patient With Aphasia.* Washington D.C., Government Printing Office, 1969.

Van Buren, J. M. Confusion and Disturbance of Speech from Stimulation in Vicinity of the Head of the Caudate Nucleus. *J. Neurosurg.*, **20**:148–157,

1963.

Van Pelt, D., Wepman, J. M., et al. *Differential Disruption of the Symbolic Process in Aphasic Language Disorders*. Chapel Hill Press, University of North Carolina, 1958.

Van Thal, J. H. Polyglot Aphasics. *Folia Phoniat.*, **12**:123–128, 1960.

Vega, Jr., A., Parsons, O. A. Relationship Between Sensory-Motor Deficits and WAIS Verbal and Performance Scores in Unilateral Brain Damage. *Cortex*, **5**: 229–241, 1969.

Vignolo, L. A. Evolution of Aphasia and Language Rehabilitation: A Retrospective Exploratory Study. *Cortex*, **1**:344–367, 1964.

—— Factors Underlying Impairment of Visual Figure-Ground Discrimination and Sorting Tasks in Hemisphere-Damaged Patients. *J. Learn. Disabil.*, **1**:230–241, 1968.

Vigotsky, L. S. *Thought and Language*. Cambridge, M.I.T., 1962.

Wada, J., Rasmussen, T. Intracarotid Injection of Sodium Amytal for the Lateralization of Cerebral Speech Dominance. *J. Neurosurg.*, **17**:266–282, 1960.

Warrington, E. K., James, M. Tachistoscopic Number Estimation in Patients With Unilateral Cerebral Lesions. *J. Neurol. Neurosurg. Psychiat.*, **30**:468–474, 1967.

Wechsler, L. Excision of the Speech Area Without Resultant Aphasia. *AMA Arch. Neurol. Psychiat.*, **38**:430–437, 1937.

Weinberg, B., Bosma, J. F., et al. Myotonic Dystrophy Initially Manifested by Speech Disability. *J. Speech Hearing Dis.*, **33**:51–58, 1968.

Weinstein, E. A. Affections of Speech with Lesions of the Non-Dominant Hemisphere. In: Rioch, D. M., Weinstein, E. A., (eds.), *Disorders of Communication*. Baltimore, Williams and Wilkins, 1964. Pp. 220–228.

——, Cole, M., et al. Anosognosia and Aphasia. *Arch. Neurol.*, **10**:376–386, 1964.

——, Kahn, R. L. Non-Aphasic Misnaming (Paraphasia) in Organic Brain Disease. *AMA Arch. Neurol. Psychiat.*, **67**:72–79, 1952.

——, Keller, N. J. A. Linguistic Patterns of Misnaming in Brain Injury. *Neuropsychol.*, **1**:79–90, 1963.

——, Lyerly, O. G., et al. Meaning in Jargon Aphasia. *Cortex*, **2**:165–187, 1966.

Weinstein, S. Experimental Analysis of an Attempt to Improve Speech in Cases of Expressive Aphasia. *Neurology*, **9**:632–635, 1959.

—— Deficits Concomitant With Aphasia or Lesions of Either Cerebral Hemisphere. *Cortex*, **1**:154–169, 1964.

——, Sersen, E. A., et al. Phantom and Somatic Sensation in Cases of Congenital Aphasia. *Cortex*, **1**:276–290, 1964.

Weisenburg, T. H., McBride, K. E. *Aphasia: A Clinical and Psychological Study*. New York, Hafner, 1964.

Wepman, J. M. The Organization of Therapy for Aphasia: The In-Patient Treatment Center. *J. Speech Hearing Dis.*, **12**:405–409, 1947.

—— *Recovery from Aphasia*. New York, Ronald, 1951.

—— A Conceptual Model for the Processes Involved in Recovery from Aphasia. *J. Speech Hearing Dis.*, **18**:4–13, 1953.

—— Aphasia and the "Whole-Person" Concept. *Amer. Arch. Rehab. Ther.*, **6**:1–7, 1958.

—— The Relationship between Self-Correction and Recovery from Aphasia. *J. Speech Hearing Dis.*, **23**:302–305, 1958.

—— *A Selected Bibliography on Brain Impairment, Aphasia, and Organic Psychodiagnosis*. Chicago, Language Research Associates, 1961.

—— Language Disorders. In: Levine, E., Garrett, J. (eds.), *Psychological Practices with the Physically Disabled*. New York, Columbia University, 1962. Pp. 197–231.

—— Language: A Perspective from the Study of Aphasia. In: Rosenberg, S. (ed.), *Directions in Psycholinguistics*. New York, Macmillan, 1965.

—— Aphasia. *Hearing Speech News*, **36**:3–5, 22–24, 26, 1968.

——Aphasia Therapy: Some "Relative" Comments and Some Purely Personal Prejudices. In: Black, J. W., Jancosek, E. G. (eds.), *Proceedings of the Conference on Language Retraining for Aphasics*. Columbus, Ohio State University, 1968.

——, Bock, R. D., et al. Psycholinguistic Study of Aphasia: A Revision of the Concept of Anomia. *J. Speech Hearing Dis.*, **21**:468–477, 1956.

——, Jones, L. V. *The Language Modalities Test for Aphasia*. Chicago, Education-Industry Service, 1961.

——, —— *Studies in Aphasia: An Approach to Testing*. Chicago, Education Industry Service, 1961.

——, —— Five Aphasias: A Commentary on Aphasia as a Regressive Linguistic Phenomenon. In: Rioch, D. M., Weinstein, E. A. (eds.), *Disorders of Communication*. Baltimore, Williams and Wilkins, 1964. Pp. 190–203.

——, —— Studies in Aphasia: Classification of Aphasic Speech by the Noun-Pronoun Ratio. *Brit. J. Disord. Commun.*, **1**:46–54, 1966.

——, ——, et al. Studies in Aphasia: Background and Theoretical Formulations. *J. Speech Hearing*

Dis., **25**:323–332, 1960.

——, Morency, A. Filmstrips as an Adjunct to Language Therapy for Aphasia. *J. Speech Hearing Dis.*, **28**:191–194, 1963.

——, Van Pelt, D. A Theory of Cerebral Language Disorders Based on Therapy. *Folia Phoniat.*, **7**:233–235, 1955.

Werner, H. Microgenesis and Aphasia. *J. Abnorm. Soc. Psychol.*, **52**:347–353, 1956.

Wertz, R. T., Porch, B. E. Effects of Masking Noise on the Verbal Performance of Adult Aphasics. *Cortex*, **6**:399–409, 1970.

West, R., Ansberry, M., et al. *The Rehabilitation of Speech.* New York, Harper, 1957. Pp. 132–157, 498–520.

——, Stockel, S. The Effect of Meprobamate on Recovery from Aphasia. *J. Speech Hearing Res.*, **8**:57–62, 1965.

Whitty, C. W. M. Cortical Dysarthria and Dysprosody of Speech. *J. Neurol. Neurosurg. Psychiat.*, **27**:507–510, 1964.

Wild, S. D., Hooker, E. H., et al. A Study of Aphasic Individuals Predicting Letters of Graded Material. *J. Commun. Disord.*, **2**:336–339, 1969.

Wilson, S. A. K. *Aphasia.* London, Kegan Paul, Trench, Trubner, 1926.

Winchester, R. A., Hartman, B. T. Auditory Dedifferentiation in the Dysphasic. *J. Speech Hearing Dis.*, **20**:178–182, 1955.

Wint, G. *The Third Killer.* New York, Abelard-Schuman, 1967.

Wohlfart, G., Lindgren, A., et al. Clinical Picture and Morbid Anatomy in a Case of "Pure Word Deafness." *J. Nerv. Ment. Dis.*, **116**:818–827, 1952.

Wyke, M. Experimental Study of Verbal Association Learning in Patients with Severe Dysphasia. *J. Neurol. Neurosurg. Psychiat.*, **29**:171–175, 1966.

Yin, R. K. Face Recognition by Brain-Injured Patients: A Dissociable Ability. *Neuropsychol.*, **8**:395–402, 1970.

Zangwill, O. L. Agraphia Due to a Left Parietal Glioma in a Left-Handed Man. *Brain*, **77**:510–520, 1954.

—— Speech and the Minor Hemisphere. *Acta Neurol. Psychiat. Belg.*, **67**:1013–20, 1969.

Zentay, P. J. Motor Disorders of the Central Nervous System and Their Significance for Speech. *J. Speech Hearing Dis.*, **2**:131–138, 1937.

Ziegler, D. Word Deafness and Wernicke's Aphasia. *AMA Arch. Neurol. Psychiat.*, **67**:323–331, 1952.

Zucker, K. An Analysis of Disturbed Function in Aphasia. *Brain*, **57**:109–127, 1934.

Zurif, E. B., Carson, G. Dyslexia in Relation to Cerebral Dominance and Temporal Analysis. *Neuropsychol.*, **8**:351–361, 1970.

Zurif, E. B., Sait, P. E. The Role of Syntax in Dichotic Listening. *Neuropsychol.*, **8**:239–244, 1970.

Appendix 2

SUGGESTED READINGS

THE HISTORY OF APHASIA

1. Bay, E. The Lordat Case and Its Import on the Theory of Aphasia. *Cortex,* **5**: 302–308, 1969.
2. Benton, A. L. Contributions to Aphasia before Broca. *Cortex,* **1**: 314–327, 1964.
3. ——, Joynt, R. J. Early Descriptions of Aphasia. *Arch. Neurol.,* **3**: 205–222, 1960.
4. Geschwind, N. The Paradoxical Position of Kurt Goldstein in the History of Aphasia. *Cortex,* **1**: 214–224, 1964.
5. —— Wernicke's Contribution to the Study of Aphasia. *Cortex,* **3**: 449–463, 1967.
6. Joynt, R. J. Centenary of Patient "Tan." *Arch. Intern. Med.,* **108**: 197–200, 1961.
7. —— Paul Pierre Broca: His Contribution to the Knowledge of Aphasia. *Cortex,* **1**: 206–213, 1964.
8. ——, Benton, A. L. The Memoir of Marc Dax on Aphasia. *Neurology,* **14**: 851–854, 1964.
9. Kann, J. A Translation of Broca's Original Article on the Location of the Speech Center. *J. Speech Hearing Dis.,* **15**: 16–20, 1950.
10. Riese, W., Hoff, E. C. A History of the Doctrine of Cerebral Localization: The History of Aphasia. *J. Hist. Med.,* **6**: 457–470, 1951.
11. Stookey, B. Jean-Baptiste Bouillaud and Ernest Auburtin: Localization and the Speech Center. *J.A.M.A.,* **184**: 1024–1029, 1963.

THEORIES OF CLASSIFICATION

1. Bay, E. The Classification of Disorders of Speech. *Cortex,* **3**: 26–31, 1967.
2. Schuell, H. M., Jenkins, J. J. The Nature of Language Deficit in Aphasia. *Psychol. Rev.,* **66**: 45–67, 1959.
3. Wepman, J. M., Jones, L., et al. Studies in Aphasia: Background and Theoretical Formulations. *J. Speech Hearing Dis.,* **25**: 323–332, 1960.

NEUROLOGICAL ASPECTS

1. Benson, D. F. Fluency in Aphasia. Correlation with Radioactive Scan Localization. *Cortex,* **3**: 373–394, 1967.
2. ——, Patten, D. H. The Use of Radioactive Isototopes in the Localization of Aphasia-Producing Lesions. *Cortex,* **3**: 258–271, 1967.
3. Brain, R. The Neurology of Language. *Brain,* **84**: 147–166, 1961.
4. Brown, J. R., Simonson, J. A Clinical Study of 100 Aphasic Patients. 1. Observations on Lateralization and Localization of Lesions. *Neurology,* **7**: 777–783, 1957.
5. De Renzi E., Faglioni, P., et al. The Influence of Aphasia and of the Hemispheric Side of the Cerebral Lesion on Abstract Thinking. *Cortex,* **2**: 399–420, 1966.

6. Ettlinger, G., Jackson, G. V., et al. Dysphasia Following Right Temporal Lobectomy in a Right-Handed Man. *J. Neurol. Neurosurg. Psychiat.*, **18**: 214–217, 1955.
7. Geschwind, N. Disconnexion Syndromes in Animals and Man. *Brain,* **88**: Part II, 237–294, 1965.
8. —— Disconnexion Syndromes in Animals and Man. *Brain,* **88**: Part III, 585–644, 1965.
9. Goodglass, H., Quadfasel, F. A. Language Laterality in Left-Handed Aphasics. *Brain,* **77**: 521–548, 1954.
10. Hécaen, H., Piercy, M. Paroxysmal Dysphasia and the Problem of Cerebral Dominance. *J. Neurol. Neurosurg. Psychiat.*, **19**: 194–201, 1956.
11. Holmes, J. E., Sadoff, R. L. Aphasia Due to a Right Hemisphere Tumor in a Right-Handed Man. *Neurology,* **16**: 392–397, 1966.
12. Humphrey, M. E., Zangwill, O. L. Dysphasia in Left-Handed Patients with Unilateral Brain Lesions. *J. Neurol. Neurosurg. Psychiat.*, **15**: 184–193, 1952.
13. Luria, A. R. The Directive Function of Speech in Development and Dissolution: Part II. Dissolution of the Regulative Function of Speech in Pathological States of the Brain. *Word,* **15**: 453–464.
14. —— Neuropsychology in the Local Diagnosis of Brain Damage. *Cortex,* **1**: 3–18, 1964.
15. Penfield, W. Conditioning the Uncommitted Cortex for Language Learning. *Brain,* **88**: 787–798, 1965.
16. Piercy, M. The Effects of Cerebral Lesion on Intellectual Function: A Review of Current Research Trends. *Brit. J. Psychiat.*, **110**: 310–352, 1964.
17. Russell, W. R. Some Anatomical Aspects of Aphasia. *Lancet,* **1**: 1173–1177, 1963.
18. Serafetinides, E. A. Speech Findings in Epilepsy and Electro-Cortical Stimulation: An Overview. *Cortex,* **2**: 463–473, 1966.
19. Sklar, M. Relation of Psychological and Language Test Scores and Autopsy Findings in Aphasia. *J. Speech Hearing Res.*, **6**: 84–90, 1963.
20. Smith, A. Certain Hypothesized Hemispheric Differences in Language and Visual Functions in Human Adults. *Cortex,* **2**: 109–126.
21. Subirana, A. The Relationship between Handedness and Language Function. *Int. J. Neurol,* **4**: 215–234, 1964.
22. Wada, J., Rasmussen, T. Intracarotid Injection of Sodium Amytal for the Lateralization of Cerebral Speech Dominance. *J. Neurosurg.*, **17**: 266–282, 1960.
23. Weinstein, S. Deficits Concomitant with Aphasia or Lesions of Either Cerebral Hemisphere. *Cortex,* **1**: 154–169, 1964.

Name Index

Subject Index